# Hyperlipidaemia

*To Patricia and the children*

# Hyperlipidaemia Diagnosis and Management

Second edition

**Paul N. Durrington** BSc, MD, FRCP, FRCPath
*Reader in Medicine, University of Manchester;*
*Honorary Consultant Physician to the Manchester Royal Infirmary, UK*

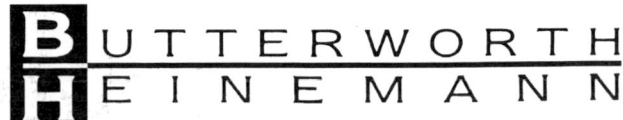

Butterworth-Heinemann
Linacre House, Jordan Hill, Oxford OX2 8DP
225 Wildwood Avenue, Woburn, MA 01801-2041
A division of Reed Educational and Professional Publishing Ltd

 A member of the Reed Elsevier plc group

OXFORD   BOSTON   JOHANNESBURG
MELBOURNE   NEW DELHI   SINGAPORE

First published 1989
Second edition 1995
Reprinted 1998

**British Library Cataloguing in Publication Data**
Durrington, Paul N.
  Hyperlipidaemia: Diagnosis and
  Management. - 2Rev.ed
  1. Title
  616.3997

ISBN 0 7506 0876 5

**Library of Congress Cataloguing in Publication Data**
  Durrington, Paul N.
  Hyperlipidaemia : diagnosis and management/Paul N. Durrington. -
  2nd ed.
  p.  cm.
  Includes bibliographical references and index.
  ISBN 0 7506 0876 5
  1. Hyperlipidemia.  I. Title
  [DNLM: 1. Hyperlipidemia-diagnosis.  2. Hyperlipidemia-therapy.
  WD 200.5.H8 D965h 1994]
  RC632.H87D87  1994                                          94-33682
  616.3'997-dc20                                                CIP

Printed in Great Britain by The University Press, Cambridge
Composition by Scribe Design, Gillingham, Kent

# Contents

'One man is measuring the lengths of the feelers of 2,000 beetles; another the amount of cholesterol in 100 samples of human blood; each in the hope, but not in the certainty, that his series of numbers will lead him to some definite law.'

J. B. S. Haldane, 1927
*The Future of Biology*

# Foreword to the first edition

Hypercholesterolaemia, while certainly not the only cause of coronary heart disease, is equally certainly one of its major correctable causes. The evidence supporting this conclusion has grown steadily in recent years, and best medical practice now requires that hypercholesterolaemia be treated. The United Kingdom has been somewhat slow to accept and act on the evidence, but now even the more vocal sceptics agree that treatment is indicated. There is still room for discussion of the cholesterol level at which treatment is called for and of just how vigorously it should be pursued. Now, however, rather similar guidelines have been proposed at the national level in a number of countries, including the United States, Europe (with concurrence of the UK representatives) and Canada. Dr Durrington's book, then, is timely. It offers the physician and the student a comprehensive discussion of hyperlipidaemia, beginning with the basic chemistry and physiology of the lipoproteins and continuing through to the most practical aspects of diagnosis and treatment. The evidence justifying the recommended therapies is reviewed in a careful, balanced manner. This clinically oriented book should allow the physician to reach a wise decision on when and how to intervene with diet and/or drugs to control his patients' hyperlipidaemias.

**Daniel Steinberg** MD PhD
Professor of Medicine
Division of Endocrinology and Metabolism
University of California, San Diego

# Preface to the first edition

Attempts to contain within a single volume the knowledge necessary for the clinical management of the hyperlipidaemias have been remarkably few, despite the indisputable need for a wider awareness of that aspect of medical care and for specialist physicians with a particular knowledge of the subject. There has been an enormous increase in our understanding of lipoproteins and their physiology in recent years. Epidemiological aspects of lipids continue to occupy much journal space and to generate as much heat as they do light. Most clinical research publications centre on therapeutic trials. Little attention is paid, however, to the diagnosis, natural history and practical management of the hyperlipidaemias. The purpose of this book is to provide a review of those aspects of the subject against the background of physiology and epidemiology.

I doubt that the book contains much of an original nature, although some of the material presented required a considerable amount of reworking in order that it might have some relevance to the clinician. Many of the views expressed will be identifiable as belonging to others. I hope I have adequately acknowledged that fact in the text and apologize if, on any occasion, this does not appear to be the case. It would be impossible not to have drawn heavily on the views and experiences of all those who have been mentors and colleagues since my interest in lipoproteins was first aroused in 1973. In particular, I should like to thank Peter Adams, Deepak Bhatnagar, Colin Bolton, Mike Davies, Eric Gowland, Martin Hartog, Paul Miller, Roger Newton, Dan Steinberg, Maurice Stone, David Weinstein and Peter Winocour. I am grateful also to my patients, who have told me more about the hyperlipidaemias than I have been able to tell them and whose common sense has preserved them from my worst vagaries, and to Mrs J. Heydon for invaluable secretarial assistance. The main burden of writing this book has fallen on my family and it is to them that I owe my greatest thanks.

Originally the book was to have been part of John Wright's medical list. That list was acquired by my present publisher, Butterworths, while I was in the process of writing. I have found the encouragement and help which I received from the staff of both companies of the greatest value.

## Figure acknowledgement

I am indebted to the University of Manchester Department of Medical Illustration for their permission to use all the figures in this book not otherwise acknowledged in the captions.

**Paul Durrington**

# Preface to the second edition

In the half decade since the publication of the first edition of this book, there have been spectacular advances on several fronts. In particular, there has been a rapid expansion of our knowledge of lipoprotein physiology and of the cellular and biochemical events in atherogenesis. In addition, therapy has advanced to the point where effective regulation of abnormal lipoprotein levels is a realistic objective in the great majority of patients requiring it. Sadly many at high risk continue to be robbed of that opportunity, because of the reactivation of controversy surrounding the management of clinically less important hyperlipidaemias. This might be seen as a welcome restraint against therapeutic recommendations which go beyond both scientific credibility and practicability. However, 'over-the-top' recommendations for treatment are common in medicine and in no other field have they excited the degree of what the author of the Foreword of the first edition of this book has called 'negatively negative criticism'. Many of those engaged in being vocally critical could by virtue of their own knowledge and experience have created more enduring and scientifically valid guidance, instead of which they seem content simply to maraud.

This book continues to focus on the diagnosis, natural history and practical management of the hyperlipidaemias and to place these in the context of the latest advances and the most recent controversies in this fascinating area of medicine. I have continued to draw heavily on the views and experience of colleagues and am especially grateful to Peter Adams, Deepak Bhatnagar, Mike Davies, John Dean, Mike France, Eric Gowland, Sudesh Kumar, Ian Laing, Mike Mackness, Tony MBewu, Paul Miller, Peter Selby, Colin Short and Peter Winocour. The second edition has in many ways been a greater torment than the first, because I could never find any undisturbed island in the tide of events upon which to write it. This has meant that an even greater debt of gratitude is due to Mrs J. Heydon and Miss C. Price for coping with secretarial matters. Again the most important contribution has been the wonderful support and forbearance of my family.

I have found the encouragement and help which I have received from the staff of Butterworth-Heinemann invaluable.

## Acknowledgements

I am yet again indebted to the University of Manchester Department of Medical Illustration not only for permission to use all the figures in this book not otherwise acknowledged, but also for the cheerful and sterling service provided by its staff.

**Paul Durrington**

# Abbreviations

| | |
|---|---|
| ABFA | albumin-bound fatty acid |
| ACAT | acyl-CoA:cholesterol acyl transferase |
| AGE | advanced glycosylation |
| apo | apolipoprotein |
| ATP | adenosine triphosphate |
| cAMP | cyclic adenosine monophosphate |
| CAPD | chronic ambulatory peritoneal dialysis |
| cDNA | complementary deoxyribonucleic acid |
| CETC | cholesteryl ester transfer complex |
| CETP | cholesteryl ester transfer protein |
| DTNB | dithiobisnitrobenzoic acid |
| EDTA | ethylenediamine tetra-acetic acid |
| EGF | epithelial growth factor |
| FCH | familial combined hyperlipidaemia |
| FCR | fractional catabolic rate |
| FFA | free fatty acids |
| FH | familial hypercholesterolaemia |
| HABL | hyperapobetalipoproteinaemia |
| HDL | high density lipoprotein |
| HMG-CoA | 3-hydroxy, 3-methyl-glutaryl-CoA reductase |
| IDDM | insulin dependent diabetes mellitus |
| IDL | intermediate density lipoprotein |
| IHD | ischaemic heart disease |
| ISA | intrinsic sympathomimetic activity |
| LCAT | lecithin: cholesterol acyltransferase |
| LDL | low density lipoprotein |
| Lp | lipoprotein |
| LTP | lipid transfer protein |
| MCV | mean corpuscular volume |
| mRNA | messenger ribonucleic acid |
| MSH | melanocyte-stimulating hormone |
| NEFA | non-esterified fatty acids |
| NIDDM | non-insulin dependent diabetes mellitus |
| PHLA | post-heparin lipolytic activity |
| RFLP | restriction-fragment length polymorphism |
| TSH | thyroid-stimulating hormone |
| VHDL | very high density lipoprotein |
| VLDL | very low density lipoprotein |

# Introduction

To many doctors, the metabolism of lipoproteins and its disorders must appear as a rather new and complex area. This, coupled with the various controversies surrounding clinical trials of lowering plasma cholesterol, which have raged over the years between various people who claimed to understand the subject, did little to convince the clinician that it was worthy of his attention. In fact, much of our knowledge of lipoproteins is neither new nor complex. Worse still, the identification and management of many patients has never been in question and sadly they have suffered because of frequently held misconceptions. Not surprisingly, few medical schools have given adequate tuition in the lipoprotein disorders, and because of the small number of clinicians with an interest in them the opportunity of postgraduate education in the subject is small. Few doctors will be aware that familial hypercholesterolaemia is our most common genetic disease, having about the same frequency as insulin dependent diabetes. It is an entirely genetic condition and has nothing to do with the so-called diet–heart controversy. It is frequently identifiable by simple physical signs and has a high mortality: almost 60% of male heterozygotes die before the age of 60 without treatment.

Thankfully, now that there is good evidence that treating the even more common and, in themselves, less risky hyperlipidaemias is beneficial, there is an increasingly rapid growth of concern by various national bodies, by the general public and by general practitioners and their hospital colleagues. Many general practices are beginning to identify patients, and hospital clinical services for those more difficult to diagnose and more resistant to treatment are being developed.

Our knowledge of lipoproteins is already vast and has as venerable a history as any other part of medicine. The first clearly recognizable description of the lipoproteins was by Hewson in 1771[1], who was one of the discoverers of the lymphatic system. He was able to observe the appearance of chylomicrons in the lymph following a fatty meal and subsequently their entry into the circulating blood. He demonstrated their fatty nature and rightly deduced that they were one means by which fat energy was distributed around the body. In most people he found that they were not present in fasting serum, but he did observe that in a few the plasma remained whey-like (vaguely opalescent) for much longer and rarely was persistently milky. He was thus the first to recognize and observe not only the chylomicrons, but also the other circulating triglyceride-rich lipoproteins now known as very low density lipoproteins (VLDL).

Credit for the first description of cholesterol is usually given to Chevreul in France, in 1816[2]. In 1830 Christison, working in the University of Edinburgh, discovered the cholesterol-carrying lipoproteins by recognizing cholesterol as one of the fats present in ether extracts of perfectly clear serum[3]. The discovery that cholesterol was a major constituent of atheromatous plaques was made by Vogel (1845) in Leipzig[4].

The earliest written accounts of xanthelasmata and xanthomata were those of Addison and Gull[5,6] of Guy's Hospital. Their report is beautifully illustrated. One of their patients with tuberoeruptive xanthomata and diabetes clearly had type III hyperlipoproteinaemia and another with xanthelasmata had chronic obstructive jaundice. Gull was physician to Queen Victoria and Addison's name has, of course, become eponymous with hypoadrenalism and pernicious anaemia. Tendon xanthomata and 'a kind of universal atheromatous change' were first described by Fagge (1873) at post-mortem examination[7].

The experimental study of blood lipids and atherosclerosis was started by Anitschkow in 1913[8]. He confidently stated that 'there can be no atheroma without cholesterol', neatly upstaging all subsequent work in the area. Familial hypercholesterolaemia was first clearly described in life with serum cholesterol measurements by Burns in 1920[9], although earlier attempts had been made to study the genetic transmission of xanthomata[10]. Even before that the nutritional debate had been initiated by de Langen (1916), who had observed a much lower blood cholesterol in the Javanese than in the Dutch, Germans and French and attributed this to diet[11].

In terms of basic research, cholesterol has become 'the most highly decorated small molecule in biology'[12]: since 1928 13 Nobel Prizes have been awarded to scientists, major parts of whose careers had been devoted to cholesterol. The most recent of these and probably the most significant in terms of clinical practice was to M. S. Brown and J. L. Goldstein in 1985 for their work in Dallas identifying the LDL-receptor defect in familial hypercholesterolaemia and defining the nature of that receptor[12].

Suffice it to say, by way of conclusion, that for the clinician and the clinical scientist the hyperlipidaemias offer an exciting challenge: much is known and much can be achieved with current knowledge, but there is also the challenging prospect of uncharted waters in abundance.

## References

1. Hewson, W. *An experimental enquiry into the properties of the blood with remarks on some of its morbid appearances and an appendix relating to the discovery of the lymphanc system in birds, fish and the animals called amphibious*, T. Cadell, London (1771)
2. Chevreul, M. E. Examen des grasses d'homme de mouton, de boeuf, de jaguar et d'oie. *Ann. Chimie. Phys.*, **2**, 339–372 (1816)
3. Christison, R. On the cause of the milky and whey-like appearances sometimes observed in the blood. *Edinb. Med. Surg. J.*, **33**, 276–280 (1830)
4. Vogel, J. *Patholog. Anat. des menschlischen*, Korpers, Leipzig (translated from the German with additions by G. E. Day 1847). *The Pathological Anatomy of the Human Body*, H. Bailliere, London, (1845)
5. Addison, T. and Gull, W. On a certain affection of the skin. *Guy's Hosp. Rep.*, ser. II, **7**, 265–270 (1851)
6. Gull, W. Vitiligoidea; α-plana, ß-tuberosa. *Guy's Hosp. Rep.*, ser. II, **8**, 149–151 (1852)
7. Fagge, C. H. General xanthelasma or vitiligoidea. *Trans. Path. Soc. Lond.*, **24**, 242–250 (1873)
8. Klimov, A. N. and Nagornev, V. A. N. N. Anitschkow and his contribution to the doctrine of atherosclerosis (in commemoration of the centennial of his birth). In *Atherosclerosis*, vol. VII (eds N. H. Fidge and P. J. Nestel), Elsevier Science, Amsterdam, pp. 371–374 (1986)
9. Burns, F. S. A contribution to the study of the etiology of xanthoma multiplex. *Arch. Derm. Syph.*, **2**, 415–429 (1920)
10. Jensen, J. The story of xanthomatosis in England prior to the First World War. *Clio. Medica*, **2**, 289–305 (1967)

11. de Langen, C. D. Cholesterine metabolism and pathology of races. *Meded. burg. geneesk. Dienst Ned.-Indië*, **1**, 1–35 (1918)
12. Brown, M. S. and Goldstein, J. L. A receptor-mediated pathway for cholesterol homeostasis. *Science, NY*, **232**, 34–47 (1986)

Chapter 1

# Lipids and their metabolism

A little knowledge of lipid metabolism is a considerable help in understanding some of the more clinical aspects of the disorders of lipoprotein metabolism which are the main theme of this book.

## What are lipids?

Definitions are seldom easy, but the definition of a lipid is more than usually difficult. The question 'What is a lipid, doctor?', well meant and coming from a patient attending a busy lipid clinic for the first time, can, if met unprepared, lead to a response which does little to inspire confidence in the expertise of the doctor. A lipid is, of course, a fat (also an oil or wax), and that explanation may well satisfy the patient. In more biochemical terms there is, however, no unifying structure, as in the case of proteins or sugars, to provide any satisfactory definition. Included among lipids are substances in which fatty acids are an essential component such as triglycerides, glycerophospholipids, sphingophospholipids and waxes, but also substances as structurally diverse as cholesterol and other steroids, terpenes and prostaglandins. Thus the only possible definition is that they are a heterogeneous group of substances which have in common their low solubility in water, but which are more readily soluble in a mixture of chloroform and methanol (2:1 v/v). They are also soluble in other non-polar (organic) solvents such as hydrocarbons, alcohols or ether. The difference between an oil and a fat is determined by the melting point.

Lipids are not in themselves bad, indeed they are essential to life, and certainly in the case of animals, the more complex the living form the more important lipids become.

The lipids with which this book is principally concerned are cholesterol, cholesteryl ester, triglycerides and phospholipids. Because a unifying feature of the structure of the last three of these is the presence of long-chain fatty acids and because of the importance of fatty acids in metabolism, it is appropriate to consider them first.

## Fatty acids

### Structure

These acids all possess a hydrocarbon group attached to a carboxyl group (Figure 1.1). Generally the hydrocarbon part is present as a long chain. Occasionally this may contain a hydroxyl group, a side chain or part of it may even be cyclic, but such rarities need not concern us here. Some important fatty acids are shown in

**Table 1.1 Examples of fatty acids***

| Fatty acid | Structure | Source | Melting point (°C) |
|---|---|---|---|
| **SATURATED** | | | |
| Lauric | C12 : 0 | Coconut fat, palm kernel oil | 44 |
| Myristic | C14 : 0 | Milk, coconut fat | 54 |
| Palmitic | C16 : 0 | Palm oil, milk, butter, cheese, cocoa | 63 |
| Stearic | C18 : 0 | butter, beef, pork, mutton and lamb | 69 |
| Behanic | C22 : 0 | Some seed oils, especially peanut | 80 |
| Lignoceric | C24 : 0 | | 84 |
| **UNSATURATED** | | | |
| Oleic | C18 : 1 | Olive oil, rapeseed oil, most ubiquitous dietary fatty acid | 11 |
| Linoleic | C18 : 2 | Corn oil, soyabean oil, sunflower oil, sunflower seed oil | − 5 |
| Linolenic | C18 : 3 | Linseed oil | −11 |
| Arachidonic | C20 : 4 | Fish oils | −50 |
| Eicosapentaenoic | C20 : 5 | Cod, salmon, pilchard, mussel, oyster | −54 |
| Docosahexaenoic | C22 : 6 | | |

* Those most frequently mentioned will be palmitic, stearic, oleic, linoleic and eicosapentaenoic acid (EPA).

Table 1.1. With the exception of some bacterial ones, naturally occurring fatty acids possess an even number of carbon atoms.

The carbon groups in the hydrocarbon chain may be linked by single or double bonds. Fatty acids containing double bonds in their carbon chains are described as unsaturated and those containing only single bonds as saturated. If only one double bond is present, as in oleic acid, the fatty acid is described as mono-unsaturated. Fatty acids with more than one double bond are described as polyunsaturated. Each double bond creates the possibility of two isomers, according to whether the hydrogen atoms bonded to the two carbon atoms at either end of the double bond are both on the same side (*cis*) or on opposing sides (*trans*) (Figure 1.2).

$$CH_3 - CH_2 - CH_2 - CH_2 - CH_2 - CH_2 - CH_2 - CH_2 - COOH$$

**Figure 1.1**   Structure of a fatty acid

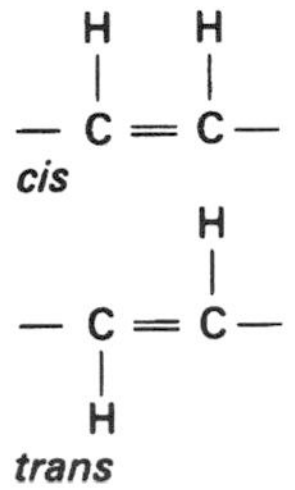

**Figure 1.2**   *Cis* and *trans* isomers of unsaturated fatty acids are possible

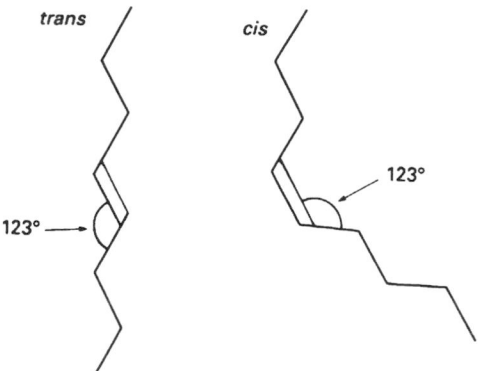

**Figure 1.3**  *Cis* isomers of unsaturated fatty acids have a kink at the double bond, whereas *trans* isomers are straight

   The usual naturally occurring isomers are *cis*. Single bonds leave the carbon atoms on either side free to rotate and are thus less rigid than double bonds. Furthermore in the case of the *cis* isomers, the presence of two hydrogen atoms on one side of the double bond induces a kink in the hydrocarbon chain (Figure 1.3). Polyunsaturated *cis* fatty acids have several of these kinks. There are thus structural reasons why the *cis* unsaturated fatty acids might be bulkier, more rigid and thus less easy to accommodate in lipoproteins or in the binding sites of enzymes. They are also more difficult to pack tightly together in crystal form, which accounts for their lower melting point than saturated fatty acids.
   As already stated, *trans* isomers are not generally found in natural fats. They are, however, produced by certain bacteria some species of which reside in the cow's rumen. *Trans* fatty acids are thus present as a minor component of the fat in milk, cheese and butter. They may also be present in the diet when hydrogenated polyunsaturates in, for example, margarines, are consumed. Hydrogenation involves the reaction of unsaturated oils with hydrogen so that the double bonds are removed, and the melting point is raised creating a solid spread such as margarine, etc. However, at many double bonds the process may be incomplete and they are simply changed from *cis* to *trans* bonds. This also has the effect of straightening the kinks, which has the intended effect of raising the melting point, although the bond remains rigid. The possibility that *trans* isomers behave more like saturated fatty acids in their influence on serum cholesterol or may even be toxic has been raised (see Chapter 9).

**Fatty acid nomenclature**

Individual fatty acids frequently have common names relating to substances from which they are easily extractable or to the use to which they have been put. These are the names by which they are usually known and which will be used in this book (Table 1.1). A more logical and informative nomenclature based on their structure also exists, but this is not widely used outside biochemical textbooks except for the more highly polyunsaturated fatty acids from fish oils. The fish oil fatty acids most frequently mentioned in this text are eicosapentaenoic acid (eicosa = 20, pentaenoic = 5 double bonds), docosahexaenoic (docosa = 22, hexaenoic =

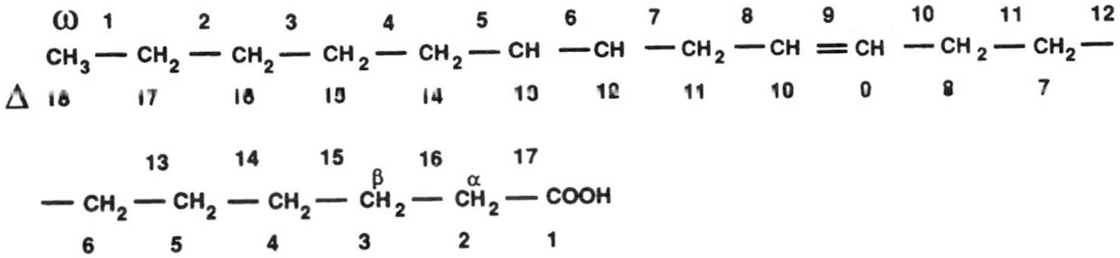

ω   1        2          3          4         5         6        7         8        9        10         11          12

CH₃ — CH₂ — CH₂ — CH₂ — CH₂ — CH — CH — CH₂ — CH ═ CH — CH₂ — CH₂ —

Δ 18     17       16       15       14       13      12      11      10      0        8          7

            13        14        15        16        17
                                      β         α
— CH₂ — CH₂ — CH₂ — CH₂ — CH₂ — COOH

       6         5          4          3          2          1

**Figure 1.4** The two classifications of unsaturated fatty acids are based on either the position of the double bond nearest the methyl carbon, which is denoted as omega and the bond involving it is the first (omega classification), or the position of all the double bonds relative to the carboxyl carbon which is counted as the first (delta classification) e.g. linoleic acid is classified as 18 : 2 Δ9, 12 or 18 : 2 ω6

6 double bonds) and docosapentaenoic (docosa = 22, pentaenoic = 5 double bonds). The adoption here of mixed terminology does not imply that the author endorses it, but the acceptance that, if this text is to be accessible to doctors and nutritionists, it must recognize what is common usage.

Notational systems for naming fatty acids also exist. The total number of carbon atoms in the fatty acid molecule are designated as C16, C18 etc. The total number of double bonds in the fatty acid molecule are then shown following a colon. Thus palmitic acid is C16 : 0, oleic acid C18 : 1, linoleic acid C18 : 2, etc.

A further refinement is to identify where any double bonds occur in the carbon chain. Usually their position is stated in relation to the methyl end of the carbon chain (Figure 1.4). The carbon atom of the terminal methyl group is the omega carbon. In this system the carbon atom attached to the carboxyl group carbon (i.e. the first carbon in the hydrocarbon chain at the carboxyl end) is called alpha, the next carbon beta and so on through the Greek alphabet. Hence the term beta oxidation when a two-carbon unit is split off the carboxyl end by oxidation of the beta carbon, i.e. carbon 3 in the delta clarification. Because few of us are gifted with the ability to remember the Greek alphabet, the last (i.e. methyl carbon) is always referred to by the last letter of the alphabet, omega (ω). A fatty acid in which the first double bond from the omega carbon occurs between the 9th and 10th carbons is referred to as omega 9, between the 6th and 7th as omega 6, between 3rd and 4th as omega 3 and so on. Thus oleic acid is omega 9, C18 : 1 and linoleic and linolenic acids are omega 6, C18 : 2 and omega 3, C18 : 3, respectively. Nutritionists and biochemists often refer to omega 3 fatty acids, meaning the highly polyunsaturated fatty acids of fish oils, i.e. eicosapentaenoic (omega 3, C20 : 5), docosahexaenoic (omega 3, C22 : 6), etc. To those unfamiliar with this terminology it can lend discussions a certain mysticism and make those taking part appear to have a greater knowledge of the subject than actually exists. Further confusion is sometimes created because many nutritionists disgruntled by the absence of an omega key on their typewriter started to replace 'ω' with 'n'. It seems pointless to continue this now that most word processors have an omega symbol. The alternative to the omega system (the Geneva system which is the official one and sadly not much used outside textbooks!) numbers the carbon atoms from the carboxyl carbon, which is one in that system. The β carbon in the omega system is thus carbon 3 in the delta classification. Double bonds are numbered according to their distance from carbon one. In the system, a capital delta (Δ) is used to indicate distance (Figure 1.4).

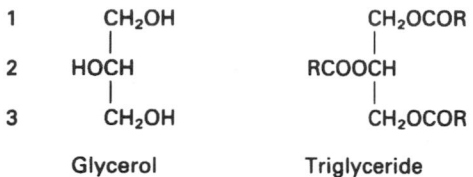

| 1 | CH₂OH | | CH₂OCOR |
| 2 | HOCH | | RCOOCH |
| 3 | CH₂OH | | CH₂OCOR |
| | Glycerol | | Triglyceride |

**Figure 1.5**  Triglycerides (triacylglycerols) are formed by esterifying the hydroxyl groups of glycerol to fatty acids. The position of the fatty acyl groups (R) is denoted as 1, 2, or 3, according to which of the carbon atoms of the glycerol they occupy

# Glycerides

### Triglycerides (triacylglycerols)

*Structure*

Triglycerides are formed by the esterification of glycerol (Figure 1.5) with fatty acids.

*Properties*

Triglycerides are the major storage form of fatty acids and, indeed, the major energy store in mammals. They are highly efficient as an energy store. Adipose cells consist of a large triglyceride droplet surrounded by a small rim of cytoplasm.

Very little water is thus required for the storage of fat. Triglycerides yield about 9 kcal/g* on respiration and since only about 10% of adipose tissue is cytoplasm, some 8 kcal is available from every gram of adipose tissue. This compares favourably with carbohydrate, which is an unsatisfactory energy store for a mobile animal. Carbohydrates, as every medical student knows, yield some 4 kcal/g. However, what is not so well appreciated is that this figure refers to refined carbohydrates. When present in living tissue even as glycogen, its storage form in animals, there is a large amount of cytoplasm also present, so that each gram of glycogen-containing liver or muscle yields less than 1 kcal.

Triglycerides are thus the major energy store to maintain humans during food deprivation. This is true of all mobile animals, and because fat is light in relation to its energy yield it is essential for hibernation and migration. In a healthy, non-obese, 70 kg man the triglyceride stores comprise some 15 kg, representing 140 000 kcal of stored energy (compare this to 6 kg of protein equivalent to 24 000 kcal and 225 mg of glycogen representing 900 kcal). In mammals, such as man, triglycerides also have a special significance, because they are the major means by which energy is transferred from mother to baby during breast feeding. Indeed, breast milk consists of lipoproteins in many respects similar to the triglyceride-rich lipoproteins produced by the gut and liver (see later). Triglycerides are also essential to mammals for thermoregulation. The subcutaneous adipose tissue acts as a heat insulator and the energy from the oxidation of fat contributes to the body's heating. In young mammals, specialized adipose tissue (brown adipose tissue) rich

---

* 1 kilocalorie  (kcal) (1000 calories) = 4.2 megajoules (MJ). In clinical practice, a kilocalorie is often written as 'Calorie', i.e. with a capital 'C' and without the 'kilo' prefix..

in mitochondria permits the rapid production of heat by fat oxidation regulated via the sympathetic nervous system.

The temperature of an animal's habitat has an important effect on the fatty acids present in its body fat. If the body is not to become a rigid structure incapable of movement, fats must be liquid at body temperature. The melting point of triglycerides is thus in general below that of the body temperature. The saturated fatty acids have higher melting points than unsaturated fatty acids and the more highly unsaturated they are the lower are their melting points. This is also true of triglycerides, which is why butter and lard are hard when stored in a refrigerator, whereas margarines high in polyunsaturates remain soft. In the case of warm-blooded animals, such as mammals, with a core temperature in the region of 37 °C, even triglycerides containing saturated fats can be stored internally in fluid form. Thus the deposition of fat around vital organs, rather than a rigid casing, provides a fluid cushion to protect them. This is, of course, evident from the feel of the tissues during a surgical operation. The subcutaneous adipose tissue, however, more closely approximates to the temperature of the environment. In animals adapted to live in a cold climate, the presence of saturated fatty acids in their subcutaneous tissues would give them a rigid carapace making movement impossible, an effect which would be heightened because it is these very animals which require the thickest layers of subcutaneous adipose tissue (blubber) for insulation. Animals such as seals, therefore, have polyunsaturated, frequently highly polyunsaturated, fatty acids in the triglycerides of their blubber. In the case of cold-blooded animals such as fish, where the whole body tends to assume the temperature of the habitat, survival in a cold climate dictates that triglyceride fatty acids throughout the body fat be unsaturated. The fats of fish, for example the liver oils of fish which live in cold water, contain large quantities of highly polyun saturated fatty acids. It is thus clearly the case that high animal fat diets consisting of blubber and fish are very different from those containing large amounts of carcass fat from pigs, cows and sheep.

### Monoglycerides and diglycerides (monoacylglycerols and diacylglycerols)

These are glycerides in which only one or two of the carbon atoms of glycerol are esterified with fatty acids. They are usually present only in tissues where triglycerides are being broken down to release fatty acids (lipolysis) and are thus present in high concentration in the gut during fat digestion (see page 20).

### Triglyceride biosynthesis

Many tissues have the capacity to synthesize triglycerides, particularly the gut, the liver, the adipose tissue and muscle.

In most tissues the reaction proceeds via glycerol-3-phosphate (Figure 1.6), which is itself synthesized via a dehydrogenase reaction from dihydroxyacetone phosphate, an intermediate in the glycolytic pathway. Liver, but not adipose tissue, also possesses a kinase, permitting the synthesis of glycerol-3-phosphate.

Glycerol-3-phosphate is esterified with fatty acids in the form of fatty acyl-CoA to form phosphatidic acid (Figure 1.6). Its 1 position is the first to be acylated and the enzyme catalysing this reaction has a preference for saturated fatty acids. The enzyme catalysing the acylation of the 2 position has a preference for unsaturated fatty acids.

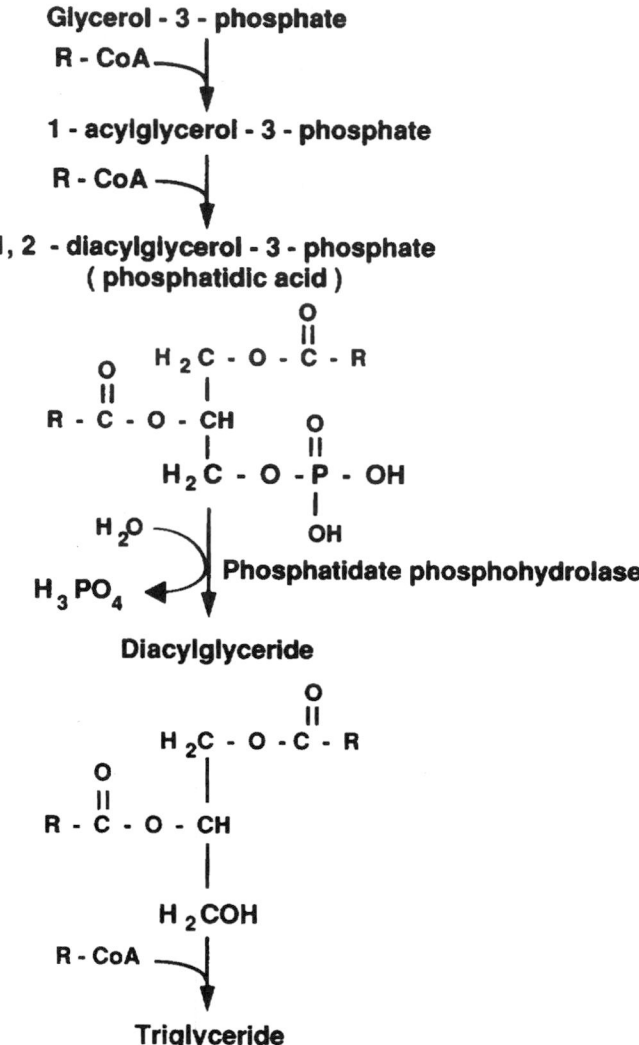

**Figure 1.6**  The synthesis of triglycerides from glycerol-3-phosphate. Phosphatidate phosphohydrolase is the rate-limiting enzyme

An enzyme, phosphatidate phosphohydrolase, then removes the phosphate group to produce diglyceride. This enzyme is rate-limiting for triglyceride biosynthesis. Diglyceride may also be formed in the gut from monoglyceride absorbed after the digestion of fat. The final stage of triglyceride synthesis involves the esterification of the free hydroxyl group of the diglycerides with fatty acyl CoA. Both saturated and unsaturated fatty acids participate in this reaction equally well.

Fatty acids for triglyceride synthesis may be supplied in several ways. In tissues such as muscle, adipose tissue and lactating breast, a major source may be from lipolysis of circulating triglycerides by the enzyme lipoprotein lipase (see Chapter 2, page 56). The major source of fatty acids for the enterocytes is from the digestion of fats. In the liver, circulating non-esterified fatty acids (NEFA) are an important source of fatty acid for triglyceride synthesis as well as for ketone body synthesis. Indeed in many conditions the rate of delivery of NEFA to the liver will be the major influence on both hepatic triglyceride synthesis and very low density lipoprotein secretion.

In addition, a major source of fatty acids for triglyceride synthesis is *de novo* fatty acid synthesis from acetyl-CoA derived from carbohydrates, such as glucose. This is the fate of most dietary carbohydrate, which is not immediately used as respiratory substrate, allowing its storage as triglycerides. The enzyme, which is rate limiting for fatty acid synthesis, is acetyl-CoA carboxylase, which permits the formation of malonyl-CoA. A series of molecules of malonyl-CoA is then combined with acetyl-CoA to form palmitic acid by an array of enzymes in a highly organized complex known as fatty acid synthetase. Further elongation and desaturation reactions may then take place to produce the great versatility of fatty acids in different tissues.

### Mobilization of fatty acids from triglyceride stores

Adipose tissue contains two triglyceride lipase enzymes. One, termed lipoprotein lipase, has many features in common with the lipoprotein lipase of muscle and lactating breast and serves to remove the triglyceride component from the circulating triglyceride-rich lipoproteins (see Chapter 2, page 56). It is located on the vascular endothelium. The other triglyceride lipase is located within the adipose cell and its function is to hydrolyse the stored triglycerides (Figure 1.7) so that their fatty acids can enter the circulation when they are required as energy substrates. During fasting, the respiratory quotient is low and these NEFA are the predominant metabolic substrate. The two triglyceride lipases are not only functionally distinct, but also structurally and immunologically so.

The intracellular triglyceride lipase of adipose tissue is sometimes called hormone sensitive lipase. This is probably a bad name for it, since lipoprotein lipase is also regulated by hormones. Regulatory factors, however, frequently have opposite effects on the two triglyceride lipases. Nevertheless, because of the very different physiological roles of these lipase enzymes this produces an overall effect which is concerted. The action of insulin, for example, is to activate lipoprotein lipase while simultaneously inhibiting the intracellular adipose tissue triglyceride lipase. Lipoprotein lipase located on the vascular endothelium of adipose tissue releases fatty acids from the triglycerides of circulating lipoproteins. These are largely taken up by the adipocytes, where the activity of the intracellular lipase,

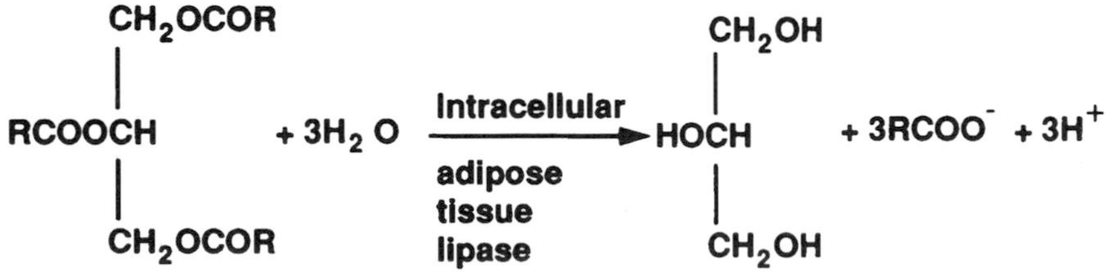

$$
\begin{array}{l}
CH_2OCOR \\
| \\
RCOOCH \qquad + 3H_2O \xrightarrow[\substack{\text{Intracellular} \\ \text{adipose} \\ \text{tissue} \\ \text{lipase}}]{} \quad
\begin{array}{l}
CH_2OH \\
| \\
HOCH \qquad + 3RCOO^- + 3H^+ \\
| \\
CH_2OH
\end{array} \\
| \\
CH_2OCOR
\end{array}
$$

**Figure 1.7**   Lipolysis: the hydrolysis of triglyceride mobilizes long-chain fatty acids from stored triglycerides

is low, and are resynthesized into triglycerides. Thus the action of insulin released, for example postprandially, is in this respect to promote the storage of triglycerides in adipose tissue. During fasting, when insulin levels are low, the intracellular triglyceride lipase becomes active and the stored triglycerides within the adipocytes are released as NEFA to fulfil the body's energy requirements – directly in the case of muscle and following their partial oxidation to ketone bodies by the liver in the case of other tissues such as brain.

A bewildering galaxy of other hormones can activate the intracellular lipase of adipose tissue, at least *in vivo*. These include catecholamines, glucagon, vasopressin, serotonin, fat mobilizing pituitary peptides and MSH. They all act on membrane receptors to activate adenylate cyclase and increase the intracellular concentration of cyclic AMP (cAMP). Thyroxine and corticosteroids also activate lipolysis, perhaps by making the adipocyte more sensitive to the lipolytic hormones possessing cell surface receptors. As already indicated, these lipolytic hormones are opposed by insulin, which decreases intracellular lipolysis, although its detailed action is less clearly understood. Certainly its effect in increasing glucose uptake will favour triglyceride synthesis, but other mechanisms directly opposing catecholamine effects may also be involved. More readily explicable is the action of β-adrenoreceptor blocking drugs which also inhibit intracellular lipolysis. Prostaglandins too inhibit the release of fatty acids from adipocytes, but the physiological significance of this observation is uncertain.

Besides hormone-sensitive triglyceride lipase, adipocytes contain other acyl hydrolase activities, such as diglyceride lipases and monoglyceride lipases and cholesterol esterases. These do not, however, appear to be rate-limiting for the release of NEFA.

The term free fatty acids has frequently been used for NEFA. The free fatty acids released into the circulation are only free in the sense that they are non-esterified. They are, in fact, very largely bound to albumin, with only the minutest quantities actually being truly free. The term non-esterified fatty acids (NEFA) is therefore to be preferred to free fatty acids (FFA) and probably even better is albumin-bound fatty acids (ABFA). The concentration of NEFA in the plasma is about 300–800 µmol/1 (7.5–20 mg/dl). The apparently low concentration of NEFA in the circulation hides their major importance as a lipid transport system. This is revealed by their very rapid circulating half-life, which is as low as 2–3 min, meaning that one-third or more of the NEFA in the plasma compartment are removed each minute. Assuming a concentration of 10 mg/dl and a plasma volume of 3 litres this represents a turnover of more than 100 mg/min or 144 g/day. Compare this with the dietary triglycerides transported in the circulation (about 70 g/day) and hepatic triglycerides transported in the circulation (20–50 g/day).

## Starvation

To understand the biological purpose of triglycerides (and for that matter to comprehend the pathophysiology of diabetic ketoacidosis (see Chapter 11)) it is important to consider what happens during fasting. Fasting leads to declining insulin secretion and the release of stress hormones such as catecholamines, glucagon, growth hormone and corticosteroids. These act on hormone-sensitive triglyceride lipase to accelerate the release of NEFA from the adipose organ, as has been previously described. Some tissues such as muscle can oxidize these fatty acids directly as an energy substrate. Other tissues are unable to do so and in the non-fasting state must oxidize glucose for their energy requirements. When, however, the very modest store of glycogen has been used up (within a few hours of commencing the fast), glucose is only available from gluconeogenesis. This occurs mainly from amino acids (principally alanine) released from the protein of muscle.

With the exception of the glycerol released during lipolysis, no component of fat can be converted to glucose in man. Man has no store of protein which does not perform some structural or functional role. If his vital proteins are to be spared, some energy substrate other than glucose, preferably derived from fatty acids, is therefore required for those tissues which cannot themselves directly oxidize fatty acids. This need is met by the ketone bodies. These are produced in the liver by a partial oxidation process, which progressively cleaves off two carbon units from the fatty acid chain by oxidizing the $\beta$ carbon thus breaking the bond between the $\alpha$ and $\beta$ carbon atoms. Hence this process is known as $\beta$-oxidation. The two carbon units are produced as acetyl-CoA, which can be released as acetone or paired together in a condensation reaction to produce acetoacetate or $\beta$-hydroxybutyrate (3-hydroxybutyrate). These ketone bodies are extremely valuable as energy substrates since they are readily soluble in water and thus easily transportable, for example, across the blood–brain barrier. Most tissues can adapt to convert ketone bodies back to acetyl-CoA, which is then fed into Krebs' (tricarboxylic acid) cycle. The brain can reduce its glucose utilization to less than 40% of its energy requirements during prolonged fasting and this, together with the requirement of red blood cells for glucose, then represents almost the sole energy requirement not met by fat. In evolutionary terms, the development of a larger brain seems to be paralleled by the capacity to generate ketone bodies.

One further advantage, usually claimed, for respiring fat during starvation is that it reduces the requirement for an external supply of water, since more water is produced by oxidation of fat than by oxidation of carbohydrate (Figure 1.8). Since food and water supplies are often in jeopardy simultaneously, this again aids survival. It can be seen from Figure 1.8 that oxidizing fat produces more water (1.1 ml/g) than the same weight of carbohydrate (0.6 ml/g). However, in terms of the energy produced, the quantity of water is rather more for carbohydrate than fat (0.15 ml/kcal against 0.12 ml/kcal).

Nevertheless, the camel's hump contains fat and not water. The advantage of this must be that fat provides a means of transporting the hydrogen to make water without the heavier oxygen which is unnecessary since it is all around him in the desert anyway. I leave the reader to speculate on whether the energy produced in oxidizing the fat to release this water is going to be surplus to his requirements,

$$5.6\ C_6H_{12}O_6 \xrightarrow{\quad O_2 \quad} 34\ CO_2 + 34\ H_2O + 4000\ kcal$$

1000 g glucose                                            612 g

$$1.2\ (C_{18}H_{33}O_2)_3\ CH_2CHCH_2 \xrightarrow{\quad O_2 \quad} 68\ CO_2 + 62\ H_2O + 9000\ kcal$$

1000 g triolein                                          1116 g

**Figure 1.8**    Energy and water produced when 1000 g of carbohydrate and 1000 g of fat are oxidized

leaving him the problem of avoiding overheating! Perhaps Kipling still has the last word:

> 'Do you see that?' said the Djinn, 'That's your very own humph that you've brought upon your very own self by not working.'
> 'How can I,' said the camel, 'with this humph on my back?'
> 'That's made a-purpose,', said the Djinn, '.... You will be able to work now for three days without eating, because you can live on your humph. ....'

[Just-So Stories]

## Phospholipids

### Structure and function

The phospholipids in plasma are largely glycerophospholipids. Like the triglycerides they are all derived from glycerol. They differ in that phosphoric acid is esterified to the glycerol (usually at the 3 position) (Figure 1.9). This phosphate is in turn ester linked to another small molecule, generally an organic base, amino acid or alcohol. Fatty acids are esterified to the glycerol backbone at one or both

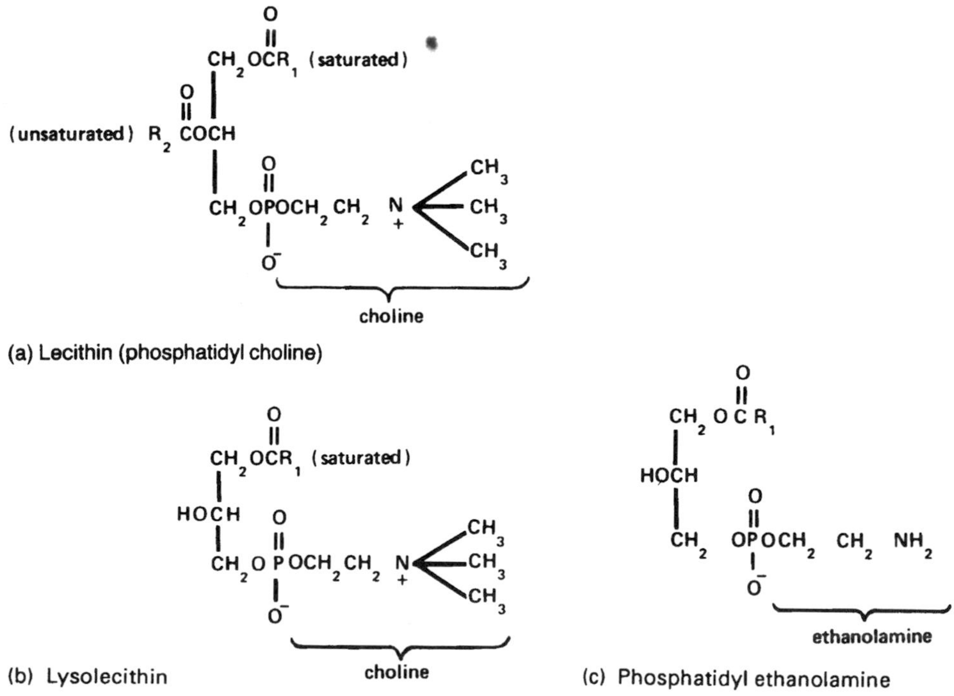

**Figure 1.9**  Some examples of glycerophospholipids. The choline-containing glycerophospholipids are the lecithins, abundant in lipoproteins and cell membranes. Phosphatidyl ethanolamine is one of the cephalins (alcohol-insoluble glycerophospholipids) which are widely distributed in cell membranes

of its other positions. The presence of the non-polar hydrocarbon chains of these fatty acids and the polar phosphate group means that glycerophospholipids have one extremity which eschews water (hydrophobic) and another which is attracted to water (hydrophilic). A great variety in the structure and properties of phospholipids is possible because of the wide range of compounds which may be esterified to the phosphate group and differences in the chain length and saturation of the fatty acyl groups.

The lecithins (phosphatidyl cholines) are the most commonly occurring glycerophospholipids in plasma and the extracellular fluids and are also abundant in cell membranes (Figure 1.9). In plasma, the fatty acyl group attached to the middle carbon of the glycerol (2 position) may be transferred to plasma cholesterol to produce cholesteryl ester, a reaction catalysed by the enzyme lecithin: cholesterol acyl transferase (see Chapter 2, p. 57). The resulting monoacyl glycerophospholipid (or lysophospholipid) is called lysolecithin. Lysophospholipids are so called because they have powerful detergent properties, which if their concentration were permitted to build up would lead to membrane lysis. In addition to the lecithins, other phospholipids are widely distributed in cell membranes. One example is the glycerophospholipids, the cephalins (having in common insolubility in alcohol), which also occur commonly. These include phosphatidyl ethanolamine (Figure 1.9), phosphatidyl serine and phosphatidyl inositol. Also widely distributed in cell membranes are phospholipids derived from the alcohol, sphingosine, rather than glycerol (sphingophospholipids). Sphingomyelins (Figure 1.10) are a commonly occurring example.

The importance of phospholipids lies in their ability to form a bridge between hydrophobic non-polar lipids and water, which is polar. They can thus act as emulsifying agents. Without an emulsifying agent, oil and water, after being mixed together, rapidly separate into two layers. If soap (the sodium salt of a long-chain fatty acid) is added, then, on shaking, the oil forms an emulsion, which is a suspension of tiny droplets. Each droplet consists of a central core of oil with a surrounding envelope, in which the hydrocarbon chains of the fatty acids have buried themselves in the oil, leaving their negatively charged carboxyl groups exposed to the ionized water to which they are attracted. Such a droplet is known as a micelle. These are basic to an understanding of lipid physiology. Because they are similarly charged, micelles repel each other and do not coalesce, thus preventing the

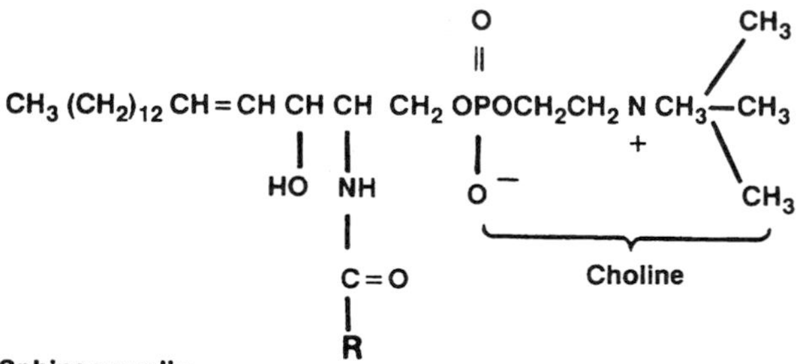

$$CH_3\,(CH_2)_{12}\,CH=CH\ CH\ CH\ CH_2\ OPOCH_2CH_2\ N\ CH_3{-}CH_3$$

with substituents: HO, NH on the glycerol carbons; C=O then R below NH; $O^-$ and $\overset{+}{N}$ on the phosphate; and CH$_3$ groups on the nitrogen labelled **Choline**.

**Sphingomyelin**

**Figure 1.10**  Sphingomyelin is an example of a sphingophospholipid in which the fatty acyl group (R) is linked to the amino groups of the alcohol spingosine and choline esterified to its phosphate group

Water

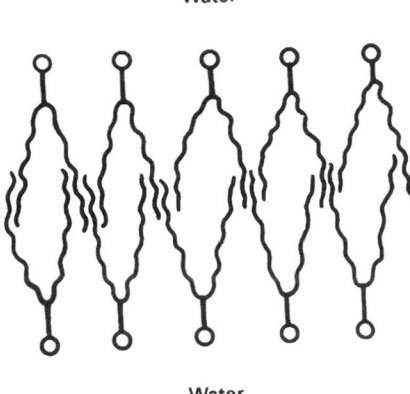

Water

**Figure 1.11**  Phospholipid bilayer

hydrophobic oil droplets uniting to form a single layer. Phospholipids behave in exactly the same way as soaps do. Their ability to form an outer charged envelope with a hydrophobic interior is the basis of the structure of the lipoproteins (see Chapter 2, page 37). The same property is partly responsible for maintaining cholesterol in micellar solution in bile and in the gut lumen.

An essential and even more fundamental role of phospholipids is in the formation of cell membranes. Just as in the formation of micelles the hydrophobic hydrocarbon chains of the phospholipid arrange themselves in contact with other non-polar lipids, so they will with the hydrocarbon chains of other phospholipids. They thus line up together with their outer phosphate groups exposed to the water and form the bilayer, which is the basis of the structure of the cell membrane (Figure 1.11).

Membrane physiology has been the subject of considerable scientific enquiry and it is beyond the scope of this book to dwell on this aspect of lipid physiology. However, the considerable variation in fatty acid structure and in the groups linked directly to the phosphate groups of the glycerophospholipids sphingophospholipids must make an important contribution to the enormous repertoire of these membranes in living organisms. Because of their ubiquity in cell membranes, phospholipids should be regarded as structural lipids (see also cholesterol below), whereas triglycerides serve principally as energy stores.

## Cholesterol

### Structure and function

Cholesterol is the predominant sterol in vertebrate animals. It may exist as free cholesterol or be esterified, usually with a fatty acyl group (Figure 1.12). It is an essential component of cell membranes, where it is present as free cholesterol. Thus most of the cholesterol in the body is free cholesterol. Cholesteryl esters may be present in cytoplasm as droplets. They are regarded as representing a storage form prevented from interacting with cell membranes because of their hydrophobicity.

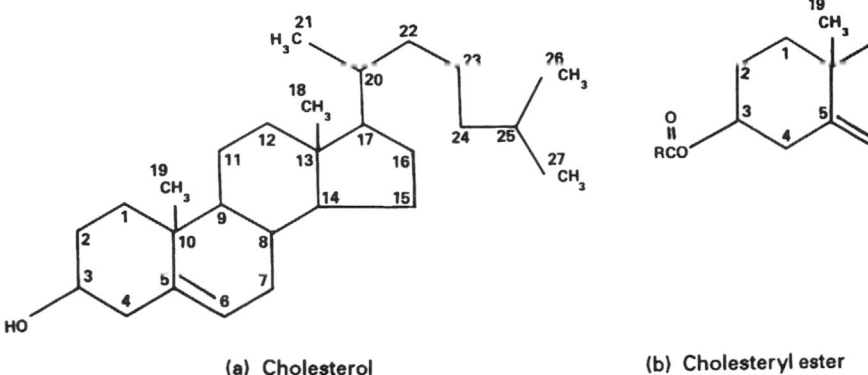

**(a) Cholesterol**

**(b) Cholesteryl ester**

**Figure 1.12**  Cholesterol and cholesteryl ester

In the plasma and extracellular fluids, where cholesterol is present in the lipoproteins, it is largely present as cholesteryl ester. In mammals, the nervous system is the tissue richest in cholesterol. During infancy there is a considerable increase in the cholesterol content of the white matter.

The role of cholesterol within the phospholipid bilayer of cell membranes appears to be to regulate and to stabilize their fluidity, which may influence important properties such as permeability. The hydroxyl groups of free cholesterol molecules are attracted to water and so within the membrane they are orientated with their hydroxyl groups adjacent to the phospholipid phosphate groups. The hydrocarbon rings of cholesterol are buried among the hydrocarbon chains of the phospholipids (Figure 1.13). This has the effect of reducing the range of movement of the first part of the hydrocarbon chains of the phospholipids and thus modifies the fluidity of the membrane in its outer region. Cholesterol also extends the temperature range over which a membrane is in a gel phase. If phospholipids alone were present in membranes, the different melting points of their fatty acids would

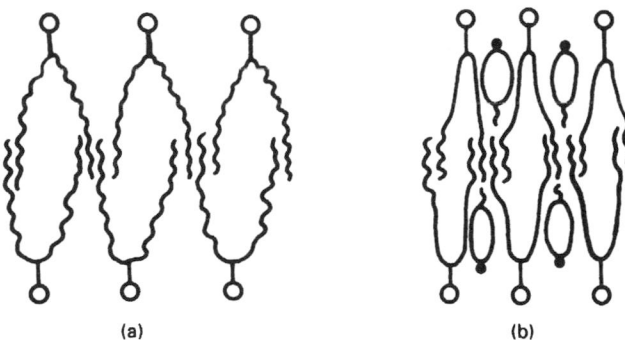

**(a)**

**(b)**

**Figure 1.13**  (*a*) A cell membrane without cholesterol and (*b*) a cell membrane with cholesterol. The presence of cholesterol makes it more rigid. Cholesterol arranges itself with its hydroxyl groups close to the phosphate groups of the phospholipid and its hydrocarbon tail tucked in towards the ends of the hydrophobic ends of the hydrocarbon chains of the phospholipid (After Myant, 1981)

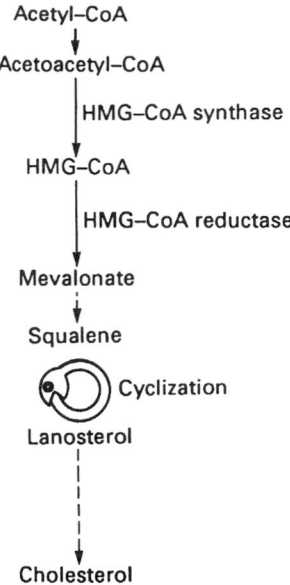

Acetyl–CoA

Acetoacetyl–CoA

HMG–CoA synthase

HMG–CoA

HMG–CoA reductase

Mevalonate

Squalene

Cyclization

Lanosterol

Cholesterol

**Figure 1.14**    Brief outline of the biosynthetic pathway of cholesterol

produce abrupt changes in fluidity. Where membrane cholesterol concentration is low, as in some leukaemic cells, there is an increase in membrane fluidity, whereas in some types of liver disease, red cell membrane cholesterol is increased and fragility decreased (see Chapter 11).

Two other major functions of cholesterol are as the precursor for bile salt synthesis and as the precursor of all the steroid hormones, including vitamin D. It is also secreted as a component of sebum.

## Cholesterol biosynthesis

The immensely complex cholesterol molecule is constructed from acetyl-CoA obtained from β-oxidation of fatty acids or from carbohydrate breakdown (Figure 1.14). A full description of the process which involves more than 30 enzymes is beyond the scope or purpose of this book. In the initial stages, three molecules of acetyl-CoA are condensed to form mevalonic acid. Further condensations then take place to give compounds of progressively increasing carbon content: isopentenyl pyrophosphate, farnesyl pyrophosphate and finally squalene. The long hydrocarbon chain of squalene then undergoes cyclization to give lanosterol, which is then converted to cholesterol. The rate-limiting stage in the process occurs in the formation of mevalonic acid from acetyl-CoA and involves the enzyme 3-hydroxy 3-methylglutaryl-coenzyme A reductase (HMG-CoA reductase).

### 3-Hydroxy, 3-methylglutaryl-coenzyme A reductase

This key enzyme (EC 1.1.1.34) is situated on the endoplasmic reticulum and catalyses the conversion of HMG-CoA to mevalonic acid. It has a molecular weight of 97 300 and its gene is located on chromosome 5.

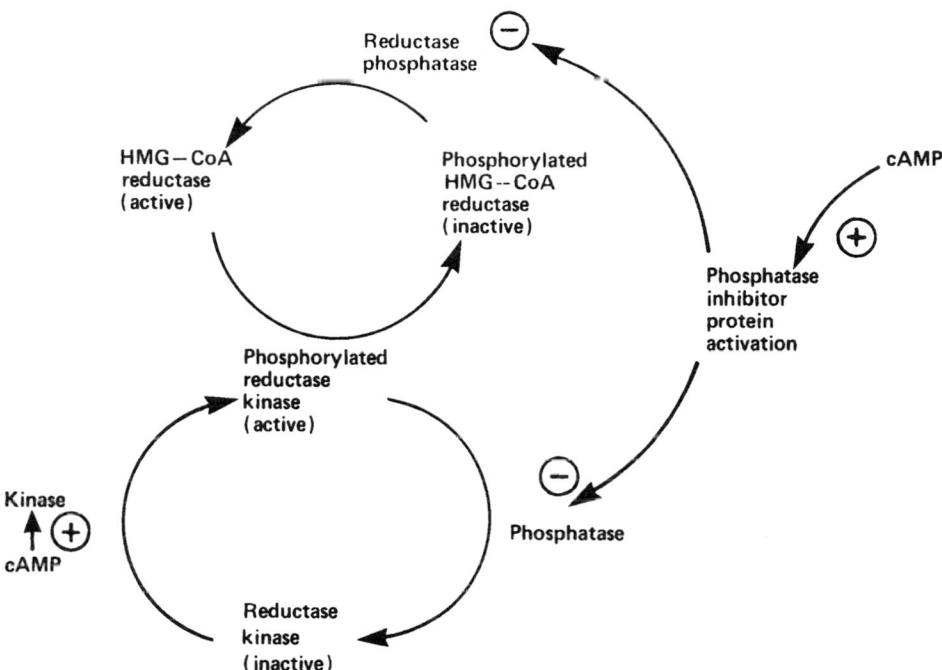

**Figure 1.15**   The reversible phosphorylation of HMG-CoA reductase may regulate its short-term activity, the dephosphorylated reductase enzyme being active. It has been proposed that this is important in the physiological regulation of the enzyme, as outlined in this chapter

HMG-CoA reductase is subject to both short-term and long-term control. Long-term effects are mediated through alterations in its rate of synthesis and degradation. Short-term effects probably involve allosteric effects and also alterations in its state of phosphorylation. In its active form the enzyme is not phosphorylated (Figure 1.15). The kinase enzyme, which maintains HMG-CoA reductase in its phosphorylated inactive state, must itself, however, be phosphorylated to be active. It has been proposed that cAMP may modify the state of phosphorylation of these proteins, perhaps via the intermediary of a phosphatase inhibitor protein, but the nature and physiological significance of these events is controversial. What is certain, however, is that cholesterol entering the liver from the diet (chylomicron remnants) has a major influence in suppressing hepatic HMG-CoA reductase and thus cholesterol synthesis. The effect is mediated by an increase in intracellular free cholesterol.

A similar inhibition of cholesterol synthesis occurs in cells such as fibroblasts in tissue culture when low density lipoprotein (LDL) cholesterol enters by the apo $B_{100}$ receptor route, and it is assumed that such a mechanism also exists in extrahepatic tissues *in vivo*. There is evidence that the effect of free cholesterol is mediated through suppression of transcription of the HMG-CoA reductase gene and an acceleration of degradation of the enzyme protein. Other factors believed to influence cholesterol biosynthesis in liver and possibly other tissues are summarized in Table 1.2.

**Table 1.2  Some factors which influence the rate of cholesterol biosynthesis\* in animal experiments**

| Cholesterol biosynthesis | |
| --- | --- |
| *Increased* | *Decreased* |
| Cholesterol malabsorption β-sitosterol | Dietary cholesterol |
| Interruption of enterohepatic circulation, e.g. biliary fistula, ileal bypass, cholestyramine | Portacaval shunt |
| Hormones insulin thyroxine catecholamines | Hormones glucagon glucocorticoids |
| Phenobarbitone | Clofibrate Nicotinic acid HMG-CoA reductase inhibitors, e.g. lovastatin |
| Dark | Light |

\* All are believed to operate by modulating the activity of the enzyme HMG-CoA reductase.

## Intestinal fat absorption

Dietary fat consists largely of triglycerides, lesser amounts of phospholipids and even smaller quantities of cholesterol (mostly free cholesterol). This is discussed in detail in Chapter 9. Within the stomach, digestion of proteins releases fats from their lipid–protein interactions and they are churned up into a loose oil–water emulsion of coarse droplets, in which the only significant surface-active materials are the dietary phospholipids. In the duodenum, mixing with bile salts leads to the formation of an emulsion of smaller oil globules, with a diameter of the order of l0 000 Å\* (Figure 1.16). The bile salts are detergents synthesized by the liver from cholesterol and released into the duodenum with bile. The primary bile salt acids are cholic acid and chenodeoxycholic acid (Figure 1.17). In the bile they are usually conjugated with glycine and taurine, but later in the lower small intestine and colon as a consequence of the activity of anaerobic bacteria (principally bacteroides) they undergo a variety of transformations. These include deconjugation, and the removal of the 7 alpha-hydroxyl groups resulting in the formation of deoxycholic acid from cholic acid and lithocholic acid from chenodeoxycholate. These are the so-called secondary bile acids. More than 20 different bile acids can be detected in the faeces. The primary bile acids and some of the secondary bile acids, deoxycholate in particular, are absorbed through the terminal ileum. They are extracted from the blood circulation by the liver, conjugated and secreted back into the bile. Bile salts emulsify fats by virtue of their polar carboxyl and hydroxyl groups which are hydrophobic, and their lipophilic hydrocarbon rings which interface with lipids.

\* 1 Angstrom (Å) = 0.1 nanometre.

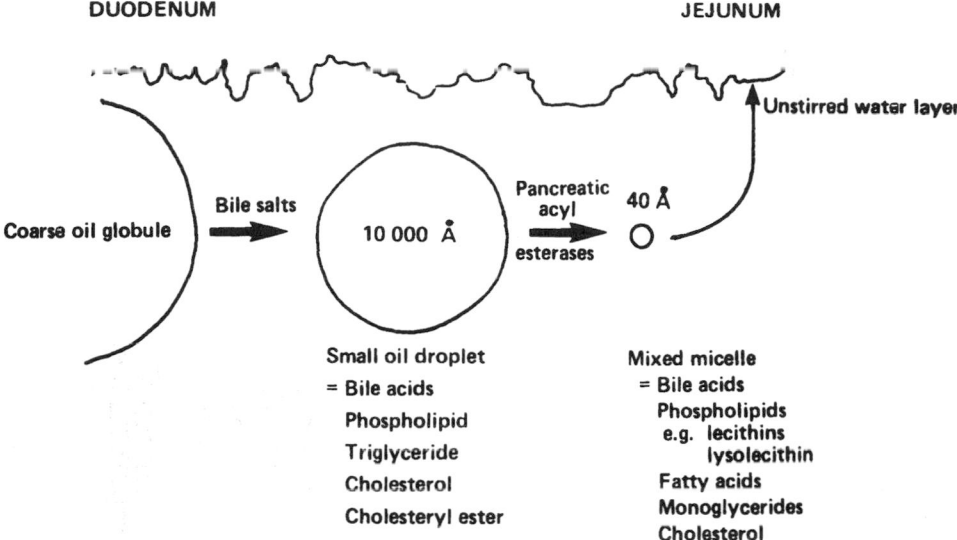

**DUODENUM**

**JEJUNUM**

Unstirred water layer

Coarse oil globule

Bile salts

10 000 Å

Pancreatic acyl esterases

40 Å

Small oil droplet
= Bile acids
  Phospholipid
  Triglyceride
  Cholesterol
  Cholesteryl ester

Mixed micelle
= Bile acids
  Phospholipids
  e.g. lecithins
     lysolecithin
  Fatty acids
  Monoglycerides
  Cholesterol

**Figure 1.16** Fat digestion relies on the formation of a progressively finer emulsion, in which bile salts, together with the products of fat digestion themselves, are essential

In the duodenum, pancreatic lipase acts on the emulsified fats, rapidly removing the fatty acid in the 3 position of the triglycerides to produce 1,2-diglycerides and then 2-monoglycerides by removal of the fatty acid in the 1 position. Some of the glycerophospholipids such as lecithin are also partially hydrolysed to lysoglycerophospholipids. Pancreatic cholesteryl ester esterase converts esterified cholesterol to free cholesterol. The combination of conjugated bile acids, phospholipids such as lecithin and lysolecithin, fatty acids, monoglycerides and small quantities of diglycerides, produces mixed micelles. These are much smaller particles, with an average diameter of 40 Å. Their formation is essential for efficient fat absorption. Mixed micelles permit intimate contact between the products of fat digestion and the microvilli. The conceptual barrier between the gut lumen and the luminal surface of the enterocyte across which the relatively insoluble molecules like the products of fat digestion must pass in order to be absorbed, is known as the

Glycine

$-CO\ NH\ CH_2\ COOH$

Taurine

$-CO\ NH\ CH_2\ CH_2\ SO_3\ H$

HO

12

HO

3

7

OH

**Cholic**

HO

3

7

OH

**Chenodeoxycholic**

**Figure 1.17** The primary bile salts: cholic acid and chenodeoxycholic acid. They are synthesized from cholesterol in the liver. Here they are shown conjugated to glycine and taurine as they occur in the bile

unstirred water layer. Although this layer is equivalent to a distance of less than 0.5 mm, it is a major barrier. In the absence of bile salts (total biliary obstruction), mixed micelles are not formed and cholesterol absorption is virtually non-existent.

Fatty acids, monoglycerides, phospholipids and cholesterol enter the enterocytes from the mixed micelles. Cholesterol absorption, unlike that of triglycerides and phospholipids, is incomplete, only 30–60% of dietary cholesterol entering the body. This is because, in addition to bile salts, the detergent properties of phospholipids and fatty acids are essential for the mixed micelles. Since these are rapidly absorbed in the jejunum, cholesterol absorption cannot therefore occur to any significant extent thereafter. Sterols other than cholesterol are also incorporated into mixed micelles. Plant sterols (phytosterols), such as β sitosterol, are present in the diet in significant amounts. However, they do not cross the enterocytes to any significant extent (other than in the exceptionally rare condition called β sitosterolaemia). The administration of large amounts of β sitosterol orally has been shown to interfere with cholesterol absorption, presumably by displacing it from mixed micelles. Neomycin, too, owes its hypocholesterolaemic action to disruption of mixed micelles (see Chapter 10).

Once in the enterocytes, long-chain fatty acids and monoglycerides are resynthesized into triglycerides and cholesterol is re-esterified. These are complexed with phospholipids and apolipoproteins, the synthesis of which is closely linked to fat absorption. The chylomicrons are the lipoprotein particles thus formed. They are secreted into the lymphatic system and are considered in detail in the next chapter. The more water-soluble short-chain fatty acids and to some extent medium-chain fatty acids up to around C14, enter the portal blood stream directly. The short-chain fatty acids are not present in substantial quantities in normal diets, but attempts are sometimes made to use them to provide nutritional support for patients in whom chylomicron formation is compromised or to be avoided (Chapter 9).

## Essential fatty acids and eicosanoids

Certain fatty acids derived from plant sources are essential components of the diet of animals. The deficiency syndrome which develops in rats fed a fat-free diet can be corrected with small quantities of linoleic acid (C18 : 22, ω6,9) and alpha linolenic acid (C18 : 3, ω3,6,9). Animals lack the desaturase enzyme which can insert double bonds in the ω6 and ω3 position of the methylene chain of saturated fatty acids. Thus the human liver can convert stearic acid (C18 : 0) to oleic acid (C18 : 1, ω9), but cannot produce the ω3 or ω6 series of fatty acids. Linoleic acid and alpha linolenic acid are termed essential fatty acids. Their particular importance is that they are the simplest substrates, from which, in animals, C20 unsaturated fatty acids can by synthesized (Figure 1.18). These are essential for the synthesis of the eicosanoids, a group of important locally active regulatory factors (autocoids) which includes prostaglandins, thomboxanes, prostacyclins and leukotrienes. The term eicosanoid means a C20 fatty acid derivative.

The eicosanoids are produced from dihomo-alpha-linolenic acid, arachidonic acid and eicosapentaenoic acid (Figure 1.18). These fatty acids have a U-bend in the middle of their hydrocarbon chains. The first eicosanoids discovered were the prostaglandins. A bond between carbon 8 and 12 makes a five-membered ring, creating the familiar hairpin structure of the prostaglandins (Figure 1.19). The ring

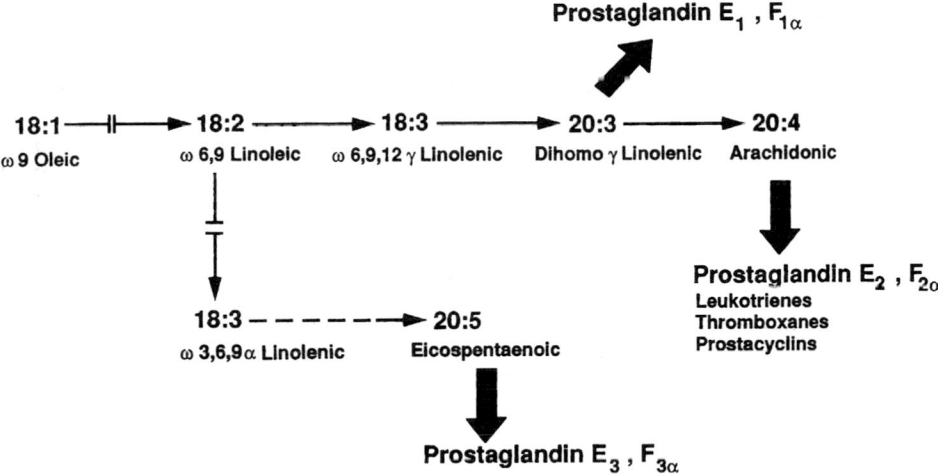

Prostaglandin E$_1$ , F$_{1\alpha}$

18:1 —||—► 18:2 ————————► 18:3 ————————► 20:3 ————————► 20:4
ω 9 Oleic      ω 6,9 Linoleic    ω 6,9,12 γ Linolenic    Dihomo γ Linolenic    Arachidonic

18:3 – – – – – ►  20:5
ω 3,6,9α Linolenic    Eicospentaenoic

Prostaglandin E$_2$ , F$_{2\alpha}$
Leukotrienes
Thromboxanes
Prostacyclins

Prostaglandin E$_3$ , F$_{3\alpha}$

**Figure 1.18**   Linoleic acid and alpha linolenic acids are essential nutrients in higher animals which lack the enzymes to convert oleic acid to linoleic acid and linoleic acid to alpha linolenic acid. Linoleic and alpha linolenic acids are precursors for eicosanoid synthesis

**Arachidonic and**

**Prostaglandin E$_2$**

**Leukotriene B$_4$**

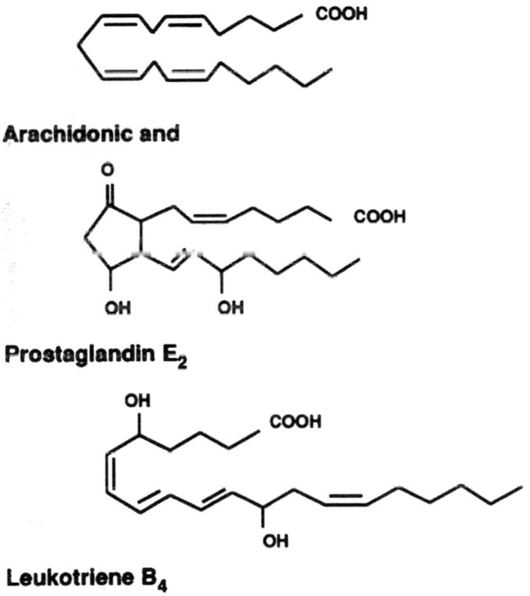

**Figure 1.19**   Structure of the fatty acid arachidonic acid and two of the eicosanoids synthesized from it

may have had a keto group or a hydroxy group at carbon 9 (PGE series and PGF series respectively). Prostacyclin and the thromboxanes, which like prostaglandins E$_2$ and F$_{2\alpha}$, are formed from arachidonic acid by cyclooxygenase activity, have a similar 5-membered ring whereas leukotrienes, hydroxy- and hydroperoxy fatty

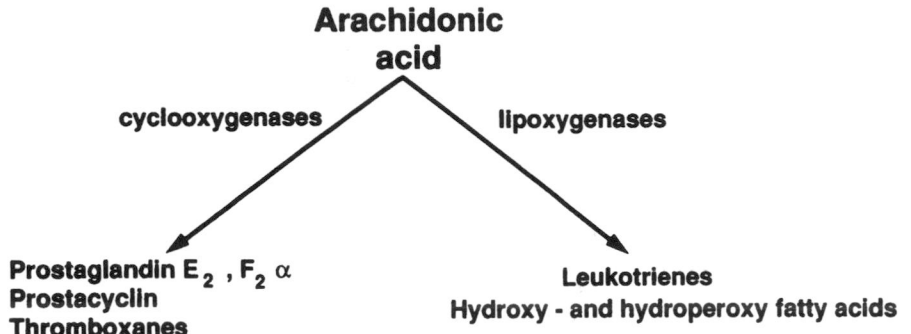

**Figure 1.20**   Eicosanoids formed from arachidonic acid by two different series of oxidation reactions catalysed by cyclooxygenases and lipoxygenases respectively

acids are formed by a different oxidation reaction of arachidonic acid catalysed by lipoxygenases and do not have the closed ring at their U-bend (Figure 1.20).

## Further reading

Applequist, D., De Puy, C.H. and Rinehart, K.L. *Introduction to Organic Chemistry*, John Wiley, New York (1982)

Cahill, G.F. Starvation in man. *N. Engl. J. Med.*, **282**, 668–675 (1970)

Coultate, T. *Food. The Chemistry of its Components*, 2nd edn, Royal Society of Chemistry, London (1989)

Gibbons, G.F., Mitropoulos, K.A. and Myant, N.B. *Biochemistry of Cholesterol*, 4th edn, Elsevier Biomedical Press, Amsterdam (1982)

Gurr, M.I. and James, A.T. *Lipid Biochemistry: An Introduction*, Chapman and Hall, London (1991)

Hilditch, T. P. and Williams, P. N. *The Chemical Constitution of Natural Fats*, Chapman and Hall, London (1964)

Lehninger, A. L. *Biochemistry*, Worth Publishers, New York (1975)

Mahler, R. F. Fat: the good, the bad and the ugly. *J. R. Coll. Phys.*, **12**, 107–121 (1977)

Mangold, H. K., Zweig, G. and Shermaeds, J. (eds). *CRC Handbook of Chromatography: Lipids*, vols I and II, CRC Press, Boca Raton (1984)

Myant, N. B. *The Biology of Cholesterol and Related Steroids*, Heinemann Medical, London (1981)

Vergroesen, A. J. (ed.). *The Role of Fats in Human Nutrition*, Academic Press, London (1975)

# Chapter 2

# Lipoproteins and their metabolism

## Outline of lipoprotein metabolism (Figure 2.1)

### Lipid transport to the tissues

The products of fat digestion (fatty acids, monoglycerides, lysolecithin and free cholesterol) enter the enterocytes from the mixed micelles. They are re-esterified in the smooth endoplasmic reticulum of these cells. Long-chain fatty acids (>14 C) are esterified with monoglycerides to form triglycerides and with lysolecithin to form lecithin. Free cholesterol is esterified by the enzyme acyl-CoA:cholesterol O-acyltransferase (ACAT). The esterified lipids are then formed into lipoproteins.

Lipoproteins are the macromolecular complexes of lipid and protein, a major function of which is to transport lipids through the vascular and extravascular body fluids (Figures 2.2, 2.3). The triglycerides, phospholipids and cholesteryl ester are rapidly combined with an apolipoprotein known as apo $B_{48}$ produced in the rough endoplasmic reticulum of the enterocyte (apolipoprotein is the term used for the protein components of lipoproteins other than enzymes). The lipoproteins thus formed are further processed in the Golgi complex, where the apo $B_{48}$ is glycosylated and actively transported to the cell surface for secretion into the lymph (chyle). These lipoproteins are large (>750 Å) and are rich in triglycerides, but contain only relatively small amounts of protein (Figure 2.4). They travel through the lacteals to join lymph from other parts of the body and enter the blood circulation via the thoracic duct. In addition to cholesterol absorbed from the diet, they may also receive cholesterol newly synthesized in the gut and cholesterol transferred from other lipoproteins present in the lymph and plasma. The newly secreted or nascent chylomicrons receive C apolipoproteins from the high density lipoproteins (HDL) (Figure 2.5), which in that respect appear to act as a circulating reservoir, since later in the course of the metabolism of the chylomicron the C apolipoproteins are transferred back. The chylomicrons also receive apolipoprotein E (apo E), although the manner in which they do so is unclear. Unlike other apolipoproteins, which are synthesized either in the liver or gut or both, apo E is exceptional in that it is synthesized (and perhaps secreted) by a large number of tissues: liver, brain, spleen, kidney, lungs and adrenal. In part, apo E may come from HDL, but also it may be acquired directly as the chylomicrons circulate through the tissues.

Once the chylomicron has acquired the apolipoprotein, apo CII, it is capable of activating the enzyme lipoprotein lipase (see Chapter 1 and page 56). This enzyme is located on the vascular endothelium of tissues with a high requirement for triglycerides, such as skeletal muscle and cardiac muscle (for energy), adipose tissue (for storage) and lactating breast (for milk). This enzyme releases triglycerides from the core of the chylomicron by hydrolysing them to fatty acids and

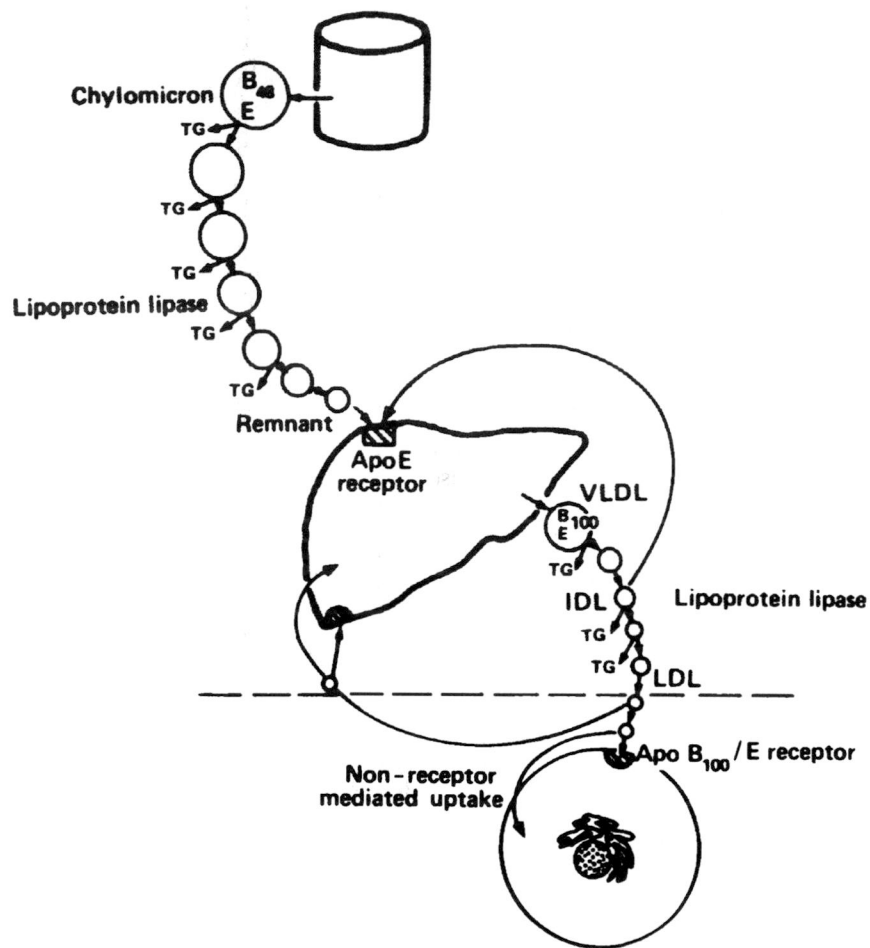

**Figure 2.1**   Metabolism of the triglyceride-rich lipoproteins secreted by the gut (chylomicrons) and liver (VLDL). Lipolysis of their triglycerides during their circulation through tissues such as adipose tissue and muscle leads to the formation of chylomicron remnants and LDL. These, together with some partially metabolized LDL (IDL) are cleared by the liver and peripheral cells which thus receive their cholesterol. Cellular uptake is probably mediated by two receptors on the liver and one in peripheral cells. Non-receptor entry also occurs. High density lipoproteins, not shown, may participate in the return of excess cholesterol from peripheral tissues to the liver (reverse cholesterol transport). Also not shown, some LDL may be secreted directly by the liver

monoglycerides, which are taken up by the tissues locally. In this way the circulating chylomicron becomes progressively smaller. Its triglyceride content decreases and it becomes relatively richer in cholesterol and protein. As the core shrinks, its surface materials (phospholipids, free cholesterol, C apolipoproteins) become too crowded and there is a net transfer of these to HDL. The apo $B_{48}$, present from the time of assembly, remains tightly secured to the core throughout. The apo E also remains and regions of its structure are exposed, which are

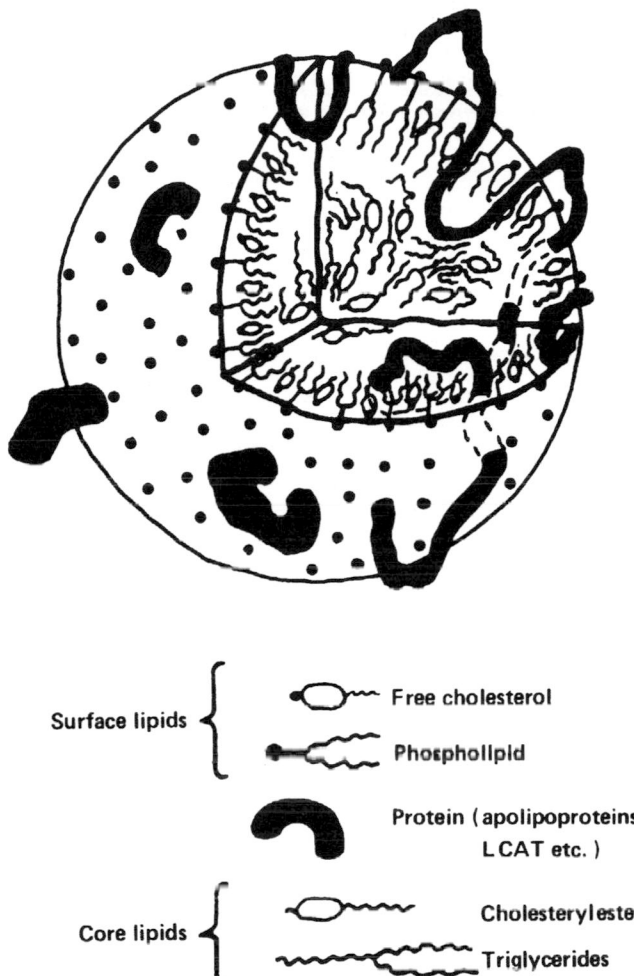

Surface lipids
- Free cholesterol
- Phospholipid

Protein (apolipoproteins
LCAT etc. )

Core lipids
- Cholesterylester
- Triglycerides

**Figure 2.2** Lipoprotein structure. The most hydrophobic lipids (triglycerides, cholesteryl esters) from a central droplet-like core, which is surrounded by lipids with popular groups (phospholipids, free cholesterol) which are directed towards the water. Apolipoproteins are anchored by their more hydrophobic regions with more polar regions exposed at the surface

recognized by the binding sites of two specialized cell surface lipoprotein receptors. These receptors are the remnant or apo E receptors (see page 41), which are present solely in the liver, and the LDL or apo $B_{100}$/E receptors (see page 38), which can be expressed by virtually every cell in the body. It is possibly the case that apo E is inhibited from binding to its receptors earlier in the metabolism of chylomicrons because its receptor-binding domain is covered by the apolipoprotein apo CIII.

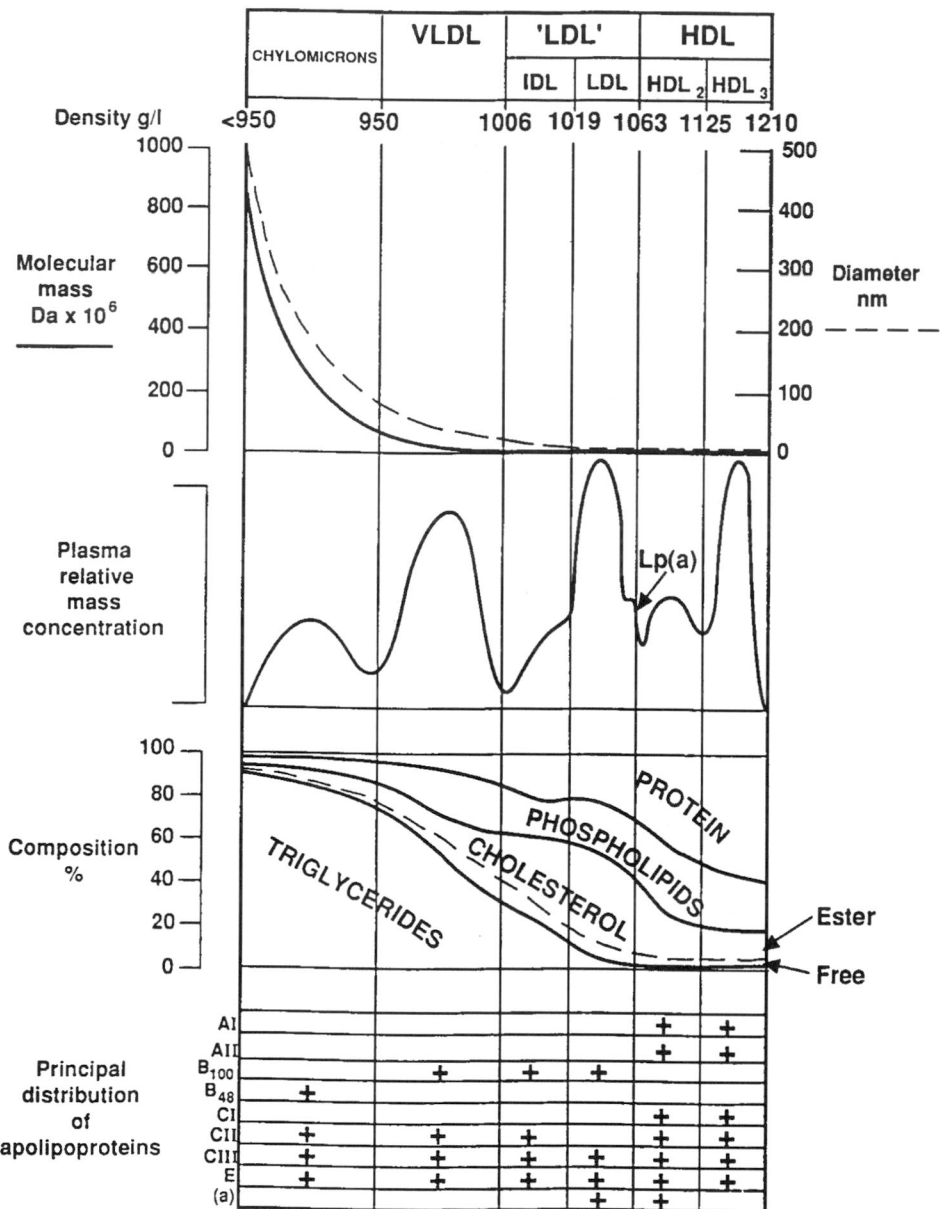

**Figure 2.3** Some properties of plasma lipoproteins: hydrated density, molecular mass, molecular diameter, relative plasma concentration, composition and location of the major apolipoproteins

The cholesterol-enriched, relatively triglyceride-depleted product of chylomicron metabolism is known as the chylomicron remnant. It is largely removed from the circulation in the liver by cellular uptake of the bound apo E receptor complex. Although its clearance via the apo $B_{100}$/E receptor is theoretically possible, this is

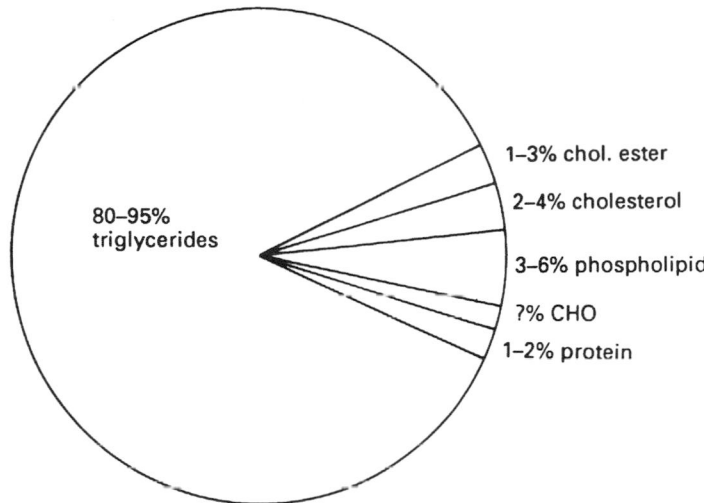

**Figure 2.4**  Chylomicron composition

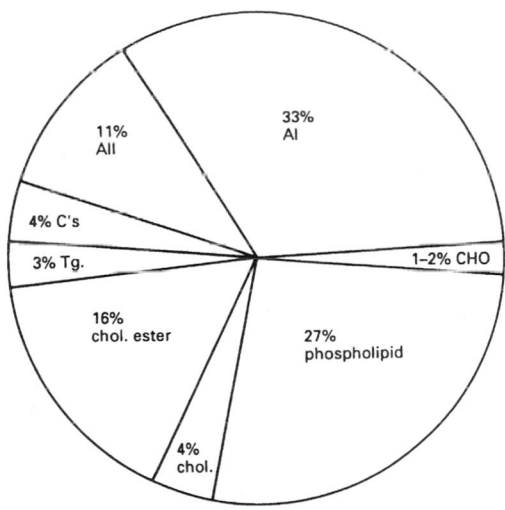

**Figure 2.5**  HDL composition

not likely to contribute greatly in the adult since the binding affinity of the hepatic apo E receptor for apo E is greater and it must compete for binding with low density lipoprotein (LDL) at the apo $B_{100}$/E receptor (see later), the particle concentration of which is much higher than that of the chylomicron remnants (even

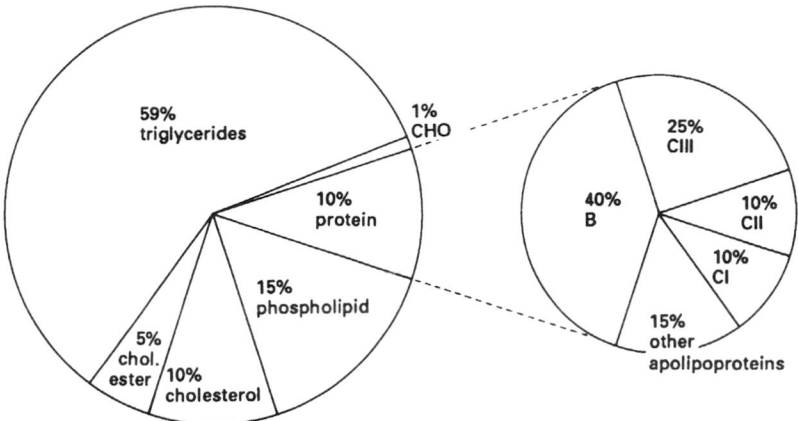

**Figure 2.6**   VLDL composition

more so in the tissue fluid than in the plasma). Also the apo $B_{100}/E$ receptor is rapidly down-regulated by the lysosomal release of free cholesterol into the cell, which follows the entry of lipoprotein-receptor complexes into the cell, whereas expression of the apo E receptor is unaffected by entry of cholesterol into the liver.

The liver also secretes a triglyceride-rich lipoprotein known as very low density lipoprotein (VLDL) (Figure 2.6). Teleologically this serves to supply triglycerides to tissues in the non-fasting as well as the fasting state. VLDL particles are somewhat smaller than the chylomicrons (300–450 Å in diameter). Once secreted, they undergo exactly the same sequence of changes as chylomicrons: that is, the acquisition of apolipoproteins and the progressive removal of triglycerides from their core by the enzyme lipoprotein lipase. There are, however, some additional metabolic transformations involved in their metabolism in the human. In man, the liver, unlike the gut, does not esterify cholesterol before its secretion. This is different from other species such as the rat. In the human, most of the cholesterol released from the liver each day into the circulation is secreted in the VLDL as free cholesterol and it undergoes esterification in the circulation. Free cholesterol is transferred to HDL along a concentration gradient. There it is esterified by the action of the enzyme lecithin: cholesterol acyltransferase (LCAT), which esterifies the hydroxyl group in the 3 position of cholesterol to a fatty acyl group. This it selectively removes from the 2 position of lecithin to give lysolecithin (Figure 2.7). The fatty acyl group in this position is generally unsaturated and the cholesteryl esters thus formed are frequently cholesteryl oleate or cholesteryl linoleate. Once formed, the cholesteryl ester is transferred back to VLDL. This cannot take place by simple diffusion because cholesteryl ester is intensely hydrophobic and because the concentration gradient is unfavourable. A special protein called cholesteryl ester transfer protein (CETP) or lipid transfer protein is present, which transports cholesteryl ester from HDL to VLDL. It does this partly in exchange for some of the triglycerides in VLDL and thus also contributes to the removal of core triglycerides from VLDL. The major mechanism for the removal of triglycerides from VLDL is, however, the lipolysis catalysed by lipoprotein lipase.

The other major difference between VLDL and chylomicrons is that the apolipoprotein B produced by the liver in man is not apo $B_{48}$, but apo $B_{100}$. As in

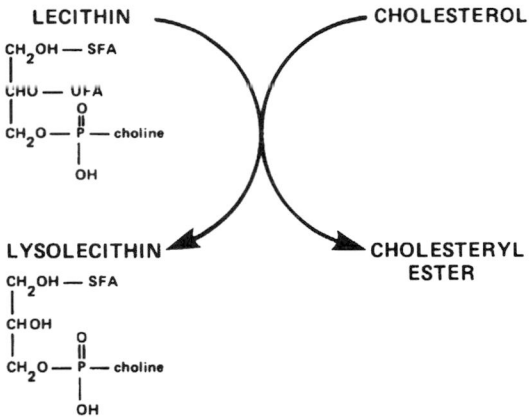

**Figure 2.7**  Cholesterol esterification reaction catalysed by lecithin: cholesterol acyltransferase (LCAT)

the case of the chylomicron, the quantum of apo B packaged in the VLDL remains tightly associated with the particle until its final catabolism and its amount does not vary after secretion. It is probable that each molecule of VLDL contains one molecule of apolipoprotein B (see page 48).

The circulating VLDL particles become progressively smaller as their core is removed by lipolysis and surface materials are transferred to HDL. The remnant particles thus formed are termed the low density lipoprotein (Figure 2.8). These particles are relatively enriched in cholesterol, but are small enough (190–250 Å)

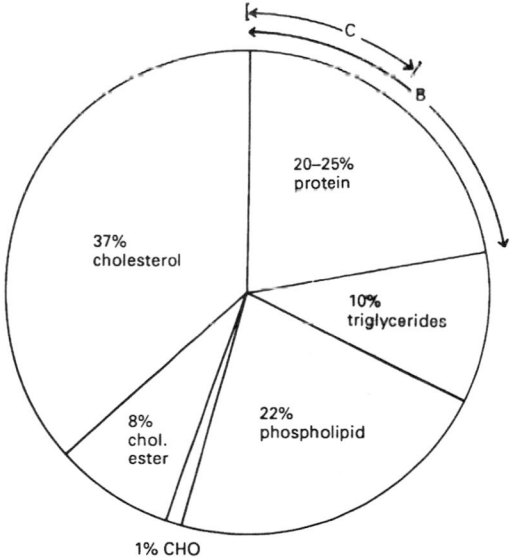

**Figure 2.8**  LDL composition. The mass of apolipoprotein B remains constant in each lipoprotein particle, whereas apolipoprotein C is present only in the less dense LDL in the process of conversion from VLDL and IDL

to cross the vascular endothelium and enter the tissue fluid so that they are able to come in contact with virtually every cell of the body. Their major function is to deliver cholesterol to the tissues. Their concentration in the extracellular fluid is probably about 10% of that in the plasma. The major role of LDL is to deliver cholesterol to cells for membrane repair and growth and, in the case of specialized tissues such as the adrenals, gonads and skin, as a precursor for steroid hormone and vitamin D synthesis. LDL is able to enter cells by two routes: one which is regulated according to the cholesterol requirement of each individual cell and one which appears to depend almost entirely on the extracellular concentrations of LDL and to serve no physiological purpose except perhaps in tissues where cholesterol is excreted, such as the liver.

The first of these two routes is by a cell surface receptor which specifically binds to lipoproteins that contain apolipoprotein $B_{100}$ or E. This is the apo $B_{100}$/E receptor. As has been mentioned previously, the receptor, although capable of binding apo E-containing lipoproteins, in practice binds largely to apo B containing lipoproteins of which LDL is the most widely distributed. After binding, the LDL-receptor complex is internalized within the cell where it undergoes lysosomal degradation (Figure 2.9). Its quantum of apo B, present since its secretion as

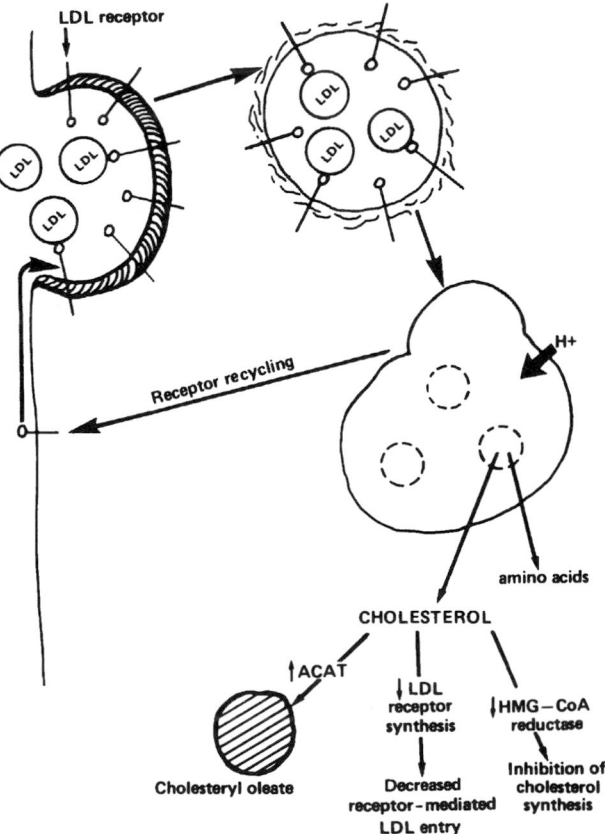

**Figure 2.9**    Metabolism of the LDL receptor (apo $B_{100}$/E receptor)—see text

nascent VLDL, is hydrolysed to its constituent amino acids and cholesteryl ester hydrolysed to free cholesterol. The release of this free cholesterol is the signal by which the cellular cholesterol content is precisely regulated by three coordinated reactions. The enzyme which is rate-limiting for cholesterol biosynthesis (3-hydroxy, 3-methylglutaryl-CoA reductase or HMG-CoA reductase) is repressed, thus effectively centralizing cholesterol biosynthesis to organs such as the liver and gut. Secondly, the synthesis of the apo $B_{100}$/E receptor itself is suppressed. Thirdly, an enzyme, acyl CoA: cholesterol O-acyltransferase (ACAT), is activated so that any cholesterol surplus to immediate requirements can be converted to cholesteryl ester, which because of its hydrophobic nature forms into droplets within the cytoplasm and is thus conveniently stored. The effect of lysosomal release of free cholesterol on the apo $B_{100}$/E receptor in both hepatic and extrahepatic tissues contrasts with its effect on the hepatic apo E receptor which is not subject to any similar regulatory process. It is widely assumed, however, that although free cholesterol released by lysosomal digestion of cholesterol-rich apo E-containing lipoproteins entering the hepatocyte via the apo E receptor does not influence the expression of the apo E receptor, it will nevertheless down-regulate the hepatic apo $B_{100}$/E receptor.

The other mechanism by which LDL cholesterol may enter the cell is by a non-receptor-mediated pathway. LDL binds to cell membranes at sites other than those where the apo $B_{100}$/E receptors are located and some of it passes through the membrane. Having regard to the structure of LDL, which in many respects is not unlike that of cell membranes, such a phenomenon is perhaps not altogether surprising. Other lipoproteins such as HDL are thus able to compete with LDL for this type of cell membrane binding. The absence of a receptor means that the binding is of low affinity and thus at low concentrations LDL entry by this route may have little significance. However, unlike receptor-mediated entry, non-receptor-mediated LDL uptake is not saturable, but continues to increase with increasing extracellular LDL concentrations. When LDL levels are relatively high, entry of cholesterol into cells by this route may thus assume greater quantitative importance than that via the apo $B_{100}$/E receptor, which will be both saturated and down-regulated. This appears to be the circumstance in adult man, whose LDL cholesterol is high relative to most animal species and in whom only about one-third of LDL is catabolized by receptors and two-thirds by non-receptor-mediated pathways. In hypercholesterolaemia, even more is catabolized via the non-receptor pathway (four-fifths in patients heterozygous for familial hypercholesterol-aemia), giving rise to speculation that non-receptor-mediated catabolism is unphysiological and that the pathways into which cholesterol leaving the circulation by this means are directed lead to atheroma.

### Transport of cholesterol from tissues back to liver (reverse cholesterol transport) (Figure 2.10)

In the human, cholesterol is transported out of the gut and liver in quantities which greatly exceed its conversion to steroid hormones and its loss through the skin in sebum. Therefore, except when the requirement for membrane synthesis is high, for example during growth or active tissue repair, the greater part of the cholesterol transported to the tissues (if it is not to accumulate there) must be returned to the liver for elimination in the bile, conversion to bile salts or reassembly into lipoproteins. The return of cholesterol from the tissues to the liver is termed

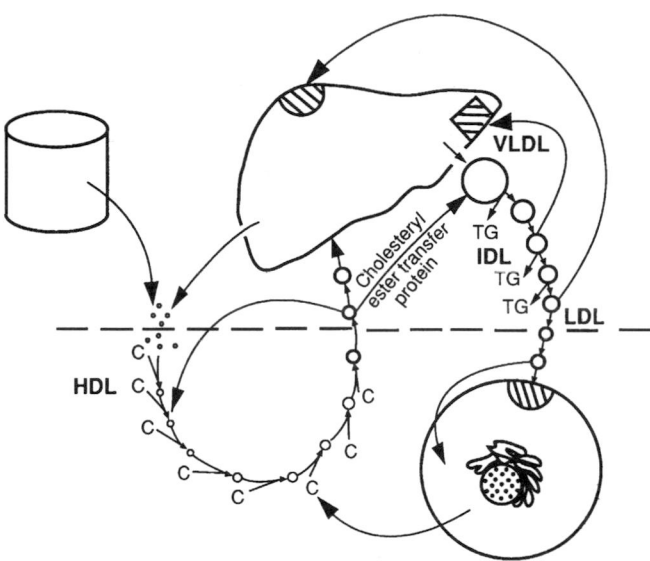

**Figure 2.10**   Reverse cholesterol transport: cholesterol surplus to cellular requirements can leave cells to enter HDL whence it can be transported to VLDL and be converted to LDL or be returned to the liver during hepatic uptake of IDL. The HDL pool is maintained by secretion of apolipoproteins AI and AII from the liver and gut and by transfer of surface materials from triglyceride-rich lipoproteins undergoing lipolysis

'reverse cholesterol transport'. It is less well understood than the pathways by which cholesterol reaches the tissues, but it may well be critical to the development of atheroma, which after all is in essence an excess accumulation of cholesterol in the arterial wall. HDL has many features which make it very likely that it is intimately involved in the reverse transport process.

The precursors of the mature circulating HDL molecules are probably disc-shaped bilayers composed largely of protein and phospholipid secreted by the gut and liver. Apolipoproteins AI and AII comprise the major protein component of the nascent HDL. Its other apolipoproteins and the bulk of its lipid (Figure 2.5) are acquired as it circulates through the vascular and other extracellular fluids. In this respect the transformation of HDL from its lipid-poor precursor to a relatively lipid-rich molecule is the opposite of that which the other lipoproteins undergo following their secretion.

HDL is a small molecule compared with the other lipoproteins (45–120 Å) and easily crosses the vascular endothelium so that its concentration in the tissue fluids is much closer to its intravascular concentration than is the case for LDL. Because the serum HDL cholesterol concentration is only about one-quarter to one-fifth that of the LDL cholesterol concentration, it is often wrongly assumed that its particle concentration is lower. In fact, the particle concentrations of HDL and LDL in human plasma are often similar, and in the tissue fluids there are several times as many HDL molecules as those of other lipoproteins present. Thus the cells are in contact with higher concentrations of HDL molecules than of any other

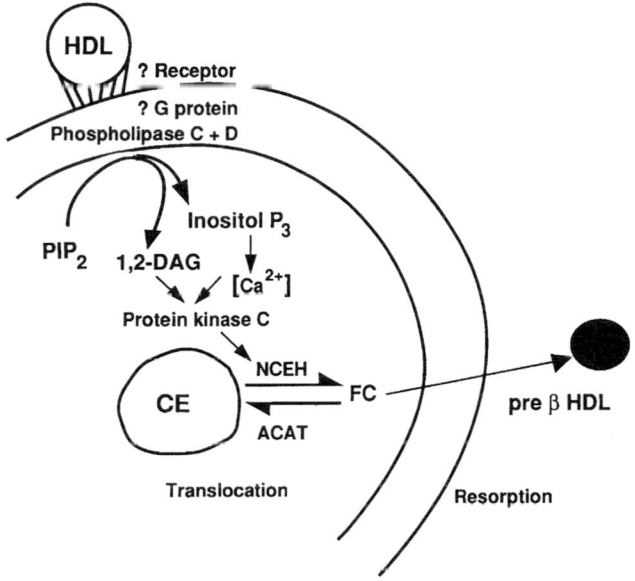

**Figure 2.11**   Interaction between HDL and the cell membrane promotes the hydrolysis of intracellular cholesteryl ester to form free cholesterol and its passage to cell membrane (translocation). Thence it can cross to become incorporated in preβ HDL (resorption). G protein, GTP-binding protein; PIP$_2$, phosphatidylinositol 4,5-biphosphate; 1,2-DAG, 1,2-diacylglycerol; inositol P$_3$, inositol 1,4,5 triphosphate; CE, cholesteryl ester; FC, free cholesterol; NCEH, neutral cholesteryl ester hydrolase; ACAT, acyl-CoA: cholesterol O-acyltransferase

lipoprotein. In man, HDL serves no apparent function in transporting cholesterol to cells. Recently it has been suggested that cells when loaded with cholesteryl ester express receptors for HDL, which might permit the transfer of cholesterol out of the cell (Figure 2.11). Cholesterol excess to cellular requirements for membranes or as a synthetic substrate is packaged as droplets of the intensely hydrophobic cholesteryl ester (page 33). In order to cross the cell membrane, cholesterol leaving cells must be unesterified (unless CETP can cross the cell membrane to bind with it or possibly apo E synthesized within the cell transports it out). Thus, critical to the passage of cholesterol out of the cell are therefore likely to be the factors regulating the intracellular neutral cholesterol esterase (neutral cholesteryl ester hydrolase). It is termed neutral to distinguish it from acid cholesterol esterase which hydrolyses the cholesteryl ester of LDL in lysosomes (page 33). The interaction of HDL with the outer cell membrane (whether or not it involves a specific receptor) alters membrane phospholipase C and D activity (Figure 2.11). Phospholipase C regulates the production of diglyceride (1,2 diacylglycerol) and inositol from phosphatidyl inositol. The physiological action of phospholipase D is less certain. Nonetheless, the release of 1,2 diacylglycerol activates a protein kinase, protein kinase C. The same kinase may also be activated by calcium ions released in response to an increase in the concentration of inositol triphosphate also produced in the phosphokinase C-mediated hydrolysis of phosphatidyl inositol diphosphate. The effect of protein kinase C activation is thought to shift the balance between cholesterol esterification and cholesteryl ester hydrolysis in favour of free cholesterol mobilization. The movement of free cholesterol out of storage droplets of cholesteryl ester is termed translocation. Free cholesterol can efflux from the cell in a process termed resorption. There has been much speculation as to what is the initial acceptor molecule for the free cholesterol as it leaves the outer cell membrane. One candidate is preβ HDL.

Preβ HDL has a molecular weight in the range 45 000–80 000 daltons. It is terminologically incorrect to call it HDL, because it does not float in the same density range as HDL. It is recovered in the infranatant on ultracentrifugation of plasma at a density of 1.21 g/ml. It does, however, have two molecules of apo AI per particle and is clearly therefore related to HDL, to which it is readily converted by the action of LCAT when free cholesterol is supplied. Preβ HDL itself is lipid-deficient containing small amounts of phospholipid and very little cholesterol as cholesteryl ester. As such it has sometimes been termed free apo AI. It comprises some 5–15% of total serum apo AI.

Preβ HDL is probably released in tissues where lipoprotein lipolysis is active by the action of their lipoprotein lipase on either triglyceride-rich lipoproteins, high density lipoproteins or both. It is small enough to enter the tissue fluid readily. Free cholesterol entering the preβ HDL particle is the preferred substrate for LCAT, which is especially active on preβ HDL. The intensely hydrophobic cholesteryl ester produced as a result forms a central droplet in preβ HDL decreasing the concentration of free cholesterol at its surface allowing further uptake of free cholesterol from its surroundings along a favourable concentration gradient. This process converts preβ HDL to larger $HDL_3$ particles. Whether or not HDL is involved as the initial acceptor molecule, cholesterol must at some stage on its return journey to the liver reside on HDL, because it is the site of LCAT activity.

To add a further complication, cholesterol cannot simply be taken up by HDL, be esterified and packed into its core and then be cleared by the liver with the whole lipoprotein particle. This is because LDL equivalent to 1500 mg of cholesterol is catabolized each day, whereas the rate of catabolism of the HDL apolipoproteins AI and AII would permit only 165 mg of HDL cholesterol to be returned to the liver each day, even assuming that the liver is the only site of HDL catabolism. Therefore: (a) the liver must be capable of selectively removing cholesterol from HDL and then returning the particle to the circulation with most of its apolipoproteins intact, or (b) the cholesterol in HDL must be transferred to another lipoprotein class which is capable of being cleared in quantity by the liver, or (c) a class of HDL which contains little apo AI or AII must be cleared by the liver at a much greater rate than the bulk of HDL.

In support of (a) there is some evidence that hepatic lipase (page 57), which is most active as a phospholipase, might punch a hole in the phospholipid envelope of HDL during its passage through hepatic sinusoids and release the cholesteryl ester contained in its core for uptake by either hepatocytes or Kupffer cells. On the other hand, in support of (b) there is a well-established mechanism for the transfer of cholesteryl ester from HDL to VLDL through the agency of CETP (see page 58). Once on VLDL the cholesteryl ester might then arrive at the liver via the binding of IDL to hepatic apo E (remnant) receptors or when LDL enters the liver after binding to the apo $B_{100}$/E receptor or by the non-receptor-mediated route. Evidence for the third possibility, pathway (c), for the return of cholesterol to the liver from HDL by a rapidly metabolized form of HDL present at low concentration in serum, is at present largely lacking.

It is incorrect to regard HDL as a single molecular species. At least two peaks are seen in the analytical ultracentrifuge, the less dense of which is designated $HDL_2$ (d = 1.063–1.125 g/ml) and the more dense, $HDL_3$ (d = 1.125–1.21 g/ml). Also, whereas antisera to apo AI precipitate virtually all of HDL, antisera to AII do not, suggesting that some molecules of HDL contain AI and AII, whereas others contain AI only. There is some evidence to support the view that $HDL_3$ is converted to $HDL_2$ by the acquisition of cholesterol, $HDL_3$ thus being a precursor form of $HDL_2$. The AI-only HDL molecules which predominate in $HDL_2$ may arise from very different metabolic channels from the AI/AII particles. Furthermore, HDL may contain other molecular species with overlapping density ranges such as Lp(a) (page 53). HDL thus represents a rather heterogeneous entity.

A small shoulder evident in the analytical ultracentrifuge at the upper end of the spectrum of LDL in the density range 1.053–1.063 g/ml was originally designated $HDL_1$. There remains, however, no certainty that it is related to HDL metabolism and its composition and identity have not been clearly established. It might represent Lp(a) or some large, possibly aggregated, product of $HDL_2$.

## Lipoprotein structure

The lipoproteins are macromolecular complexes of lipids and protein (see Figure 2.2). Great diversity of composition and physical properties are possible, particularly in disease but also in health. As such, their classification and definition is particularly difficult. Each lipoprotein has a wide range of components, each with its own metabolic origin and fate. Lipoprotein components undergo a complex metabolic interplay with receptors and with enzymes located on the lipoproteins, and on the capillary endothelium and between the circulating lipoproteins themselves, both in the vascular compartment and within the tissue fluid space. It is thus naive in the extreme to try to think of serum cholesterol or triglycerides in the same way as serum sodium or glucose, which are transported simply as solutes. The very existence of lipids within the circulation is dependent on lipoproteins.

The general structure of lipoprotein molecules is globular (Figure 2.2). The physicochemical considerations, which govern the arrangement of their constituents, are similar to those discussed in the context of mixed micelles (pages 15 and 20). Thus, within the outer part of the lipoprotein are found the more polar lipids, namely the phospholipids and free cholesterol, with their charged groups pointing out towards the water molecules. In physical terms, however, the role of the bile salts is assumed by proteins, so that the outer layer of a lipoprotein structurally resembles the outer layer of a cell membrane (pages 16 and 17). The protein components of lipoproteins are the apolipoproteins (Table 2.1), a group of proteins of immense structural diversity, some of which have a largely structural role, others of which are major metabolic regulators and yet others of which may influence immunological and haemostatic responses apparently unconnected with lipid transport. In addition, enzymes are found as components of lipoproteins. The leading example is LCAT (page 57) which is located on the high density lipoproteins, which are also its site of action, cholesterol being transported to and from its location for esterification.

Tucked away in the core of the lipoprotein particle are the more hydrophobic lipids, the esterified cholesterol and the triglycerides. These form a central droplet to which are anchored by their hydrophobic regions the surface coating of

**Table 2.1 Characteristics of the apolipoproteins**

| Apolipoprotein | Molecular weight (Da) | Chromosomal location of gene | Plasma concentration (mg/dl) |
|---|---|---|---|
| AI | 28 016 | 11 | 60–160 |
| AII | 17 414 ?8 000 | 1 | 25–55 |
| AIV | 44 500 | 11 | 15 |
| $B_{48}$ | 264 000 | 2 ⎤ | |
| $B_{100}$ | 550 000 | 2 ⎦ | 60–160 |
| CI | 6 600 | 19 | 3–10 |
| CII | 8 750 | 19 | 1–6 |
| CIII | 8 800 | 11 | 4–20 |
| D | 33 000 | 3 | ~6–10 |
| E | 34 100 | 19 | 2–7 |
| F | 28 000 | ? | 2 |
| G | 72 000 | ? | ? |
| H | 43 000 (54 000) | ? | 20 |
| J | 70 000 | 8 | 10 |
| (a) | 300 000–700 000 | 6 | 1–100 |

phospholipid, cholesterol and protein. The exception to this general structure is the newly formed or nascent HDL, which it has been suggested lacks the central lipid droplet and appears to exist as a disc-like bilayer, consisting largely of phospholipid and protein.

## LDL receptor (apo $B_{100}$/E receptor)

This receptor was first discovered by J. L. Goldstein and M. S. Brown in 1974 when they found that whereas LDL would inhibit cholesterol synthesis in cultured fibroblasts, HDL would not, and that the inhibitory effect of LDL was absent in fibroblasts from patients who were homozygotes for familial hypercholesterol-aemia (Chapter 5). They and other workers then went on to reveal in detail the fascinating biochemistry of the receptor, which has contributed not only to our knowledge of lipoprotein metabolism, but also led to advances in our general understanding of receptors and molecular genetics.

The gene for the LDL receptor is located on chromosome 19 and contains some 45 000 base pairs, and includes 18 exons (translated sequences) and 18 introns (untranslated intervening sequences). The receptor protein itself contains 839 amino acids. Its apparent molecular weight immediately after synthesis is about 120 000 daltons, but it subsequently acquires carbohydrate in the Golgi appara-tus and undergoes changes in its molecular conformation, altering its electrophoretic mobility, and thus the estimated molecular weight of the mature protein is in the region of 160 000 daltons. The receptor migrates to the cell surface (Figure 2.9), the interval between synthesis and arrival in the coated pit averaging 45 min. There it enters a cycle in which it enters the cell by invagina-tion of coated pits and closure of their necks to form coated endocytic vesicles. These rapidly lose their clathrin coat and fuse to form larger vesicles (endosomes or receptorsomes). ATP-dependent proton pumps in their walls lower the pH of the enclosed fluid and the LDL receptor–LDL complex dissociates. The released

LDL receptor leaves the endosome and migrates back to the surface, linking up with other receptors in the coated pit region. The whole cycle is believed to take approximately 10 min

The LDL receptor undergoes the cycle whether or not it has bound to a lipoprotein, and it is also known that the coated pits contain receptors for other ligands and so therefore must the vesicles produced by endocytosis of the coated pits. The endosomes deliver their contents to the lysosomes where LDL undergoes acid hydrolysis. This process is rapid since, when cells in culture are incubated with LDL labelled in its protein moiety with radioactive iodine, the iodine is released into the culture medium within 60 min. Chloroquine, which raises the pH of lysosomes, inhibits this process. There is no mechanism for sucrose to be released from lysosomes and thus by linking radioactive sucrose to lipoproteins it has been possible by the presence of trapped sucrose to identify tissues in which lipoprotein degradation is active. The receptor-binding sites of apo B and apo E can be blocked by chemical modifications such as methylation, cyclohexanedione treatment and glycosylation. Since the receptor-binding sites do not appear to be important for non-receptor-mediated LDL uptake (page 33), this has made it possible to quantitate in vivo the relative amounts of LDL catabolized by the receptor-mediated and the non-receptor-mediated routes.

The complex nature of the events from the synthesis of the LDL receptor to the successful entry of the receptor into the recycling process and the completion of that process, means that the clinical syndrome of familial hypercholesterolaemia can be produced by a variety of gene mutations (Chapter 5).

The receptor has at its amino end (first domain) (Figure 2.12) the region which binds to apo B and apo E. It contains seven repetitive sequences, each of 40 amino acids. Of these, about seven are cysteine residues, which form disulphide bridges retaining a rigidly crosslinked structure in their part of the molecule. Negatively charged clusters of amino acids are displayed which complement the positively charged receptor-binding sites of apo E and apo B.

The binding site region of the receptor molecule is adjacent to a long sequence of amino acids homologous to part of the epithelial growth factor (EGF) precursor. It should be noted that there is no homology with the portion of EGF released. Thus, although the homology may be informative about how different proteins have evolved, it does not suggest that there is a functional link between the two proteins. The same is probably true of the sequences in the receptor-binding part of the molecule which have similarities with the C9 component of complement.

The next sequence of amino acids is rich in sugar and this leads on to a hydrophobic region of the molecule, which spans the cell membrane. The final carboxyl end of the molecule extends into the cytoplasm and its interaction with clathrin is essential for the arrival of the receptor in the coated pit region of the cell membrane.

Synthesis of the LDL is suppressed when the cell is replete in cholesterol. In this regard LDL receptor-mediated catabolism differs from that of chylomicron remnants for which there appears to be a hepatic receptor-mediated pathway for their removal from the circulation, which is not down-regulated by entry of cholesterol into the liver. Similarly, entry of cholesterol into cells by the non-receptor route (page 33) continues even after they are replete in cholesterol, so long as the extracellular LDL cholesterol concentration is sufficiently high. In tissue culture the LDL receptor is saturated when the concentration of LDL cholesterol in the

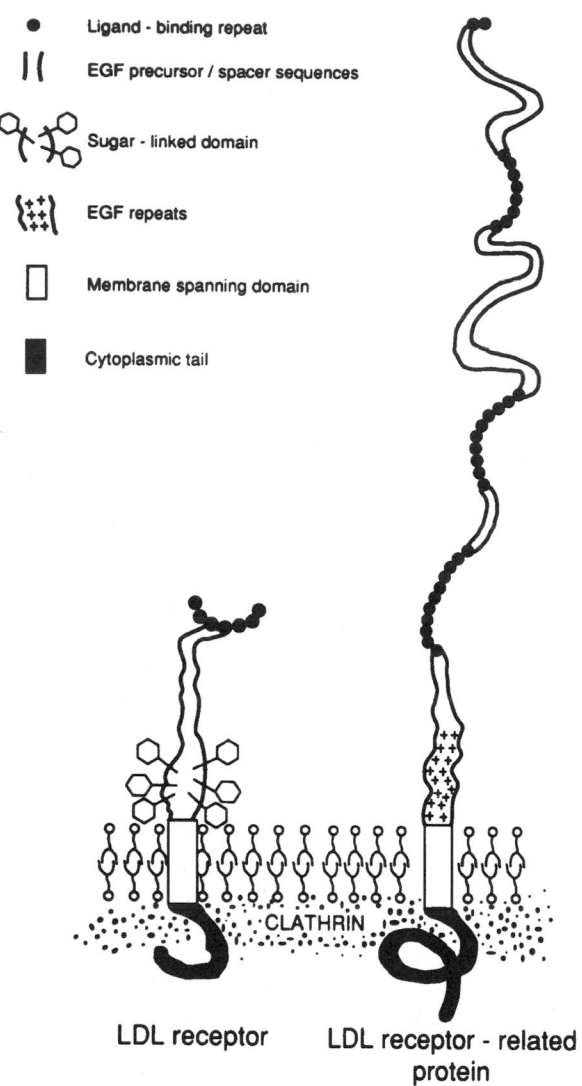

- ● Ligand - binding repeat
- EGF precursor / spacer sequences
- Sugar - linked domain
- EGF repeats
- Membrane spanning domain
- Cytoplasmic tail

CLATHRIN

**LDL receptor**    **LDL receptor - related protein**

**Figure 2.12**   The low density lipoprotein receptor (LDL receptor, apo $B_{100}$/E receptor) and the LDL receptor-related protein receptor (LRP receptor). The LRP receptor is currently believed to serve the function of the apo E receptor or remnant receptor

medium is 2.5 mg/dl (0.065 mmol/l)*. The concentration of LDL cholesterol in the extracellular fluid of most tissues is about one-tenth of that in the plasma. Thus, if the behaviour of cells in tissue culture can be extrapolated to whole man, a plasma LDL cholesterol of 25 mg/dl (0.65 mmol/1) should saturate the LDL receptor and provide all the cell's cholesterol requirement. It has been pointed out by

* The unit 'mg/dl' is commonly used in the USA and in parts of Europe, whereas the SI unit 'mmol/l' has been widely adopted in the UK. This book gives the conversion in each case.

Goldstein and Brown that in mammalian species which do not develop atherosclerosis, serum LDL cholesterol seldom exceeds 80 mg/dl (2 mmol/l) and that in the newborn human the serum LDL cholesterol concentration is about 30 mg/dl (0.8 mmol/l). In humans, who have always subsisted on a diet low in fat serum, LDL cholesterol is also generally in the range 50–80 mg/dl (1.3–2 mmol/l). The serum LDL cholesterol concentration of much of the population of countries with a Northern European diet, however, exceeds 150 mg/dl (3.8 mmol/l) and it can be argued that in large part their LDL must be catabolized by the non-receptor-mediated route, which would be expected to be active at this concentration of LDL. That this is the case has been shown in experiments in which the catabolic rates of unmodified LDL and cyclohexanedione-treated LDL have been compared (page 33). This has led to speculation that the non-receptor-mediated route may be linked with atherogenesis. However, it should be remembered that much of the non-receptor-mediated catabolism may be through the liver and therefore not contribute to cholesterol deposition in the arterial wall and elsewhere. This is because the blood vessels of the liver have a fenestrated endothelium and thus the concentration of LDL in the hepatic extracellular fluid will be substantially higher than in peripheral tissues and a correspondingly much higher rate of non-receptor-mediated uptake of LDL may therefore occur in the liver. Also there is evidence that, although HDL does not compete with LDL for receptor-mediated uptake, it does interact with LDL to inhibit its non-receptor-mediated uptake. The concentration of HDL in extracellular fluid is closer to that in plasma. Thus, in whole man, non-receptor-mediated LDL catabolism may be substantially in the liver. Even so, local conditions may be such in the arterial wall and some other tissues that excess cholesterol does accumulate.

## The chylomicron remnant receptor (apo E receptor)

Experimentally it can be shown that the liver avidly removes chylomicron remnants from the circulation by a process which is mediated through the binding of apo E, but which continues to be active when LDL receptors are down-regulated and for which apo $B_{100}$-containing lipoproteins, like LDL, do not compete. The apo E-rich HDL subfraction does, however, compete with chylomicron remnants for hepatic uptake. Unlike the LDL receptor, hepatic chylomicron remnant uptake is not down-regulated as intrahepatic cholesterol levels rise. It is, however, blocked by the presence of C apolipoproteins in the remnant particles. These apolipoproteins are lost from chylomicrons as they undergo lipolysis and exchange their surface components with HDL. Their apo E component, however, is unaffected by lipolysis and remains present in the chylomicron remnants. It has thus been suggested that this process may operate as a mechanism to prevent the uptake of chylomicrons by the liver until their triglyceride component has been distributed to peripheral tissues, principally skeletal muscle and adipose tissue.

The great problem with the chylomicron receptor concept has been the failure to isolate it and to be able to perform the definitive experiments that have been possible with the LDL receptor. In the first edition of this book I discussed at some length how it might be possible to explain most of the experimental observations supporting the concept of a chylomicron receptor on the basis of there being only one receptor, the LDL receptor, if that receptor had an substantially greater affinity for chylomicron remnants than for LDL. In fact, it does prove to be the case that the LDL receptor does have a high affinity for chylomicron remnants partly because only the fifth cysteine-rich repeat out of the seven in the ligand-binding domain of the LDL receptor has to be intact for binding to apo E to occur whereas cysteine-rich repeats 3–7 must be intact for binding to apo B. Furthermore there is only one apo B molecule per LDL molecule (and thus only one LDL receptor-binding site) whereas in chylomicron remnants there are several apo E molecules. This combined with the larger size of the remnant particle means that frequently they may bind not just to a single LDL receptor, but to two simultaneously, increasing their likelihood of internalization

On the other hand patients who are homozygous for familial hypercholesterolaemia (Chapter 5) have only small increases in intermediate density lipoprotein and their clearance of chylomicron remnants is relatively normal, particularly if compared to people with type III hyperlipoproteinaemia in whom polymorphism or mutation of apo E decreases receptor binding. This argues very much for there being a second receptor for chylomicron remnants, which is unaffected by the LDL receptor mutation, and which has the capacity to catabolize chylomicron remnants including those that would normally be removed by the LDL receptor.

The most likely candidate for the chylomicron receptor is another recently discovered member of the LDL supergene family, termed the LDL receptor-related protein (LRP) (see Figure 2.12). This is an enormous protein of 4525 amino acids with an initial molecular mass of 600 000 daltons which after proleolytic shortening in the Golgi complex appears as a membrane receptor with a molecular mass of 515 000 daltons.

The LRP resembles four LDL receptors joined together. Instead of a single negatively charged ligand-binding domain, consisting of seven cysteine-rich repeats, homologous to complement situated at its amino end, LRP has four of these ligand-binding sites. One at the amino terminal end has two cysteine-rich repeats. Three others are then strung out along the molecule consisting of 8, 10 and 11 cysteine-rich repeats respectively. In between the ligand-binding sites are sequences resembling EGF precursor. LRP lacks the sugar-rich domain. Instead a sequence closer to EGF itself links it to its hydrophobic membrane-spanning region. This in turn leads to a cytoplasmic tail. Like that of the LDL receptor this anchors the molecule to the clathrin of the coated pit region of the cellular membrane, but in the case of the LRP it is twice as long, perhaps because its size demands a more secure anchorage. LRP appears to undergo a similar recycling process to LDL. LRP and the LDL receptor are part of a family of molecules with certain features in common which have evolved from a common ancestral gene, which includes the vitellogenin receptor of egg-laying birds and reptiles and glycoprotein 330, the function of which is unknown, but which is the antigen for an autoimmune nephritis in rats.

Herz and colleagues first suggested in 1988 that the LRP was the chylomicron receptor. At the time of writing there is a good case for this, but it is not proven. There is binding of chylomicron remnants to isolated LRP if they are first experimentally enriched in apo E. Fibroblasts from homozygotes for familial hypercholesterolaemia (Chapter 5) will take up the cholesterol from similar apo E-enriched remnant lipoproteins. It has, however, proved impossible to demonstrate apo E degradation in the same way that this was shown for apo B at the LDL receptor. This may be for technical reasons or possibly because the LRP allows cellular cholesterol uptake, but does not allow degradation of the apolipoprotein moiety of lipoproteins. Binding of remnants to LRP is inhibited by

C apolipoproteins, particularly apo CI and II. There is *in vivo* evidence that C apolipoproteins inhibit chylomicron remnant catabolism, but CIII was reported to be most active in this respect. So this is inconsistent.

The LRP is found in a wide variety of tissues and cultured cells, yet chylomicron remnant catabolism is targeted to the liver. Perhaps the fenestrated capillary endothelium of the liver means that the large chylomicron remnant particles come in contact with hepatocytes whereas they less readily cross other vascular endothelia to come in contact with other cell types. Recently it has been shown that the binding of chylomicron remnants to hepatocytes is enhanced by the presence of lipoprotein lipase. It is known that some of this enzyme detaches itself from the capillary endothelium during the passage of chylomicrons through adipose tissue and skeletal muscle and attaches to the chylomicrons. It is possible therefore that binding of lipoprotein lipase to the LRP is a mechanism for increasing the likelihood of remnants binding to it by creating an additional site for remnant binding besides that which binds to apo E. Perhaps also the liver showers the remnants with apo E during their passage through it, thus enhancing LRP binding, or has some trapping mechanism, possibly involving extracellular glycosaminoglycans or hepatic lipase.

LRP is certainly not a receptor dedicated to the clearance of lipoproteins. It has a major function in clearing alpha$_2$-macroglobulin from the circulation. This is a protein which scavenges serine proteases and certain growth factors and cytokines leaking into the plasma compartment. Its circulating concentration (200–400 mg/dl) is much higher than that of remnants except in say type III hyperlipoproteinaemia (Chapter 8). The LRP also appears to bind other molecules such as lipoprotein lipase and plasminogen activator/plasminogen activator inhibitor complexes. Not all the ligands binding to LRP compete with each other, suggesting that the ligand-binding sites may each be specific for different molecular complexes. A protein, receptor associated protein (RAP), has been identified which can competitively block all ligand binding. A single receptor possessing a range of binding sites for catabolizing a range of molecular complexes, either partially or wholly, is a fascinating concept, but whether LRP is the putative chylomicron remnant receptor requires further confirmation.

In man, some VLDL remnants (IDL) appear to be catabolized by the liver rather than be converted to LDL. In the rat, most of the VLDL is removed by this route, short-circuiting its conversion to LDL, so that in that species cholesterol transport to the tissues is subserved not by LDL but by HDL. This should be kept in mind when attempting to extrapolate rat research to the human condition. The rat is not susceptible to atherosclerosis, even when made grossly hyperlipidaemic.

It is known that phospholipid complexes containing apo E$_2$ as opposed to apo E$_3$ or apo E$_4$ bind less well to the fibroblast LDL receptor (page 51). Although this has not been directly demonstrated for the putative hepatocyte remnant receptor, it is nevertheless widely believed to apply and to account at least in part for the accumulation of chylomicron remnants and IDL in type III hyperlipoproteinaemia (Chapter 8). It is of great interest that in type III hyperlipoproteinaemia LDL cholesterol levels are low. It might be thought that decreasing uptake of IDL at the remnant receptor would allow more to enter the pathway leading to LDL and that the levels of LDL would increase. This is far from the case. Indeed, the influence of the apo E genotype extends beyond patients with type III hyperlipoproteinaemia to the general population. Thus apo E$_2$ homozygotes, who do not have the type III phenotype, have lower LDL levels on average than heterozygotes who are $E_{2/3}$, and theirs is lower than $E_{3/3}$ and these in turn than $E_{3/4}$ and $E_{4/4}$. This could suggest that binding to the hepatic remnant receptor is important in the conversion of IDL to LDL and that degradation of IDL does not inevitably follow binding. Possibly, binding at the hepatic remnant (apo E) receptor brings IDL in contact with some factor which is rate-limiting for the metabolism of IDL to LDL, for example hepatic lipase (page 57), after which it may be released back into the circulation. If on the other hand a separate hepatic remnant receptor was less important than the hepatic LDL receptor, then the low LDL cholesterol in apo $E_2$ homozygotes might be explained because their remnants should compete less favourably with LDL, allowing increased LDL catabolism via the LDL receptor. On the same reasoning high LDL levels in apo $E_4$ homozygotes would be due to the greater competition between LDL and $E_4$-containing IDL at the LDL receptor because of the higher affinity of $E_4$ for that receptor. Other possibilities are discussed later (page 51).

# Other lipoprotein receptors

### β-VLDL receptor

Because fatty streaks and atheromatous plaques contain macrophages the cytoplasm of which is rich in lipid droplets (foam cells) (page 60), there has been much interest in the lipoprotein receptors of those cells. The lipoprotein β-VLDL binds to a receptor on the cultured macrophage, which is a modified LDL receptor which is not down-regulated allowing large amounts of lipid to build up in the cytoplasm of macrophages exposed to β-VLDL. β-VLDL is present at high concentration in the plasma of patients with type III hyperlipoproteinaemia (see Chapter 8). Its hydrated density is in the same range as normal VLDL, but it is a cholesterol-rich lipoprotein. It is derived from the metabolism of chylomicrons and VLDL and probably represents the chylomicron remnants and IDL. These are normally rapidly cleared from the circulation by the hepatic remnant receptor or, in the case of IDL, converted to LDL, but in type III hyperlipoproteinaemia those events are impaired.

The β-VLDL receptor, despite its potential involvement in atherogenesis, has been rather neglected in recent years while the search for the remnant receptor has intensified. Undoubtedly the discovery of the LRP (page 42) and the even more recent discovery of the VLDL receptor in adipose tissue and skeletal muscle (next section) will renew interest in the exact nature of the β-VLDL receptor.

### VLDL receptor

Recently the cDNA of a receptor with sequence homology with the LDL receptor was isolated from a cDNA library from which the LDL receptor genes had been removed by restriction enzyme digestion. This receptor when expressed in LDL receptor-deficient cells bound the apo E-containing lipoproteins VLDL, β-VLDL and IDL, but not LDL. It was termed the VLDL receptor. Its mRNA is most abundant in heart, skeletal muscle and adipose tissue. These are tissues in which there is also high activity of the enzyme lipoprotein lipase (page 56) and which have a high requirement for triglyceride either for respiration or for storage.

The receptor predicted from the cDNA is clearly part of the LDL receptor supergene family. It thus has five domains: an amino-terminal ligand-binding domain, an EGF precursor homologous domain, an O-linked sugar domain, a transmembrane domain and a cytoplasmic domain mediating clustering into coated pits. The ligand-binding domain comprises eight cysteine-rich repeat sequences whereas the LDL receptor has only seven (page 38).

It has been suggested that the physiological function of the VLDL receptor is to assist in the uptake of the small apo E-rich lipoprotein particles formed when lipoprotein lipase located on the capillary endothelium hydrolyses the triglycerides on VLDL, itself too large to cross into the tissue space.

## Acetyl-LDL receptor (scavenger receptor)

When LDL is incubated with macrophages *in vitro* very little uptake occurs. This is rather disappointing, if an interaction between LDL crossing the arterial intima and stimulating foam cell formation is to be the starting point of atheroma (page 60). Yet LDL in epidemiological terms is the lipoprotein most conspicuously associated with premature atheroma. Certain chemical modifications of LDL, however, make it avidly taken up by macrophages in culture to form foam cells. Acetylation, which increases the negatively charged residues on LDL, was the first chemical modification shown to do this. Thus the receptor involved is often called the acetyl-LDL receptor. Oxidized LDL is readily taken up at this receptor and it is now more commonly referred to as the scavenger receptor. Great interest centres on whether oxidation of LDL by cells in the arterial wall   for example, smooth muscle and endothelial cells or macrophages themselves – proceeds at such a rate as to lead to foam cell formation *in vivo*.

Oxidized LDL competes with acetyl-LDL for macrophage uptake, but also appears to undergo receptor mediated uptake independent of the acetyl LDL receptor at receptors termed oxidized LDL receptors. Whether either of these processes has aetiopathological relevance to atherosclerosis has yet to be established. The acetyl-LDL receptor has been most extensively studied. It has a molecular mass of 220 000 daltons and probably consists of three strands. Their cytoplasmic tails are at the amino-terminal and lead to membrane-spanning regions. The three protein strands after a short intervening sequence are then wound together first in an alpha helix and then in collagen-like coils. This fibrous section probably means that the receptor protrudes some 400 Å from the cell surface. It leads either to a cysteine-rich domain of 110 amino acids (type I acetyl-LDL receptor) or simply to a terminal sequence of only six amino acids (type II acetyl-LDL receptor). Like the LRP, the acetyl-LDL receptor binds to a variety of ligands including acetylated and oxidized LDL, maleylated bovine serum albumin and polyvinyl sulphate, which are subsequently taken up by the macrophage. Both type I and II receptors appear to be active in this respect so the binding site for these ligands may be the fibrous part of the molecule rather than the cysteine-rich C-terminal domain absent from the type II receptor. Acetyl-LDL receptors seem to be expressed only by macrophages. Unanswered question are: What is (are) the nature of the other macrophage receptor(s) for oxidized LDL; how do endothelial and smooth muscle cells take up modified LDL?

### HDL receptor

It has been suggested that HDL may have a membrane binding site, which allows it to remove cholesterol from a variety of cells (page 35). Evidence for this is currently somewhat circumstantial. The interaction between HDL and cell membranes, whether or not it involves a receptor, does, however, appear to enhance the mobilization and efflux of free cholesterol from cells.

## Apolipoproteins

### Structure and evolutionary origin

The apolipoproteins can be classified according to the similarities of their structure and that of their genes. Apolipoproteins AI, AII, AIV, CI, CIII, CII and E have much in common. In particular they are of relatively low molecular weight and can transfer easily between lipoproteins. Their genes reveal that they have a common ancestral origin (Figure 2.13). Clearly, however, apolipoprotein B and apolipoprotein (a), which are massive by comparision, each have their own unique origin. Apolipoprotein D has structural homology with a family of ligand-binding proteins which includes some lipid transport proteins such as retinol-binding protein. Its function is unknown, but it also clearly cannot be classified with the major group of apolipoproteins. Apolipoprotein J too is from a different protein family from that of the majority of the apolipoproteins.

The apo CI gene was probably the first to spring from the primordial apolipoprotein gene and to be conserved (Figure 2.13). Apo CII probably arose next, to

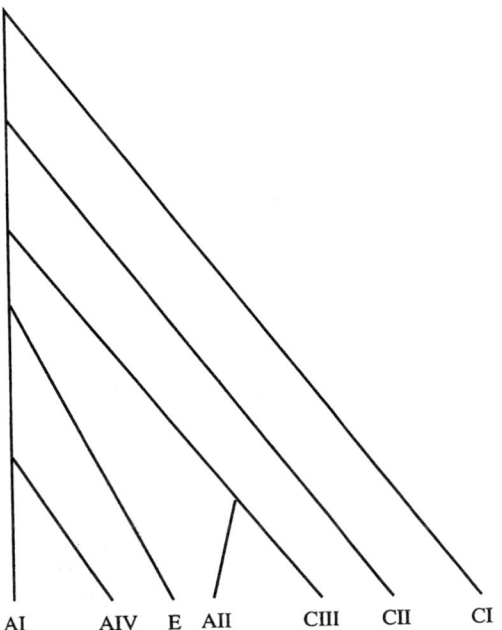

**Figure 2.13**   Evolution of certain apolipoproteins from a common apolipoprotein  AI-like ancestral gene

be followed by another apolipoprotein which itself duplicated to give apo CIII and AII. There then followed apo E and subsequently AIV. Apo AI with its high mutation rate is probably the descendant of the main lineage of the ancestral gene

## Apolipoprotein AI

The principal apolipoproteins of HDL are the A apolipoproteins, so called because the old name for HDL was alpha-lipoprotein. In man, the two major A apolipoproteins are AI and AII. Apo AI is the most abundant. Indeed it is present in plasma in health at mass concentrations, which generally exceed those of apo B, the major apolipoprotein of LDL, and in the tissue fluid AI is the apolipoprotein present at the greatest concentration.

Apo AI originates from both the gut and the liver, whence it is secreted with apo AII as phospholipid-rich discs called nascent HDL. The gene for apo AI is located on chromosome 11, where it occurs in close proximity to the genes for apo CIII and apo AIV. In common with many of the other apolipoprotein genes, it consists of four translated regions (exons) with three intervening untranslated regions (introns). These exons code for a 267 amino acid precursor known as preproapo AI. The prepeptide at the N-terminal end of this molecule is 18 amino acids long and is cleaved cotranslationally leaving the proapo AI, which is the form secreted. The six amino acid N-terminal propeptide is then removed in the circulation by a specific calcium-dependent protease. This results in the mature 243 amino acid apo AI. The residence time of proapo AI in the circulation is approximately 4.5 h, whereas the half-life of mature AI is of the order of 5–6 days. Proapo AI comprises 4% of the total fasting serum apo AI, but increases transiently after meals.

Most of the C terminal 200 amino acids of the mature apo AI are coded for by the 4th exon, which is the largest. In this part of the molecule are six repeated sequences each of 22 amino acids, each ending with proline. In between the prolines is an alpha helical structure with polar and non-polar faces. This confers upon the AI molecule powerful detergent properties, the non-polar groups being directed towards the hydrophobic core lipids and the polar groups interfacing with water molecules outside. Besides its structural role, apo AI is the major activator of the enzyme, LCAT (page 57). Most apo AI is present in plasma and extravascular tissue fluid in HDL. There is, however, a small percentage of apo AI which is not present in lipoproteins and which is generally referred to as free apo AI, although it is associated with some phospholipids. It is also called prebeta HDL, which accurately describes its electrophoretic mobility, but wrongly describes its hydrated density which is greater than that of HDL (page 36).

Apo AI has six polymorphic isoforms designated 1–6, of which 4 and 5 are the most common. In addition, there are genetic mutants of apo AI referred to as apo $AI_{Tangier}$, apo $AI_{Milano}$, apo $AI_{Marburg}$ etc. (Chapter 12). Apo AI is unusual among the apoliproteins in the absence of carbohydrate as a component of its mature form.

## Apolipoprotein AII

Apolipoprotein AII is one of the more abundant apoliproteins in plasma and tissue fluid. It originates in the liver and intestine, where it is synthesized as preproapolipoprotein AII which contains 100 amino acids. The 18 amino acid preprotein is cleaved cotranslationally. The propeptide, which contains five amino acids, is present in less than 1% of plasma apo AII, indicating a rapid removal either immediately before secretion or in the circulation. The mature apo AII contains 77 amino acids, but exists mainly as a dimer, the two molecules being linked by a disulphide bridge between the cysteine at position 6 of the primary sequence. Apo AII can also disulphide link to other apolipoproteins such as apo E which it does in a small proportion of human HDL, designated HDLC, which appears in plasma during the feeding of high cholesterol diets. A specific role for apo AII has yet to be cast.

## Apolipoprotein AIV

In the human apolipoprotein IV is generally recovered from the ultracentrifuge infranatant, even at densities of greater than HDL (1.21 g/ml), suggesting that *in vivo* it is either unassociated with plasma lipoproteins or only loosely so. It has been of most interest in the rat, where it occurs as a major apolipoprotein of lymph chylomicrons.

## Apolipoprotein B

As previously discussed (pages 25–33), apo B is central to the lipoprotein transport system. It acquires its name because it is the most abundant protein in LDL, which was formerly known as β lipoprotein. Its serum concentration in Northern European and American populations is in the range 50–180 mg/dl. More than 90% of this is in the low density lipoproteins and the rest in very low density lipoproteins. In conditions associated with a raised serum concentration of LDL, serum apolipoprotein B is generally also raised, even when increased LDL concentrations are not accompanied by hypercholesterolaemia (hyperapobetalipoproteinaemia; see Chapter 6). It has long been realized that many of the hyperlipoproteinaemias leading to premature atherosclerosis are those in which serum apolipoprotein B levels are high. In 1974, D. S. Fredrickson commenting about apo B wrote: 'Its resistance to characterization, its seeming essentiality for glyceride transport, and perhaps the added suspicion that it has something to do with atherogenesis have all transformed apo B into one of the central mysteries of lipoprotein physiology.'

Since that time, evidence has progressively accumulated for a close association between serum apo B and premature coronary atheroma (Chapters 6 and 12). Until recently, the structure and properties of the apo B molecule remained a mystery because its enormous size, insolubility even when only partially delipidated and tendency to aggregate make it resistant to many biochemical techniques. Now, as a result of advances in immunochemistry, the study of specific proteolytic fragments and molecular genetic techniques, fascinating details of its biochemistry have emerged. The apo B gene is situated on chromosome 2. Its messenger RNA (mRNA) contains 14 121 nucleotides and is thus the largest mRNA known. It codes for a 4563 amino acid protein, the N-terminal 27 amino acids of which are cleaved resulting in a 4536 amino acid native apo $B_{100}$. The 27 residue terminal portion is hydrophobic and large enough to span a biological membrane. It may thus be important in the membrane transport and anchoring of the apo B during the synthesis and secretion of the apo B-containing lipoproteins. Apo B is synthesized in the rough endoplasmic reticulum, and triglycerides and phospholipids are synthesized in the smooth endoplasmic reticulum, becoming bound to the apo B before its appearance in the Golgi complex. There carbohydrate is acquired before secretion of the nascent VLDL. N-linked oligosaccharides comprise some 8–10% of the mass of apo B.

The primary sequence of apo $B_{100}$ is unlike that of other apolipoproteins such as the As and Cs. It is a much larger molecule. Estimates of its molecular weight from the amino acids present are around 500 000 daltons which, allowing for the additional presence of carbohydrate, would suggest an actual mass as high as 550 000 daltons. From our knowledge of the protein content of LDL, there can therefore be only one molecule of apo $B_{100}$ per molecule of LDL. Typically, apolipoproteins consist largely of alpha helices and little beta structure. They bind to lipid through amphipathic sequences in the classical detergent-style. Apo B is different. It is very much more hydrophobic. Long hydrophobic sequences interspersed with hydrophilic ones characterize much of its structure, which is only 43% alpha helix with the rest comprising about equally beta sheet, beta turn and random structures. About 11 hydrophobic regions are thus strung out along the apo B molecule and these probably bury themselves in the triglycerides and cholesteryl esters of the lipoprotein core, leaving the more hydrophilic intervening sections at the surface or within the outer phospholipid, free cholesterol- and apo C-containing regions of the VLDL (Figure 2.2). There are several points in the apo B structure where disulphide bonds could occur either internally or with another protein such as the (a) apolipoprotein of LP(a) (see page 53).

Despite its enormous size, apo B, like apo E, has only one receptor-binding site per molecule. It is in a region about one-quarter of the way from the C-terminal of the apo B molecule, which is rich in basic amino acids, homologous with the receptor-binding site of apo E. However, because of the smaller size of apo E, lipoprotein particles frequently contain several apo E molecules and thus several binding sites for apo E receptors. If the apo E receptor requires binding at several sites in a lipoprotein particle before cellular internalization can occur, this may be a reason why apo $B_{100}$ is not cleared through the apo E receptor. It is assumed that during the removal of the lipid core from VLDL in its conversion to LDL, conformational changes occur in the apo B, which allow the receptor site to bind to the LDL (apo $B_{100}/E$) receptor. The removal of VLDL from the circulation is thus prevented until it has shed its triglyceride load. Perhaps during the conversion of VLDL to LDL some of the hydrophobic regions of apo B become less deeply embedded in the diminishing lipid core and the surface parts of the molecule crowd closer together and project out further, allowing the receptor binding site to become more prominently exposed and to assume its most active shape.

Apo $B_{48}$ is the apo B produced by the gut in man, but not the liver. It is estimated to have about 48% of the molecular weight of apo B (hence its name). It does not bind to lipoprotein receptors. Both apo $B_{100}$ and apo $B_{48}$ appear to arise from an identical gene. Apolipoprotein $B_{48}$ consists of the N-terminal 2152 amino acids of apo $B_{100}$. Examination of the genome shows that it terminates in about the middle of the largest exon, meaning that transcription of the message is unlikely to be broken at this point. However, in the RNAs from gut and liver, codon 2153 is different. In that codon, cytosine is present in hepatic mRNA, whereas uracil is present in intestinal mRNA. This makes the codon read CAA in the liver, which translates as glutamine, and UAA in the gut, an order to terminate translation. The intestine proves to possess a highly specific enzyme which changes the cytosine (perhaps by deamination) in codon 2153 of apo B mRNA. Such an arrangement had not previously been contemplated by molecular geneticists. The effect of the two types of apo B produced in the liver and gut is of fundamental importance to lipoprotein metabolism. Because the receptor-binding site of apo $B_{100}$ is in the C-terminal half not present in apo $B_{48}$, the triglyceride-rich lipoproteins from the gut are dependent on apo E (page 27) for their clearance from the circulation.

It is also becoming clear that apo $B_{100}$ is highly polymorphic. This has been demonstrated by the variety of restriction fragment length polymorphisms of apo B, and by individual variation in the binding affinities of apo B-containing lipoproteins to monoclonal antibodies directed at different parts of the apo B molecule. The present interest in that area of research focuses on whether these polymorphisms have any influence on the metabolism of apo B-containing lipoproteins and thus their serum concentration and their involvement in atherogenesis (Chapter 5 and Chapter 12).

## Apolipoprotein CI

The C apolipoproteins are a group of apolipoproteins initially isolated from VLDL, where they are most abundant, although they are also constituents of the protein moieties of chylomicrons and HDL. They all lack cysteine residues. They have been shown to originate from the liver and to a lesser extent from the gut. Other tissues have not been exhaustively ruled out as a source. As has been described for apo AI and AII, C apolipoproteins may have prepro forms but the sequence of events from gene translation to the appearance of the mature proteins in the circulation is less clear. The genes for apo CI and CII, like those for apo E (page 51), are located on chromosome 19, whereas the gene for apo CIII is part of the gene cluster incorporating the genes for AI and AIV on chromosome 11. Whether this has any functional significance and whether there should be any reclassification as a result of this knowledge remains to be seen.

Apo CI is a protein of 57 amino acids, which as yet has no certain role in lipoprotein metabolism.

## Apolipoprotein CII

Apolipoprotein CII, although present in plasma at lower concentrations than either CII or CIII, is the only C apolipoprotein with a definitely assigned major role in lipoprotein metabolism. It is the activator of lipoprotein lipase. Thus without apo CII the triglycerides of circulating triglyceride-rich lipoproteins could not be removed by lipolysis by tissues such as skeletal muscle and adipose tissue, which are their major sites of clearance. The autosomal recessive condition in which apo CII is deficient produces hypertriglyceridaemia as extreme as the inherited deficiency of the lipoprotein lipase enzyme itself (Chapter 7). Apo CII is thought to be largely absent from newly secreted chylomicrons or VLDL, but to be transferred to them from HDL, which acts as a circulating reservoir. As a result of the subsequent apo CII-activated lipolysis, an imbalance is created between the shrinking core of the triglyceride-rich lipoproteins and their surface materials, including apo CII, which are shed and transferred back to HDL.

The mature apo CII protein has 79 amino acids. The lipoprotein lipase activating portion of apo CII is located in its C-terminal third.

## Apolipoprotein CIII

This 79 amino acid glycoprotein is the most abundant of the circulating C apolipoproteins. Although no definite function has been assigned for it, the possibility that it might, in some way, obscure the apo E of triglyceride-rich lipoproteins, preventing their premature uptake by remnant receptors, has been proposed.

The carbohydrate moiety is linked to a threonine residue at position 74. Galactose and galactosamine are present in all apo CIII molecules, but they differ according to whether no sialic acid is present or one or two molecules are incorporated. In this respect, apo CIII is sometimes referred to as apo CIII-0, apo CIII-1, or apo CIII-2.

## Apolipoprotein E

The major role of apo E is in the hepatic catabolism of chylomicron remnants and other apo E-containing lipoproteins, as discussed on pages 25 and 41.

Three isoforms of apo E are commonly produced by genetic polymorphism. They are identifiable by isoelectric focusing of delipidated triglyceride rich lipoproteins (Plate 1) and are referred to as apo $E_2$, apo $E_3$ and apo $E_4$. The corresponding gene polymorphisms are termed $\epsilon_2$, $\epsilon_3$ and $\epsilon_4$. There is one allele on each chromosome containing the apo E gene, so that an individual may possess two similar (homozygotes) or two different (heterozygotes) apo E gene polymorphisms. The following genotypes are thus possible: $\epsilon_2/\epsilon_2$, $\epsilon_2/\epsilon_3$, $\epsilon_3/\epsilon_3$, $\epsilon_3/\epsilon_4$ and $\epsilon_4/\epsilon_4$. The corresponding lipoprotein phenotypes are $E_2/E_2$, $E_2/E_3$, $E_3/E_3$, $E_3/E_4$ and $E_4/E_4$. The most frequently occurring gene is $E_3$, and most people are $E_3/E_3$ homozygotes or $E_2/E_3$ heterozygotes (Table 2.2).

**Table 2.2 Frequency of different apolipoprotein E phenotypes in the general population***

| Phenotype | $E_2/E_2$ | $E_2/E_3$ | $E_3/E_3$ | $E_3/E_4$ | $E_4/E_4$ | $E_2/E_4$ |
|---|---|---|---|---|---|---|
| Frequency in population | <2% | 23% | 60% | 12% | <1% | <2% |

* Based on averages of several studies in Europe, Canada, New Zealand and the USA. Apo $E_4$-containing phenotypes tend to be commoner in Finland and less common in Japan than the average.

Homozygotes for $E_2$ are least common (less than 1% of the population) and it is in this group that most of the patients with type III hyperlipoproteinaemia occur (Chapter 8). The apo E polymorphisms presumably arose as mutations of apo $E_3$. They are the result of variation in arginine and cysteine composition. Thus, apo $E_3$ has a cysteine residue as the 114th amino acid and arginine as its 158th (Figure 2.14). In $E_2$, the arginine at position 152 is substituted by cysteine, whereas in apo $E_4$ the arginine at 158 is preserved and an additional arginine is present in place of the cysteine at position 114.

The avidity of the binding of the apo E isoforms to receptors recognizing apo E is $E_4 > E_3 > E_2$. The apo E phenotype not only determines the likelihood of type III hyperlipoproteinaemia, but also influences the concentration of serum LDL cholesterol. Serum LDL cholesterol tends to be lowest in $E_2$ homozygotes and then increases progressively through $E_2/E_3$ to $E_3/E_3$ to $E_3/E_4$ to the highest concentration in $E_4/E_4$ individuals (Table 2.3). Intravenously injected apo $E_3$ is distributed evenly between VLDL and HDL, whereas apo $E_2$ attaches principally

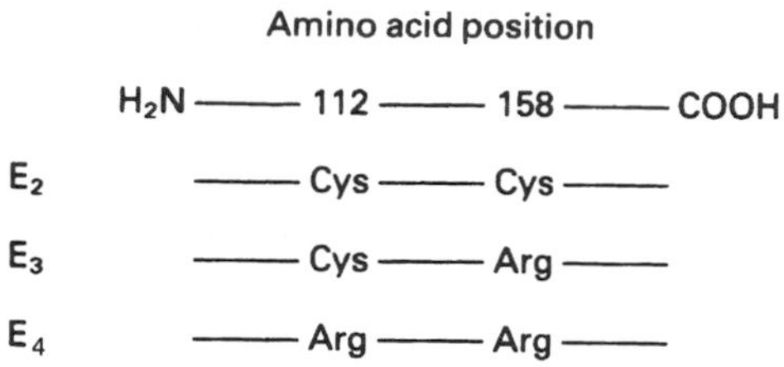

Amino acid position

H₂N ——— 112 ——— 158 ——— COOH

E₂        ——— Cys ——— Cys ———

E₃        ——— Cys ——— Arg ———

E₄        ——— Arg ——— Arg ———

**Figure 2.14**  Amino acid substitutions in the commonly occurring genetic polymorphisms of apolipoprotein E

to HDL and $E_4$ to VLDL. Apo $E_4$ is catabolized fastest (FCR = 2.5/day), apo $E_3$ at an intermediate rate (FCR = 1.43/day) and $E_2$ slowest (FCR = 1.25/day). If hepatic uptake of cholesterol-rich apo E-containing lipoproteins, such as chylomicron remnants via the apo E receptor, is also more rapid when the apo E is $E_4$, then a higher concentration of cholesterol might result in hepatocytes and lead to a down-regulation of the LDL (apo $B_{100}$/E receptor). This down-regulation of the apo $B_{100}$/E receptor might then reduce LDL catabolism, accounting for the higher serum LDL cholesterol concentrations associated with apo $E_4$ expression. Slower rates of hepatic clearance of remnants containing $E_3$ and $E_2$ might lead to lower hepatic cholesterol levels and thus more expression of LDL (apo $B_{100}$/E) receptors, increasing LDL catabolism and thus lower serum LDL cholesterol levels. Alternatively, or in addition, if binding of IDL to the remnant (apo E) receptors is important for its conversion to LDL, a decrease in the affinity of apo E for its receptor would be expected to slow down the rate of formation of LDL, giving rise to lower plasma levels. The hepatic (apo E) receptor is not down-regulated by cholesterol. This is also discussed on pages 41–44 and 219–220.

The gene for apo E is on chromosome 19 adjacent to that of apo CI, with the CII gene being nearby. The gene has the familiar apolipoprotein gene structure of four exons and three introns. Apo E has an 18 amino acid prepeptide, which is cleaved cotranslationally to leave the 299 amino acid apolipoprotein, which has no propeptide. The significance of this is at present speculative. The receptor-binding sequence is in the middle of the molecule between amino acids 140 and 150, although as has been discussed previously, the charge on the amino acid at position 158 has a critical effect on its affinity, presumably via an effect on its conformation.

**Table 2.3 Example of the influence of apolipoprotein E phenotype on the serum concentration of cholesterol, LDL cholesterol and apolipoprotein B in 120 insulin-treated diabetics (From Winocour, P.H. et al., 1989, Atherosclerosis, 75, 167–173)\***

| Phenotype | | $E_2/E_2$ $E_2/E_3$ | $E_3/E_3$ | $E_4/E_4$ $E_3/E_4$ |
|---|---|---|---|---|
| Serum cholesterol | (mg/dl) | 212 ± 22 | 219 ± 6 | 242 ± 22 |
| | (mmol/l) | (5.43 ± 0.56) | (5.61 ± 0.16) | (6.21 ± 0.56) |
| LDL cholesterol | (mg/dl) | 120 ± 16 | 140 ± 6 | 157 ± 20 |
| | (mmol/l) | (3.07 ± 0.41) | (3.60 ± 0.16) | (4.02 ± 0.52) |
| Apolipoprotein B | (mg/dl) | 97 ± 11 | 106 ± 3 | 123 ± 16 |

\* The same effect has been repeatedly demonstrated in the general population.

Apo E is the only apolipoprotein known to be synthesized outside the liver or gut. A large number of tissues contain mRNA for apo E such as liver, brain, spleen, kidney, lung and adrenal. Its role in most of these tissues is speculative. The concentration in the brain is about one-third that of the liver, which is the only tissue possessing a greater concentration. Astrocytes contain apo E, which may be important in transporting lipids along their cytoplasmic processes to the cells they nourish. Neurons, myelin-forming cells (oligodendroglia) and microglia do not contain mRNA for apo E. Macrophages in tissue culture have been shown to secrete apo E. It has been suggested that apo E may assist in the transport of cholesterol out of cells such as macrophages and thus be important at an early stage in reverse cholesterol transport. The accumulation of cholesterol in macrophages may lead to the development of fatty streaks in arterial walls, which may go on to produce atheromatous plaques (page 60). Apo E synthesis in response to a high intracellular free cholesterol content might be a mechanism for preventing its accumulation. The secretion of apo E by cells replete in cholesterol might also produce levels in the tissue fluid cells adjacent to the cell surface sufficient to block the apo LDL ($B_{100}$/E) receptor and prevent further receptor-mediated entry of cholesterol-rich lipoproteins. Apo E is present in HDL, principally the $HDL_2$ subfraction. Possibly some of this results from apo E cholesterol complexes escaping from cells such as macrophages. The apo E-containing HDL is referred to as $HDL_C$ (note the c used as a subscript differentiates $HDL_C$ from HDL-C which some authors use as an abbreviation for HDL cholesterol). $HDL_C$ may transport cholesterol to the liver, where it may be cleared by the hepatic remnant (apo E) receptor or release its cholesterol by some mechanism involving hepatic lipase (page 57), for which it is the preferred substrate.

The possible involvement of apo E in Alzheimer's disease is discussed on page 376.

## Apolipoprotein (a)

Apolipoprotein (a) is present in a lipoprotein called Lp(a). This was first identified as a blood group variant occasionally responsible for transfusion reactions. Initially it was thought to be an inherited factor, which was either present or absent. It is now realized, as the result of sensitive immunoassays for the apo(a) antigen, that it is detectable in virtually all individuals, but that its concentration varies over an enormous range (1–>100 mg/dl) and its frequency distribution is markedly positively skewed. Its concentration, however, has been confirmed to be substantially genetically determined, more so than any other apolipoprotein thus far studied.

Lp(a) is a lipoprotein, which when present in high concentrations can be seen on agarose gel or cellulose acetate chromatography as a band (pre-$\beta_1$ band) migrating in advance of VLDL (pre-$\beta$ lipoprotein) and LDL ($\beta$-lipoprotein). This faster mobility is because its content of sialic acid is higher than the other apo B-containing lipoproteins. The mean hydrated density of Lp(a) is 1.085 g/ml, but its range of particle sizes means that it is present both in LDL, particularly that part with a density greater than 1.053 g/ml, and in $HDL_2$. Lp(a) contains both apo(a) and apo B in addition to lipid, particularly cholesterol and phospholipid. The apo B is probably disulphide linked to the apo(a) protein. In people with high plasma concentrations of apo(a), as much as 20% of their apo B may be in Lp(a). Because of its cholesterol content, Lp(a) may make a substantial contribution to the HDL cholesterol concentration, particularly that of $HDL_2$. Some methods for isolating HDL, such as ultracentrifugation, will include some Lp(a), whereas others, such as the phosphotungstate–magnesium method, will precipitate it.

Lp(a), unlike most of the LDL present in the circulation, does not appear to have a triglyceride-rich lipoprotein precursor and is probably directly secreted by the liver. In patients with cirrhosis or in people who habitually consume large amounts of alcohol, even in the absence of liver disease, plasma levels of Lp(a) are low. The average level of Lp(a) is higher in people whose ancestors originated in Africa or the Indian subcontinent than in Europids, suggesting an ethnic difference. Europids with a family history of premature ischaemic heart disease do, however, have on average high levels of plasma Lp(a). The clearance of Lp(a) from the circulation is only slightly delayed compared with LDL-apo B, and it has been demonstrated *in vitro* that Lp(a) binds to fibroblast apo LDL ($B_{100}$/E) receptors, albeit with lower affinity than LDL. Cholestyramine and HMG-CoA reductase inhibitor drugs which up-regulate LDL (apo $B_{100}$/E) receptors do not, however, influence the serum levels of Lp(a). This supports the conclusions from kinetic studies that a major influence on serum Lp(a) is its rate of hepatic production.

The apo(a) protein is large. Its molecular weight has been reported to vary greatly over a range between 300 000 and 700 000 daltons. The variation in its molecular weight is due to a series of 20 or more isoforms of apo(a), which are inherited in an allelic manner (Chapter 12 page 364). There is marked homology between the cDNA of apo(a) and the genetic sequence of plasminogen.

Plasminogen is a much smaller protein of 791 amino acids, which is the precursor of plasmin, the protease enzyme responsible for lysing fibrin in clots. Its primary structure contains a series of five similar cysteine-rich sequences which each curl themselves up into a Pretzel- or Danish pastry-like structure ('kringle') (*kringlos* = hoop in old Norse) held together by three internal disulphide bonds. Conversion to the smaller plasmin, its active form, is achieved by cleavage at a particular arginine residue. Other proteins in the coagulation system, such as tissue plasminogen activator and prothrombin, have similar structures, suggesting how a blood clotting cascade capable of increasingly sophisticated amplification and modulation may have evolved. Apo(a) also consists of kringle-like structures, but one of these, kringle 4, is repeated over and over again: 37 times in the case of the DNA polymorphism studied in most detail, which coded for a protein predicted to have 4529 amino acids (Figure 2.15). An additional cysteine residue is incorporated in the 36th of these and this may be the one which is linked to apo B in Lp(a). Thus apo(a) appears to be a gigantic deformed relative of plasminogen. Its evolutionary conservation suggests some selective advantage, at least during some stage of man's evolution. In our present condition, however, it may increase the likelihood of thrombosis occurring on atheromatous plaques. Thus apo B-containing lipoproteins and remnant-like lipoproteins may be the major biochemical factor leading to the formation of atheroma, whereas apo(a) may be a major determinant of whether thrombosis occurs on the atheromatous plaques, leading to clinical events such as myocardial infarction. Increased levels of apo(a) may not, however, be a disadvantage in racial groups whose genetic make-up or nutrition does not otherwise predispose them to develop atheroma.

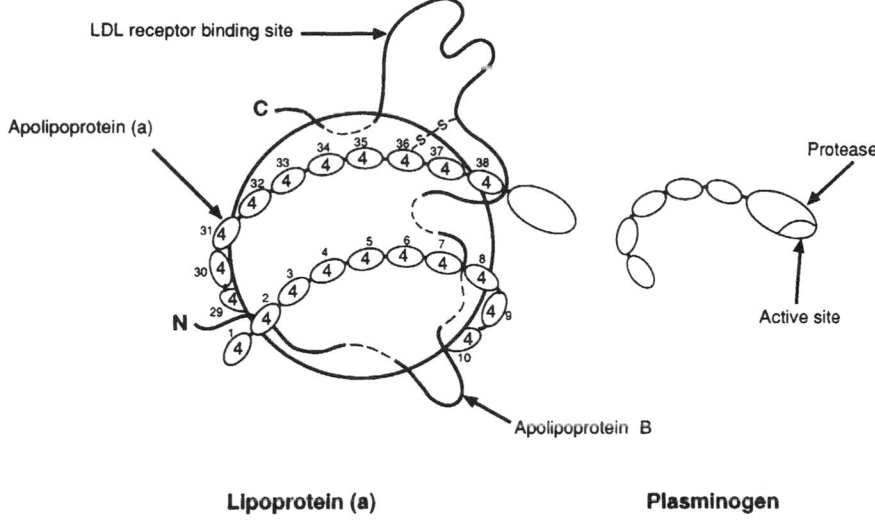

Lipoprotein (a)                              Plasminogen

**Figure 2.15**   Apolipoprotein (a) has evolved from a mutation of a plasminogen-like molecule in which the fourth kringle is repeated many times. It is present in Lp(a) probably disulphide linked to apolipoprotein B at the penultimate kringle 4 repeat

## Apolipoprotein J (Clusterin)

Apo J is distributed in HDL and VHDL. HDL containing apo J has alpha$_2$ electrophoretic mobility. Apo J circulates as a heterodimer comprising two subunits, J alpha (34 000–36 000 daltons) and J beta (36 000–39 000 daltons) joined by 5 disulphide bonds. It is markedly glycated, carbohydrate accounting for 30% of its molecular mass. There are three polymorphisms of apo J, termed apo J-1, J-2 and J-3 of which apo J-1 is the commonest. Apo J-2 is present in 20–30% people of African descent and apo J-3 is uncommon. Apo J is present in a wide variety of body fluids: plasma, urine, cerebrospinal fluid, milk and seminal fluid and is expressed by all tissues with the exception of adult lung and the intestine derived from the mid- and hind gut. Concentrations of apo J mRNA are especially high in the stomach, testis, brain and liver. It is particularly associated with epithelial cells in mucosal linings.

The exact role of apo J is uncertain. However, it is a good candidate for a role outside that of lipoprotein metabolism. It has heparin-binding domains which would permit attachment to the heparan and other glycosaminoglycans on cell surfaces. It has an amphipathic helical domain which would allow it to bind to lipids and other hydrophobic molecules. It inhibits complement-mediated cell lysis and could protect mucosal cells against the toxic biproducts of antibacterial and antiviral mucosal defence processes, digestive enzymes, bile acids and phospholipids. This might explain its presence in the lining of the stomach, duodenum, pancreas, gall bladder, bile ducts and urinary tract.

## Other apolipoproteins

A variety of proteins besides those discussed in detail are found in the delipidated residues of the lipoproteins, especially VLDL and HDL. Some of these may also be present in plasma unassociated with lipoproteins. Apo D, F and H have already been classified as apolipoproteins and have been partially characterized. At present they do not contribute to our understanding of lipoprotein metabolism, which is, of course, also the case for many of the apolipoproteins discussed in detail in earlier parts of this chapter. Lipoproteins and their apolipoproteins, however, almost certainly have major biological roles quite apart from the transport of lipids in extracellular fluids. Their likely involvement in immunology, haemostasis and membrane physiology spring immediately to mind. They may be important too in toxicology, and the presence of apolipoprotein E in cells of the central nervous system suggests an intracellular transport function. The apolipoproteins afford us one of the most exciting frontiers in biology and medicine for future exploration.

# Endothelial lipases

### Lipoprotein lipase

Lipoprotein lipase (EC 3.1.1.34) is the enzyme responsible for stripping triglycerides from the triglyceride-rich lipoproteins (chylomicrons and VLDL) during their passage through the circulation. It is a glycoprotein, which in its active form exists as a dimer of molecular weight 63 000 daltons. It has a binding site for sulphated glycosaminoglycans and another for apolipoprotein CII. The first of these sites allows it to be anchored to the capillary endothelium by attachment to heparan sulphate on the cell surface. The enzyme protrudes from that attachment into the current of circulating blood, where it comes into contact with lipoproteins. It hydrolyses their triglycerides to 2-monoglycerides and fatty acids. The fatty acids released diffuse into cells in the vicinity of the capillaries, and the monoglycerides are hydrolysed by locally active monoglyceridase enzymes to glycerol and fatty acids. Lipoprotein lipase is present in substantial amounts in tissues that have a high requirement for triglycerides: for storage in the case of adipose tissue, for energy in skeletal or cardiac muscle and for milk in the lactating breast. The enzyme is thought to originate in the cells of these tissues and then migrate to its functional site on the capillary endothelium. The glycosaminoglycan-binding site has a higher affinity for heparin than for heparan sulphate. It is thus released into the circulation following the intravenous injection of even small amounts of heparin.

Lipoprotein lipase requires apolipoprotein CII as a cofactor, if it is to be active. Its activity also increases with increasing lipoprotein size. Thus it is more active against chylomicrons than VLDL and preferentially hydrolyses triglycerides in even larger lipid complexes, such as those of Intralipid (after its exposure to apolipoprotein CII). It is inhibited by salt solutions such as 1 molar NaCl and by protamine, which usefully distinguishes it from hepatic triglyceride lipase.

Lipoprotein lipase is active in all mammalian species and the great similarity of its structure indicates that it has been well conserved during evolution. It has a central role in lipoprotein metabolism in releasing triglycerides from their transporting lipoproteins. In so doing, the core of these lipoproteins shrinks leading also to the release of surface materials, such as apolipoproteins, phospholipids and free cholesterol. A substantial part of HDL is therefore the result of the action of lipoprotein lipase.

## Hepatic triglyceride lipase

This enzyme is probably also a glycoprotein and has an ancestral gene in common with lipoprotein lipase. It is, however, active in its monomeric form, the molecular weight of which is 67 500 daltons. It is not readily inhibited by concentrated salt solutions or by protamine. It is bound to glycosaminoglycan components of the endothelium of the hepatic microcirculation. Like lipoprotein lipase it is released from this attachment by preferential binding to heparin and together with lipoprotein lipase contributes to the lipolytic activity of plasma collected after the intravenous injection of heparin (post-heparin lipolytic activity or PHLA).

Hepatic triglyceride lipase is not active in all mammalian species. Also in contradistinction to lipoprotein lipase, it is most active against smaller, denser, cholesteryl ester-rich lipoproteins, showing most marked catalytic activity against HDL. Its place in lipoprotein metabolism has not yet been established with certainty and it is thus an enzyme looking for a role.

Some evidence exists that it may be important in the release of cholesteryl ester from HDL molecules circulating through the liver (page 36), perhaps by producing a hole in their outer phospholipid coat. As such it may allow the regeneration of the smaller $HDL_3$ from $HDL_2$. This $HDL_3$ may then be released back into the systemic circulation to acquire further cholesterol, and so on, in a cyclical process, allowing the return of cholesterol to the liver. It is also possible that hepatic triglyceride lipase might participate in the conversion of IDL to LDL (page 44).

# Lecithin: cholesterol acyltransferase (LCAT)

Lecithin: cholesterol acyltransferase (LCAT, EC2.3.1.43) catalyses the transfer of a fatty acid from the 2 position of lecithin (phosphatidyl choline) to the 3-beta-hydroxyl group of cholesterol to form cholesteryl ester (see Figure 2.7). It has a molecular weight of approximately 68 000 daltons. Its carbohydrate component comprises some 24%. LCAT has its gene on chromosome 16 and its principal source is the liver. Within the circulation, LCAT is localized to HDL and this is its site of action. An essential cofactor for LCAT activity is apolipoprotein AI. It has also been shown that in vitro, using artificial micelles, other apolipoproteins such as apo E, AIV and CI also exhibit some ability as activators. Conversely, apo AII, CII, CIII and D inhibit the enzyme, probably by displacing AI from the micelles. It is doubtful that these observations have any major physiological significance, although they may account for LCAT activity in patients with apo AI deficiencies. Sulphydryl groups are important for LCAT activity, as is demonstrated by the profound inhibitory effect of sulphydryl blocking agents such as dithiobisnitrobenzoic acid (DTNB).

In man, although the liver possesses a cholesterol esterifying enzyme, the cholesterol transported into the circulation from the liver is largely free cholesterol. Esterification of this cholesterol takes place after its transfer from VLDL to HDL. The esterified cholesterol is then transferred back to VLDL by cholesteryl ester transfer protein (CETP). The gut, unlike the liver, secretes esterified cholesterol. It is, however, also likely that much, if not all, of the cholesterol transported out of peripheral cells, as part of the process of reverse cholesterol transport, is in the form of free cholesterol. Certainly in vitro the passage of free cholesterol across the outer membrane of cells in tissue culture is much more readily accomplished than that of cholesteryl ester. If this also obtains *in vivo*, then this cholesterol too will require to be esterified by LCAT if it is to become a core component of lipoproteins and thus be transported efficiently.

Variation in the activity of LCAT itself has never been shown to have any direct link with atherogenesis. This is despite its important role in cholesterol metabolism in species such as man. Events following the esterification of circulating free cholesterol by LCAT, for example the transfer of cholesteryl ester out of HDL by CETP, may be more crucial in atherogenesis (page 59).

## Acyl-CoA: cholesterol O-acyltransferase (ACAT)

In contrast to LCAT, much less is known about acyl-CoA: cholesterol O-acyltransferase (ACAT). In the gut, free cholesterol absorbed as a product of digestion and newly synthesized cholesterol is esterified before its secretion in chylomicrons. Inhibitors of ACAT, for example synthetic fatty acids capable of binding to the enzyme, but not of being esterified to cholesterol, are currently attracting interest, because of their potential as hypocholesterolaemic drugs.

Enzymes with cholesterol esterifying ability are widely distributed. Although present in liver, the esterification of cholesterol, which is to be exported into either the bile or plasma, does not occur to any substantial extent in man, unlike for example the rat.

The major role of ACAT in tissues other than the gut is to esterify free cholesterol released from lysosomes (page 33). The storage of this cholesterol in the cytoplasm is facilitated by esterification. Because of the hydrophobic nature of cholesteryl ester, esterification leads to the formation of storage droplets. The fatty acid to which the cholesterol is esterified in this reaction is generally oleic acid. Synthetic ACAT inhibitors have also attracted interest as potential anti-atherogenic drugs discouraging the accumulation of intracellular cholesterol deposits in atheromatous plaques.

Entry of LDL into the cell, certainly by the receptor-mediated route, leads to the activation of ACAT. Unlike free cholesterol, cholesteryl ester cannot move along concentration gradients in aqueous media without a specific transport protein. Transport of cholesterol out of storage droplets when it is required is therefore likely to require its conversion to free cholesterol. This is accomplished by a neutral cholesteryl ester hydrolase (esterase). In some *in vitro* experiments this enzyme is rate-limiting for egress of excess cholesterol out of cells, free cholesterol migrating through cytoplasm and crossing the outer membrane with much more facility than cholesteryl ester which is non-polar (page 35).

## Cholesteryl ester transfer protein (CETP)

Cholesteryl ester transfer protein (CETP; synonym: lipid transfer protein, LTP) is a glycoprotein of molecular weight approximately 64 000 daltons. Another lipid transfer protein of lower molecular weight may also be present in plasma, but its significance is uncertain. CETP circulates as part of a complex containing cholesteryl ester and triglycerides (cholesteryl ester transfer complex, CETC). The origin of CETP is uncertain. It is absent from the circulation of several species, for example the rat, the dog and the pig.

The role of CETP is to transfer cholesteryl ester out of HDL to triglyceride-rich lipoproteins. A reciprocal exchange of triglycerides out of the triglyceride-rich lipoproteins to HDL occurs (considerably more of their triglycerides are removed by the enzyme lipoprotein lipase). Both chylomicrons and VLDL may act as acceptor molecules for the cholesteryl ester. CETP shows preference for lipoproteins richest in triglyceride. In man, the greater part of the cholesteryl ester formed on HDL is transported to other lipoproteins by this route. It is estimated that some 1500 mg of free cholesterol is esterified in the circulation each day. There is thus clearly a very active role for CETP in cholesterol metabolism. Free cholesterol, although insoluble in water (critical micelle concentration approximately $3 \times 10^{-8}$ molar) is nevertheless, by virtue of its polar hydroxyl group, able to move along a concentration gradient from cell membranes or from lipoproteins such as VLDL or LDL to HDL. The influence of LCAT and CETP is dramatically illustrated by an old observation from the 1920s that cholesterol, while being virtually insoluble in water, nevertheless dissolves in plasma particularly when incubated at 37 °C. We now know that the cholesterol which dissolves is converted to cholesteryl ester, and although there may be some small increase in the quantity in HDL, the bulk of it is found in VLDL.

After esterification on HDL by LCAT, cholesteryl esters are transported out of HDL by CETP thus allowing LCAT to esterify fresh free cholesterol entering the HDL molecule along the concentration gradient. The cholesteryl ester on CETP is then transferred to chylomicrons or VLDL whence it may be cleared by the liver through the remnant (apo E) receptor with the chylomicron remnants or IDL. It may then be eliminated by the liver as biliary cholesterol or converted to bile salts. In the case of cholesteryl ester entering VLDL, some will also remain with IDL during its conversion to LDL. Some of this LDL will be removed by the liver via the hepatic LDL (apo $B_{100}/E$) receptor or by non-receptor-mediated uptake, for which the liver is well adapted by virtue of its fenestrated endothelium. All these processes constitute what has been termed reverse cholesterol transport (page 33). It is also, however, the case that cholesteryl ester which enters the LDL pool will be contributing to an atherogenic lipoprotein pool. High rates of cholesteryl ester transfer from HDL to VLDL result in low serum HDL cholesterol levels and increased likelihood of coronary heart disease. A genetic deficiency of CETP has been described associated with relative freedom from coronary disease (Chapter 12, page 372). Furthermore the expression of simian CETP in transgenic mice is associated with susceptibility to atherosclerosis and diminished HDL. The reason for the association of high cholesteryl ester transfer rates with coronary heart disease may be more subtle than simply that the cholesteryl ester it transports contributes to the LDL cholesterol. It is possible that a similar mechanism involving CETP also permits the movement of cholesteryl ester out of LDL itself back to VLDL in exchange for triglyceride (Figure 2.16) Heightened activity in such a process would lead to a small, cholesteryl ester-depleted, triglyceride-rich LDL as has been described in a variety of clinical conditions associated with increased coronary risk (Chapter 7, page 192). This LDL appears to be particularly susceptible to oxidative modification which has been implicated in atherogenesis (next section).

CETP itself is not the only rate-limiting factor in determining the rate at which cholesteryl ester is transferred into the VLDL pool from either HDL or LDL. The size of the VLDL and chylomicron pool also influences the rate which thus increases in hypertriglyceridaemia and post prandially. Also the free cholesterol

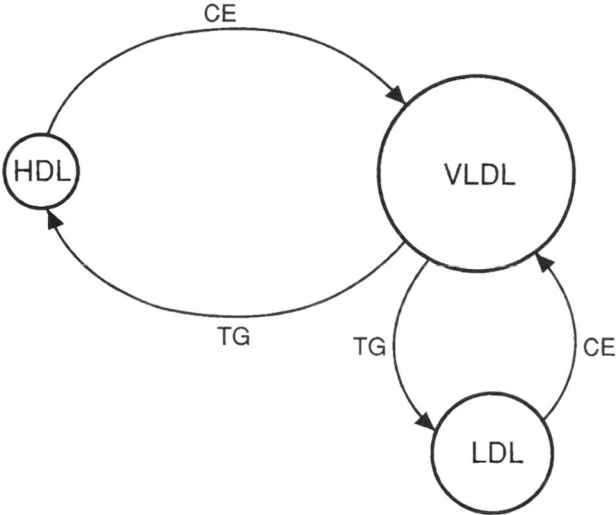

**Figure 2.16**   The movements of cholesteryl ester complexed with cholesteryl ester transfer protein (CETP) which can occur in plasma between HDL and LDL and VLDL (and chylomicrons). A reciprocal movement of triglyceride also occurs. Increased transfer results in low plasma HDL cholesterol levels and the formation of small, dense LDL which may make little contribution to the plasma cholesterol concentration

content of the VLDL increases the rate of transfer. This may account for the increased CHD risk associated with states of hypertriglyceridaemia, increased hepatic VLDL production and low serum HDL cholesterol levels.

## Atherogenesis

A major discussion of the pathological processes that lead to atheroma is outside the scope of this book. However, there would be little point in reviewing the physiology of lipids and lipoproteins and then going on to debate the clinical aspects of their disordered metabolism without an appraisal of their involvement in atherogenesis at the cellular level. Recently, studies in primate models and of cells *in vitro* have led to a much clearer picture of events in the development of atheroma.

The initiating event in atherogenesis appears to be the formation of the fatty streak (Figure 2.17). This is formed when the arterial endothelium becomes excessively permeable, as it may do from time to time particularly at sites of bifurcation due to local minor trauma, anoxaemia or hypertension. There follows an increased entry of lipoproteins and other blood components into the arterial subintima. Blood monocytes migrate through the endothelium at the same sites and there engulf the lipoproteins. The lipid-laden macrophages so formed (foam cells) constitute the main cellular element of the fatty streak, which may either resolve or go on to form an atheroma. Which of these two courses is followed is determined by whether or not proliferation of the smooth muscle cells of the arterial walls occurs. Factors which stimulate smooth muscle cell proliferation probably include growth factors from the foam cells, platelet factors from any overlying thrombus (platelets may

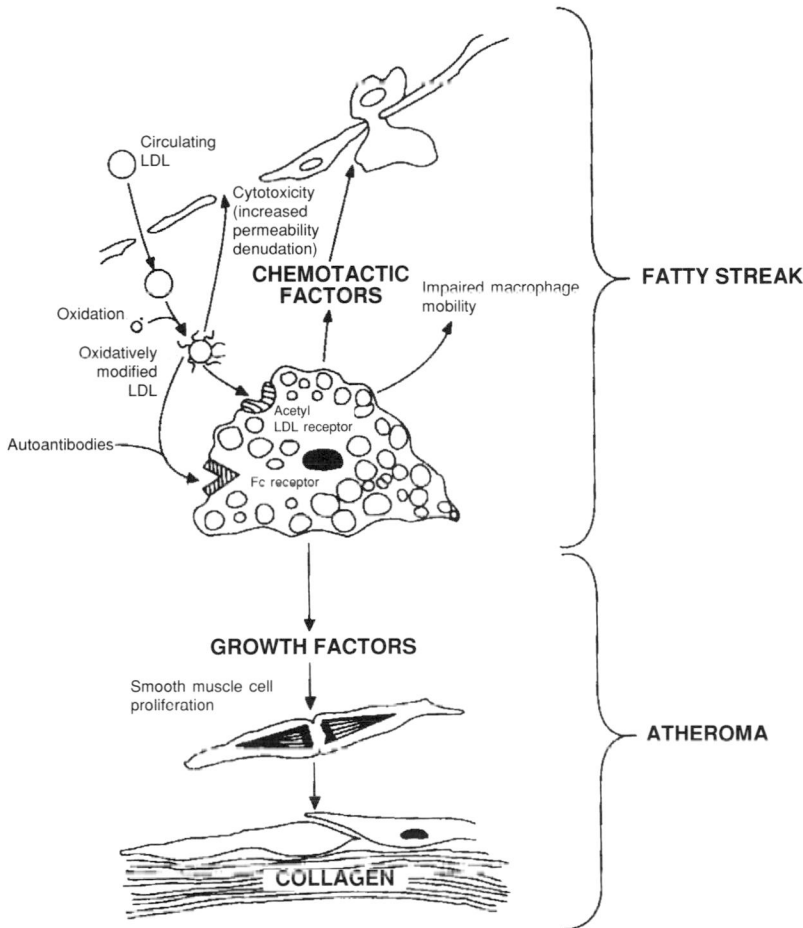

**Figure 2.17**    Atherogenesis. The fatty streak is characterized by lipid-laden macrophages (foam cells) derived from blood monocytes attracted to the arterial subintima where they engulf lipoproteins such as oxidatively modified low density lipoprotein (LDL). Conversion of the fatty streak to atheroma depends on the proliferation and differentiation of smooth muscle cells into fibroblasts, the elaboration of collagen and repetition of the whole process. As the lesion progresses necrosis of foam cells leaves behind extracellular lipid deposits and an overlying fibrous cap develops

also be attracted to the damaged endothelium) and lipoproteins themselves. The resulting new smooth muscle cells behave rather like fibroblasts and lay down collagen which traps foam cells. Repetition of the process leads to the development of the mature atheroma with its layers of fibrous tissues and cholesterol. Frequently the final event leading, for example, to myocardial infarction may be an acute occlusion or critical narrowing of the artery by the formation of thrombus overlying the atheromatous plaque. Often this may be precipitated by rupture of that plaque. Plaque rupture frequently occurs through the overlying fibrous cap in the region adjacent to where it joins the normal arterial wall. Interestingly, even at this stage

LDL oxidative-modification may be important in weakening tissues because intense macrophage activity and foam cell formation is often evident in this region of the mature lesion. The likelihood of thrombosis on the damaged surface once the rupture has occurred may be increased by coagulation factors or platelet activation and decreased fibrinolytic activity. This tendency may be heightened by genetic factors (possibly apo(a)), diet, smoking etc., and other less well-defined factors.

As was described earlier in this chapter (page 44), macrophages have receptors for chylomicron-remnant-like lipoproteins (β-VLDL receptors) and for modified LDL (acetyl-LDL receptor, oxidized LDL receptor). Low density lipoprotein can also enter macrophages via their Fc receptor as a component of an immune complex. The two primary lipoprotein disorders associated with premature atheroma about which most is known are type III hyperlipoproteinaemia (Chapter 8) and familial hypercholesterolaemia (Chapter 5). In type III hyperlipoproteinaemia, excessive quantities of remnant particles accumulate in the circulation and these are exactly the type of lipoproteins which rapidly enter macrophages via the β-VLDL receptor *in vitro*, converting them to foam cells (Figure 2.18). In familial hypercholesterolaemia, LDL accumulates in the circulation. LDL from normal people when incubated *in vitro* with macrophages does not lead to the

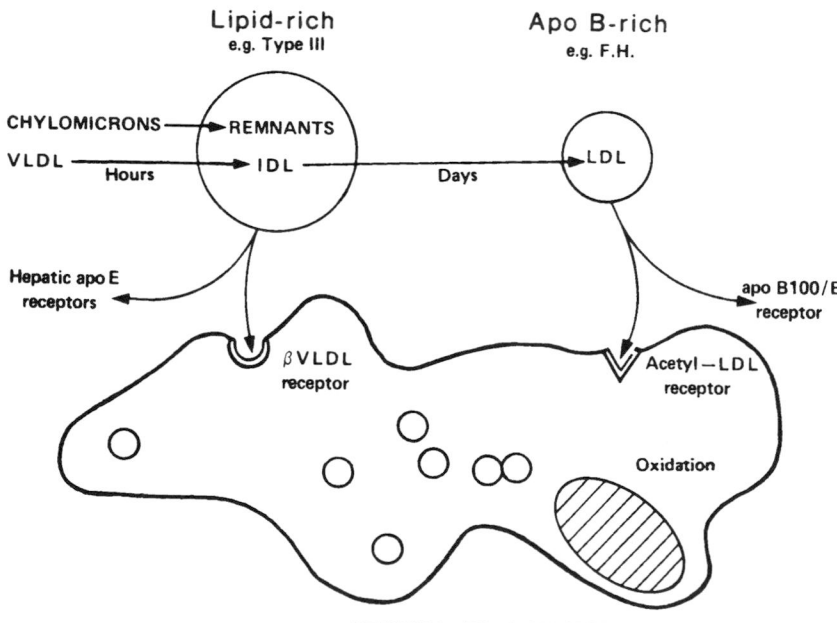

**Figure 2.18**  *In vitro* chylomicron remnants and IDL readily induces macrophages to become foam cells, whereas LDL requires some chemical modification such as oxidation before it will do so. *In vivo*, however, clearance of remnants and IDL normally occurs within a few hours (except, for example, in type III hyperlipoproteinaemia). Clearance of IDL normally takes 2–3 days, even longer in FH (familial hypercholesterolaemia), and thus the potential for chemical modifications within the circulation or the arterial wall exists

formation of foam cells. If, however, it is oxidized before addition to macrophages, it is rapidly internalized and foam cells are formed. Thus local oxidation in the arterial wall perhaps secondary to free radical formation may be important in the modification of LDL to an atherogenic lipoprotein.

# Oxidative modification of lipoproteins

Despite the epidemiological and clinical trial evidence that LDL is closely involved in the development of atherosclerosis and the obvious early involvement in the fatty streak of foam cells derived principally from monocyte-macrophages, the uptake of LDL by macrophages in tissue culture is disappointingly poor. In the course of experiments to block the uptake of LDL at the LDL receptor its lysine groups were acetylated with acetic anhydride in Goldstein and Brown's laboratory. The acetyl-LDL produced was not taken up at the fibroblast LDL receptor, but was avidly taken up by macrophages to form foam cells resembling those in the arterial wall. This uptake did not involve the LDL receptor, but took place at another receptor, the acetyl-LDL receptor subsequently also termed the scavenger receptor (page 45). Acetyl-LDL is not a naturally occurring modification of LDL. Fogelman in 1980, however, found that treatment of LDL with malonyldialdehyde modified it so that it was taken up by macrophages to form foam cells and would compete with acetyl-LDL for macrophage uptake. Malonyldialdehyde-LDL could occur naturally, because malonyldialdehyde is a product of lipid peroxidation. Steinberg and other workers then showed that incubation of LDL with cells such as smooth muscle cells, macrophages or endothelial cells in tissue culture modified LDL so that it was taken up by macrophages at the acetyl-LDL receptor and that the modification appeared to be an oxidative one similar to that produced when LDL was incubated under oxidizing conditions with ions of copper or iron or with the oxidizing enzyme lipoxygenase. This led to the theory that oxidative modification of LDL might be fundamental to atherogenesis.

## Oxidative mechanisms

The oxidation of molecular oxygen to water requires the addition of four electrons and this occurs stepwise.

(i) $O_2 + e + H^+ \longrightarrow HO_2 \cdot \longleftarrow \longrightarrow H^+ + O_2 \cdot$
      Hydroperoxyl                  Superoxide
      radical                       radical

(ii) $HO \cdot_2 + e + H^+ \longrightarrow H_2O_2$
       Hydroxyl peroxide

(iii) $H_2O_2 + e + H^+ \longrightarrow H_2O + OH \cdot$
        Hydroxyl radical

(iv) $OH \cdot + e + H^+ \longrightarrow H_2O$

The process produces three free radicals: hydroperoxyl, superoxide and hydroxyl. A free radical is an atom, molecule or ion, which has a single electron orbital containing only one electron. They are highly reactive and usually exist only as short-lived intermediates. They are strong oxidizing agents because they strongly attract electrons from other molecules (thus undergoing reduction themselves). Once they have acquired an electron to fill their single unpaired orbital they are energetically extremely stable, having acquired an outer electron shell resembling that of an inert (group 8) atom. Fluorine ($F_2$) for example, can break down to two free radicals F· and F·. The · indicates a single unpaired electron orbital. F· is an extremely reactive free radical. Once it acquires an electron in a chemical reaction this will enter its outer electron shell which is then complete with four pairs of electrons and thus it resembles neon with an inner shell of two electrons and an outer one of eight. Oxygen has two electrons in its inner shell and six electrons in its outer shell (two pairs and two unpaired electrons). In the first stage of the reduction of oxygen it acquires one electron so that it now has seven electrons in its outer shell (three pairs and one unpaired) and in this respect it has a similar electron structure to F· and is written O·. It is a free radical, almost as reactive as fluorine. Generally O· does not exist in isolation and remains bonded with other atoms on molecules with which it shares its extra electron. This affects its reactivity. Thus superoxide, $O_2$·, is not a particularly active free radical whereas the hydroxyl radical, OH·, is particularly reactive.

The reduction of molecular oxygen occurs in several biochemical pathways. Most oxygen is utilized in the mitrochondria in which successive oxygen reductions are tightly linked so that oxygen radicals are extremely unlikely to migrate into the cytoplasm and even less to leave the cell. Oxygen free radicals are probably also unlikely to leak out of the cell when they are produced in the peroxisomes. They may, however, do so when oxygen is reduced in the cytoplasm (e.g. cytochrome P450 system linked to glucuronidation of drugs) or in tissues recovering from hypoxia in which xanthine oxidase is active because AMP levels are high and the pathways for the salvage of purine bases are overloaded. Undoubtedly too, certain cell types secrete free radicals. The macrophage employs oxygen free radicals to kill bacteria. The system which does this employs NADPH oxidase located on the outside of the cell, which catalyses the reaction of free oxygen from the tissue fluid with NADPH to produce superoxide and hydrogen peroxide. The macrophage may not confine its attentions to bacteria and may well oxidatively modify macromolecular complexes, which come in contact with its cell surface, to compromise their activity or to facilitate their uptake. Macrophage production of oxygen free radicals is defective in chronic granulomatous disease.

Arachidonic acid metabolism during inflammation may also lead to the escape of oxygen free radicals. 15-Lipoxygenase catalyses the production of hydroxy-eicosa-tetraenoic acid, which in part mediates the inflammatory response (page 22). The enzyme activity occurs in smooth muscle cells and also in monocytes stimulated by interleukin-4. Interleukin-4 is produced almost exclusively by T-lymphocytes which account for about one-fifth of the cells in early atherosclerotic lesions and persist in the active shoulder region of older plaques which is liable to plaque rupture (page 61). In hypercholesterolaemic rabbits, but not normal rabbits, lipoxygenase is expressed in the artery wall. The conversion of arachidonic acid to prostaglandins and thromboxanes involving cyclooxygenase may also lead to the formation of oxygen free radicals.

Another source of free radicals may be reduced thiol compounds, such as cysteine, which escape from smooth muscle cells. These and compounds such as superoxide may have little effect in oxidizing LDL, but when iron or copper ions are present the lipid peroxidation process is dramatically increased, the transition metals acting as catalysts in this respect.

Peroxidation is potentially harmful and has been implicated in a wide range of diseases apart from atherosclerosis. Not surprisingly, there are systems to combat it. These include superoxidase dismutase (most effective in inhibiting LDL oxidation by smooth muscle cells, less so by macrophages or endothelial cells), catalase and glutathione peroxidase. Also tissue copper and iron are normally tightly bound to caeruloplasmin, transferrin or other proteins to prevent their involvement in oxidation. Factors within LDL itself also contribute to resistance to peroxidation. These include fat soluble antioxidants (antioxidants are compounds which react rapidly with free radicals) such as tocopheral (vitamin E), carotenoids and ubiquinone. Vitamin C is a powerful reducing agent present widely in tissue fluid and plasma, and although not fat soluble may none the less be important in replenishing the antioxidant capacity of vitamin E present in LDL, i.e.

$$\text{Vitamin E} + \text{OH} \cdot \longrightarrow \text{Vitamin E} \cdot + H_2O$$

$$\text{Vitamin E} \cdot + \text{Ascorbate} \longrightarrow \text{Vitamin E} + \text{Dehydroascorbate}$$

In addition the fatty acid composition of LDL lipids is a determinant of how readily it is peroxidized. The greater the number of double bonds (particularly those with a *cis* configuration) in a hydrocarbon the more readily it undergoes peroxidation. Thus saturated fatty acids do not undergo peroxidation and oleic acid (C18 : 1) is less likely to do so than linoleic (C18 : 1) or arachidonate (C20 : 4) and the highly polyunsaturated fatty acids in fish oil such as eicosapentaenoiate (20 : 5) and docosahexaenoiate (22 : 6). This has excited some controversy about the wisdom of recommending unsaturated fats in diets aimed at coronary disease prevention. However, it should not be overlooked that the best way of preventing LDL peroxidation in the arterial wall is probably to decrease its circulating level. The least unsaturated fatty acid which, when it replaces saturated fat, will lower LDL cholesterol levels would be the healthiest dietary fat on this reckoning and it would thus be oleic acid (Chapter 9).

It has been known for many years that LDL is highly susceptible to peroxidation upon exposure to transition metal contains such as copper and iron and that EDTA can prevent the artificial oxidation of lipoproteins during their isolation from plasma or serum. The process of lipid peroxidation has been extensively investigated because it is an important cause of the deterioration of stored food.

Oxidation of unsaturated fatty acyl groups of both the phospholipids and the cholesteryl esters on LDL is particularly likely to produce products that will modify the receptor-binding characteristics of apolipoprotein B and produce other tissue changes likely to contribute to atherogenesis. The peroxidation of triglycerides in, for example, chylomicrons or VLDL, may, however, be important in the aetiology of acute pancreatitis (Chapter 7, page 203).

Lecithin frequently has an unsaturated fatty acyl group in the 2 position. Let us imagine this is linoleate. The first stage is the abstraction of hydrogen from the methylene group in the ω8 position (Figure 2.19). This produces a free radical due to the loss of a proton at carbon 8. This undergoes rearrangement by the formation of a more stable *trans* double bond between C8 and C9. Now the structure has alternating double and single bonds (conjugated diene) and thus resonates absorbing ultraviolet of wavelength 234 nm. The lipid free radical is highly reactive

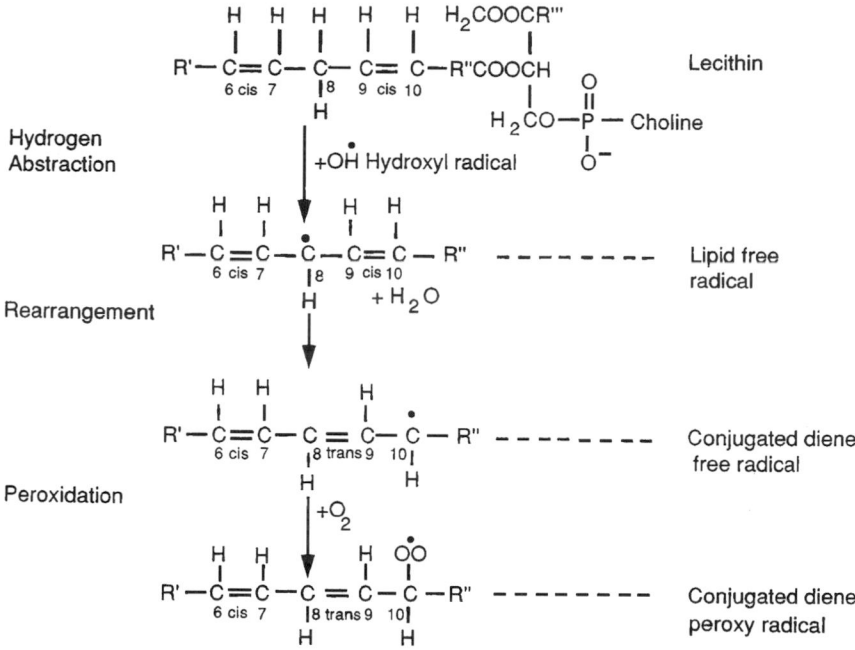

**Figure 2.19** The likely reactions in lipid peroxidation (in this case the linoleyl group in lecithin). The oxygen radical which initiates the process is uncertain. Because of the rearrangement of the position of one of the double bonds a conjugated diene is formed, i.e. double and single bonds now alternate with each other (this obviously cannot occur with a monounsaturated fatty acid such as oleate although hydrogen abstraction and the formation of lipid free radicals etc. can still proceed)

and can react with low-energy ground state oxygen to form a peroxy radical. Peroxy radicals react with other fatty acyl groups by hydrogen abstraction resulting in more lipid free radicals and themselves becoming lipid peroxides (Figure 2.20). Lipid peroxides react together to form peroxy radicals and alkoxy radicals. Transition metal cations essentially catalyse the reaction between lipid peroxides (Figure 2.21). This is frequently used as an experimental device to produce oxidatively modified LDL in experiments. The presence of iron and copper in atherosclerotic lesions has led to speculation that they may have a role in atherogenesis. The peroxy radicals thus formed abstract hydrogen from other fatty acyl groups and thus a chain reaction has been initiated which generates alkoxy radicals. Hydrocarbon chains containing alkoxy groups readily break to yield aldehydes or ketones. This would leave lecithin, for example, with a short chain fatty acyl group in the 2 position, the portion of the fatty acid hydrocarbon chain distal to the site of peroxidation having gone. There is an enzyme on LDL termed phospholipase A2 (synonymous with platelet-activating factor lipase) which hydrolyses the ester bond at the 2 position if a short chain fatty acyl group is present, but not a long chain fatty acyl group such as the original linoleate. This reaction can now take place and leads to the formation of the lysolecithin which is cytotoxic. A bewildering array of ketones, aldehydes, hydroxylipids and lysolipids are also formed during the peroxidation of unsaturated fatty acyl groups. Oxidation of fatty acyl groups in cholesteryl esters and of cholesterol itself is also possible by lipid free

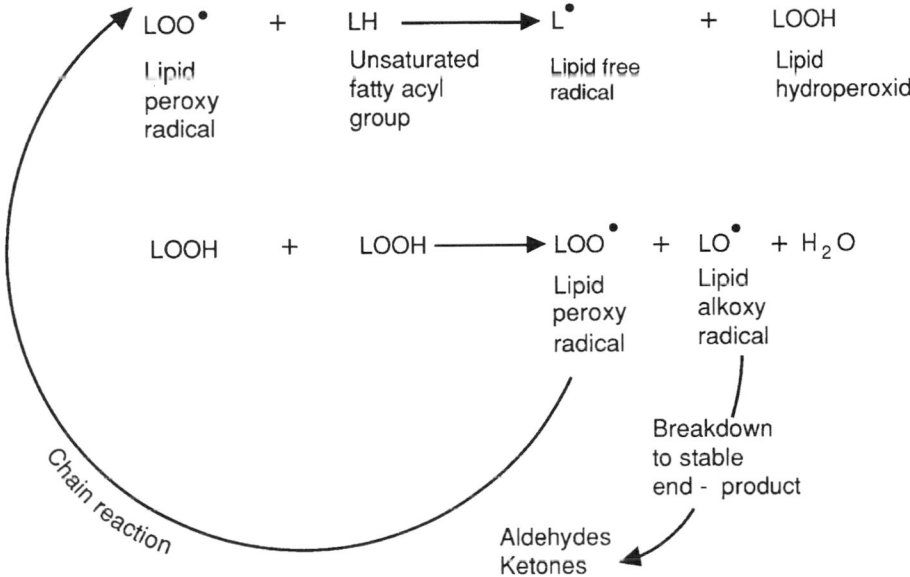

**Figure 2.20**   Once lipid peroxy radicals have been formed a chain reaction can develop generating more lipid peroxy radicals and yielding alkoxy radicals which break down to aldehydes and ketones which will directly damage proteins, such as apolipoprotein B

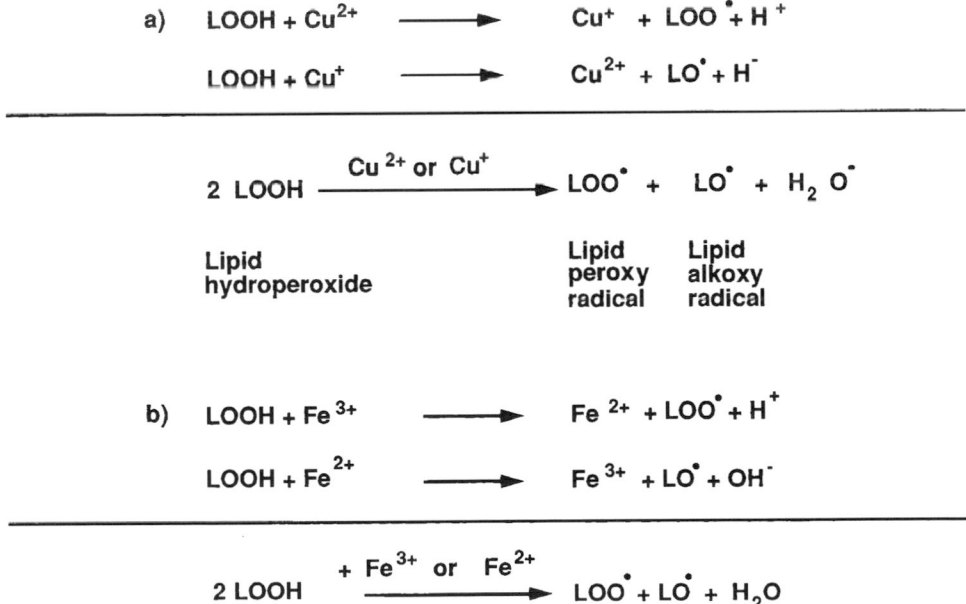

**Figure 2.21**   Iron and copper ions catalyse the production of peroxy and alkoxy radicals from lipid peroxides

**Table 2.4 Lipid oxidation products of low density lipoprotein After Rice-Evans and Bruckdorfer, 1992**

1.  From fatty acyl groups:
    malondialdehyde
    4-hydroxynonenal, 4-hydroxyoctenal, 4-hydroxyhexenal
    hexanal, pentanal, butanal, propanal
    hydroxydienoic acid, hydroxytetraenoic acids their hydroperoxy derivatives
2.  From phosphatidylcholine:
    lysophosphatidylcholine
3.  From cholesterol:
    cholesterol oxides

radicals (Table 2.4). In some experimental systems half of the lecithin in LDL is converted to lysolecithin. This urges some caution in the interpretation of whether some of the effects of oxidatively modified LDL demonstrated *in vitro* could actually take place in the arterial wall. Furthermore one has to ask whether oxidation of LDL in the arterial wall could conceivably occur to any significant extent. When LDL is incubated *in vitro* with copper ions and conjugated diene formation follows there is a long phase before conjugated dienes begin to accumulate, which is highly variable from individual to individual, but which on average may last 60–90 minutes. It is during this phase that the fat soluble vitamins in LDL are being oxidized in preference to the unsaturated acyl groups. *In vivo*, however, it would be expected that protection might be more prolonged because of the presence of vitamin C and the enzyme systems protective against oxygen radicals. Furthermore HDL present in the tissue fluids in higher concentration than LDL also appears to prevent lipid peroxides accumulating in LDL. On the other hand it is possible that local factors in the arterial subintima may increase the likelihood of LDL oxidation: in particular, factors which might prolong the residence time of LDL in the arterial subintima or which may bring LDL into contact with the macrophage NADPH oxidase or lipoxygenase systems. Glycation of LDL may increase the likelihood that it will persist in the arterial wall and come in contact with macrophages. Furthermore some workers have reported that apolipoprotein B-containing lipoproteins retained within lesions are predominantly in Lp(a). Lp(a) binds to a variety of connective tissue proteins including glycosaminoglycans which would explain its persistence in the arterial wall. Like LDL it is susceptible to oxidative damage and uptake by macrophages. Intriguingly too lipoprotein (a) will bind to plasminogen receptors through its apolipoprotein (a) moiety. This might bring it into close contact with macrophages because they have such receptors, and then it may be subjected to deliberate oxidation. There is also increasing interest in the concept that oxidatively modified LDL may excite an immune response, particularly the production of antibodies against it. This would not only provide another means of macrophage LDL uptake via the Fc receptor, but could also be the basis of an immune basis for some of the inflammatory element of atherogenesis.

In addition to foam cell formation and the production of toxic substances such as lysolipids LDL lipid peroxidation may contribute to atherogenesis and to myocardial ischaemia in other ways. Thus it is chemotactic to monocytes, potentially attracting them to areas where fatty streaks are developing, and inhibits the migration of macrophages, possibly interfering with their movement out of the artery wall once they have taken up LDL. It may also act on endothelial cells to cause them to produce growth factors important in the development of the atheromatous plaque such as granulocyte and monocyte colony stimulating factors. It also appears to inhibit the release of endothelial derived relaxing factor (nitric oxide) from the arterial endothelium which might contribute to arterial spasm.

The *in vivo* evidence for involvement of oxidized LDL in atherogenesis is:

1. Epidemiological evidence showing an inverse relation between dietary/plasma antioxidants and CAD.
2. Immunocytochemical evidence of oxidized LDL in atherosclerotic lesions.
3. Evidence that LDL extracted from lesions has physiochemical, immunological, and biological properties of oxidized LDL.
4. Presence in serum of autoantibodies with specificity for epitopes of oxidized LDL.
5. Presence in lesions of IgG with specificity for epitopes of oxidized LDL.
6. Presence in serum of subfractions of LDL with properties similar to early stages of oxidized LDL.
7. Ability of antioxidants to inhibit atherosclerosis in animal models.

The hypothesis which thus emerges is that there are two atherogenic classes of lipoproteins in man: (a) the lipid-rich lipoproteins resembling chylomicron remnants or IDL, which are normally rapidly removed by the remnant (apo E) receptor of the liver or converted to LDL, and (b) apo B-containing lipoproteins characterized by a relatively long circulating half-life, which are consequently relatively small, and have had a longer exposure to oxidative processes. The former circumstance appears to operate in type III hyperlipoproteinaemia and also perhaps in, for example, diabetes mellitus (page 62). The latter condition exists in familial hypercholesterolaemia, where apo B-containing lipoproteins accumulate as a result of the LDL receptor defect, but oxidatively modified LDL may also be particularly relevant in familial combined hyperlipidaemia and hyper-apobetalipoproteinaemia, in both of which apo B-containing lipoproteins are over-produced and a small, dense LDL, susceptible to oxidation, circulates.

## Further reading

LIPOPROTEIN TRANSPORT AND LIPID TRANSFER

Barter, P. High-density lipoproteins and reverse cholesterol transport. *Current Opinion in Lipidology.*, **4** 210–217 (1993)

Durrington, P.N. and Mackness, M.I. Lipoprotein transport and metabolism. In *Oxidative Stress, Lipoproteins* and *Cardiovascular Disease.* (eds C.A. Rice-Evans and K.R. Bruckdorfer) Portland Press, London (in press)

Eisenberg, S. High density lipoprotein metabolism. *J. Lipid Res.*, **25**, 1017–1058 (1984)

Fielding, C. J. Factors affecting the rate of catalyzed transfer of cholesteryl esters in plasma. *Am. Heart J.*, **113**, 532–537 (1987)

Gotto, A. M., Pownall, H. J. and Havel, R. J. Introduction to the plasma lipoproteins. In *Methods in Enzymology*, vol. 128, *Plasma Lipoproteins. A Preparation, Structure and Molecular Biology* (eds J. P. Segrest and J. J. Albers), Academic Press, Orlando, Ca, pp. 3–41 (1986)

Grundy, S. M. Cholesterol and coronary heart disease. A new era. *J. Am. Med. Assoc.*, **256**, 2849–2858 (1986)

Havel, R. J., Goldstein, J. L. and Brown, M. S. Lipoproteins and lipid transport. *In Metabolic Control and Disease*, 8th edn (eds P. K. Bondy and L. E. Rosenberg), W. B. Saunders, Philadelphia, pp. 393–494 (1980)

Kesaniemi, Y. A., Farkkila, M., Kerviner, K., Koivisto, P., Vuoristo, M. and Miettinen, T. A. Regulation of low-density lipoprotein apolipoprotein B levels. *Am. Heart J.*, **113**, 508–513 (1987)

Myant, N. B. *The Biology of Cholesterol and Related Steroids*, Heinemann Medical, London (1981)

Nikkila, E. A., Taskinen, M-R. and Sane, T. Plasma high-density lipoprotein concentration and subfraction distribution in relation to triglyceride metabolism. *Am. Heart J.*, **113**, 543–548 (1987)

Neary, R., Bhatnagar, D., Durrington, P.N., Ishola, M., Arrol, S. and Mackness, M.I. An investigation of the role of lecithin: cholesterol acyl transferase and triglyceride-rich lipoproteins in the metabolism of pre-beta high density lipoproteins. *Atherosclerosis*, **85**, 34–48 (1991)

Reichl, D. and Miller, N. E. The anatomy and physiology of reverse cholesterol transport. *Clin. Sci.*, **70**, 221–231 (1986)

Shepherd, J. and Packard, C. J. Metabolic heterogenicity in very low density lipoproteins. *Am. Heart J.*, **113**, 503–508 (1987)

Vega, G. L. and Grundy, S. M. Mechanisms of primary hypercholesterolaemia in humans. *Am. Heart J.*, **113**, 493–502 (1987)

## LIPOPROTEIN RECEPTORS

Beisiegel, U. Apolipoproteins as ligands for lipoprotein receptors. Chapter 10 in *Structure and Function of Apolipoproteins* (ed. M. Rosseneu) CRC Press, Boca Raton, pp. 269–294 (1992)

Bierman, E. L. and Oram, J. F. The interaction of high-density lipoproteins with extrahepatic cells. *Am. Heart J.*, **113**, 549–550 (1987)

Brown, M. S. and Goldstein, J. L. A receptor-mediated pathway for cholesterol homeostasis. *Science*, **232**, 34–47 (1986)

Brown, M.S., Herz, J., Kowal, R.C. and Goldstein, J.L. The low-density lipoprotein receptor-related protein: double agent or decoy? *Current Opinion in Lipidology*, **2**, 65–72 (1991)

Brown, M. S., Kovanen, P. T. and Goldstein, J. L. Evolution of the LDL receptor concept – from cultured cells to intact animals. *Ann. NY Acad. Sci.*, **348**, 549–550 (1980)

Havel, R. J. Functional activities of hepatic liprotein receptors. *Ann. Rev. Physiol.*, **48**, 119–134 (1986)

Shepherd, J. and Packard, C. H. Lipoprotein receptors and atherosclerosis. *Clin. Sci.*, **70**, 1–6 (1986)

Yamamoto, T., Takahashi, S., Sakai, J. and Kawarabayasi, Y. The very low density lipoprotein receptor. A second lipoprotein receptor that may mediate uptake of fatty acids into muscle and fat cells. *Trends Cardiovasc. Med.*, **3**, 144–148 (1993)

## APOLIPOPROTEINS AND LIPOPROTEINS

Breslow, J. L. Genetic regulation of apolipoproteins. *Am. Heart J.*, **113**, 422–427 (1987)

Brown, M. S. and Goldstein, J. L. Teaching old dogmas new tricks. *Nature*, **330**, 113–114 (1987)

Jordan-Starck, T.C., Witte, D.P., Aronow, B.J. and Harmony, J.A.K. Apolipoprotein J: a membrane policeman? *Current Opinion in Lipidology.*, **3**, 75–85 (1992)

Kostner, G. M. Apolipoproteins and lipoproteins of human plasma. Significance in health and in disease. *Adv. Lipid Res.*, **20**, 1–43 (1983)

Luo, C-C., Li, W-H., Moore, M.N. and Chan L. Structure and evolution of the apolipoprotein multigene family. *J. Mol. Biol.*, **187**, 325–334 (1986)

Mahley, R. W. Apolipoprotein E. Cholesterol transport protein with expanding role in cell biology. *Science*, **240**, 622–630 (1988)

MBewu, A. and Durrington, P.N. Lipoprotein (a): structure, properties and possible involvement in thrombogenesis and atherogenesis. *Atherosclerosis*, **85**, 1–14 (1990)

Olofsson, S-O., Bjursell, G., Bostrom, K., Carlsson, P., Elovson, J. *et al.* Apolipoprotein B. Structure, biosynthesis and role in the lipoprotein assembly process. *Atherosclerosis*, **68**, 1–17 (1987)

Utermann, G. Apolipoprotein E polymorphisms in health and disease. *Am. Heart J.*, **113**, 433–440 (1987)

ENZYMES

Bell, R. A. and Cameron, R. A. Enzymes of glycerolipid synthesis in eukaryotes. *Ann. Rev. Biochem.*, **49**, 459–487 (1980)

Quinn, D., Shirai, K. and Jackson, R. L. Lipoprotein lipase: mechanisms of action and role in lipoprotein metabolism. *Prog. Lipid Res.*, **22**, 35–78 (1982)

Suckling, K. E. and Stange, E. F. Role of acyl-CoA: cholesterol acyltransferase in cellular cholesterol metabolism. *J. Lipid Res.*, **26**, 647–671 (1985)


ATHEROGENESIS AND LIPOPROTEIN OXIDATION

Esterbauer, H., Gebicki, J., Puhl, H. and Jurgens, G. The role of lipid peroxidation and antioxidants in oxidative modification of LDL. *Free Radical Biol. Med*, **13**, 341–390 (1992)

Rice-Evans, C. and Bruckdorfer, K.R. Free radicals, lipoproteins and cardiovascular dysfunction. *Molec. Aspects Med.*, **13**, 1–111 (1992)

Ross, R. The pathogenesis of atherosclerosis. An update. *N. Engl. J. Med.*, **314**, 488–500 (1986)

Steinberg, D. Lipoprotein and atherosclerosis. A look back and a look ahead. *Arteriosclerosis*, **6**, 283 301 (1983)

Steinberg, D., Parthasarathy, S., Carew, T. E., Khoo, J. C. and Witztum, J. L. Beyond cholesterol. Modifications of low-density lipoprotein that increase its atherogenicity. *N. Engl. J. Med.*, **320**, 915–924 (1989)

# Chapter 3

# Normal serum lipid and lipoprotein concentrations

## What are normal serum lipid levels?

Although a concept of normal serum lipid values is central to the identification and management of hyperlipidaemia, the definition of normality is complex. The reader anxious to reach the later sections of this book dealing directly with diagnosis and management might be persuaded to pause to read this chapter. This is because the interpretation of what is an acceptable cholesterol level either before or after therapy is very much dependent on the individual patient. There has been an altogether excessive arbitrariness in many of the recommendations about the interpretation of serum lipid levels. Biology is not like that. Whoever heard of a horse-race where all the runners had the same odds!

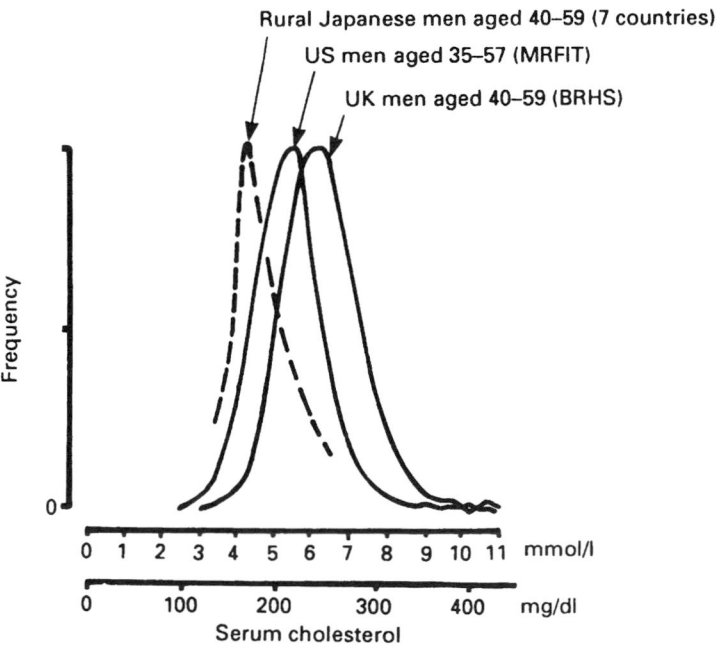

**Figure 3.1** Frequency distribution curves for serum cholesterol in men in rural Japan[10], the USA[8] and the UK[15]

# Serum lipid and lipoprotein concentrations in different populations

## Serum cholesterol and LDL cholesterol

The largest and most informative population studies relating to serum cholesterol and lipoprotein concentrations in apparently healthy (free of clinical disease at the time of examination) populations have been in the USA. This has been as a result of three major investigations: the Cooperative Lipoprotein Phenotyping Study[l], the Lipid Research Clinics (LRC) Program Prevalence Study [2–7] and the Multiple Risk Factor Intervention Trial (MRFIT) [8,9]. The MRFIT involves men aged 35–57, whereas the Cooperative Lipoprotein Phenotyping Study and the LRC Program Prevalence Study cover a wider age range and also include women and, in the latter study, children. These studies establish that the frequency distribution of serum cholesterol is almost Gaussian, with a slight tendency to a positive skew (Figure 3.1). They also provide a great deal of information useful in the diagnosis and management of patients with hyperlipidaemia.

For plasma cholesterol, the 75th and 90th percentiles for the US white population are given in Tables 3.1 and 3.2. These percentiles are quoted because the National Institutes of Health (NIH) Consensus Conference chose to define moderate risk as above the 75th percentile and high risk as exceeding the 90th

**Table 3.1  Plasma cholesterol concentration in 24 425 white males in the USA (After Rifkind and Segal[7])**

| Age (yr) | Plasma cholesterol (mg/dl; mmol/l) | | |
|---|---|---|---|
|  | Mean | 75th percentile | 90th percentile |
| 0–19 | 155 (4.0) | 170 (4.4) | 185 (4.7) |
| 20–24 | 165 (4.2) | 185 (4.7) | 205 (5.3) |
| 25–29 | 180 (4.6) | 200 (5.1) | 225 (5.8) |
| 30–34 | 190 (4.9) | 215 (5.5) | 240 (6.2) |
| 35 39 | 200 (5.1) | 225 (5.8) | 250 (6.4) |
| 40–44 | 205 (5.3) | 230 (5.9) | 250 (6.4) |
| 45–69 | 215 (5.5) | 235 (6.0) | 260 (6.7) |
| 70+ | 205 (5.3) | 230 (5.9) | 250 (6.4) |

**Table 3.2  Plasma cholesterol concentration in 24 057 white females in the USA (After Rifkind and Segal[7])**

| Age (yr) | Plasma cholesterol (mg/dl; mmol/l) | | |
|---|---|---|---|
|  | Mean | 75th percentile | 90th percentile |
| 0–19 | 160 (4.1) | 175 (4.5) | 190 (4.9) |
| 20–24 | 170 (4.4) | 190 (4.9) | 215 (5.5) |
| 25–34 | 175 (4.5) | 195 (5.0) | 220 (5.6) |
| 35–39 | 185 (4.7) | 205 (5.3) | 230 (5.9) |
| 40–44 | 195 (5.0) | 215 (5.5) | 235 (6.0) |
| 45–49 | 205 (5.3) | 225 (5.8) | 250 (6.4) |
| 50 54 | 220 (5.6) | 240 (6.2) | 265 (6.8) |
| 55+ | 230 (5.9) | 250 (6.4) | 275 (7.1) |

**Table 3.3 Plasma low density lipoprotein cholesterol concentration in 3524 white males in the USA (After Rifkind and Segal[7])**

| Age (yr) | Plasma LDL cholesterol (mg/dl; mmol/l) | | |
|---|---|---|---|
| | Mean | 75th percentile | 90th percentile |
| 5–19 | 95 (2.4) | 105 (2.7) | 120 (3.1) |
| 20–24 | 105 (2.7) | 120 (3.1) | 140 (3.6) |
| 25–29 | 115 (2.9) | 140 (3.6) | 155 (4.0) |
| 30–34 | 125 (3.2) | 145 (3.7) | 165 (4.2) |
| 35–39 | 135 (3.5) | 155 (4.0) | 175 (4.5) |
| 40–44 | 135 (3.5) | 155 (4.0) | 175 (4.5) |
| 45–69 | 145 (3.7) | 165 (4.2) | 190 (4.9) |
| 70+ | 145 (3.7) | 165 (4.2) | 180 (4.6) |

**Table 3.4 Plasma low density lipoprotein cholesterol concentration in 3364 white females in the USA (After Rifkind and Segal[7])**

| Age (yr) | Plasma LDL cholesterol (mg/dl; mmol/l) | | |
|---|---|---|---|
| | Mean | 75th percentile | 90th percentile |
| 5–19 | 100 (2.6) | 110 (2.8) | 125 (3.2) |
| 20–24 | 105 (2.7) | 120 (3.1) | 140 (3.6) |
| 25–34 | 110 (2.8) | 125 (4.2) | 145 (3.7) |
| 35–39 | 120 (3.1) | 140 (3.6) | 160 (4.1) |
| 40–44 | 125 (3.2) | 145 (3.7) | 165 (4.2) |
| 45–49 | 130 (3.3) | 150 (3.8) | 175 (4.5) |
| 50–54 | 140 (3.6) | 160 (4.1) | 185 (4.7) |
| 55+ | 150 (3.8) | 170 (4.4) | 195 (5.0) |

percentile. Corresponding values for plasma LDL cholesterol are given in Tables 3.3 and 3.4.

The LRC Program Prevalence Study provides considerable information about the influence of age on plasma lipids and lipoproteins. In childhood there is a tendency for plasma cholesterol to be marginally higher in girls (Figure 3.2). In both boys and girls there is an increase from birth until late childhood which is followed by a decline during early adolescence before it begins its major rise from the mid-teens onwards. Men overtake women in terms of their plasma cholesterol during their early twenties. However, there is a fairly abrupt increase in women from their late forties (presumably at the menopause) and by their early fifties it is they who on average have the higher plasma cholesterol, and that obtains thereafter. A parallel increase in plasma LDL cholesterol occurs in women following the menopause (Figure 3.3). However, in general, that increase is only sufficient to give levels marginally greater than men of corresponding age. Part of the reason for the higher levels of total plasma cholesterol in post-menopausal women must also be the tendency for VLDL cholesterol to continue to rise with age in women, whereas in men it declines from middle age onwards [3,4].

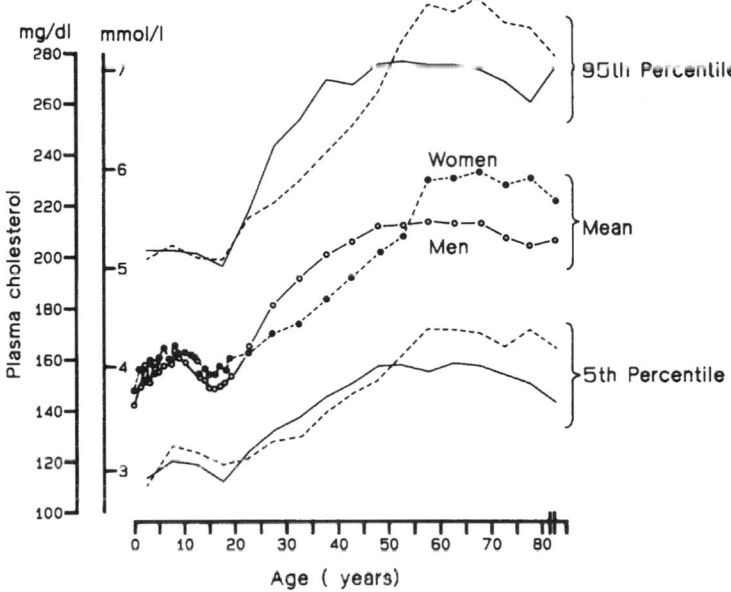

**Figure 3.2**  Plasma cholesterol concentration as a function of age in men and women living in the USA (Lipid Research Clinics Prevalence Program  see text for references)

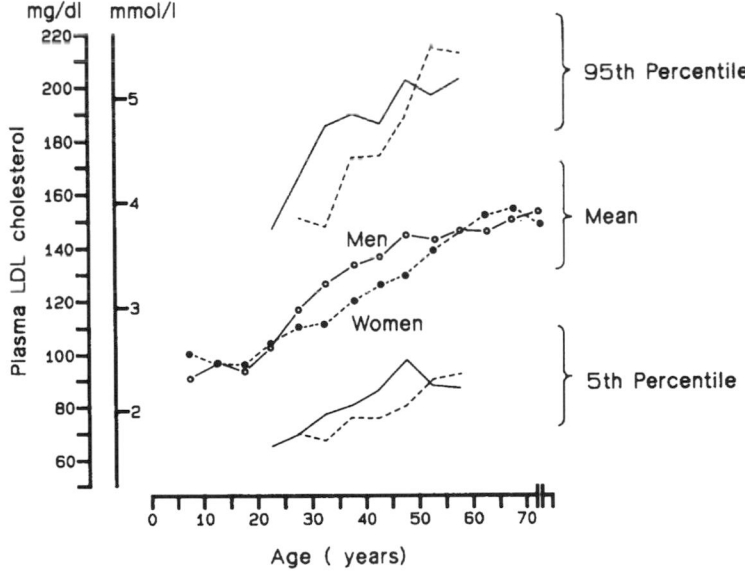

**Figure 3.3**  Plasma low density lipoprotein (LDL) cholesterol concentration in men and women in the USA at various ages (Lipid Research Clinics Prevalence Program – see text for references)

**Table 3.5 Serum cholesterol concentration in 157 men and women aged 30–39 years in Uppsala, 276 aged 20–69 in London, 314 aged 20–69 in Geneva and 238 aged 20–59 in Naples (After Lewis *et al.*[11])**

| | *Mean serum cholesterol* (mg/dl; mmol/l) | | | |
| --- | --- | --- | --- | --- |
| | *Uppsala* | *London* | *Geneva* | *Naples* |
| Men | 254 (6.50) | 234 (5.99) | 228 (5.85) | 193 (4.95) |
| Women | 238 (6.11) | 225 (5.78) | 202 (5.18) | 191 (4.90) |

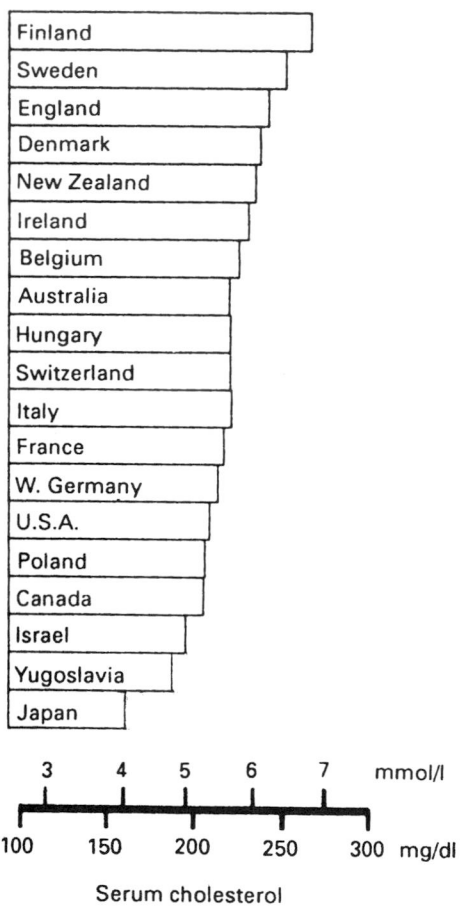

**Figure 3.4**   Average serum cholesterol concentration of men living in different countries, showing great variation

The importance or otherwise of considering age in the definition of normal serum lipids is considered on pages 85–87 of this chapter.

That the average concentration of serum cholesterol varies enormously between different racial groups and different nations dependent largely upon diet has been known since de Langen first compared the serum cholesterol of Japanese stewards on Dutch ships with that of Japanese living at home[10]. Ancel Keys's Seven Countries study[10] clearly demonstrated major differences between men in nations such as Finland, the USA and the Netherlands, more than 30% of whom had serum cholesterol levels exceeding 250 mg/dl (6.4 mmol/l) and those in Japan, Greece, Italy and Yugoslavia, where fewer than 15% did. More recently the difference between Northern and Southern Europe was confirmed in a study[11] which compared Londoners with citizens of Uppsala, Geneva and Naples (Table 3.5).

Comparison of cholesterol values from large population studies in individual nations has also repeatedly pointed to the same conclusion (Figure 3.4). Thus the high cholesterol nations tend to be those whose population and traditions derive largely from Northern Europe, and nations with lower serum cholesterol are those of Southern Europe, rural Africa and the Orient.

In comparing cholesterol levels in different reports, differences in laboratory methods and whether serum or plasma was used must be taken into account. However, the differences between many populations are substantially greater than can be explained by such factors.

The mean serum cholesterol of middle-aged men throughout Britain is between 234 and 257 mg/dl (6.0 and 6.6 mmol/l) with an average of 246 mg/dl (6.3 mmol/l) [12–17]. The results of these studies are summarized in Tables 3.6 and 3.7. Serum cholesterol in Britain thus appears to be higher in Britain than in the USA (see Figure 3.1). However, it is likely that part of this difference is due to different standardization of the cholesterol assays used in British and US studies, the British standard being higher. Thus, as recently as 1993 a positive bias of around 4% at the clinically important level of 7.8 mmol/l (300 mg/dl) was revealed when results from laboratories in Scotland in the British quality control scheme were compared

**Table 3.6 Serum cholesterol concentration in men in London and other parts of Britain***

| Age (yr) | Serum cholesterol (mg/dl; mmol/l) | | |
|---|---|---|---|
| | Mean | 75th percentile | 90th percentile |
| 18–29[a] | 192 (4.9) | 218 (5.6) | 242 (6.2) |
| 25–29[d] | 203 (5.2) | 232 (5.9) | 258 (6.6) |
| 30–34[d] | 215 (5.5) | 243 (6.2) | 269 (6.9) |
| 30–39[a] | 214 (5.5) | 243 (6.2) | 269 (6.9) |
| 20–39[b] | 214 (5.5) | 230 (5.9) | 245 (6.3) |
| 35–39[d] | 226 (5.8) | 258 (6.6) | 286 (7.3) |
| 40–44[d] | 234 (6.0) | 266 (6.8) | 294 (7.5) |
| 40–49[a] | 233 (6.0) | 262 (6.7) | 288 (7.4) |
| 45–49[d] | 238 (6.1) | 269 (6.9) | 300 (7.6) |
| 50–54[d] | 238 (6.1) | 269 (6.9) | 300 (7.6) |
| 50–59[a] | 231 (5.9) | 260 (6.7) | 285 (7.3) |
| 40–59[c] | 246 (6.3) | 279 (7.1) | 308 (7.9) |
| 55–59[d] | 238 (6.1) | 269 (6.9) | 300 (7.6) |
| 60–64[a] | 236 (6.1) | 267 (6.9) | 296 (7.6) |
| 40–69[b] | 234 (6.0) | 256 (6.6) | 276 (7.1) |

* The data in this table are partly recalculated from those in [a] References 12 and [b] 13, which reported on 1027 and 140 men, respectively, in London; [c] Reference 15 in which 7690 men in different British towns were studied; and [d] Reference 17, which screened 5481 men in Oxford, London, Leicester and Glasgow.

**Table 3.7 Serum cholesterol concentration in women in London***

| Age (yr) | Serum cholesterol (mg/dl; mmol/l) | | |
|---|---|---|---|
| | Mean | 75th percentile | 90th percentile |
| 18–29[a] | 185 (4.7) | 204 (5.2) | 222 (5.7) |
| 25–29[c] | 200 (5.1) | 225 (5.8) | 249 (6.4) |
| 30–34[c] | 203 (5.2) | 229 (5.9) | 253 (6.5) |
| 20–39[b] | 211 (5.4) | 230 (5.9) | 248 (6.4) |
| 30–39[a] | 200 (5.1) | 224 (5.7) | 246 (6.3) |
| 35–39[d] | 207 (5.3) | 233 (6.0) | 257 (6.6) |
| 40–44[c] | 218 (5.6) | 247 (6.3) | 273 (7.0) |
| 40–49[a] | 227 (5.8) | 253 (6.5) | 276 (7.1) |
| 45–49[c] | 230 (5.9) | 262 (6.7) | 290 (7.4) |
| 50–54[c] | 250 (6.4) | 279 (7.1) | 305 (7.8) |
| 50–59[c] | 261 (6.7) | 293 (7.5) | 321 (8.2) |
| 50–59[a] | 247 (6.3) | 277 (7.1) | 303 (7.8) |
| 40–69[b] | 245 (6.3) | 269 (6.9) | 291 (7.5) |

* Data partly recalculated from those in [a] References 12 and [b] 13, which reported on 577 and 136 women, respectively, living in the London area, and [c] Reference 17, which screened 6251 women in Oxford, London, Leicester and Glasgow.

with results using the standard from the Centre for Disease Control, Atlanta based on the Abell-Kendell method [18]. This bias would mean that instead of 10% of the UK having serum cholesterol levels exceeding 7.8 mmol/l perhaps as few as 5–6% do. The percentage may be even smaller, because there is some reason to believe that the positive bias in British cholesterol assays was even higher when the surveys were done.

## Serum triglycerides

Serum triglyceride concentrations behave similarly to those of cholesterol during childhood, but the adolescent rise in men overtakes that of women earlier, around the mid-teens (Figure 3.5). Serum triglyceride levels are then persistently higher in men until old age. In men, serum triglyceride concentrations peak in middle age, whereas in women they continue to rise until the age of about 70 years.

Serum triglycerides have not generally been found to correlate with the risk of ischaemic heart disease as closely as serum cholesterol. The NIH Consensus Conference therefore chose the 95th percentile to define hypertriglyceridaemia [19]. The mean and 95th percentile for the US white population from the LRC Program Prevalence Study are shown in Tables 3.8 and 3.9.

There have been few studies of triglycerides in other nations, and such large-scale studies as there have been have sometimes measured serum triglycerides in the non-fasting state [15].

Both in the fasting and non-fasting state the frequency distribution of the serum triglyceride concentration is positively skewed (Figure 3.6). It may be converted to a near Gaussian distribution by logarithmic transformation. Perhaps a better reflection of the typical levels for a population would, therefore, be represented by the geometric mean (the antilog of the mean of logarithmically transformed data), rather than the arithmetic mean which is often quoted. When comparing

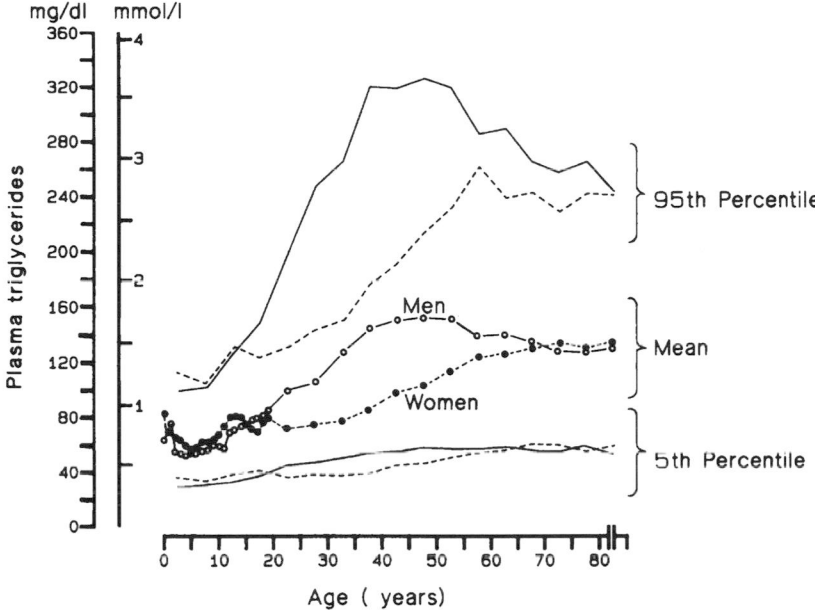

**Figure 3.5**  Fasting plasma triglyceride concentrations as a function of age in men and women in the USA (Lipid Research Clinics Prevalence Program – see text for references)

different populations, serum triglyceride values must be logarithmically transformed unless non-parametric statistical tests are employed.

Some data for the UK populations comparable with the US were, however, obtained by Slack and co-workers[12] in the London area (Table 3.10). These suggest that the UK population is fairly similar to the US population with regard to serum triglycerides. This view is also supported by a study of 81 healthy men aged 40–60 years in Manchester whose geometric mean serum triglyceride concentration was 116 mg/dl (1.30 mmol/l), the 95th percentile being 270 mg/dl (3.0

**Table 3.8 Fasting plasma triglyceride concentration of 24 425 white males in the USA (After Rifkind and Segal[7])**

| Age (yr) | Plasma triglycerides (mg/dl; mmol/l) | |
| --- | --- | --- |
| | Mean | 95th percentile |
| 0–9 | 55 (0.6) | 100 (1.1) |
| 10–14 | 65 (0.7) | 125 (1.4) |
| 15–19 | 80 (0.9) | 150 (1.7) |
| 20–24 | 100 (1.1) | 200 (2.2) |
| 25–29 | 115 (1.3) | 250 (2.8) |
| 30–34 | 130 (1.5) | 265 (3.0) |
| 35–39 | 145 (1.6) | 320 (3.6) |
| 40–54 | 150 (1.7) | 320 (3.6) |
| 55–64 | 140 (1.6) | 290 (3.3) |
| 65+ | 135 (1.5) | 260 (2.9) |

**Table 3.9 Fasting plasma triglyceride concentration of 24 057 white females in the USA (After Rifkind and Segal[7])**

| Age (yr) | Plasma triglycerides (mg/dl; mmol/l) | |
| --- | --- | --- |
| | Mean | 95th percentile |
| 0–9 | 60 (0.7) | 110 (1.2) |
| 10–19 | 75 (0.8) | 130 (1.5) |
| 20–34 | 90 (1.0) | 170 (1.9) |
| 35–39 | 95 (1.1) | 195 (2.2) |
| 40–44 | 105 (1.2) | 210 (2.4) |
| 45–49 | 110 (1.2) | 230 (2.6) |
| 50–54 | 120 (1.3) | 240 (2.7) |
| 55–64 | 125 (1.4) | 250 (2.8) |
| 65+ | 130 (1.5) | 240 (2.7) |

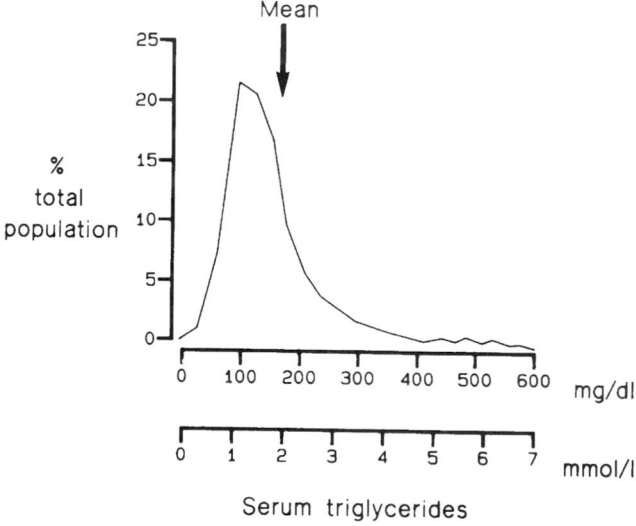

**Figure 3.6**    The frequency distribution curve for fasting serum triglyceride concentrations is typically positively skewed, as in this example from the USA (From Castelli et al.[1])

mmol/l)[16]. The published results of a study in Oxford, London, Leicester and Glasgow of approximately 10 000 patients aged 25–59 years were unfortunately reported as arithmetic mean and standard deviation [17]. However, the 95th percentile for men was 340 mg/dl (3.8 mmol/l) and for women 230 mg/dl (2.6 mmol/l) (A. F. Winder, personal communication), which is again similar to US white women.

It is frequently suggested that the different communities tend to vary in their average serum triglyceride concentrations in a rather similar way to cholesterol. There is remarkably little solid evidence for such a contention. For example, in the Cooperative Lipoprotein Phenotyping Study[1], men in Albany and Framingham

**Table 3.10 Serum triglyceride concentration in white males in London***

| Age (yr) | Serum triglycerides (mg/dl; mmol/l) | |
| --- | --- | --- |
| | Mean | 95th percentile |
| 20 | 85 (1.0) | 190 (2.1) |
| 30 | 110 (1.2) | 240 (2.7) |
| 40 | 125 (1.4) | 285 (3.2) |
| 50 | 130 (1.5) | 300 (3.4) |
| 60 | 125 (1.4) | 285 (3.2) |

* Based on data presented in Reference 12 from a study of 1027 men.

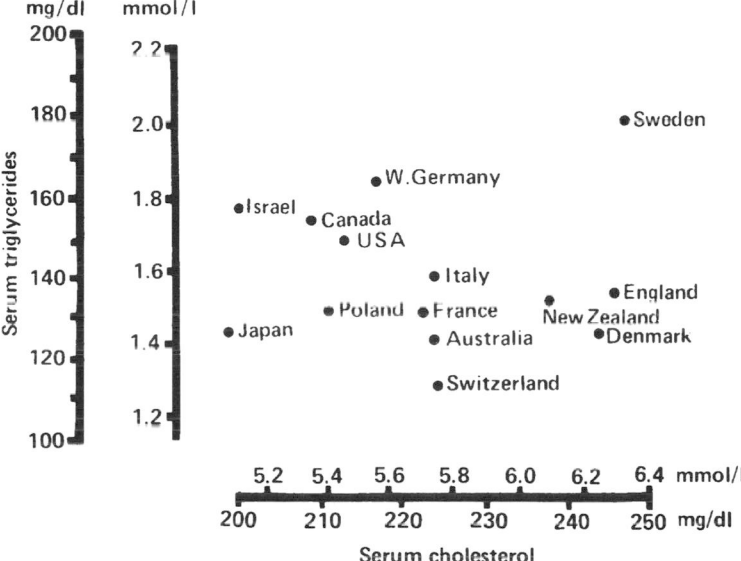

**Figure 3.7**   There is commonly held misconception that nations with high serum cholesterol levels also have high triglyceride values. The mean serum cholesterol concentration as shown in this example of middle-aged men are, in fact, unrelated to their triglycerides (From Simons[20])

had on average serum cholesterol levels about 30 mg/dl (0.8 mmol/l) higher than Puerto Rican men, but their serum triglyceride concentrations were virtually identical. The average concentrations of serum cholesterol and triglycerides in men aged 40–64 years from 14 different nations collected by Simons[20] showed no correlation (Figure 3.7). Much of the interpopulation variation in serum cholesterol is due to differences in fat intake, particularly in saturated fat (Chapter 9). Whereas diets low in saturated fat would also be expected to lower serum triglycerides, it is generally the case that populations whose fat intake is low have a substantially greater carbohydrate intake. Since serum triglycerides tend to show a stronger increase with dietary carbohydrate than does cholesterol, the triglyceride-lowering effect of the low saturated fat intake of nations with low serum cholesterol levels may be counteracted by their high carbohydrate intake (see Chapter 9).

## High density lipoprotein cholesterol

Plasma HDL cholesterol levels are similar in boys and girls before puberty (Figure 3.8). In boys, however, there is a marked decrease following puberty, whereas no change is apparent in girls during adolescence. From the age of about 25 there is a progressive rise in plasma HDL cholesterol in women; whereas in men the level stays constant until between 50 and 65 years of age, when it increases steeply but its average concentration never achieves that of women. It is more than likely that the changes in plasma HDL and LDL cholesterol concentrations (Figures 3.3 and 3.8) occurring at around puberty and the climacteric are due to endocrine changes (Chapter 11). Because premature mortality is associated with low plasma HDL and high LDL cholesterol levels, there must be some tendency for HDL to rise and LDL to decrease with age in the surviving population. However, only a small proportion of the population perish before the age of 60, so that this effect is probably small until old age. Cohort studies indicate that individuals retain levels of lipids and lipoproteins in the same part of the frequency distribution as they get older [21].

The frequency distribution of plasma serum HDL cholesterol is essentially Gaussian. The most extensive data available for plasma HDL are those from the LRC Program Prevalence Study[3 ,4]; the median values in both men and women at all ages were never more than 2 mg/dl (0.05 mmol/l) less than the mean values.

The concentration of plasma HDL cholesterol is inversely related to the risk of developing ischaemic heart disease[4,22,23]. In clinical practice the 10th percentiles for the plasma or serum HDL cholesterol might therefore be considered important,

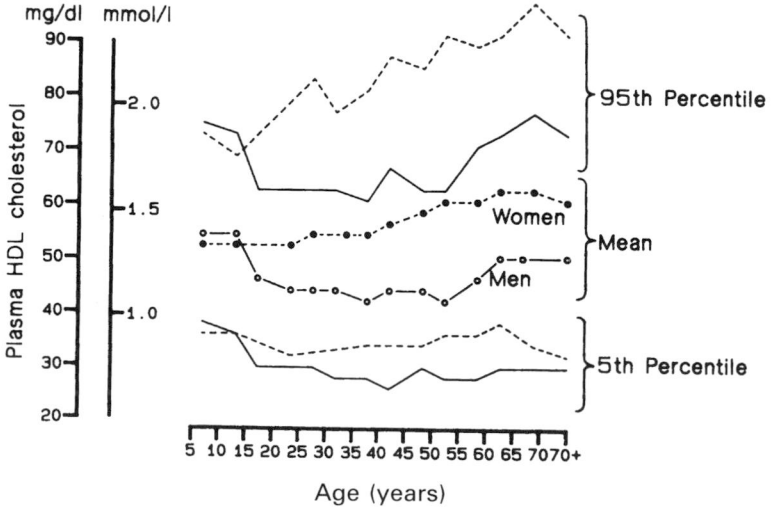

**Figure 3.8** Plasma high density lipoprotein (HDL) concentrations in US men and women at various ages (Lipid Research Clinics Prevalence Program – see text for references)

**Table 3.11 Plasma high density lipoprotein cholesterol concentrations in 3546 white males in the USA (After Rifkind and Segal[7])**

| Age (yr) | Plasma HDL cholesterol (mg/dl; mmol/l) | |
| --- | --- | --- |
| | Mean | 10th percentile |
| 5–14 | 55 (1.4) | 40 (1.0) |
| 15–19 | 45 (1.2) | 35 (0.9) |
| 20–44 | 45 (1.2) | 30 (0.8) |
| 45–69 | 50 (1.3) | 30 (0.8) |
| 70+ | 50 (1.3) | 35 (0.9) |

**Table 3.12 Plasma high density lipoprotein cholesterol concentrations in 3382 white females in the USA (After Rifkind and Segal[7])**

| Age (yr) | Plasma HDL cholesterol (mg/dl; mmol/l) | |
| --- | --- | --- |
| | Mean | 10th percentile |
| 5–19 | 55 (1.4) | 40 (1.0) |
| 20–24 | 55 (1.4) | 35 (0.9) |
| 25–44 | 55 (1.4) | 40 (1.0) |
| 45–54 | 60 (1.5) | 40 (1.0) |
| 55+ | 60 (1.5) | 40 (1.0) |

and these are shown in Tables 3.11 and 3.12 for the US population. In Britain there has been only one substantial survey of serum HDL cholesterol employing adequate laboratory control[15]. The mean serum HDL cholesterol concentration of 7735 men aged 40–59 years in 24 towns throughout England and Wales was 45 mg/dl (1.15 mmol/l). From the results of that report, the 10th percentile can be estimated to be around 32 mg/dl (0.82 mmol/l). The phosphotungstate/magnesium method was used to isolate HDL, which tends to give lower results than the heparin/manganese method employed in the LRC Program Prevalence Study. Nevertheless, British men would seem to have levels of serum HDL cholesterol similar to their US counterparts. There are no British data to allow a similar comparison of women.

Serum HDL cholesterol concentrations do show quite marked variation between certain communities. However, the inverse relationship with ischaemic heart disease, which is evident within virtually all populations studied, is less evident when different populations are compared[20]. Certain populations with a low incidence of ischaemic heart disease have on average lower HDL cholesterol levels than populations with a high rate of ischaemic heart disease. In general such populations, despite their low HDL cholesterol levels, also have low total serum cholesterol or LDL cholesterol levels, presumably explaining their low ischaemic heart disease risk. Perhaps the most striking example of this is the Mexican Tarahumara Indians[24]. This observation gives rise to the thought that the most appropriate definition of a normal HDL cholesterol value would depend on the prevailing concentration of serum total or LDL cholesterol. Thus the use of a ratio between total serum cholesterol and HDL cholesterol has been advocated. This ratio is more closely related to ischaemic heart disease rates in different nations than HDL cholesterol or even total cholesterol alone[20]. It should be emphasized that neither this nor other evidence for the superiority of the ratio as a predictor of risk when compared with total cholesterol or HDL cholesterol alone can be interpreted as showing that HDL is an independent predictor of risk. The reason is that even supposing HDL were irrelevant, such a ratio would be expected to be more closely related to risk than total serum cholesterol because it is a measure of non-HDL cholesterol[25].

## Factors important in the interpretation of normal serum lipid levels

It is important to recognize all the sources of variation in plasma lipids in defining normal levels, in planning cut-off points for screening programmes and in assessing therapeutic responses.

### Fasting versus non-fasting serum lipid levels

Fasting has little effect on serum cholesterol levels in normal healthy individuals[26] (Table 3.13). For population screening, where triglyceride determination is considered unnecessary, at least in the initial examination, non-fasting specimens are probably adequate. In practical terms, the removal of the restraint of fasting is a considerable advantage.

Unlike serum cholesterol, the concentration of serum triglycerides is affected by meals. This is because the total serum triglyceride concentration represents triglycerides secreted into the serum both by the gut, principally in the form of chylomicrons, and by the liver as VLDL (Chapter 2). The contribution from the gut to total serum triglycerides is dependent on the interval since the last meal, on the fat content of the meal and on various other factors, such as the rate of intestinal absorption and the efficiency of the catabolism of the chylomicrons entering the plasma compartment. In most healthy subjects, fasting for 6 hours is usually sufficient to produce a steady triglyceride level. Usually, however, fasting from 2200 hours the night before, with the blood sample being taken the next morning, is the practice in clinics and research protocols.

**Table 3.13 Serum lipids and apolipoprotein B in 11 normal subjects in the fasting and non-fasting states (From Durrington et al.[26])**

| | Fasting (mg/dl; mmol/l) | 3 hours after breakfast (mg/dl; mmol/l) | 3 hours after lunch (mg/dl; mmol/l) |
|---|---|---|---|
| Serum cholesterol | 211 ± 12 (5.4 ± 0.3) | 207 ± 12 (5.3 ± 0.3) | 207 ± 12 (5.3 ± 0.3) |
| Serum triglycerides | 100 ± 10 (1.12 ± 0.11) | 131 ± 13 (1.47 ± 0.15) | 149 ± 13 (1.67 ± 0.15) |
| Serum apolipoprotein B | 110 ± 8 | 110 ± 8 | 112 ± 8 |

Conventionally, serum triglycerides are determined in the fasting state, because this produces a more reproducible level. It is sometimes suggested that this is an essentially unphysiological approach and does not reflect the average level during the day[27]. It has been proposed, too, that gut lipoproteins, or at least their remnants, are atherogenic. In that case there would be some purpose in estimating their levels. Presumably this would require multiple sampling throughout the day or at some defined interval following a standard meal. However, at the present time, the fact remains that such data as there are relating serum triglyceride concentrations to disease are based on fasting levels and fasting levels are what we must measure in current clinical practice. The situation is not unlike that with blood pressure, where we choose to base clinical decisions on a resting level rather than on the casual level or on the level during exercise. Meals have very little effect on HDL cholesterol. The cholesterol secreted by the gut is largely esterified and any increased flux of free cholesterol through HDL is probably matched by an increase in LCAT and cholesteryl ester transfer protein activity[28], so that the overall HDL cholesterol level fluctuates little, although some small change in the relative cholesterol content of its subfractions may be evident [29].

## Drugs

Concurrent administration of drugs frequently affects the concentration of serum lipids and lipoproteins. This is considered more fully in Chapter 11.

## Age (see also pages 74–76)

Low concentrations of cholesterol are present in the serum of cord blood, usually 50–95 mg/dl (1.3–2.4 mmol/l)[30]. During infancy there is a rise in serum cholesterol, rapidly until 6 years and thereafter more gradually[6,31] (Figure 3.2). It falls during adolescence, but then in Northern Europe and the Northern European based cultures of North America, Australia and South Africa, there is a clear tendency for the serum cholesterol concentration to increase during adult life, with women overtaking men in their late forties or early fifties. In rural black South African men and Bushmen consuming their traditional low fat, high carbohydrate diet, no increase in serum cholesterol occurs during adult life, whereas those living in urban areas, probably due to their adoption of a more European diet, show the familiar rise in serum cholesterol with age[32]. This has given rise to speculation that it is unphysiological for serum cholesterol to rise with age. This may indeed be correct: it is quite plausible that diets rich in saturated fat and cholesterol lead to increased hepatic cholesterol secretion which is better tolerated by the growing, more energetic young, who are less frequently obese and who catabolize cholesterol-rich lipoproteins more rapidly[33].

It has further been argued that the increase in serum cholesterol with age should, therefore, be regarded not as a normal effect of ageing, but rather as a progressive increase in the frequency of hypercholesterolaemia with age. As such, it is suggested that normal ranges for serum cholesterol should not be age-related. Although it is accepted here that this is probably true; it is certainly not true to conclude further that age is not of considerable importance in deciding how to treat the patient suspected of having a raised serum cholesterol. Although it may be unphysiological for serum cholesterol to rise with age, it is nevertheless the case that its importance as a risk factor which distinguishes individuals at risk of

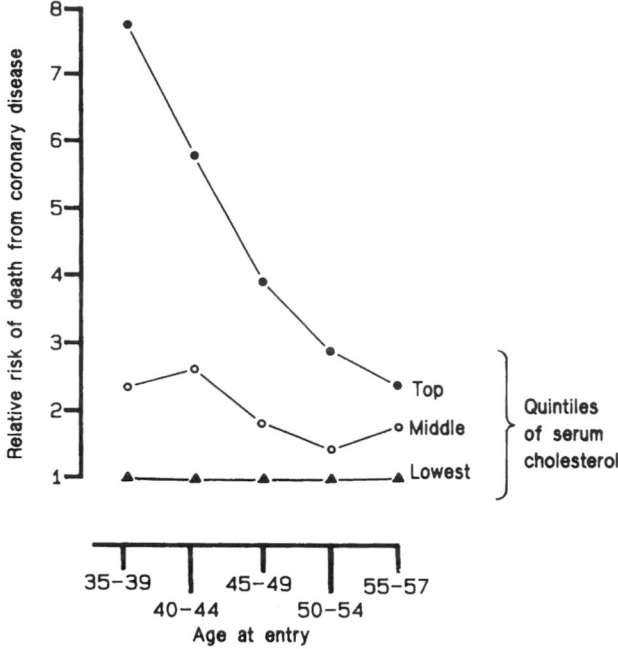

**Figure 3.9**    Risk of men in the upper fifth of the population for plasma cholesterol relative to that of the middle and lowest fifths at different ages (From Stamler *et al.*[9])

ischaemic heart disease declines with age. Thus in the town of Framingham a serum cholesterol of 310 mg/dl (7.9 mmol/l) in a 35-year-old man increased his risk of having a myocardial infarction by 5.5 times over a similar man whose serum cholesterol was 185 mg/dl (4.7 mmol/l). Two 60-year-olds, however, with those serum cholesterol levels, differed only 1.5 times in risk[34]. Similar conclusions regarding diminishing relative risk from serum cholesterol with age may be drawn from the more recent MRFIT study[9]. The relevant findings are illustrated in Figure 3.9.

Interestingly the explanation for the diminution in the slope of the curve relating IHD to cholesterol with advancing age is that a greater decrease in relative risk from cholesterol with age occurs in the section of the population with the highest serum cholesterol, whereas in those whose serum cholesterol is in the middle range the relative risk due to cholesterol is reasonably constant with increasing age. This effect is also observed in people with familial hypercholesterolaemia who are from the very top part of the serum cholesterol concentration distribution. There are astronomic increases in their relative risk of IHD whilst they are young and middle-aged but the more elderly patients have a similar rate of IHD to that of the general populations[35].

All this is true of relative risk, but in clinical practice it is the absolute risk which must most often be considered. Consideration of absolute risk in the elderly leads to a different conclusion from that of relative risk. In an elderly person whose annual IHD risk might, for example, be 40/1000 an increase in relative risk of only 1.5 times would increase the number of people suffering an IHD event each year from 40/1000 to 60/1000, an increment of 20, whereas in a younger age group with an annual IHD risk of 1/1000 an increase in relative risk of 6 times would only increase the number of preventable deaths by 5/1000.

## Illness, surgery and trauma

Illness, surgical operations and trauma have the effect of reducing serum cholesterol concentrations and elevating serum triglycerides. The effect on serum cholesterol can be profound, the level in patients with familial hypercholesterolaemia decreasing from 400 mg/dl (10–11 mmol/l) to perhaps 225 mg/dl (5–6 mmol/l). Serum cholesterol decreases[36,37] following myocardial infarction or surgical procedures such as coronary artery bypass surgery[38] or abdominal operations. This effect may be quite rapid; certainly within 48 h of the onset of the illness or operation. After acute myocardial infarction the decrease in serum cholesterol is due to a decrease in both LDL and HDL cholesterol. Serum apolipoprotein B and AI also decline. Recovery takes place over 4–6 weeks or longer if illness persists. The slowest recovery is in apolipoprotein AI. There is more variable rise in serum triglyceride concentration.

Other major illnesses such as cancer are also believed to result in decreases in serum cholesterol[39,40]. It is difficult to be as certain about the effects of more minor illness on serum cholesterol, but the author has on several occasions suspected that intercurrent infections such as gastroenteritis and influenzal-type illnesses can have a marked effect on serum cholesterol. One recalls seeing patients with definite tendon xanthomata, who were reported to have relatively normal serum cholesterol levels on their biochemistry profile during what was presumably an acute viral illness, but who a few weeks later are shown to be grossly hypercholesterolaemic. This is one reason why the suggestion that general practitioners can screen for hypercholesterolaemia by determining the serum cholesterol in patients attending their surgery for some other purpose may not be a good one, unless account is taken of why the patient is attending.

The reason for the decrease in serum cholesterol during physical stress is unknown, but is probably the result of decreased synthesis and intake. In the case of low cholesterol associated with tumours the elaboration of humoral substances accelerating LDL catabolism may also be important. Whether serum cholesterol increases or decreases with mental stress is uncertain. In the case of serum triglycerides, an increase certainly occurs with physical stress concurrently with the decline in serum cholesterol. An increase in hepatic triglyceride synthesis due to a catecholamine-induced increase in the release of non-esterified fatty acids from adipose tissue is a possible mechanism. However, the reason for the persistence of the elevation of the serum triglycerides for several weeks when the patients have apparently regained their health is difficult to explain.

The most important practical lesson is that serum lipids should not be determined within 6 weeks of a surgical operation, myocardial infarction or major illness. Also, when hypercholesterolaemia is suspected and the serum cholesterol is unexpectedly low, enquiry should be made regarding recent illness. In the case of patients presenting with myocardial infarction, it has been suggested that the serum cholesterol value will truly represent the pre-infarction level if blood is taken within 24 h of the onset of symptoms[41]. The evidence for this is that the cholesterol level at this stage is similar to that 3 months later (when it has presumably risen to approach earlier levels unless a diet has been introduced). However, most of the patients in studies of this type had normal serum cholesterol levels and the rapidity and magnitude of the change in patients with preceding hypercholesterolaemia remains unclear. Secondly, it is extremely difficult to time the onset of myocardial infarction and in any event the cholesterol may start to fall before this when there is a pre-infarction syndrome. Thirdly, even when serum cholesterol is requested by the clinician the practicalities of hospital practice are such that it is seldom possible to know whether the sample was taken at the correct time. By waiting until 6 weeks after a heart attack, it is true that the diagnosis of hypercholesterolaemia will be missed in patients who die in the meantime and that the opportunity to screen their relatives may thus be missed. However, this need not be of great practical significance, since the relatives of any young patient dying of a myocardial infarction should in any well-regulated medical practice have their serum lipids checked.

## Biological variation in serum lipids in individuals

In a study of eight men and six women on six occasions over 10 days, the coefficient of variation for fasting serum cholesterol within individuals after allowing for variation due to laboratory error was 4.8% and for fasting serum triglycerides was 25%[42]. The variation in triglyceride concentration appeared to be more marked when the levels were high.

## Variation in serum lipids during the menstrual cycle

Serum lipid concentrations vary during the phases of the menstrual cycle. Both cholesterol and triglycerides tend to build up to a peak around mid-cycle at the time of ovulation and to fall away during the subsequent progestogenic phase, probably until about the time of the menses[43]. The rise in serum cholesterol is predominantly due to an increase in HDL cholesterol[44].

## Female menopause and male climacteric

The LRC Prevalence Program showed a fairly abrupt rise in serum cholesterol concentration in women in their late forties and early fifties (Figure 3.2). It is difficult in that study to be certain which of the lipoproteins is responsible for the rise, because there was a more gradual increase in VLDL, LDL and HDL during the same ages. Other studies have, however, attributed the rise largely to an increase in LDL cholesterol[45,46]. Some studies have reported small increases in HDL following the menopause[45] and others decreases[46]. It is important for the clinician to be aware that many women maintain a high serum HDL cholesterol after the menopause (Figure 3.8) and that despite an apparently high total serum cholesterol their serum cholesterol to HDL cholesterol ratio reveals them not to be at any substantially increased risk of myocardial infarction. This was demonstrated in a population survey in the Oxford region of England[47].

In the case of men the climacteric is less consistent in its timing and its effects can only be inferred. Certainly, however, the LRC Prevalence Program results would tend to suggest that the male increase in cholesterol with age reaches a plateau in the late forties and may drift downwards from around 60 years of age (Figure 3.2). Serum triglyceride levels probably behave similarly but there is an earlier tendency for them to decline (Figure 3.5). The HDL cholesterol on the other hand, which decreases abruptly in male adolescence, climbs from the mid-fifties to the mid-sixties (Figure 3.8).

## Pregnancy

There is a progressive rise in both serum cholesterol and triglyceride concentrations during pregnancy. The increment in serum cholesterol probably averages 30–40 mg/dl (1 mmol/l), but even greater increases in serum triglycerides of around 150 mg/dl (1.7 mmol/l) occur[48–54]. The maximum concentration of both lipids is usually reached by the 36th–39th week. There is an increase in the lipid concentration in all three major lipoproteins (VLDL, LDL and HDL).

## Seasonal variation in serum lipids

It is generally agreed that serum cholesterol concentrations are highest in the winter and lowest in the summer[55]. The magnitude of individual fluctuations has been variously reported between 0 and 100 mg/dl (2.5 mmol/l) and probably averages around 20–30 mg/dl (0.5–0.8 mmol/l). Information is only available for US and European populations, and such variation may reflect seasonal changes in diet and body weight.

## Laboratory methods and sampling conditions

In the diagnosis of indisputable hyperlipidaemia, small inaccuracies in lipid determinations introduced either by virtue of inaccuracies in the laboratory or by the method of venous blood sampling employed by the clinician may be of little consequence. Even so, it behoves the clinician to recognize that such errors occur and to avoid basing major decisions, such as the introduction of drug therapy, on single determinations of serum lipids. Variations in the accuracy of serum lipid determinations are, however, of the greatest significance in the institution of screening programmes for the detection of hyperlipidaemia and are relevant to the definition of normal serum lipids (Chapter 13). With the recent trend to decrease the cut-off points for the detection of hypercholesterolaemia towards the middle range, the number of people whose serum cholesterol falls within 5% on either side becomes enormous. Adequate allowance must be made for this because screening frequently involves only a single cholesterol determination and cholesterol measurements in the same individual may vary by considerably more than ±5%.

Hospital laboratories have generally nowadays adopted automated enzymic methods for the determination of serum cholesterol. Of relevance to the definitions of normal lipid levels, it should be realized that these methods may give higher serum cholesterol levels than the adaptations of the Liebermann–Burchardt and ferric chloride/sulphuric acid methods, which were used in the studies describing the concentration of serum cholesterol in the US population[1,7,8]. In one study, comparing methods in routine use in hospital laboratories with the LRC method, the hospital methods gave results from 20 to 55 mg/dl (0.5 to 1.4 mmol/l) higher at the critical 75th and 90th percentiles advocated as the levels defining moderate and high risk[56]. Also, most hospital laboratories assay lipids in serum. Values for cholesterol in plasma employed, for example, in the LRC Program Prevalence Study[7], are about 3% lower[57].

The concentration of cholesterol in plasma or serum may also vary with body position, with venous stasis (particularly if prolonged) and when red blood cells or their membranes are not properly removed from the sample by centrifugation (there is a considerable quantity of cholesterol in red cell membranes, which is why the term 'blood cholesterol' should be abandoned). Ideally, venous blood should be obtained with the patient lying down, with minimal venous occlusion and without haemolysis[58].

The introduction of rapid methods for cholesterol analysis, particularly those employing capillary blood on dry reagent strips, although offering many potential advantages in community health care, is not likely to improve the accuracy of cholesterol measurements. These methods are mostly intended for screening and, as such, will require the use of lower cut-off limits than conventional laboratory methods, because of their greater error.

Any criticism of the accuracy of cholesterol measurement pales into insignificance beside the variation which is encountered in serum triglyceride determinations. This is probably because serum triglyceride levels are less stable within individuals (page 84). In many hospital laboratories, HDL cholesterol determinations are also likely to be highly variable. This, however, is not because HDL concentrations are inherently variable within the individual, but rather because the methods generally used in hospital laboratories are based on poorly validated commercial kits and idiosyncratic combinations of precipitants and methods for lipid determination. In particular, the phosphotungstate/magnesium method is widely used, whereas the epidemiological investigations, which have defined normal ranges and the value of HDL as a risk factor, have generally employed the heparin/manganese method[3,4]. The phosphotungstate method tends to give lower results, particularly in the upper part of the HDL cholesterol distribution[22,59]. HDL cholesterol levels obtained with it have not been shown to be as closely inversely correlated with coronary disease risk[24]. In other laboratories where the heparin/manganese method is employed, it is often not realized that the manganese interferes with the enzymatic methods for cholesterol determination[22,60]. Also many laboratories issue results for HDL cholesterol in patients whose serum triglyceride concentration is too high to permit complete precipitation of the apolipoprotein B-containing lipoproteins[22,61]. Very often, therefore, little reliance can be attached to HDL cholesterol values reported by routine laboratories or, by the same token, on LDL cholesterol levels when these are obtained, as they generally are, by calculations employing the HDL value[62]. The same, of course, must apply to ratios such as HDL:total cholesterol and HDL:LDL cholesterol.

Patients and their doctors are frequently frustrated and perplexed by what appear to be inexplicable changes in serum lipid levels. This may be the reason for the patient's referral to the lipid clinic. Generally the source of these variations is to be found in the foregoing section.

# Definition of hyperlipidaemia

### Statistical definition of normal serum lipid concentration

The normal range for most variables measured in the clinical chemistry laboratory is based on the assumption that 95% of the population are normal and the range

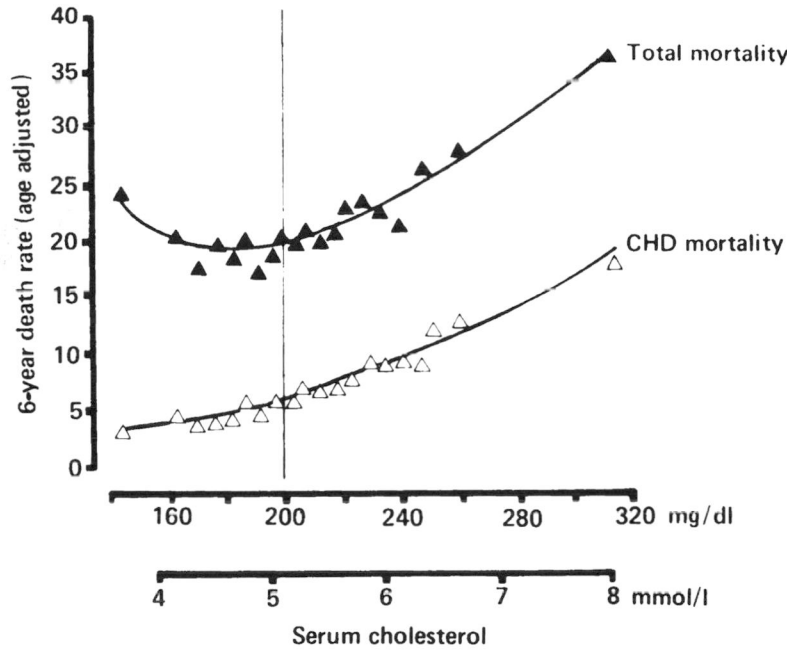

**Figure 3.10**   Total mortality and coronary heart disease (CHD) mortality relative to the initial serum cholesterol concentration in US men (From Martin *et al.*[8])

of normality is from the 2.5 to the 97.5 percentile[63]. The use of the word 'normal', however, also implies a state of health or that a variable within the range described as normal is acceptable in the sense that no action is required. In the case of serum cholesterol and probably also serum triglycerides, lipoproteins and certain apolipoproteins, an upper limit of normality based on the 97.5 percentile cannot, in a society where ischaemic heart disease is prevalent, have any practical value. The usual purpose in measuring a patient's serum cholesterol is to assist in establishing the risk of premature atherosclerosis in that particular individual. It is well established that cholesterol operates as a risk factor not only at levels above its 97.5 percentile, but also at much lower concentrations (Figure 3.10). Such a definition would also lead to the anomaly that what was normal, in for example the UK or USA, would be grossly abnormal in Japan or Southern Europe (Figures 3.1 and 3.4 and Table 3.5).

The definition of normality in the case of serum cholesterol must therefore be linked to some concept of health or of therapeutic benefit.

### Definition of the ideal serum cholesterol concentration

Another approach is to define hypercholesterolaemia as a serum or plasma cholesterol concentration associated with a significantly increased risk of ischaemic heart disease. This has the conspicuous advantage that it relates the cholesterol concentration to clinical risk rather than to its frequency distribution within any particular population. The NIH and European Atherosclerosis Society Consensus Conference both adopted this approach in their original recommendations[19,64]. However, the problem with this definition is that the relationship between serum cholesterol and ischaemic heart disease risk is graded. Indeed, cholesterol continues to be related to IHD risk even in communities with the very lowest IHD rates such as China[65]. There is no threshold for serum cholesterol below which the risk of IHD does not exist. Thus a definition of normality based on IHD risk[8,9] leaves the question of what constitutes a significantly increased risk unanswered.

An alternative way of defining the ideal serum cholesterol concentration would be to base the definition on the cholesterol distribution of a population which has a desirably low incidence of ischaemic heart disease. This still leaves unanswered the question of what constitutes a desirably low risk of ischaemic heart disease and also raises two further important considerations. First, it implies that a universal definition of hypercholesterolaemia is possible. This has been assumed by the European Atherosclerosis Society which has on two occasions attempted to set guidelines for the management of hypercholesterolaemia using common reference levels of cholesterol for nations whose IHD risk varies several fold[64,66]. It is more than possible, however, that different populations may vary in their susceptibility to ischaemic heart disease caused by hypercholesterolaemia, either because of their genetic make-up or because of the prevalence of other risk factors. A statistical overview of the three international studies comparing IHD rates between communities suggests that this may be the case with the IHD rates associated with a particular cholesterol value being higher in cohort studies within communities at high IHD risk than in communities at low IHD risk, particularly at the lower end of the cholesterol concentration distribution[67]. Secondly, and perhaps more importantly, populations with low rates of ischaemic heart disease may be more subject to other diseases. Thus in Japan, for example, cerebral haemorrhage and certain types of cancer may be more common than in North America or Europe. In Africa, those populations with low ischaemic heart disease rates are frequently more prone to infectious diseases, particularly in infancy. It is, of course, perfectly possible to argue that there are other reasons unrelated to the lower serum cholesterol for the increased risk of diseases other than ischaemic heart disease in each of these populations. Nevertheless, if one examines the curve relating serum cholesterol to death from all causes in a single population such as US men (Figure 3.10), it is evident that at serum cholesterol levels below 160 mg/dl (4.0 mmol/l) the likelihood of death from causes other than ischaemic heart disease increases. This has been the subject of much recent debate. Similar findings to those of the MRFIT study, which itself had some 350 000 participants, emerged from a meta-analysis of 18 other smaller prospective cohort studies involving a total of 150 000 men[68]. There was an increasing gradient of risk of IHD death and all cardiovascular deaths with increasing cholesterol. In 11 studies of 120 000 women on the other hand, whilst a similar gradient existed for IHD, cholesterol was unrelated to all causes of cardiovascular disease pooled together. In women as opposed to men IHD constituted only about half the total cardiovascular mortality. It is likely that cholesterol was positively related to non-haemorrhagic stroke, but inversely to haemorrhagic stroke which may have made up a greater proportion of strokes in women, perhaps explaining the overall relatively flat relationship with cardiovascular disease.

## Low serum cholesterol and non-IHD death

In both men and women the relationship between all non-cardiovascular deaths and serum cholesterol showed an upturn in the group with serum cholesterol levels <160 mg/dl (4.0 mmol/l), but did not show an inverse relationship at higher levels. Currently the aim of cholesterol-lowering treatment in clinical practice is not to achieve levels as low as this, so perhaps the argument about whether low cholesterol is a cause of non-cardiovascular disease is irrelevant. The increase in cancer deaths in the cohort studies largely disappears during the early years of the studies. Neoplastic diseases such as carcinoma of colon and prostate and leukaemia are well known to lower cholesterol[40], indeed it may be prognostic. It may be concluded that much of the excess cancer mortality is associated with pre-existent sub-clinical cancer present at the time of entry into the trial. However, for some diseases such as lung cancer, there is a graded inverse relationship with cholesterol across its whole concentration range, which appears to antedate any cholesterol-lowering effect of cancer itself. This may be explained because the antecedent causes of both low cholesterol and cancer or suicide or accident may co-exist well before the development of cancer. Examples would be low body weight due to cigarette-smoking, emphysema, mental illness such as depression, poor nutrition, alcoholism, low socioeconomic status leading to low cholesterol, but each of them related to other causes of increased mortality. This is made likely by four lines of evidence. First there is an important difference between the results from prospective studies in employed populations and those in whole communities[69]. There is no excess mortality from non-IHD causes relative to the rest of the study population associated with low cholesterol in employed people. The implication is that in studies of whole communities those too sick to work already have a tendency to low cholesterol and their non-IHD mortality is high. Secondly, in studies with the largest follow-up the excess mortality associated with low cholesterol eventually disappears entirely[70,71]. If it were causal it should persist, as does the relationship between high cholesterol and IHD incidence. Thirdly, in the genetic condition hypobetalipoproteinaemia in which low LDL cholesterol levels are present throughout life longevity with relative freedom from IHD and not premature death from malignancy or suicide is the rule (Chapter 12)[72]. Finally, in the Whitehall study the effect of taking into account confounding factors associated with increased mortality and low cholesterol was to markedly attenuate or abolish the associations between low cholesterol and non-IHD mortality[73].

## Serum cholesterol and stroke

The overall relationship between serum cholesterol and stroke is a positive one[74]. However, the relationship is not as strong as that between cholesterol and IHD and has often been more U-shaped, particularly in studies of younger age groups and women in whom haemorrhagic stroke may cause a higher proportion of cerebral infarcts. Furthermore, in the two cohort studies in which the distinction between haemorrhagic and thrombotic stroke has been made, both studies showed an excess risk of haemorrhagic stroke in the subgroup with the lowest cholesterol[75,76]. It is important not to get the observation out of proportion. In the MRFIT study, for example, the mortality in the group with the lowest cholesterol concentrations (<160 mg/dl; <4.1 mmol/l) compared to the next lowest group

(160–200 mg/dl; 4.1–5.2 mmol/l) showed that mortality from haemorrhagic stroke was 0.3 per 10 000 man years higher whereas IHD deaths were 3.3 per 10 000 man years lower and deaths from thrombotic stroke were also fewer.

The relationship between low cholesterol and haemorrhagic stroke is sometimes described as causal[69]. One reason for this is that it has been difficult for epidemiologists to uncover confounding factors to explain the association as they have done with other diseases associated with low serum cholesterol. Haemorrhagic stroke is undoubtedly positively related to blood pressure and much more strongly so than to low cholesterol. It is not clear to the author that blood pressure as a confounding factor has been adequately investigated. The same is also true of alcohol[77], which is positively related to stroke risk and could be associated with causes of low cholesterol such as respiratory disease, malnutrition and mental illness. Furthermore, there may be confounding factors which have not been taken into account because they were not measured. Coagulation factors, for example fibrinogen, may well be present at lower concentrations in people with low cholesterol levels and on low fat diets. It is also the case that with the exception of MRFIT the association between low cholesterol and haemorrhagic stroke has been largely confined to studies involving Japanese or at least oriental populations[69]. Again it is unclear whether an ethnic predisposition to haemorrhagic stroke explains some of its association with low cholesterol which is, of course, more commonly encountered in Japan and China. Experimental evidence and further epidemiological investigation is therefore required before causality can be established. In the meantime the balance of benefit from a low cholesterol so much outweighs its potential hazards that this potential hazard of cholesterol reduction is not relevant to the clinician and should also not be a restraint to public health policy to decrease serum cholesterol values in populations in which IHD is a major cause of premature mortality and morbidity. At present therefore there would appear to be little support for the view that low cholesterol levels are causally related to causes of death other than IHD[78,79].

The curve relating total mortality to cholesterol is relatively flat between 180 and 200 mg/dl (4.6 and 5.2 mmol/l). The ideal cholesterol level has generally been considered to lie somewhere within this range. But this was before the major enquiries into the causes of the association between lower cholesterol levels and non-IHD deaths had been completed. Now this could be regarded as somewhat conservative and there is certainly a tendency to push the definition of the ideal cholesterol level downwards, especially in patients who have established IHD due to exposure to higher cholesterol levels earlier in life. It is frequently proposed that a desirable public health objective would be to decrease a nation's serum cholesterol to less than 200 mg/dl (5.2 mmol/l). If, however, this were done – the ideal cholesterol thus becoming the optimal or desirable level for the whole population, for example by alterations of the national diet to such an extent that the great majority of the population had serum cholesterol concentrations of less than 200 mg/dl (5.2 mmol/l) – then the frequency distribution curve for cholesterol would have been shifted so that most of it was below 200 mg/dl (5.2 mmol/l) (Figure 3.11a). This would leave many people with serum cholesterol levels below 180 mg/dl (4.6 mmol/l). Earlier arguments that this might be undesirable are now less easy to sustain[80]. The practicality of achieving a downward shift in the cholesterol distribution was recently addressed in a randomized controlled trial of over 12 000 men and their wives and partners in 26 general practices in 13 towns in Britain[81]. Despite vigorous efforts by the general practice teams, each of

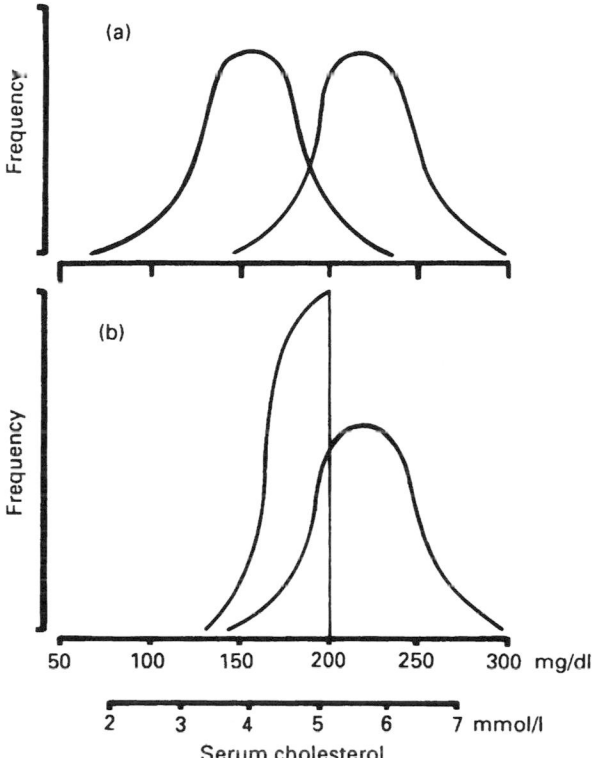

**Figure 3.11**  In both (a) and (b) the same distribution curves for serum cholesterol are shown on the right. They are typical of populations such as those of the USA or the UK. The curve on the left in (a) shows the effect of applying a strategy aimed at reducing serum cholesterol regardless of its starting value, whereas in (b) only those people whose cholesterol exceeds 200 mg/dl (5.2 mmol/l) have been advised to lower it. Policy (a), if it is not to leave large numbers of people with persistent undesirably high levels, must also result in large numbers of people with unnecessarily, and potentially harmful, low levels

which included a nurse whose whole time was devoted to the project, the cholesterol distribution curve shifted downwards only by an average of 0.1 mmol/l at one year. A greater decrease in cholesterol was, however, achieved in people at the higher end of the frequency distribution curve. There seems a case therefore for devoting medical and nursing attention to people with higher cholesterol levels. This, however, will do little to decrease a nation's death rate from IHD because most IHD deaths come from the middle part of the cholesterol distribution which would not shrink from such a high risk intervention programme (Figure 3.11b). It seems that the only means of lowering the levels in this middle range is by an alteration of public policy: a deliberate programme of governmental subsidies and other encouragement aimed at increasing the consumption of healthy foods and disincentive for the production of foods high in saturated fat and excessive energy. This is perhaps not such a radical idea, if it is considered that our present diet is largely the result of government nutritional policies from the past and not as some people believe founded in tradition (Chapter 9).

Clearly there is a case, implicit in the definition of the ideal cholesterol, for a combined public health and clinical approach to hypercholesterolaemia. The clinical approach to hypercholesterolaemia, certainly when it calls for the use of more extreme dietary regimens or lipid-lowering drugs, however, involves a further appraisal of the definition of hypercholesterolaemia. This is because such therapy may have disadvantages in terms of reduced quality of life and, in the case of drugs, perhaps harmful side-effects. The level of serum cholesterol concentration at which the advantages of therapy outweigh the disadvantages is thus critical to the clinician. This therapeutic threshold for serum cholesterol may be very different from the disease threshold discussed in this section in the context of the ideal cholesterol.

## Definition of hypercholesterolaemia based on therapeutic benefit

The curve relating serum cholesterol to ischaemic heart disease risk is not linear: it becomes progressively steeper with increasing cholesterol concentration (Figure 3.10). Thus the greater the serum cholesterol, the greater will be the benefit of treatment over any potential disadvantages. As we have already seen, age is another factor defining the advantages of treatment, since the relative risk of death from ischaemic heart disease from high cholesterol is greater in young adults than in older age groups (Figure 3.9 and page 85). In children, too, this argument may apply, but we are ignorant of the long-term side-effects, certainly of drug therapy, and so we are even less certain than in adults what quantity to weigh against the potential advantages of such treatment. The context in which hypercholesterolaemia occurs is also important in the evaluation of likely benefit from drug therapy. The risk is frequently greater when it results from familial hypercholesterolaemia (Chapter 5), the diagnosis of which almost invariably calls for lipid-lowering drugs in addition to diet. Other features potentially increasing a patient's susceptibility to ischaemic heart disease will also be important in determining the threshold of serum cholesterol at which to introduce drug therapy. A poor family history in a patient may suggest a worse prognosis from a given level of cholesterol, even in the absence of clinical features of familial hypercholesterolaemia, since genetic factors are almost certainly important in determining an individual's resistance to atheroma and to thrombosis[82]. The decision to begin cholesterol-lowering drug treatment will also depend on heightened susceptibility to atheroma due to the presence of other risk factors (Figure 3.12). Thus, whereas some of these factors, such as smoking, are best tackled by cessation, others such as diabetes and hypertension continue to influence risk despite adequate control of glycaemia and blood pressure.

Sex must also be a major consideration in establishing the therapeutic threshold for hypercholesterolaemia. The risk of ischaemic heart disease from serum cholesterol is substantially less in women than men and this continues to apply even after the menopause. It is also important to remember that there are no data for women similar to those of the MRFIT[8]. Thus their ideal cholesterol cannot be defined from the relationship between serum cholesterol and ischaemic heart disease risk on the one hand and, on the other, there have been no intervention trials on the scale of the Lipid Research Clinics Study[83,84] or the Helsinki Heart Study[85] which might allow an attempt to define the cholesterol level at which lipid-lowering drugs might be of benefit, other than by extrapolation from results in men. Such extrapolation may be inappropriate, since women are susceptible to

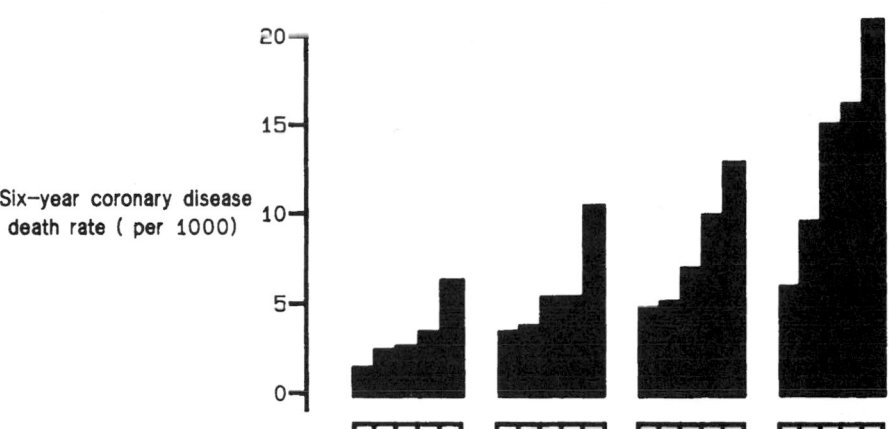

MEN AGED 35–57 YEARS AT ENTRY

**Figure 3.12**   The risk of coronary disease from cholesterol increases more steeply with increasing blood pressure and cigarette smoking (From Stamler *et al.*[9])

different cancers and immunological disorders. The definition of a therapeutic threshold in women is certainly higher than for men, but even more difficult to judge with certainty. The diagnosis of familial hypercholesterolaemia in women, however, as with men, almost invariably calls for the use of lipid-lowering drugs in addition to diet (Chapter 5). Also the presence of other risk factors continues to be important. Diabetes in particular largely abolishes the advantages of women over men in terms of ischaemic heart disease risk[86]. As the use of exogenous sex steroid preparations becomes more prevalent in women this is an additional prognostic factor operating in women which is difficult to fit into their overall risk equation (Chapter 10 and 11). The presence of premature ischaemic heart disease in female members of a family, even when the cause of the hypercholesterolaemia is not familial hypercholesterolaemia, is also a particularly important adverse factor in the author's view, probably because it indicates a particularly strong genetic susceptibility.

Many large primary prevention studies have shown no overall benefit from cholesterol reduction in terms of decreased mortality. This has provoked much interest, but the only reasonable conclusion that can be drawn is that the level of fatal IHD risk was too low in many of these studies for any decrease in its incidence to have any impact on overall mortality unless there had been huge numbers of participants (Chapter 6). There must therefore be a level of IHD risk where there is no clinical benefit even though no harm is done by therapy.

In terms of the therapeutic risk which must be set against the benefits dietary treatment has generally been exonerated[69, 87]. The incidence of adverse effects of lipid-lowering drugs on death rates has probably been exaggerated out of all proportion and present data do not allow any reliable conclusions except, if real, the frequency of such events has been small and does not relate to any specific cause of death making it likely to have arisen by change in studies which were not designed to look for it[69]. Thus, the number of such possible adverse events is so small that they are not discernible in patients with established IHD[69] or at high IHD risk[87] in whom cholesterol reduction has an overall benefit on mortality. These issues relevant to the therapeutic definition of action limits for cholesterol and IHD risk are dealt with in greater depth in Chapter 6. It should be remembered that the potential for side-effects may be greater with certain drugs and that side-effects are less well defined for those which have undergone less extensive clinical evaluation.

### Hypertriglyceridaemia

In the case of serum triglycerides, disease risk is less clearly defined and thus normality is even more imprecisely defined than for serum cholesterol. Tables 3.8–3.10 show that the 95th percentile for serum triglycerides is much higher than the upper limit of normal quoted by many hospital laboratories. The European Consensus Statement[64] was more precise in its recommendations regarding serum triglycerides than the other consensus reports. There would be general agreement that at levels exceeding 1000 mg/dl (11 mmol/l) the increased risk of acute pancreatitis is a clear indication for therapeutic intervention (Chapter 7). At levels below this, hypertriglyceridaemia increases the risk of any associated hypercholesterolaemia, most conspicuously when this cholesterol is present in VLDL (type III hyperlipoproteinaemia; Chapter 8) or in LDL (type IIb hyperlipoproteinaemia; Chapters 6 and 7). Under these circumstances levels of triglycerides of 200 mg/dl (2.2 mmol/l) should be regarded as abnormal. The great difficulty is to decide whether any level of serum triglycerides of less than 1000 mg/dl (11 mmol/l) can be regarded as abnormal in the absence of hypercholesterolaemia. The extent to which we can regard multivariate analysis as a means of establishing the independence of a risk factor in biological as opposed to mathematical terms is clearly relevant to this issue. The significance of hypertriglyceridaemia is considered in detail in Chapter 7.

In summary, moderate degrees of hypertriglyceridaemia in the absence of hypercholesterolaemia, poor family history, manifestations of ischaemic heart disease or diabetes mellitus rarely justify drug therapy. Attention should, however, always be given to diet, particularly if there is obesity, and perhaps also to the choice of anti-hypertensive agent when there is coexistent high blood pressure (Chapter 11).

### Action limits for serum HDL cholesterol

As has been previously discussed, the routine laboratory determination of HDL cholesterol does not generally have a major influence on therapeutic decisions. It should, however, always be undertaken before introducing drug therapy, for two important reasons. Occasionally levels of HDL cholesterol are high enough to take total serum cholesterol above 275 mg/dl (7.0 mmol/l) despite an LDL cholesterol of less than 200 mg/dl (5.2 mmol/l). This may be detected if the Friedewald formula is employed to calculate LDL cholesterol[62]. The formula is reasonably accurate if the serum triglyceride concentration does not exceed 400 mg/dl (4.5 mmol/l) and is as follows:

$$\text{LDL cholesterol} = \frac{(\text{Total cholesterol} - \text{HDL cholesterol}) - \text{Triglycerides}}{5 \text{ mg/dl}}$$

or

$$\text{LDL cholesterol} = \frac{(\text{Total cholesterol} - \text{HDL cholesterol}) - \text{Triglycerides}}{2.19 \text{ mmol/l}}$$

The other occasion when an HDL determination may be helpful is when a level of less than 35 mg/dl (0.9 mmol/l) is detected, since this tends to identify an 'at risk' patient and together with other adverse factors might influence therapeutic decisions[64].

## Apolipoproteins

Case control and prospective studies indicate that the serum apolipoprotein B is more closely associated with the development of ischaemic heart disease than other lipid risk factors such as total cholesterol, HDL cholesterol and triglycerides[16, 88]. Apolipoprotein AI may also be an improvement on HDL cholesterol and influence ischaemic heart disease risk independently of apolipoprotein B[16,89,90]. The same may be true of apolipoprotein (a)[88–93].

It seems probable that serum apolipoprotein B will soon become more widely available in hospital laboratories. Reference ranges and action limits are very much dependent upon individual laboratories at present. In our laboratory serum, apolipoprotein B was less than 123 mg/dl in 97% of 64 men and women whose serum cholesterol was less than 250 mg/dl (6.4 mmol/l) and triglycerides less than 170 mg/dl (1.9 mmol/l)[94]. In 11 studies, each of 40 or more normal people, which measured serum apolipoprotein B by a variety of techniques published since (summarized in reference[95]), the average 97th percentile was 135 mg/dl calculated from the mean and SD assuming a Gaussian distribution. A fuller discussion of apolipoproteins and hyperapobetalipoproteinaemia is to be found in Chapters 2 and 6.

## References

1. Castelli, W. P., Cooper, G. R., Doyle, J. T., Garcia-Palmieri, M., Gordon, T. et al. Distribution of triglyceride and total LDL and HDL cholesterol in several populations: a cooperative lipoprotein phenotyping study. J. Chron. Dis., **30**, 147–169 (1977)
2. Lipid Research Clinics Program Epidemiology Committee. Plasma lipid distributions in selected North American populations: the Lipid Research Clinics Program Prevalence Study. Circulation, **60**, 427–439 (1979)
3. Heiss, G., Tamir, I., Davis, C. E., Tyroler, H. A., Rifkind, B. M. et al. Lipoprotein-cholesterol distributions in selected North American populations: the Lipid Research Clinics Program Prevalence Study. Circulation, **61**, 302–315 (1980)
4. Heiss, G., Johnson, N. J., Reiland, S., Davis, C. E. and Tyroler, J. A. The epidemiology of plasma high-density lipoprotein cholesterol levels. The Lipid Research Clinics Program Prevalence Study Summary. Circulation, **62** (suppl. IV), 116–136 (1980)
5. Williams, O. D., Heiss, G., Beaglehole, R., Dennis, B., Bazarre, T. and Tyroler, H. A. Hyperlipidaemia and nutrition: data base and trends. In Atherosclerosis Reviews, vol. 7, Measurement and Control of Cardiovascular Risk Factors (ed. R. Hegyeli), Raven Press, New York, pp. 145–156 (1980)

6. Christensen, B., Glueck, C., Kviterovich, P., De Groot, I., Chase, G. *et al.* Plasma cholesterol and triglyceride distributions in 13,665 children and adolescents: the prevalence study of the Lipid Research Clinics Program. *Pediat. Res.*, **14**, 19202 (1980)

7. Rifkind, B. M. and Segal, P. Lipid Research Clinics Program reference values of hyperlipidaemia and hypolipidaemia. *J. Am. Med. Assoc.*, **250**, 1869–1872 (1983)

8. Martin, M. J., Hulley, S. B., Browner, W. S., Kuller, L. H. and Wentworth, D. Serum cholesterol, blood pressure and mortality: implications from a cohort of 361 662 men. *Lancet*, **ii**, 933–936 (1986)

9. Stamler, J., Wentworth, D. and Neaton, J. D. Is relationship between serum cholesterol and risk of premature death from coronary heart disease continuous and graded? Findings in 356 222 primary screenees of the Multiple Risk Factor Intervention Trial (MRFIT). *J. Am. Med. Assoc.*, **256**, 2823–2828 (1986)

10. Keys, A. Coronary heart disease – the global picture. *Atherosclerosis*, **22**, 149–192 (1975)

11. Lewis, B., Chait, A., Sigurdsson, G., Mancini, M., Farinaro, E. *et al.* Serum lipoproteins in four European communities: a quantitative comparison. *Eur. J. Clin. Invest.*, **8**, 165–173 (1978)

12. Slack, J., Noble, N., Meade, T. W. and North, W. R. S. Lipid and lipoprotein concentrations in 1604 men and women in working populations in North West London. *Br. Med. J.*, **ii**, 353–356 (1977)

13. Lewis, B., Chait, A., Wootton, I. D. P., Oakley, C. M., Wrikler, D. M. *et al.* Frequency of risk factors for ischaemic heart disease in a healthy British population with particular reference to serum-lipoprotein levels. *Lancet*, **i**, 141–146 (1974)

14. Shaper, A. G., Pocock, S. J., Walker, M., Cohen, N. M., Wale, C. J. and Thomson, A. G. British Regional Heart Study: cardiovascular risk factors in middle-aged men in 24 towns. *Br. Med. J.*, **283**, 179–186 (1981)

15. Thelle, D. S., Shaper, A. G., Whitehead, T. P., Bullock, D. G., Ashby, D. and Patel, I. Blood lipids in middle-aged British men. *Br. Heart J.*, **49**, 205–213 (1983)

16. Durrington, P. N., Hunt, L., Ishola, M., Kane, J. and Stephens, W. P. Serum apolipoproteins Al and B and lipoproteins in middle aged men with and without previous myocardial infarction. *Br. Heart J.*, **56**, 206–212 (1986)

17. Mann, J. I., Lewis, B., Shepherd, J., Winder, A. F., Fenster, S. *et al.* Blood lipid concentrations and other cardiovascular risk factors: distribution, prevalence and detection in Britain. *Br. Med. J.*, **296**, 1702–1706 (1988)

18. Packard, C.J., Bell, M.A., Eaton, R.H., Dagen, M.M., Cassidy, M. and Shepherd, J. A pilot scheme for improving the accuracy of serum cholesterol measurement in Scotland and Northern Ireland. *Ann. Clin. Biochem.* **30**, 387–393 (1993)

19. Consensus Conference (NHLBI). Lowering blood cholesterol to prevent heart disease. *J. Am. Med. Assoc.*, **253**, 2080–2086 (1985)

20. Simons, L. A. Interrelations of lipids and lipoproteins with coronary artery disease mortality in 19 countries. *Am. J. Cardiol.*, **57**, 5G–10G (1986)

21. Mellies, M. J., Laskarzewski, P. M. and Glueck, C. J. Tracking of high- and low-density-lipoprotein cholesterol from childhood to young adulthood in a single large kindred with familial hypercholesterolaemia. *Metabolism*, **34**, 747–753 (1985)

22. Durrington, P. N. High-density lipoprotein cholesterol: methods and clinical significance. *CRC Crit. Rev. Clin. Lab. Sci.*, **18**, 31–78 (1982)

23. Castelli, W. P., Garrison, R. J., Wilson, P. W. F., Abbott, R. D., Kalousdian, S. and Kannel, W. B. Incidence of coronary heart disease and lipoprotein cholesterol levels. The Framingham Study. *J. Am. Med. Assoc.*, **256**, 2835–2838 (1986)

24. Connor, W. E., Cerqueria, M. T., Connor, R. W., Wallace, R. B., Malinow, M. R. and Casdorph, H. R. The plasma lipids, lipoproteins, and diet of the Tarahumara Indians of Mexico. *Am. J. Clin. Nutr.*, **31**, 1131–1142 (1978)

25. Pocock, S. J., Shaper, A. G., Phillips, A. N., Walker, A. N. and Whitehead, T. P. High density lipoprotein cholesterol is not a major risk factor for ischaemic heart disease in British men. *Br. Med. J.*, **292**, 515–519 (1986)

26. Durrington, P. N., Whicher, J. T., Warren, C., Bolton, C. K. and Hartog, M. A comparison of methods for the immunoassay of serum apolipoprotein B in men. *Clin. Chim. Acta*, **7**, 95–108 (1976)

27. Zilversmit, D. B. Atherogenesis: a postprandial phenomenon. *Circulation*, **60**, 473–485 (1979)

28. Tall, A., Sammett, D. and Granst, E. Mechanisms of enhanced cholesteryl ester transfer from high density lipoproteins to apolipoprotein B-containing lipoproteins during alimentary lipemia. *J. Clin. Invest.*, **77**, 1163–1172 (1986)

29. Patsch, J. R., Prasad, S., Gotto, A. M. and Gentsson-Olivecrona, G. Post-prandial lipaemia. A key for the conversion of high density lipoproteins$_3$ into high density lipoproteins$_2$ by hepatic lipase. *J. Clin. Invest.*, **74**, 2017–2023 (1984)

30. Levy, R. I. and Rifkind, B. M. Diagnosis and management of hyperlipoproteinaemia in infants and children. *Am. J. Cardiol.*, **31**, 547–556 (1973)

31. Morrison, J. A., de Groot, I. M. P. H., Edwards, B. K., Kelly, K. A., Mellies, M. *et al.* Lipids and lipoproteins in 927 school children aged 6 to 17 years. *Pediatrics*, **62**, 990–995 (1978)

32. Rossouw, J. E., Van Staden, D. A., Benede, A. J. S., Jooste, P. L., Rossouw, L. J. *et al.* Is it normal for serum cholesterol to rise with age? In *Atherosclerosis*, vol . VII (eds N.H. Fidge, and P.J. Nestel), Excerpta Medica, Amsterdam, pp. 27–40 (1986)

33. Grundy, S. M., Vega, G. L. and Bilheimer, D. W. Kinetic mechanisms determining variability in low density lipoprotein levels and rise with age. *Arteriosclerosis*, **5**, 623–630 (1985)

34. Dawber, T. R. *The Framingham Study. The Epidemiology of Atherosclerotic Disease*, Harvard University Press, Cambridge, Mass (1980)

35. The Scientific Steering Committee on behalf of the Simon Broome Register Group. The risk of fatal coronary heart disease in familial hypercholesterolaemia. *Br. Med. J.* **303**, 893–896 (1991)

36. Rosenson, R.S. Myocardial injury: the acute phase response and lipoprotein metabolism. *J. Am. Coll. Cardiol.*, **22**, 933–940 (1993)

37. MBewu, A.D., Durrington, P.N., Bulleid, S. and Mackness, M.I. The immediate effect of streptokinase on serum lipoprotein (a) concentration and the effect of myocardial infarction on serum lipoprotein (a), apolipoproteins AI and B, lipids and C-reactive protein. *Atherosclerosis*, **103**, 65–71 (1993)

38. Shaukat, N., Ashraf, S.S., Mackness, M.I., MBewu, A.D., Bhatnagar, D. and Durrington, P.N. A prospective study of serum lipoproteins after coronary bypass surgery. *Q. J. Med.*, **87**, 539–545 (1994)

39. Rose, G. and Shipley, M. J. Plasma lipids and mortality: a source of error. *Lancet*, **i**, 523–526 (1980)

40. Sherwin, R. W., Wentworth, D. N., Cutler, J. A., Hulley, S. B., Kuller, L. H. and Stamler, J. Serum cholesterol levels and cancer mortality in 361 662 men screened for the multiple risk factor intervention trial. *J. Am. Med. Assoc.*, **257**, 943–948 (1987)

41. Ryder, R. E. J., Hayes, T. M., Mulligan, I. P., Kingswood, J. C., Williams, S. and Owens, D. R. How soon after myocardial infarction should plasma lipid values be assessed? *Br. Med. J.*, **289**, 1651–1653 (1984)

42. Hammond, J., Went, P., Statland, B. E., Phillips, J. C. and Winkel, P. Daily variation of lipids and hormones in sera of healthy subjects. *Clin. Chim. Acta*, **73**, 347–352 (1976)

43. Low Beer, T. S., Wicks, A. C. B., Heaton, K. W., Durrington, P. and Yeates, J. Fluctuations of serum and bile lipid concentrations during the menstrual cycle. *Br. Med. J.*, **i**, 1568–1570 (1977)

44. Lyons Wall, P.M., Choudhury, N., Gerbrandy, E.A. and Truswell, A.S. Increase of high-density lipoprotein cholesterol at ovulation in healthy women. *Atherosclerosis*, **105**, 171–178 (1994)

45. Razay, G., Heaton, K.W. and Bolton, C.H. Coronary heart disease risk factors in relation to menopause. *Q. J. Med.*, **85**, 307–308 (1992)

46. Stevenson, J.C., Crook, D.and Godsland, I.F. Effects of age and menopause on lipid metabolism in healthy women. *Atherosclerosis*, **98**, 83–90 (1993)

47. Neil, H.A.W., Mant, D., Jones, L. and Mann, J.I. Lipid screening: is it enough to measure total cholesterol concentration? *Br. Med. J.*, **301**, 584–587 (1990)

48. Oliver, M. F. and Boyd, G. S. Plasma lipid and serum lipoprotein patterns during pregnancy and puerperium. *Clin. Sci.*, **14**, 15–23 (1955)

49. Cramer, K., Aurell, M. and Pelirson, S. Serum lipids and lipoproteins during pregnancy. *Clin. Chim. Acta*, **10**, 470–472 (1964)

50. Knopp, R. H., Warth, M. R. and Carroll, C. Lipid metabolism in pregnancy I. Changes in lipoprotein triglyceride in normal pregnancy and the effects of diabetes mellitus. 1. *Reprod. Med.*, **10**, 95–101 (1973)

51. Hillman, L., Schonfeld, G., Miller, J. P. and Wuff, G. Apolipoproteins in human pregnancy. *Metabolism*, **24**, 943–952 (1975)

52. Taylor, G. O. and Akande, E. P. Serum lipids in pregnancy and socioeconomic status. *Br. J. Obstet. Gynaecol.*, **82**, 297–302 (1975)
53. Svanborg, A. and Vikrot, O. Plasma lipid fractions, including individual phospholipids at various stages of pregnancy. *Acta Med. Scand.*, **178**, 615–630 (1975)
54. van Stiphout, W. A. M. J., Hofman, A. and de Bruijn, A. M. Serum lipids in young women before, during and after pregnancy. *Am. J. Epidemiol.*, **126**, 922–928 (1987)
55. Heyden, S. Epidemiological data on dietary fat intake and atherosclerosis with an appendix on possible side effects. In *The Role of Fats in Human Nutrition* (ed. A.J. Vergroesen), Academic Press, London, pp. 45–113 (1975)
56. Blank, D. W., Hoeg, J. M., Kroll, M. H. and Ruddel, M. E. The method of determination must be considered in interpreting blood cholesterol levels. *J. Am. Med. Assoc.*, **26**, 2867–2870 (1986)
57. Laboratory Methods Committee of the Lipid Research Clinics Program. Cholesterol and triglyceride concentrations in serum/plasma pairs. *Clin. Chem.*, **23**, 60–63 (1977)
58. Koerselman, H. B., Lewis, B. and Pilkington, T. R. E. The effects of venous occlusion on the level of serum cholesterol. *J. Atheroscler. Res.*, **1**, 85–88 (1961)
59. Durrington, P. N. A comparison of three methods of measuring serum high density lipoprotein cholesterol in diabetics and non-diabetics. *Ann. Clin. Biochem.*, **17**, 199–204 (1980)
60. Steele, B. W., Koehler, D. F., Azar, M. M., Blaszkowski, T. P., Kuba, K. and Dempsey, M. E. Enzymatic determinations of cholesterol in high-density-lipoprotein fractions prepared by a precipitation technique. *Clin. Chem.*, **22**, 98–101 (1976)
61. Albers, J. J., Warwick, G. R., Johnson, N., Bachorik, P. S., Meusing, R. *et al.* Quality control of plasma high-density lipoprotein cholesterol methods. Lipid Research Clinics Program Prevalence Study. *Circulation*, **62** (Suppl. IV), 9–18 (1980)
62. Friedewald, W. T., Levy, R. I. and Fredrickson, D. S. Estimation of serum low density lipoprotein cholesterol without use of the preparative ultracentrifuge. *Clin. Chem.*, **18**, 499–502 (1972)
63. Reed, A. J., Henq, R. J. and Mason, W. B. Influence of statistical method used on the resulting estimate of normal range. *Clin. Chem.*, **17**, 275–284 (1971)
64. Recommendations of the European Atherosclerosis Society prepared by the International Task Force for Prevention of Coronary Heart Disease. Prevention of coronary heart disease: scientific background and new clinical guidelines. *Nutr. Metabol. Cardiovasc. Dis.*, **2**; 113–156 (1992)
65. Chen, Z., Peto, R., Collins, R., MacMahon, S., Lu, J. and Li, W. Serum cholesterol concentration and coronary heart disease in population with low cholesterol concentrations. *Br. Med. J.*, **303**, 276–282 (1991)
66. European Atherosclerosis Society International Task Force for Prevention of Coronary Heart Disease. Prevention of coronary heart disease: scientific background and new clinical guidelines. *Nutr. Metabol. Cardiovasc. Dis.*, **2**, 113–156 (1992)
67. Law, M.R., Wald, N.J.and Thompson, S.G. By how much and how quickly does reduction in serum cholesterol concentration lower risk of ischaemic heart disease? *Br. Med. J.*, **308**, 367–373 (1994)
68. Jacobs, D., Blackburn, H., Higgins, M., Reed, D., Iso, H. *et al.* Report of the conference on low blood cholesterol: mortality associations. *Circulation*, **86**, 1046–1060 (1990)
69. Law, M.R., Thompson, S.G. and Wald, N.J. Assessing possible hazards of reducing serum cholesterol. *Br. Med. J.*, **308**, 373–379 (1994)
70. Anderson, K.M., Castelli, W.P. and Levy, D. Cholesterol and mortality: 30 years of follow-up from the Framingham Committee. *J. Am. Med. Assoc.*, **257**, 2176–2180 (1987)
71. Klag, M.J., Ford, D.E., Mead, L.A., He, J., Whelton, P.K. *et al.* Serum cholesterol in young men and subsequent cardiovascular disease. *N. Engl. J. Med.*, **328**, 313–318 (1993)
72. Khan, J.A. and Gheck, C.J. Familial hypobetalipoproteinaemia. Absence of atherosclerosis in post-mortem study. *J. Am. Med. Assoc.*, **240**, 47–48 (1978)
73. Davey Smith, G., Shipley, M.J., Marmot, M.G. and Rose, G. Plasma cholesterol concentration and mortality: the Whitehall Study *J. Am. Med. Assoc.*, **267**, 70–76 (1992)
74. Qizilbash, N., Duffy, S.W., Warlow, C. and Mann, J. Lipids are risk factors for ischaemic stroke: overview and review. *Cerebrovasc. Dis.*, **2**, 127–136 (1992)
75. Neaton, J.D., Blackburn, H., Jacobs, D., Kuller, L., Lee, D.J. *et al.* Serum cholesterol level and mortality findings for men screened in the multiple risk factor intervention trial. *Arch. Intern. Med.*, **152**, 1490–1500 (1992)

76. Frank, J.W., Reed, D.M., Grove, J.S. and Benfarte, R. Will lowering population levels of serum cholesterol affect total mortality? *J. Clin. Epidemiol.*, **45**, 333–346 (1992)

77. Shaper, A.G., Phillips, A.N., Pocock, S.J., Walker, M. and Macfarlane, P.W. Risk factors for stroke in middle aged British men. *Br. Med. J.*, **302**, 1111–1115 (1991)

78. Schatzkin, A., Hoover, R. N., Taylor, P. R., Ziegler, R. G., Carter, C. L. *et al*. Serum cholesterol and cancer in the NHANES. 1 Epidemiologic follow-up study. *Lancet*, **ii**, 298–301 (1987)

79. Jacobs, D. Low blood cholesterol and associated mortality. Chapter I in *Cholesterol Lowering Trials. Advice for the British Physician* (eds M. Laker, A. Neil and C. Wood), Royal College of Physicians, London, pp. 5–23 (1993)

80. Marmot, M. The cholesterol papers. Lowering population cholesterol concentrations probably isn't harmful. *Br. Med. J.*, **308**, 351–352 (1994)

81. Family Heart Study Group. Randomised controlled trial evaluating cardiovascular screening and intervention in general practice: principal results of British Family Heart Study. *Br. Med. J.*, **308**, 313–320 (1994)

82. Burn, J., Durrington, P.N. and Harris, R. Genetics and cardiovascular disease. In *Recent Advances in Cardiology* (ed. D.J. Rowlands), Churchill Livingstone, Edinburgh, pp. 27–47 (1987)

83. Lipid Research Clinics Program. The Lipid Research Clinics Coronary Primary Prevention Trial Results. I. Reduction in incidence of coronary heart disease. *J. Am. Med. Assoc.*, **251**, 351–374 (1984)

84. Lipid Research Clinics Program. The Lipid Research Clinics Coronary Primary Prevention Trial Results II. The relationship of reduction in incidence of coronary heart disease to cholesterol lowering. *J. Am. Med. Assoc.*, **251**, 365–374 (1984)

85. Manninen, V., Elo, O., Frick, H., Haapa, K., Heinonen, O. P. *et al*. Lipid alterations and decline in the incidence of coronary heart disease in the Helsinki Heart Study. *J. Am. Med. Assoc.*, **260**, 641–651 (1988)

86. Fuller, J. H. Causes of death in diabetes mellitus. In *Macrovascular Disease in Diabetes Mellitus. Pathogenesis and Prevention* (eds H. U. Janka, H. Mehnert, and F. Standl) Georg Theime Verlag, Stuttgart, pp 3–9 (1985)

87. Davey Smith, G., Song, F. and Sheldon, T.A. Cholesterol lowering and mortality: the importance of considering initial level of risk. *Br. Med. J.*, **306**, 1367–1373 (1993)

88. Wald, N. J., Law, M., Watt, H., Wu, T., Bailey, A. *et al*. Apoliproteins and ischaemic heart disease, implications for screening. *Lancet*, **343**, 75–79 (1994)

89. Bhatnagar, D. and Durrington, P. N. Clinical value of apoliprotein measurements. *Ann. Clin. Biochem.*, **28**, 427–437 (1991)

90. Durrington, P. N. and Bhatnagar, D. Does measurement of apoliproteins add to the clinical diagnosis and management of dyslipidaemias. *Curr. Opin. Lipidol.*, **4**, 299–304 (1993)

91. Rhoads, G. G., Dahlen, G., Berg, K., Morten, N. E. and Dannenberg, A. L. Lp(a) lipoprotein as a risk factor for myocardial infarction. *J. Am. Med Assoc.*, **256**, 2540–2544 (1986)

92. Dahlen, G. H., Guyton, J. R., AKar, M., Fammer, J. A., Judith, A. and Gotto, A. M. Association of levels of lipoprotein Lp(a), plasma lipids, and other lipoproteins with coronary artery disease documented by angiography. *Circulation*, **74**, 758–765 (1986)

93. Durrington, P. N., Ishola, M., Hunt, L., Arrol, S. and Bhatnagar, D. Apolipoprotein(a), AI and B and parental history in men with early onset ischaemic heart disease. *Lancet*, **i**, 1071–1073 (1988)

94. Durrington, P. N., Bolton, C. H. and Hartog, M. Serum and lipoprotein apolipoprotein B levels in normal subjects and patients with hyperlipoproteinaemia. *Clin. Chim. Acta*, **82**, 151–160 (1978)

95. Rosseneu, M., Vercaerist, R., Steinberg, K. K. and Cooper, G. R. Some considerations of methodology and standardization of apolipoprotein B immunoassays. *Clin. Chem.*, **29**, 427–433 (1983)

# Chapter 4

# Classification of hyperlipoproteinaemia

The classification of the hyperlipoproteinaemias frequently gives rise to misunderstanding and confusion. There is no doubt that this has been an obstacle to diagnosis and treatment. This need not be the case.

Already the reader will be aware, from Chapters 1 and 2, that cholesterol and triglycerides are not present in the circulation to any appreciable extent, except as components of lipoproteins. The term hyperlipidaemia refers to an increase in one of the plasma or serum lipids, usually cholesterol or triglycerides. Any such increase can only be mediated through changes in one or more of the lipoproteins transporting cholesterol or triglycerides. Hypertriglyceridaemia usually results, for example, from increases in chylomicrons or VLDL or both. The term hyperlipoproteinaemia allows us to refer to an increase in a specific lipoprotein, rather than simply to a lipid, which is the limitation of the term hyperlipidaemia. The various lipoproteins are metabolically very different and an increase in cholesterol in say chylomicrons may have a very different clinical significance to that of a high concentration in LDL.

Evidence for the existence of lipoproteins dates back to the eighteenth century[1], although it was not until the 1950s that our modern definitions emerged largely as a result of the work of Gofman and co-workers at the Donner Laboratory in Berkeley, California[2] using the analytical ultracentrifuge. Essentially four classes of lipoproteins were defined (see Chapter 2). These were chylomicrons, very low density lipoproteins (VLDL), low density lipoproteins (LDL) and high density lipoproteins (HDL). Chylomicrons and VLDL are triglyceride rich and in health chylomicrons are absent from serum in the fasting state. The bulk of serum cholesterol is present in LDL and HDL, the latter only exceptionally containing more than 40% of serum cholesterol and commonly less than 30%. Rarely, an abnormal cholesterol-rich VLDL is present in serum and this is known as β-VLDL.

Because the ultracentrifuge is only rarely employed in the clinical investigation of patients, a whole range of other lipoprotein terminologies have been introduced based on more routine clinical laboratory methods, e.g. lipoprotein electrophoresis: preβ meaning VLDL, β meaning LDL, and α meaning HDL and broad β meaning β-VLDL; and from nephelometry: L particles meaning chylomicrons, M particles meaning VLDL and S particles meaning LDL. There is no justification for the use of different terminologies in either the clinical laboratory or the scientific literature. Methods for lipoprotein isolation other than ultracentrifugation and precipitation are not usually employed other than semi-quantitatively and they are now disappearing from routine use. The only terms which should commonly be used to describe the lipoproteins are, therefore, chylomicrons, VLDL, LDL, HDL and β-VLDL.

The hyperlipoproteinaemias were defined by Fredrickson, Levy and Lees in a series of articles in 1967[3]. Five phenotypes were defined according to which of

**Table 4.1 WHO classification of hyperlipoproteinaemia (After Beaumont *et al.*[4])**

| Type | Lipoprotein elevated |
|------|----------------------|
| I    | Chylomicrons |
| IIa  | LDL |
| IIb  | LDL and VLDL |
| III  | β-VLDL |
| IV   | VLDL |
| V    | Chylomicrons and VLDL |

**Table 4.2 Some of the more common causes of secondary hyperlipoproteinaemia**

Obesity
Drugs, e.g. beta-blockers, thiazide diuretics,
    oestrogens
Diabetes mellitus
Alcohol
Renal disease
Hypothyroidism
Biliary obstruction
Myeloma
Pregnancy

the lipoproteins was increased; later, type II was subdivided into IIa and IIb[4]. Table 4.1 shows this classification, which is frequently and wrongly regarded as a diagnostic classification. It cannot be overemphasized that this is not the case: it is often no more than a way of reporting which of serum lipoproteins is increased in concentration. All of the types may be either primary or secondary. The secondary causes are described in detail in Chapter 11, but for convenience some of the commoner ones are shown in Table 4.2. However, even within the primary types there may be recognizably different diseases. In particular, primary type IIa and occasionally type IIb may occur as the result of a single defective gene (monogenic) producing the clinical syndrome of familial hypercholesterolaemia (Chapter 5) with such manifestations as tendon xanthomata and a substantially decreased life expectancy, or as the result of an interaction between at least two genes (polygenic) and environmental influences, particularly nutritional influences (Chapter 6) which probably never leads to tendon xanthomata and often has a better prognosis than familial hypercholesterolaemia. As more of the molecular mechanisms underlying the different phenotypes are discovered, it is being increasingly realized that they are each a heterogeneous group of different disorders.

It should further be emphasized that the WHO phenotype (frequently referred to as the 'Fredrickson type') frequently changes as treatment with diet and drugs is introduced. This may be a source of confusion to the clinician inexperienced in the management of hyperlipoproteinaemia and repeated lipoprotein phenotyping is a totally pointless exercise on the part of the clinical laboratory. Type IIa hyperlipoproteinaemia often changes to type IIb when bile acid sequestrating drugs such as cholestyramine are given, because there is often a rise in VLDL while some elevation of LDL persists. As type III resolves with diet, some elevation of VLDL persists producing type IV hyperlipoproteinaemia. Type V almost invariably is converted to type IV by dietary treatment, and the rare type I to type V or IV. After the initial phenotyping there is therefore no point in further phenotyping and the response to therapy is best monitored by determination of serum cholesterol and triglycerides and occasionally HDL cholesterol. Indeed, these simple tests combined with visual inspection of the serum will in almost all cases allow the patient's phenotype to be established at the outset without resort to more sophisticated investigations.

Unless the serum triglycerides are markedly elevated, a raised serum cholesterol generally indicates an increased LDL cholesterol and thus a type IIa or IIb disorder. The LDL cholesterol concentration may be calculated by the Friedewald formula if HDL cholesterol is determined (Chapter 3, page 99). It is always useful to inspect the fasting plasma or serum visually for lipaemia (the presence of increased quantities of chylomicrons or VLDL, which are sufficiently large particles to scatter light). This can be done in the clinic or surgery without the need for centrifugation, if in addition to the clotted blood sample (for cholesterol, triglycerides and HDL cholesterol by precipitation) blood is also taken into an EDTA (sequestrene)-containing tube (blood counts), heparin-containing tube (biochemical profile), fluoride-containing tube (blood glucose) or citrate-containing tube (ESR bottle). If such tubes are left standing upright for a few minutes, the red cells will sediment sufficiently for a layer of plasma to be seen at the top. This will be clear in the type IIa phenotype. If chylomicrons are present (generally type V), it will be milky in appearance. The triglycerides are then generally grossly elevated >1000 mg/dl or 11 mmol/l). Serum cholesterol will also be raised, although to a lesser extent than triglycerides. This is because cholesterol present in VLDL and chylomicrons, which does not normally contribute substantially to total cholesterol, does so under these circumstances. In type IV hyperlipoproteinaemia, less marked increases in the serum triglycerides occur and the serum cholesterol is not elevated above 275 mg/dl (7.0 mmol/l). The plasma will appear opalescent in indirect light, but not milky. If the level of triglycerides does not exceed 400 mg/dl (4.5 mmol/l), the Friedewald formula may still be used to calculate LDL cholesterol. In type IIb hyperlipoproteinaemia, an increase in serum cholesterol occurs in association with increased triglycerides. Usually the increase in the concentration of the triglycerides is less than that in cholesterol. However, when the elevation of triglycerides is closer to that of cholesterol, particularly in molar terms, then the possibility of type III must be considered. This disorder is sufficiently rare that techniques for its diagnosis need to be available, say, on a regional basis and should not deter a district hospital from establishing a lipid clinic.

If lipoprotein electrophoresis is available, then the presence of a broad band adds further suspicion and the presence of striate palmar or tuberoeruptive xanthomata is virtually diagnostic (Chapters 8 and 11). The definitive test is to isolate VLDL in the ultracentrifuge, which is very easily accomplished if a preparative ultracentrifuge is available (Chapter 8). The ratio of VLDL cholesterol to total serum triglycerides, if >0.3 (if mg/dl are the units of concentration) or >0.68 (if mmol/l), indicates the presence of β-VLDL and establishes the diagnosis of type III hyperlipoproteinaemia. The presence of suspicious levels of total serum cholesterol and triglycerides in a patient whose apolipoprotein E genotype on isoelectric focusing of VLDL is E2/E2, if this is available, is equally good evidence for the diagnosis (Chapter 8).

# Hyperapobetalipoproteinaemia

It is likely that increasingly disorders will be described in which elevated levels of lipoproteins or abnormalities of lipoproteins will be identified without there being concomitant increases in total serum cholesterol or triglycerides. A potentially important example of this is hyperapobetalipoproteinaemia, in which an elevation of serum LDL is indicated by increased levels of its major protein, apolipoprotein B, but not by any increase in serum cholesterol and triglycerides (Chapter 6). The possibility that abnormal lipoproteins might be present in some people without the elevation in serum lipids or lipoproteins, has led some authors to replace the term hyperlipoproteinaemia with dyslipoproteinaemia, and it seems likely that future research may lead to further justification for the use of this term.

## References

1. Hewson, W. *An experimental enquiry into the properties of the blood with remarks on some of its morbid appearances and an appendix relating to the discovery of the lymphatic system in birds, fish and the animals called amphibious*, T. Cadell, London (1771).
2. Gofman, J. W., De Lalla, O., Glazier, F., Freeman, N. K., Nicholas, A. V., Strisower, E. H. and Tamplin, A. R. The serum lipoprotein transport system in health, metabolic disorders, atherosclerosis and coronary artery disease. *Plasma*, **2**, 413 484 (1954)
3. Fredrickson, D. S., Levy, R. I. and Lees, R. S. Fat transport in lipoproteins – an integrated approach to mechanisms and disorders. *N. Eng. J. Med.*, **276**, 34–42, 94–103, 148–156, 215–225 and 273–281 (1967)
4. Beaumont, J. L., Carlson, L. A., Cooper, G. R., Fejfar, Z., Fredrickson, D. S. and Strasser, T. Classification of hyperlipidaemias and hyperlipoproteinaemias. *Bull World Hlth Org.*, **43**, 891–915 (1970)

Chapter 5

# Familial hypercholesterolaemia

Familial hypercholesterolaemia (FH) is the most important clinical syndrome leading to premature ischaemic heart disease which we are currently able to identify. Despite this, few clinicians are attuned to its recognition. The clinical features of the condition have only recently begun to be included in textbooks of medicine, although they have been known for many years. Although it is true to say that interest in FH has received considerable impetus from the relatively recent unravelling of its pathophysiology, it is also the case that many other diseases of similar prevalence, of whose underlying causes we remain ignorant, receive a much greater share of medical attention. It seems therefore that despite the fact that patients with FH have a condition which is entirely genetic in its origin and produces a clinical syndrome often clearly recognizable at the bedside, they have been made to suffer unduly by the widespread confusion surrounding the relationship with atheroma of the more common, less severe, largely nutritionally induced hypercholesterolaemia present in societies such as ours.

## History

Undoubtedly the familial occurrence of xanthomata and atheroma were well described before the turn of the century[1,2]. It was also appreciated that both lesions contained substantial deposits of cholesterol[3]. The earliest account of FH in which all the essential elements were present including the determination of serum cholesterol was that of Burns in 1920[4]. More extensive studies appeared in the 1930s due to the work of Muller[5] and of Thannhauser[6]. These and many later studies indicated a dominant pattern of inheritance, but this was not inescapably confirmed until the 1960s when Kachadurian[7], working in the Lebanon where FH and first-cousin marriages are common, demonstrated a monogenic pattern of inheritance with expression in heterozygotes and an even more severe form of the disease in homozygotes.

Evidence that the high serum cholesterol was due to an increase in LDL was first provided by Gofman and co-workers following the introduction of the analytical ultracentrifuge[8]. That the primary defect was due to decreased catabolism of LDL was demonstrated by Langer and colleagues in 1972[9].

In 1973, Goldstein and Brown[10], as the result of studies with cultured fibroblasts, disclosed that the reason for this catabolic defect was a failure of expression of specific cell surface receptors for LDL in patients with FH. For this and their subsequent work on the LDL receptor they received the Nobel Prize for Medicine in 1985. In 1979, using native LDL and LDL in which the receptor-binding site had been blocked by chemical modification, Shepherd and co-workers[11] were able to show that the LDL receptor was active *in vivo* and that its activity was indeed decreased in patients with FH.

# Pathophysiology (Figure 5.1)

The importance of the LDL receptor or apo $B_{100}$/E receptor for entry of cholesterol into cells has previously been described in Chapter 2. It is a defect in that
receptor which leads to the clinical syndrome known as familial hypercholesterolaemia. Fibroblasts from normal people when cultured without an exogenous
source of cholesterol produce receptors at their cell surface, which avidly bind and
internalize LDL added to the culture medium. Fibroblasts from patients homozygous for FH grown under the same conditions largely fail to internalize LDL and
those from heterozygotes do so only about half as effectively as normal fibroblasts[12,13]. From studies of fibroblasts of homozygotes, two main defects have
been identified in the receptor[14]; in one of these, no receptor-mediated binding
activity can be demonstrated and such individuals are termed receptor-negative
(or $R^{b^0}$). Fibroblasts from most other homozygotes will bind LDL, but do so with
a markedly decreased affinity. Such are termed receptor-defective ($R^{b-}$). A small
number of homozygotes have been reported whose fibroblasts appear to bind
normally to LDL, but which fail to internalize the LDL-receptor complex ($R^{b+,i^0}$).
Patients who are receptor-defective can express 25–30% of normal fibroblast
receptor activity and although their clinical syndrome is similar in most respects
to the others, they are said to respond better to treatment[15].

The mutations leading to the receptor-negative and receptor-defective states
have been intensively studied in recent years following the discovery of the DNA
sequence of the LDL receptor gene and the development of methods for the isolation of the receptor itself, and investigation of intracellular events such as its
synthesis, migration to the cell surface, movement into the coated pit region, internalization and recycling (Chapter 2, pages 32 and 38)[16,17, see also 130]. The
number of mutations described in genes encoding receptor-mediated LDL catabolism leading to the clinical syndrome of FH is already approaching 200. In general

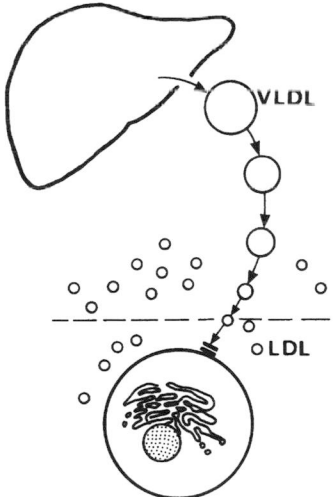

**Figure 5.1**   In familial hypercholesterolaemia the LDL receptor is defective and the concentration
of LDL in plasma and tissue fluid is increased

terms these may be categorized as having their major impact at one of four different critical stages in the receptor-mediated LDL catabolic pathway:

1. Mutations which affect receptor synthesis.
2. Mutations which affect the transport of the receptor from the endoplasmic reticulum to the Golgi complex.
3. Mutations which interfere with the binding of LDL to the receptor.
4. Mutations in which LDL binds normally, but, because of the cytoplasmic tail of the receptor, will not bind to clathrin, migration to the coated pit does not occur and internalization is defective.

Investigations using LDL and more recently VLDL labelled in their apolipoprotein moiety with $^{125}$I or $^{131}$I, have shown that in normal man LDL has a plasma half-life between 2.5 and 3 days[18,19]. Some 30–50% of LDL is catabolized every day[11,19–21], depending upon diet and probably other factors. This is the fractional catabolic rate (FCR) of LDL and represents the combined effects of receptor-mediated and non-receptor-mediated cellular LDL uptake (Chapter 2, pages 31–33). Using a technique in which the receptor-binding site of $^{131}$I-labelled LDL, is blocked by cyclohexanedione and then is injected into the circulation at the same time as unmodified $^{125}$I-labelled LDL, it has been possible to estimate that one-third of LDL is catabolized via receptors in Scottish men whose serum LDL cholesterol is not raised.

In heterozygotes for FH, the half-life of circulating LDL is prolonged by about 2 days as a result of the receptor defect. Consistent with this, the FCR is approximately half that in normal people[9,20] and one-fifth or less of LDL catabolism is due to receptors[11]. There is an even lower FCR[19] and receptor-mediated clearance in homozygotes[22].

The synthetic rate of LDL apo B in normal people averages 10 mg/kg per day[21]. There is general agreement that in homozygotes for FH this figure is doubled[18, 19,23–28], but there has been disagreement about whether there is any increase in heterozygotes. One consensus view is that their LDL apo B synthesis is increased approximately 30%[29]. Some of the increased LDL apo B produced enters the circulation as a result of direct secretion of IDL or LDL, presumably from the liver[25–27], without the normal requirement for a VLDL precursor. Despite the increase in apo B synthesis, whole body cholesterol biosynthesis seems only exceptionally to be raised even in homozygotes and then there is a tendency for it to decline towards normal as they grow older[30].

In theory mutations of apolipoprotein B affecting its receptor binding site should produce a defect in LDL catabolism resembling that in FH due to defects in the LDL receptor itself. This has been termed familial defective apolipoprotein B. Only one apolipoprotein B mutation, the apolipoprotein B3500 mutation, has been reliably shown to affect LDL catabolism to an extent approaching that in FH (see Familial defective apolipoprotein B, page 132).

## Clinical features

### Prevalence

Familial hypercholesterolaemia in its heterozygous form is the commonest genetic disease in many societies including our own. In the UK, the USA and Japan, the frequency of heterozygotes is about 1 in 500[18,31]. In the Lebanon[32], in South Africa[33], in French-speaking Canada[34] and in Lithuanian Jews[35] it is considerably more common. This is due to these populations having arisen from a relatively small number of migrants, some of whom by chance had heterozygous FH[36]. This is called a 'founder gene effect'. It also means that the range of mutations encountered in the LDL gene is small in such populations compared with societies in which open breeding has been the rule. Thus in South Africa two LDL mutations account for a great majority of FH[37] whereas in Britain and the USA no single LDL receptor mutation appears to account for more than a tiny percentage of FH[38].

The prevalence of homozygous FH is much less. Both parents must have FH for there to be any likelihood of them producing a child homozygous for the condition.

If marriage between heterozygotes is a matter of chance, then only 1 marriage in 250 000 (= $500^2$) could result in the birth of a homozygote and then by simple mendelian genetics only one-quarter of the pregnancies would be expected to produce a homozygote, and then only if intrauterine survival was unaffected by the receptor defect. In the Lebanon, first-cousin marriages are, however, common and this has given the opportunity to study the genetics of FH in detail[7]. The number of people with homozygous FH in the UK population is not at present known with certainty, but it is undoubtedly less than 50.

## Xanthomata

Xanthomata are localized infiltrates of lipid-containing histiocytic foam cells[39]. The diagnostic hallmark of FH is the presence of xanthomata in tendons (Plates 2 and 3). Frequently these appear in heterozygotes from the age of 20 onwards[7,29,32]. Exceptionally they are present in heterozygotes in their teens. In homozygotes their occurrence in childhood is the rule.

The most common sites for tendon xanthomata are in the tendons overlying the knuckles and in the Achilles tendons. Less commonly they may also be found in the extensor hallucis longus and triceps tendons and occasionally elsewhere. It is common to find xanthomata on the upper tibia at the site of the insertion of the patellar tendon (Plate 4). These should be classified as subperiosteal xanthomata rather then tendon xanthomata. Unlike tendon xanthomata, they cannot be waggled from side to side.

It is important to emphasize that the skin overlying tendon xanthomata is a normal colour and does not appear yellow. The cholesterol accumulation is deep within the tendons. Furthermore, the tendon xanthomata feel hard and not soft. This is because they contain not only foam-laden macrophages but also collagen, since they excite a fibrous reaction; hence their marked histological resemblance to atheromatous lesions[39]. Of clinical importance too is their tendency to become inflamed, particularly those in the Achilles tendons. Many patients who are heterozygotes for FH reveal on questioning a past history of Achilles tenosynovitis, particularly in the athletic, presumably where football boots or trainers rub against the tendons, or in those attempting to wear 'fashionable' shoes, especially if their occupations involve a good deal of standing, as is the case for example with hairdressers. Occasionally patients have actually ruptured their Achilles tendons previously. A number of patients attending our lipid clinic have been discovered to have xanthomata as a result of tendon biopsy, and diagnoses such as tumours of the tendon, tophi and rheumatoid nodules have all been previously entertained. The determination of serum cholesterol has its place therefore in the rheumatology and orthopaedic clinic.

There are two conditions other than FH which produce tendon xanthomata. Fortunately these are so rare that there is virtually never any diagnostic difficulty. One of these conditions is cerebrotendinous xanthomatosis in which high levels of plasma cholestanol occur, probably secondary to a block in bile acid synthesis, and lead to excessive tissue deposition of cholestanol rather than cholesterol[40]. The other is phytosterolaemia (β-sitosterolaemia) in which high levels of plant sterols, not normally absorbed from the gut, such as β-sitosterol and to a lesser extent campesterol and stigmasterol, accumulate in the plasma and tissues[40,41]. Most commonly, when a patient with tendon xanthomata and normal serum cholesterol is discovered the reason is a laboratory error or the cholesterol was determined when the patient was ill with, for example, an acute myocardial infarction (Chapter 3).

Because of the importance of tendon xanthomata in differentiating patients with FH from those with hypercholesterolaemia due to other causes, attempts have been made to refine our ability to identify xanthomata by means other than palpation. In many patients with FH, the presence of tendon xanthomata is indisputable (to those who take the trouble to look). However, there are large numbers of patients in whom detection of tendon xanthomata is a rather subjective judgement on the part of the clinician. Soft-tissue radiography, similar to mammography, and more recently, computer assisted (computed) tomography[42] (Figure 5.2), have been used, but in the author's view, although these techniques are valuable in objectively assessing changes in size of tendon xanthomata, they are not helpful in deciding their presence or absence in equivocal cases.

Patients do occasionally report decreases in the size of tendon xanthomata with treatment and it may be that obligate heterozygotes commenced on treatment early in life do not develop them as adults. There is objective evidence of a decrease in the size of Achilles tendon xanthomata with treatment with combined cholestyramine and nicotinic acid[43] with probucol[44] and anecdotally with HMG-CoA reductase inhibitors. The decrease in size is frequently not obvious in the clinic (much of the xanthoma consists of fibrous tissue and no promise should be made to the patient that the xanthomata will diminish in size). Occasionally the institution of cholesterol-lowering medication seems to be followed by an episode of discomfort in the tendons or even frank tenosynovitis, possibly analogous to an attack of gout when urate is mobilized from joints after the institution of hypouricaemic treatment in patients with hyperuricaemia. This occurs most often in patients who are treated with HMG-CoA reductase inhibitors or partial ileal bypass. Occasionally inflammation of the tendons in areas where xanthomata are not clinically detectable occurs, for example at the front of the ankles or in the tendons of muscles inserting around the wrist or elbows. Perhaps this indicates the presence of subclinical xanthomata in these regions. It is often confused with myositis, but the serum creatinine kinase activity is either unaffected or only minimally elevated. A more gradual build-up of the dose of HMG-CoA reductase inhibitor may overcome it.

Patients can be reassured that the prominence of their tendon xanthomata does not seem to be very closely related to the age of onset of clinical manifestation of arterial disease.

In homozygotes, elevated orange–yellow subcutaneous planar and tuberose xanthomata occur. These are predominantly on the buttocks, antecubital fossae

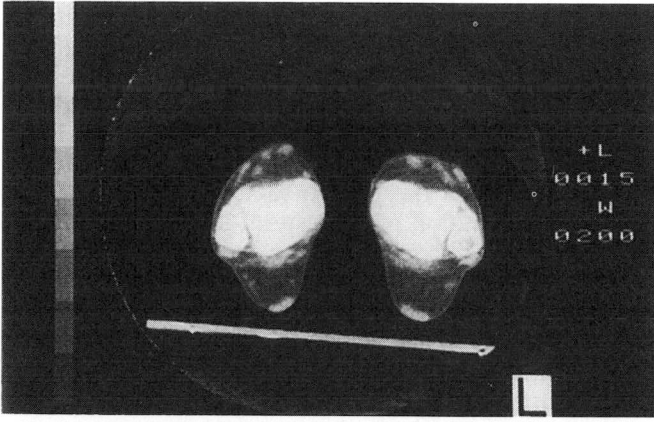

(a)

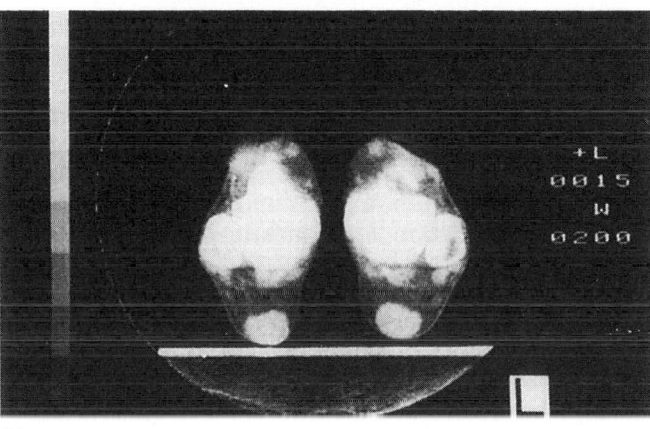

(b)

**Figure 5.2** Computed tomography of the ankle: (*a*) Normal person (note the narrow strap-like Achilles tendons; (*b*) heterozygote for familial hypercholesterolaemia (the Achilles tendons are swollen and bean-shaped in cross-section) (From Durrington *et al.*[42])

and the hands (Plate 5) after walking commences. However, they may occur in the first year of life and then may be in areas subjected to pressure during crawling, such as the knees, thenar eminences and dorsum of the feet. Xanthomata occurring so early may indicate that both of the LDL receptor mutations are of the receptor-negative type.

Xanthelasma palpebrarum (Plate 6) and corneal arcus, although they occur in FH, are not especially helpful in making the diagnosis. It is not at all uncommon to encounter a patient who is a definite heterozygote, with well-developed tendon xanthomata but no corneal arcus. Xanthelasmata are present in only a minority of patients. Both corneal arcus and xanthelasmata may occur in association with hypercholesterolaemia not due to FH (Chapter 6) and often the serum cholesterol concentration does not depart very much from the average. Corneal arcus is more closely associated with hypercholesterolaemia in younger people (arcus juvenilis), but even then the association is not invariable. With increasing age, corneal arcus becomes common (arcus senilis) and carries little clinical significance. Xanthelasma palpebrarum seems to have a predilection for overweight middle-aged women without any very marked hyperlipidaemia (if any). Occasionally there is a strong family history of xanthelasmata, often again not in association with any marked alteration in the serum lipids. It may under those circumstances develop in the early teens. Local factors within the skin seem to be as important as the serum lipids and many such patients have a tendency to keloid formation in the skin around the eyes. This is the major reason why the author does not refer such patients for plastic surgery. Occasionally when associated with obesity they resolve with weight reduction and occasionally with drug therapy to reduce plasma lipids, particularly with probucol (Plate 6 and Chapter 10). Most often they persist despite treatment and, if the patients find them disfiguring, referral to a dermatologist for cauterization or silver nitrate application seems to produce the best result. There is nevertheless some scarring and a tendency for recurrence about which the patient should be warned.

Corneal arcus never impairs vision and patients may be reassured accordingly. There is, of course, no treatment and no evidence that resolution ever occurs.

## Ischaemic heart disease

Clinical manifestations of ischaemic heart disease occur as early as the mid-twenties in heterozygotes. Men are at more risk than women. In a series of patients not presenting as a result of ischaemic heart disease[45], over half of the men had died by the age of 60 and 15% of the women (Table 5.1). In homozygotes, ischaemic heart disease develops in childhood: death before the age of 30 due to myocardial infarction, progressive heart failure or dysrhythmia was virtually certain before the advent of coronary artery bypass surgery and more recently cardiac transplantation.

Atheroma frequently produces severe left main stem or triple vessel coronary disease[46,47] and this may be present even in patients who are asymptomatic or have only relatively mild angina. Indeed many patients with severe disease, being young, are capable of considerable exertion, making exercise electrocardiography a poor means of detecting them. Symptoms of cardiac ischaemia in a young patient

**Table 5.1 Death and morbidity from ischaemic heart disease in heterozygous familial hypercholesterolaemia in a UK population not presenting as a result of ischaemic heart disease[45]. Figures in parentheses are from a compilation of reports including data from the USA and France[29]**

| Age (yr) | Incidence of ischaemic heart disease (%) | | Deaths from ischaemic heart disease (%) | |
|---|---|---|---|---|
| | Men | Women | Men | Women |
| <30 | 5 | 0 | 0 | 0 |
| 30–39 | 24 (20) | 0  (3) | 7 | 0  (0) |
| 40–49 | 51 (45) | 12  (2) | 24 (25) | 0  (2) |
| 50–59 | 85 (75) | 58 (45) | 54 (50) | 15 (15) |
| 60–69 | 100 | 74 (75) | 78 (80) | 15 (30) |

with hypercholesterolaemia and tendon xanthomata call for full investigation, including coronary angiography, at a centre experienced in the management of such patients.

The age at which ischaemic heart disease manifests itself in heterozygotes, although on average much earlier, of course, than in the general population and in many other hyperlipoproteinaemias, does vary a great deal between affected individuals. There is, however, much less variation among related individuals. In a study of Norwegian and British families, the ages at coronary death of affected siblings after allowance for the sex difference (by subtraction of 9 years, the median age difference between men and women) from the age of death of women were correlated (correlation coefficient 0.70)[48]. Thus other familial factors, perhaps genetic or owing to being brought up together, must influence the rate of development of coronary disease. Interestingly neither the untreated serum cholesterol level nor the LDL cholesterol level is related to age of onset of symptoms or of death from IHD in either heterozygotes[48–50] or homozygotes[51–53]. More information on average serum LDL cholesterol levels and perhaps more importantly apolipoprotein B concentrations in relation to prognosis is, however, required.

There is some evidence that HDL may relate to prognosis in heterozygous FH[54,55], and also that patients with a tendency to run higher serum triglyceride levels (also associated with low HDL) may fare worse[50]. It is certainly the case that a number of different mutations affecting LDL receptor expression produce the clinical syndrome of FH and these may have a bearing on the rate of development of coronary atheroma, perhaps by influencing the quantity of LDL which must leave the circulation by the non-receptor-mediated pathway (Chapter 2, page 33). Whether the apparently worse prognosis in homozygotes with receptor-negative mutations as opposed to receptor-defective ones (page 109) also applies to heterozygotes is unknown.

Smoking and hypertension are highly likely to accelerate the onset of ischaemic heart disease in FH[49,56], but there is no particular association of the FH syndrome with either of those. Higher serum fibrinogen levels may also hasten the onset of symptomatic arterial disease[57] and further work in that area is important since therapeutic reduction of serum fibrinogen is possible. In a series of Finnish patients, low rates of bile acid synthesis in FH heterozygotes were associated with early onset of ischaemic heart disease[49]. This effect did not appear to be mediated through any other risk factor and it was argued that it might be a reflection of increased LDL catabolism through non-receptor-mediated pathways.

## Other atheromatous manifestations

In addition to the proximal coronary arteries, atheromatous deposits occur in the root of the aorta and may extend into the aortic valve cusps. Extensive involvement at these sites, giving rise sometimes to funnelling of the aortic root and to abnormal pressure gradients across the aorta valve, are a feature of homozygous FH[58]. However, it is wrong to assume that these sites are spared in heterozygotes, since aortic systolic murmurs are common in heterozygotes[59] and echocardiographic evidence of valvular or supravalvular deposits, although less severe than in homozygotes, was observed in some 30% of heterozygotes[60]. Histologically the aortic root deposits contain masses of cholesterol-laden foam cells, and in the larger (and presumably older) lesion bands of fibrous tissue are also present welling off extracellular lakes of cholesterol. They thus closely resemble advanced atheromatous lesions and xanthomata.

Despite the marked increase of frequency of coronary and aortic root atheroma in FH, atheroma at other sites occurs in only a small proportion of patients. We have seen only the occasional heterozygote with symptomatic femoropopliteal atheroma. This of course is quite different from, for example, type III hyperlipoproteinaemia (Chapter 8). Cerebral atheroma is also uncommon and ischaemic syndromes due to brachial and subclavian arterial disease are exceptional.

The reason for this remarkable predilection for the coronary vessels, particularly the proximal ones, is not known with certainty, but presumably the nature of the lipoprotein particles themselves may be important (as presumably it is for the virtually diagnostic tendon xanthomata). Other risk factors such as smoking may be important when arterial disease does develop more peripherally.

## Polyarthritis

Reference has already been made to tendinitis or tenosynovitis which seems to occur as a consequence of cholesterol deposition in the tendon and is not infrequent in both homozygotes and heterozygotes for FH. There is also, however, an arthritis which is a particular feature of homozygotes[61]. It affects predominantly the ankles, knees, wrists and proximal interphalangeal joints. Fluid aspirated from the joints may contain occasional cholesterol crystals, but they are not so plentiful as to suggest that the basis of the arthritis is indisputably crystal deposition[62] and its aetiology is thus uncertain. Occasionally heterozygotes also seem to have similar episodes of joint pain[63,64], but polyarthralgias of uncertain aetiology are, of course, sufficiently common in the adult population without any specific diagnostic features that it is difficult to be certain just how frequently they are due to FH. In one study, investigations suggested that the joint symptoms were most likely due to inflammatory periarthritis and peritendinitis[64].

In homozygotes the concurrence of polyarthritis, a cardiac murmur and sometimes a raised ESR (secondary to increased serum fibrinogen) does occasionally lead to the erroneous diagnosis of acute rheumatic fever.

## Other diseases associated with familial hypercholesterolaemia

The expression of hypercholesterolaemia in FH is entirely genetic and does not require any additional nutritional or other factors. The typical patient with FH is lean and superficially appears physically well. When obesity does occur in patients with FH, it often produces a dramatic rise in the serum cholesterol (Figure 11.9), and a small increase in the serum triglycerides not usually found in FH is frequently also present (Chapter 7). There is no association between FH and diabetes mellitus and, unlike the hypertriglyceridaemias, hyperuricaemia is also not a feature.

Hypertension too is not commonly found in FH. When it does occur it may hasten the onset of ischaemic heart disease. The gene for the LDL receptor is on chromosome 19 and its inheritance would be expected to be linked with other adjacent genes, and indeed it is with the third component of complement[65–67]. As yet, however, no association with another genetic defect has been described. The gene for myotonic dystrophy is close to the LDL receptor gene, but no linkage has been reported. A proximal muscle atrophy syndrome was, however, described

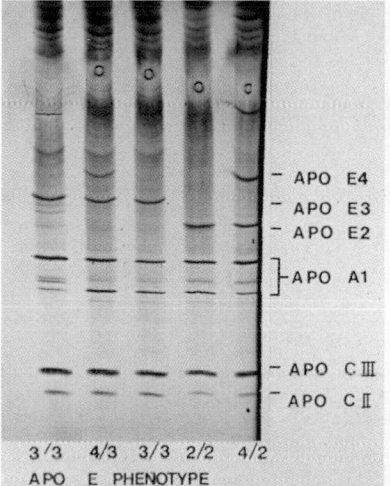

**Plate 1** Polyacrylamide isoelectric focusing of VLDL apolipoproteins from five people with different apolipoprotein E phenotypes (Courtesy of Drs J. Kane and E. Gowland)

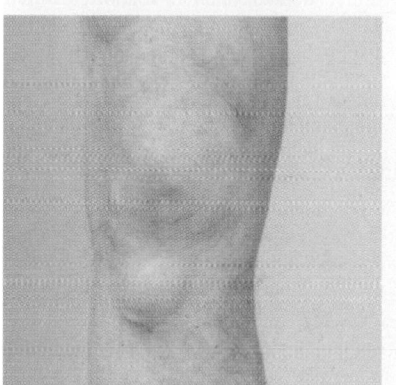

**Plate 4** Subperiosteal xanthoma over tibial tuberosity (heterozygous familial hypercholesterolaemia)

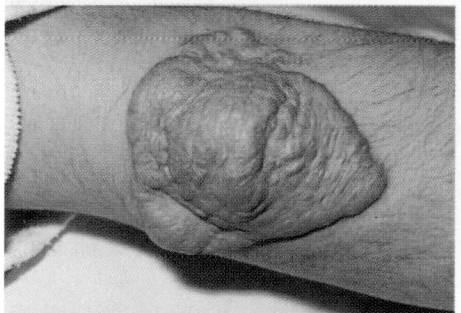

**Plate 5** Subcutaneous planar xanthoma in antecubital fossa (homozygous familial hypercholesterolaemia)

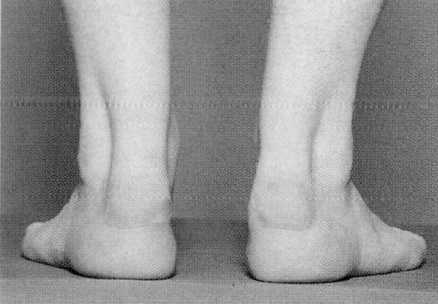

**Plate 2** Achilles tendon xanthomata (heterozygous familial hypercholesterolaemia)

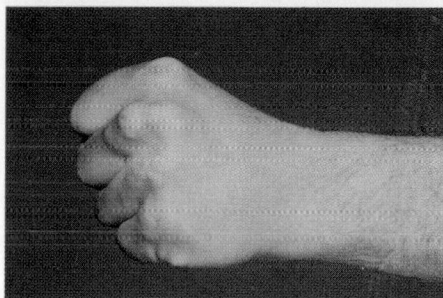

**Plate 3** Tendon xanthomata on dorsum of hand (heterozygous familial hypercholesterolaemia)

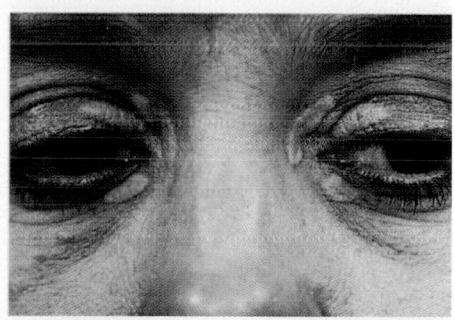

*(a)*

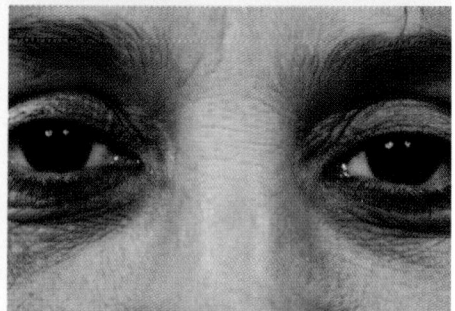

*(b)*

**Plate 6** Xanthelasma palpebrarum. Note resolution in lower plate after treatment with probucol

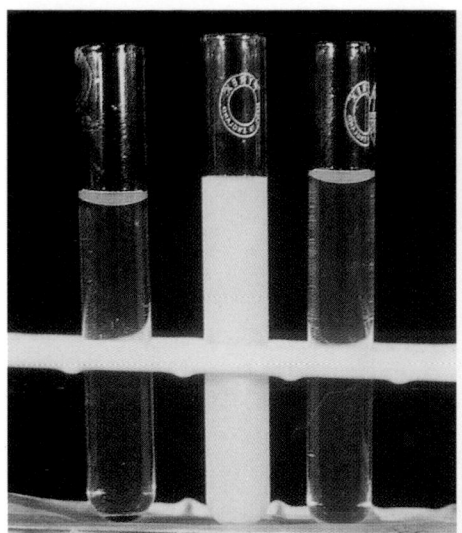

(a)

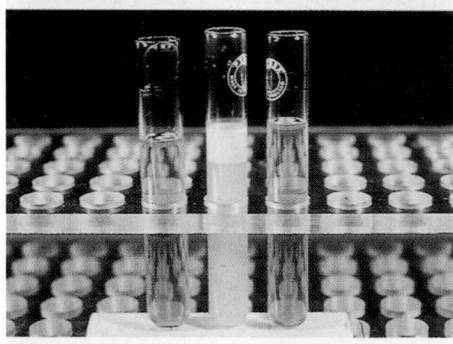

(b)

**Plate 7**   Appearance of the serum in severe hypertriglyceridaemia: *(a)* the middle tube contains fasting serum of triglyceride concentration 5000 mg/dl (50–60 mmol/l); *(b)* the chylomicrons have formed a creamy surface layer on standing

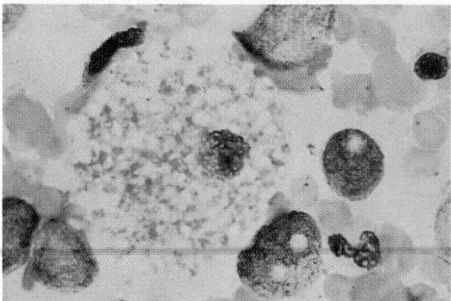

**Plate 8**   Bone marrow aspirate of a patient with familial lipoprotein lipase deficiency, showing a lipid-laden macrophage ('foam cell') (Courtesy of Dr J. E. MacIver)

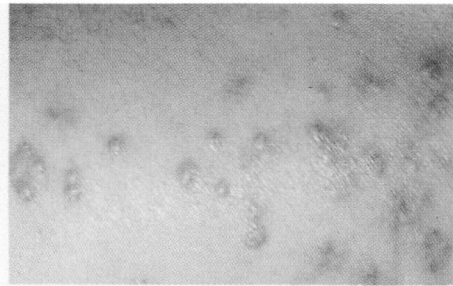

**Plate 9**   Eruptive xanthomata (type I or V hyperlipoproteinaemia)

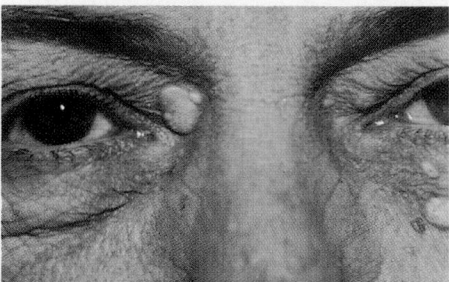

(a)

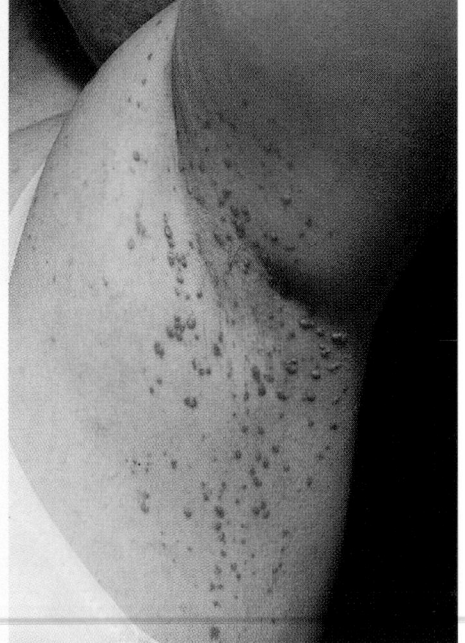

(b)

**Plate 10**   Xanthomata and skin lesions, which may not be associated with hyperlipidaemia: *(a)* epidermal cysts (Courtesy of Dr G. Auckland); *(b)* xanthoma disseminatum (see Reference 109, Chapter 7) (Courtesy of Dr R. Ead)

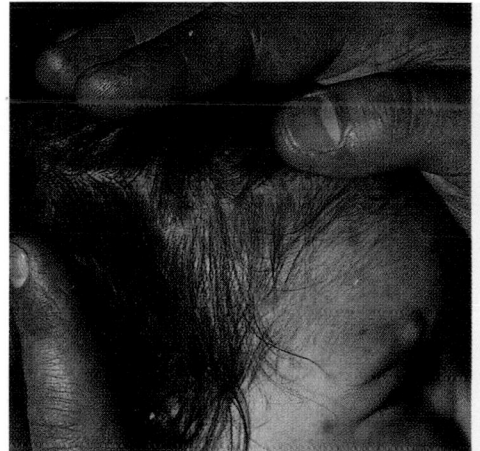

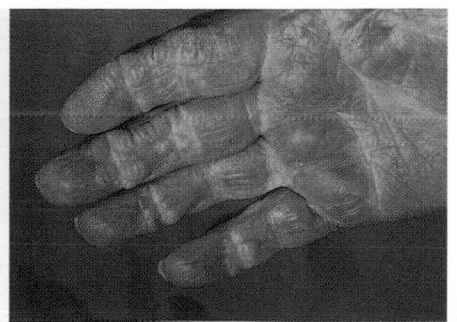

(a)

(c)

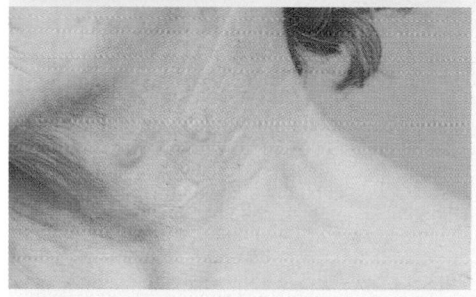

(d)

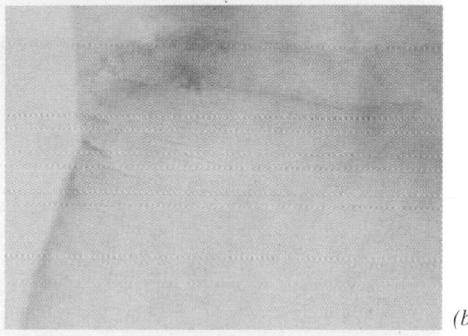

(b)

**Plate 10** *cont.* *(c)* multiple juvenile xanthogranulomata (see Reference 110, Chapter 7) (Courtesy of Dr G. Auckland); *(d)* diffuse planar xanthomata typically found on neck and often associated with myeloma (see Reference 357, Chapter 11)

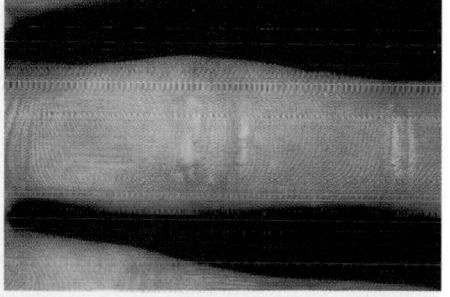

(c)

**Plate 12** Striate palmar xanthomata (type III hyperlipoproteinaemia) (Courtesy of Dr G. Auckland)

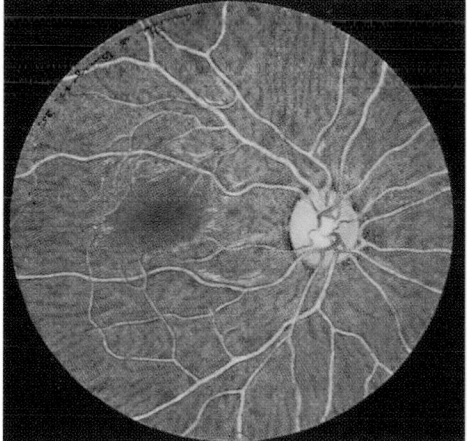

**Plate 11** Lipaemia retinalis (types I and V hyperlipoproteinaemia) (from Holt *et al.* [Reference 62, Chapter 7] by courtesy of *Johns Hopkins Hospital Bulletin)*

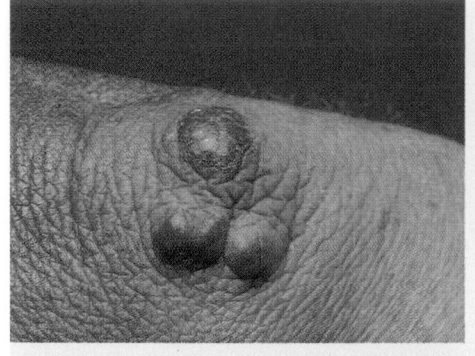

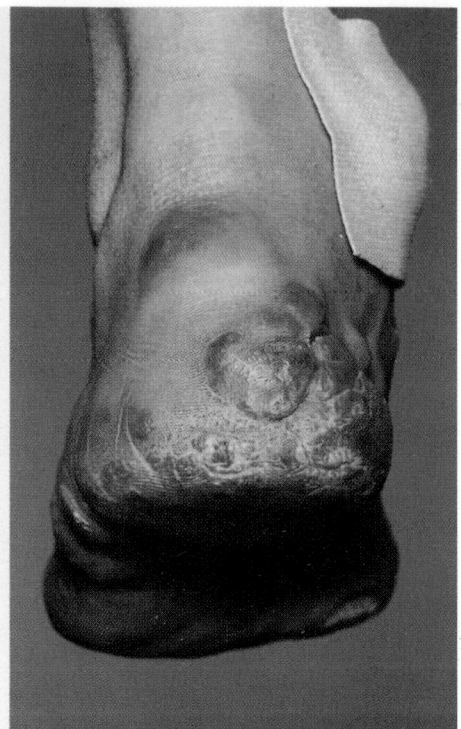

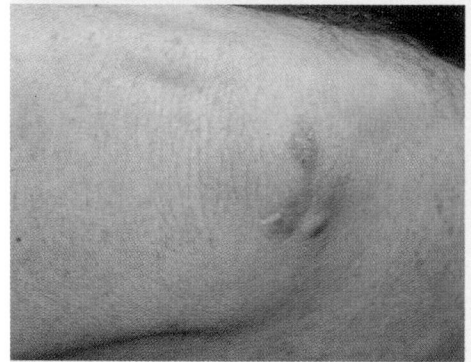

**Plate 13** *(a)* Tuberose xanthomata on the elbow; *(b)* note resolution after 8 months' therapy with diet and fibrate drug (type III hyperlipoproteinaemia)

**Plate 14** Tuberoeruptive xanthomata on heel. Note how their cutaneous location differs from that of an Achilles tendon xanthoma (type III hyperlipoproteinaemia)

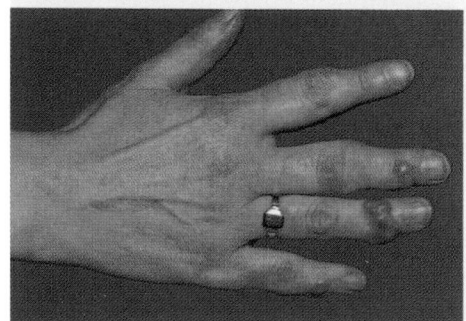

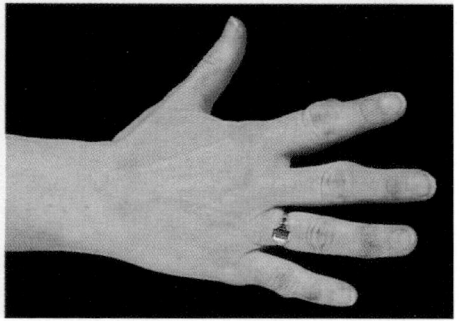

**Plate 15** *(a)* Tuberose xanthomata on knuckles; *(b)* note resolution after 11 months' treatment with diet and a fibrate drug (type III hyperlipoproteinaemia)

in the members of one family who had FH[68]. Heterozygous FH is sufficiently common that it may very occasionally occur in an individual who also has type III hyperlipoproteinaemia. Although the apo E gene is also located on chromosome 19, it is probably too far away for the genetic association to have arisen other than by chance.

## Laboratory diagnosis and phenotypic variation

The average serum cholesterol in adult heterozygotes for FII untreated is around 350 mg/dl (9.00 mmol/l). There is, however, considerable variation so that, exceptionally, in patients in whom the diagnosis is indisputable, serum cholesterol concentrations of only around 270 mg/dl (7.0 mmol/l) may occur. At the other end of the scale, levels of serum cholesterol exceeding 800 mg/dl (20 mmol/l) occasionally occur in patients who are apparently heterozygotes, rather than homozygotes. Generally, however, the serum cholesterol level is higher in homozygotes than heterozygotes and is almost invariably greater than 600 mg/dl (15 mmol/l) extending up to 1200 mg/dl (30 mmol/l). There is remarkably little variation in the average serum cholesterol in homozygotes reported from different countries such as China and Japan compared to the USA and Europe despite the wide variation in the prevalence of the more common types of hypercholesterolaemia in these countries[69]. The nature of the inherited LDL receptor defects is a much more important source of the variation in serum LDL cholesterol. Heterozygotes in societies with low background rates of hypercholesterolaemia do appear to have on average somewhat lower levels of cholesterol than heterozygotes from the USA and Europe. However, it is not known for certain whether this reflects a preponderance of mutations which themselves produce less severe hypercholesterolaemia or whether mutational differences are wholly responsible.

The increase in serum cholesterol in both heterozygotes and homozygotes is due to an increase in LDL. The concentration of serum apolipoprotein B is also greatly elevated, generally to levels exceeding 150 mg/dl but sometimes to more than 200 mg/dl even in heterozygotes. The composition of the LDL is altered from normal[18], although it has not been compared with LDL from other diseases giving rise to similar LDL elevations. It is inevitable on the basis of the one gene, one protein dogma, that the changes in LDL composition are a consequence of delayed catabolism due to the LDL receptor defect, but it has also been suggested that the abnormally high levels of Lp(a) frequently found may also contribute[70–73]. There is an increase in the quantity of cholesterol complexed to apolipoprotein B and a decrease in the quantity of triglycerides carried. Lecithin in LDL is less abundant and sphingomyelin more so, although the total quantity of phospholipid relative to both free cholesterol and apolipoprotein B is decreased[18]. In addition to the effect of FH on LDL concentration, it has been widely reported that serum HDL cholesterol tends to be low. It is not certain that in the adult patients studied there was not a bias towards those with ischaemic heart disease, which is, itself, associated with low HDL cholesterol, an effect further exacerbated if patients with FH were being treated with β-adrenoreceptor blocking drugs more often than controls. In children, however, some decrease in HDL levels is found, so that part of the decrease in adults is likely to be due to FH *per se*[50,54,74,75].

It will be evident, from a consideration of the frequency distribution of serum cholesterol levels in the general population, for example in the US and the UK (Chapter 3), that heterozygotes for FH have serum cholesterol and LDL cholesterol concentrations in the same range as the top 5% of the population (i.e. greater than 270 mg/dl or 7.00 mmol/l). Since all of the 1 in 500 heterozygotes present in the population will be in the top 5% of the cholesterol distribution, about 1 in 25 people with serum cholesterol levels greater than 270 mg/dl (7.00 mmol/l) will be heterozygotes for FH.

The FH heterozygotes will have even higher cholesterol levels on average than the rest of the people, with a serum cholesterol concentration exceeding 270 mg/dl (7.00 mmol/l), so that among those with levels over 350 mg/dl (9.00 mmol/l) (the median serum cholesterol in heterozygotes for FH), the majority will be FH heterozygotes. However, between 270 and 350 mg/dl (7.00 and 9.00 mmol/l) the great majority of people, particularly those at the lower end of this range, will not have FH. When tendon xanthomata are clearly present, the identification of patients with FH is easy. In those with higher levels of cholesterol, the diagnosis is also more likely. However, there will be a substantial number of patients whose serum cholesterol is in the appropriate range, but where the diagnosis is in doubt. Many such patients will be in the younger age range, where they may not yet be expected to have developed tendon xanthomata. If they are children, then the finding of high cholesterol makes FH the most likely diagnosis because the other common types of hypercholesterolaemia (polygenic, familial combined see Chapter 6) do not generally make their appearance until the 3rd or 4th decade.

There have been two studies of children with at least one first-degree relative heterozygous for FH[75,76]. In both studies the serum cholesterol was bimodally distributed, as would be expected if the major influence on its concentration was a single dominant gene. In the investigation in the US[75], the frequency distribution curves intersected at about 235 mg/dl (6.00 mmol/l), whereas in the British series[76] this occurred at 265 mg/dl (6.8 mmol/l). The rather lower dividing point in the US population may have been because of the older age of the group studied, there being a tendency for cholesterol to fall during adolescence (Chapter 3), differences in the criteria for diagnosis in the affected relative and differences in environmental and nutritional factors. In boys, the serum cholesterol tends to be lower than in girls and so the tendency to miss the diagnosis of FH is also greater, which is all the more worrying in view of the worse prognosis of boys and thus a greater urgency about instituting treatment in childhood. The author's policy for children of parents heterozygous for FH is to advise dietary modification, if the cholesterol exceeds 240 mg/dl (6.00 mmol/l). Stricter advice about diet should be given if the cholesterol is above 270 mg/dl (7.00 mmol/l) and if this is unsuccessful in reducing the serum cholesterol below 270 mg/dl the use of a bile acid sequestrating agent should be considered. It would be rash completely to reassure parents that their child has not inherited FH unless the serum cholesterol was less than 220 mg/dl (5.5 mmol/l) and it is also wrong to be too dogmatic about the child having inherited the condition unless the cholesterol is greater than 270 mg/dl (7.00 mmol/l).

The age at which the diagnosis of FH can be made by cholesterol determination has received much attention. It is generally agreed that one reason, at least for the particularly high risk of early onset of ischaemic heart disease in FH, is its duration. In both heterozygotes and, of course, homozygotes hypercholesterolaemia is present through childhood, unlike many of the other even more common hypercholesterolaemias, which very often do not make their appearance until the 3rd decade. It seems logical therefore that treatment will be most effective in preventing coronary atheroma if it is begun in childhood, especially in boys. There seems, however, little point in attempting to diagnose heterozygous FH before the age of 2 on the purely pragmatic grounds that it would be extraordinarily difficult to impose dietary treatment and certainly, before that age, drug treatment. It has been suggested that, when one parent is known to be affected, offspring with FH can be identified by cholesterol, or better LDL–cholesterol, determination in umbilical cord blood[74]. Against this, the identification of heterozygotes in the general population by cholesterol measurement in cord blood or blood taken even up to 1 year of age, proved impossible[77,78]. This is because of the relatively low LDL concentration, so that variations in HDL cholesterol have more impact on the total cholesterol level. When both parents are heterozygotes and there is thus the possibility that the baby may be a homozygote, there is a more urgent reason for diagnosis, because manifestations of coronary disease have been reported as early as the age of 2 in homozygotes. Total and, if possible LDL, cholesterol should thus be monitored regularly from 4 months when homozygous FH is considered a possibility[18].

It is possible to make the diagnosis of homozygous FH prenatally by culturing amniotic fluid cells and examining them for inability to degrade LDL[79]. This permitted the termination after 20 weeks' gestation of a homozygous fetus. There would, of course, be no justification for the therapeutic abortion of a fetus believed to be a heterozygote and it is unlikely that a method such as this could reliably identify a heterozygous fetus.

Receptor assay in cultured fibroblasts may be helpful in confirming the diagnosis of receptor negative homozygous FH at any age. It may also be helpful in many patients with receptor defective homozygous FH, although the decision as to whether such a child is a severe heterozygote or a receptor-defective homozygote may occasionally be impossible unless clinical criteria are employed. A major area of diagnostic imprecision is in deciding whether a patient is heterozygous for FH or has one of the more common forms of hypercholesterolaemia such as polygenic hypercholesterolaemia or familial combined hypercholesterolaemia. Receptor assays of cultured fibroblasts or more conveniently incubated blood mononuclear cells have not proved valuable since they all produced at least some overlap between the FH population and the non-FH population, which because of the enormous size of the non-FH population would lead to an unacceptably high frequency of false positives.

The possibility of discovering a genetic marker for FH which would allow the identification of heterozygotes has been considered. Using radiolabelled probes to the DNA of the receptor gene and restriction enzymes (endonucleases), mutations and polymorphisms within or adjacent to the receptor gene which would act as a marker for FH have been sought. In some families it has proved possible to identify affected individuals[80,81], but for any single restriction-fragment length polymorphism (RFLP) such families are sufficiently infrequent as to make the test of very limited value in the diagnosis of unrelated individuals. The explanation for this lies in the large number of different genetic mutations affecting the genes regulating the LDL receptor activity which produce the clinical syndrome of FH (pages 109–110) and thus there may be a large range of different polymorphisms linked with them. Thus, unless some proved common, even testing for multiple RFLPs would only prove helpful in a limited number of families. The possibility that some RFLPs might indicate a worse prognosis, however, remains to be adequately tested and this might, for example, prove useful in deciding how rigorously treatment should be pursued in childhood and for which older patients more drastic procedures such as partial ileal bypass should be considered.

In patients with a raised serum cholesterol level and tendon xanthomata, the diagnosis of FH is beyond dispute. In young children too in whom the serum cholesterol is obviously elevated the diagnosis is extremely likely because of the rarity at that age of other types of hypercholesterolaemia. There is, however, a difficult period from adolescence when tendon xanthomata may not yet have developed and other types of hypercholesterolaemia are becoming increasingly prevalent. It is very hard to know what proportion of heterozygotes for FH go through life without developing tendon xanthomata. The prevalence of xanthomata among heterozygotes does appear to increase at least until the end of the 5th decade. Available data also suggest that by the time of death some 20% of heterozygotes may not have developed tendon xanthomata[29,75,82]. However, since we rely on the presence of tendon xanthomata in at least one family member to make the diagnosis in other members of the family, we really cannot say whether there are families in whom the tendency to express xanthomata is less, but precocious coronary disease may nevertheless still feature.

For many clinical purposes the certain diagnosis of FH is not essential. For example, few would argue with the decision to give cholesterol-lowering medication to a young male patient with a serum cholesterol of 360 mg/dl (9 mmol/l) unresponsive to diet, even if a definite diagnosis of FH could not be made. The higher the serum cholesterol and the more unresponsive to diet, the more likely is the patient to have FH. The difficulty comes with patients with lower levels of cholesterol. However, even in that group most patients with FH will receive treatment if the presence of a family history of ischaemic heart disease early in life is regarded as an important indication favouring drug therapy in patients unresponsive to diet. It should be realized, however, that the family history can be misleading in the diagnosis of FH. It is not uncommon, for example, to find a middle-aged man presenting with angina or myocardial infarction, hypercholesterolaemia and tendon xanthomata, both of whose parents are alive and well with no symptoms of ischaemic heart disease. The affected parent almost invariably turns out to be the mother. A glance at Table 5.1 reveals the explanation for this: women who are heterozygotes for FH frequently live to their seventies or beyond without symptoms of ischaemic heart disease. On other occasions there may be a family history of premature death, but this is stated not to be due to a cardiac cause. For example, death of a father by drowning, a car accident or while undergoing a surgical operation should be viewed with suspicion, because it may indicate death due to an undiagnosed coronary thrombosis. In a series of 463 definite heterozygotes for FH collected for the Simon Broome register in Britain, 60% did not give a history of myocardial infarction in either parent before the age of 65 years[83]. The most common reasons for this are likely to be inheritance from a mother who has been spared CHD or an affected natural parent who is not the legal parent. It is also possible that the receptor defect is not penetrant in the affected parent.

In the USA and Europe it is probably uncommon for the LDL receptor defect not to be sufficiently penetrant to produce some manifestation of FH, usually hypercholesterolaemia. Almost invariably homozygous FH will be penetrant, usually in childhood producing the full clinical syndrome. Probably also the great majority of heterozygotes will at some stage of their lives develop xanthomata. Many, particularly women, will not manifest CHD. Some families appear to be more resistant to CHD in both men and women Perhaps they have other genetic factors protective against CHD or an absence of acquired cardiovascular risk factors as has been discussed previously (page 115). However, in societies subsisting on low energy diets expression of the FH syndrome may be impeded. There have also been other albeit rare situations described in which the rise in LDL does not occur even on Western diets. For example, the coinheritance of lipoprotein lipase deficiency[84] or of hypobetalipoproteinaemia (Chapter 12, page 370)[85] and of another as yet unidentified dominant genetic factor[86].

A relatively mild defect in LDL catabolism in both parents of twins with severe hypercholesterolaemia due to a more major decrease in the catabolism of LDL has also been reported. One parent had normal cholesterol levels and in the other these were only modestly elevated and it was suggested that the coinheritance of two relatively minor defects in LDL clearance could therefore occasionally produce a major defect[87].

In epidemiological studies and particularly in trials of lipid-lowering drugs, it is important to establish whether the study group consists of patients with FH or not because of the poorer prognosis in FH compared with many other types of hypercholesterolaemia and because of the relative unresponsiveness of patients with FH to lipid-lowering medication. Simply describing patients as having type IIa or even type IIa with a family history of early onset ischaemic heart disease is inadequate, because many such patients actually have polygenic hypercholesterolaemia or familial combined hyperlipidaemia, both of which respond better to, for example, fibrate drugs than do heterozygotes for FH. Wherever possible, the criteria of the Simon Broome register should be adopted for the diagnosis of FH:

DEFINITIVE FAMILIAL HYPERCHOLESTEROLAEMIA is defined as

(a) Cholesterol level above 260 mg/dl (6.7 mmol/l) in children under 16 or 290 mg/dl (7.5 mmol/l) in an adult

*or*

    LDL level above 190 mg/dl (4.9 mmol/l) in adults.

PLUS

(b) Tendon xanthomas in patient or in first- or second-degree relative.

POSSIBLE FAMILIAL HYPERCHOLESTEROLAEMIA is defined as

(a) Cholesterol level above 260 mg/dl (6.7 mmol/l) in children under 16 or 290 mg/dl (7.5 mmol/l) in an adult

*or*

    LDL level above 190 mg/dl (4.9 mmol/l) in adults.

PLUS ONE OF (c) or (d)

(c) Family history of myocardial infarction below age of 50 in second-degree relative or below age of 60 in first-degree relative.

(d) Family history of raised cholesterol levels above 290 mg/dl (7.5 mmol/l) in first or second-degree relative).

## Serum lipoprotein (a) in FH

It was first suggested in 1986 that serum lipoprotein (a) levels might be high in familial hypercholesterolaemia[70]. Subsequently this was confirmed in three studies of FH heterozygotes[71–73]. A possible explanation for this might be that high serum Lp(a) levels increased the likelihood of the expression of xanthomata or CHD in FH so that cases presenting to clinics with high serum Lp(a) were more frequent. Two pieces of evidence tend to discount this possibility. First, it was shown that the elevation of Lp(a) in FH was independent of the apolipoprotein(a) genotype so that the effect could not be explained by a tendency for clinically identified cases of FH to have smaller molecular weight apolipoprotein (a) which is associated with higher serum lipoprotein (a) levels[71,78]. Secondly, when FH patients were compared with their unaffected siblings there was still a two- to three-fold increase in the serum lipoprotein(a) concentration in those with FH[73]. Another possibility was that the increase in serum lipoprotein(a) was secondary to the elevation in serum LDL. Evidence against this was, however, provided by comparing FH heterozygotes with patients with similar increases in serum LDL cholesterol due to other primary causes when it was found that only in the FH heterozygotes were the serum Lp(a) levels increased[73]. It thus appears most likely that the increase in serum Lp(a) in FH is due to the inheritance of the LDL receptor defect. A contrary finding was that in one large FH kindred no difference in the serum Lp(a) concentration was observed between family members affected and unaffected by FH[89]. It is hard to draw any firm conclusion from this because all the observations were made in closely related individuals and the family in which first-cousin marriages was the rule may have been exceptional in its resistance to the effects of the LDL receptor defect on serum Lp(a) levels. Also it has not been adequately emphasized that the family originated in the Indian subcontinent and our own observations amongst normal Indians living in the same area in Britain indicate higher serum Lp(a) levels than in Europids and thus presumably different regulation of serum Lp(a) levels.

If inheritance of the LDL receptor defect does increase serum Lp(a), this might suggest that catabolism of Lp(a) via the LDL receptor makes a considerable contribution to its serum concentration. However, this has not been confirmed either in studies in normal controls or FH An alternative explanation might be that secretion of Lp(a) is increased in FH Interestingly, kinetic studies have shown that there is direct hepatic secretion of LDL without a VLDL precursor in FH (page 110) and Lp(a) is itself known to be directly secreted without a VLDL precursor.

One other factor which may have a more significant impact in regulating serum Lp(a) in FH is apo E. In normal people the apo E phenotype has little impact on serum Lp(a) levels. However, in our clinic FH heterozygotes with the highest levels of Lp(a) have the $E_{3/4}$ phenotype and those with the lowest levels have the $E_{2/2}$ or $E_{2/3}$ phenotype. Intermediate levels are seen in $E_{3/3}$ and $E_{2/4}$ phenotypes (Table 5.2). A possible explanation is that hepatic IDL uptake may be lowest in patients with the apo $E_2$ isoform and as a consequence they may have lower intrahepatic cholesterol levels than those possessing other apo E isoforms. Serum Lp(a) secretion may be boosted by high intrahepatic cholesterol concentration.

In two studies serum Lp(a) was higher in FH heterozygotes with manifest CHD[71,72,88], whereas in the other no difference was observed[73]. This may have been because of a high prevalence of subclinical CHD in the latter study and

**Table 5.2 Serum concentration of lipoprotein (a) (Lp(a)) in 170 heterozygotes for familial hypercholesterolaemia subdivided by apolipoprotein E isoform expression**

| | | Apolipoprotein E phenotype | | | |
| | 2/2 | 2/3 | 3/3 | 2/4 | 3/4 |
| --- | --- | --- | --- | --- | --- |
| n | 1 | 16 | 113 | 8 | 32 |
| Serum Lp(a) (mg/dl) | 6.0 | 18.2 | 28.0 | 29.9 | 33.5 |

*Source*: Bhatnagar, Weiringa, Durrington, MBewu, Mackness, Miller, unpublished observation

illustrates the difficulty of drawing conclusions about serum Lp(a) and its relationship to CHD without prospective data. Serum Lp(a) levels may well rise at some critical point in the development of CHD, because in non-FH patients with CHD it has been shown that the serum Lp(a) concentration is greater than would have been anticipated from the apo(a) genotype (Chapter 12, page 364). Indeed, this may be the explanation for the high serum Lp(a) levels in FH populations. This does not mean it is without clinical utility, if it indicates the presence of significant coronary disease at a stage before it is clinically evident, but this must await confirmation.

## Management

All patients with FH should be advised to keep to a diet which is low in saturated fat (Chapter 9) and to maintain their body weight close to the ideal (Chapter 11). It seems reasonable too that they should also attempt to reduce the amount of cholesterol in their diet (Chapter 9). Many young, lean, physically active people with FH will find it difficult to maintain their body weight if they genuinely do reduce their dietary saturated fat, and they will need to alter their eating habits to include foods rich in carbohydrate and mono-unsaturated and polyunsaturated fats (olive oil, sunflower oil, safflower oil, corn oil and fatty fish). It must be realized, however, that it would be unusual for dietary therapy alone to lower the serum cholesterol to the normal range in FH. Usually a decrease of about 40 mg/dl (1 mmol/l) is achieved. Thus a patient whose serum cholesterol is initially 400 mg/dl (10 mmol/l) will still have some way to go. In children where parents do impose such a diet, greater decreases in serum cholesterol are often achieved and such treatment alone may be possible. With advancing age, however, diet alone becomes less adequate.

The modes of action of drugs used to lower serum LDL in FH are discussed in Chapter 10. There is evidence that lipid-lowering drugs, when used to produce effective reductions in serum LDL cholesterol, can not only impede the progress of coronary atherosclerosis in heterozygous FH but may also produce regression[90].

In 1989 when the first edition of this book was published, the most effective and the first-line drugs for heterozygous FH were the bile-acid sequestrating agents cholestyramine and colestipol. The data in Table 5.3 from the Simon Broome register collected during the time that such treatment was the rule show that whatever its merits as far as CHD prevention were concerned, it did not cause an increase in non-CHD deaths[83].

**Table 5.3 Deaths in 526 men and women with definite familial hypercholesterolaemia followed for an average of 4.2 years during which most received lipid-lowering drugs compared to the expected deaths in the general population of similar age and sex composition**

|  | Observed | Expected |
|---|---|---|
| All deaths | 24 | 13.1 |
| CHD deaths | 15 | 3.88 |
| Non-CHD deaths | 9 | 9.22 |

Data from reference[83]

The introduction of HMG-CoA reductase (Chapter 10) in the intervening years is undoubtedly a major therapeutic advance in the management of heterozygous FH[91–94]. Although bile-acid sequestrants can produce substantial decreases in serum LDL in patients who can tolerate them[95] (Figure 5.3) such patients are exceptional. A glance through notes of patients at our Lipid Clinic reveals that the majority of patients with FH were inadequately treated before the introduction of HMG-CoA reductase inhibitors. These have proved to be well tolerated and effective in lowering serum LDL, usually by around 30–40%. Very few patients in our clinic have continued on the regimen of six or even more sachets of bile-acid sequestrating agents previously employed. Most have reduced the dose of bile-acid sequestrating agents to two sachets before breakfast and an evening dose of the HMG-CoA reductase inhibitor or have stopped the bile-acid sequestrating agent altogether in favour of HMG-CoA reductase inhibitor therapy alone. The use of other agents such as fibric acid derivatives, probucol or nicotinic is now unusual.

HMG-CoA reductase inhibitors have, of course, only been in clinical use for a relatively short period of time and so there are as yet no data concerning their long-term safety. I still, therefore, tend to limit their use to patients whose CHD risk is greatest and often spare the dose of HMG-reductase inhibitor by commencing treatment by introducing a bile-acid sequestrating agent in a dose of two sachets before breakfast before commencing the HMG-CoA reductase in the evening. The logic of this is to attempt to reduce the dose of HMG-CoA reductase inhibitor by combining its use with that of a bile-acid sequestrating agent with which it may synergize in lowering serum LDL cholesterol[92]. Such a policy is not sensible in patients who are already on complicated treatment regimens for established CHD or who may be alienated by unnecessarily complicated or unpleasant treatment. Increasingly, too, even patients who were prepared to use combined bile-acid sequestrating agents and HMG-CoA reductase therapy are asking to discontinue the sequestrating agent. A complication of the HMG-CoA reductase inhibitor therapy encountered in a small percentage of patients, particularly in the early trials and soon after the introduction of lovastatin, was myositis. This is more likely to occur in combination with fibric acid derivatives or cyclosporin, but can occasionally occur spontaneously. It is usual therefore to monitor the serum creatinine kinase activity after the introduction of HMG-CoA reductase therapy and with increases in dose and to avoid combination with fibrates. It is important to remember that excursions of serum creatinine kinase activity up to three times or even more of the upper limit of normal

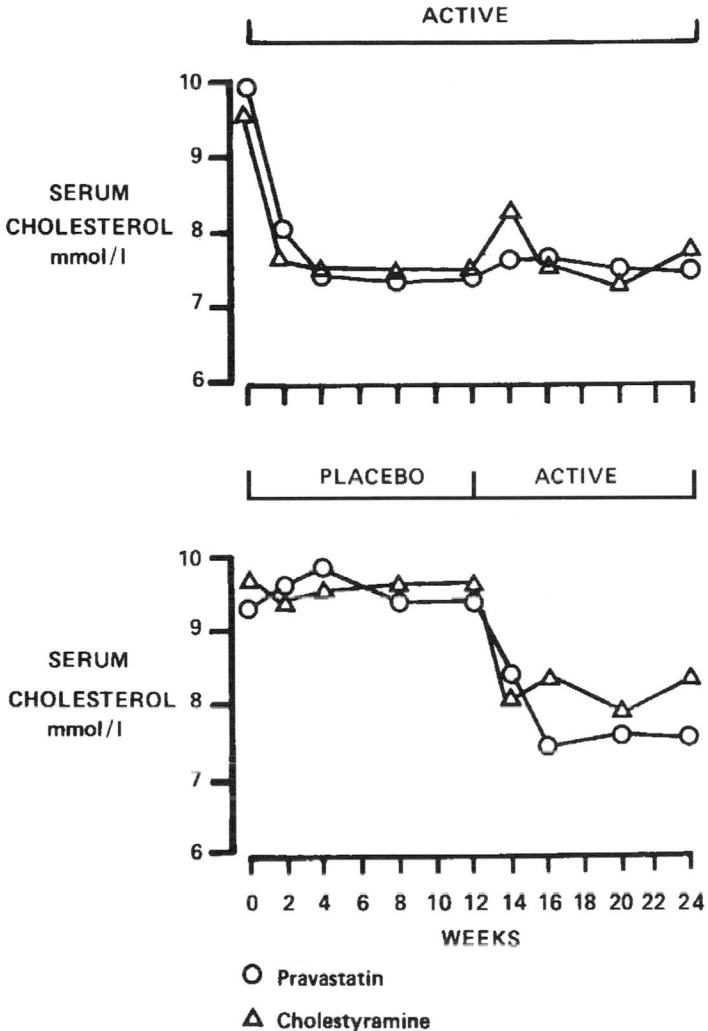

**Figure 5.3**  *Upper panel*: The response to cholestyramine four sachets or to pravastatin 40 mg daily for 24 weeks in patients with heterozygous FH who were compliant with cholestyramine. *Lower panel*: at 12 weeks a parallel placebo group were randomized to either pravastatin or cholestyramine and showed the same response as those on the active therapies from the outset (data from Ref. 95)

for hospital laboratories are not uncommon in ambulant populations and our observations in untreated FH heterozygotes[96] suggest that whilst this may be associated with unusual physical exercise or overindulgence in alcohol, more often than not no explanation is forthcoming. Often inexperienced clinicians stop HMG-CoA reductase therapy because of small asymptomatic apparent increases in serum creatinine kinase activity when it is more appropriate to monitor the levels closely for a while to establish that the increase was spontaneous rather than drug-induced.

It is also important not to confuse myositis induced by HMG-CoA reductase inhibitor therapy with the acute tenosynositis which can follow its introduction in FH. This may be confined to the Achilles tendons, but can be more generalized affecting, for example, tendons in the forearms in which xanthomata were not clinically evident. It is transient, responds to non-steroidal anti-inflammatory drugs and is probably due to the mobilization of deposits of cholesterol in tendons when a marked decrease in LDL cholesterol has occurred. Sometimes a temporary reduction in the dose of HMG-CoA reductase inhibitor is necessary. It also occurs after partial ileal bypass surgery (page 130).

There are certain groups of heterozygotes for FH in whom it is not possible to justify the use of HMG-CoA reductase therapy until more information is available about long-term safety. These include children and younger women. The decision not to use an HMG-CoA reductase inhibitor generally means that the serum cholesterol will remain largely untreated and there can be no hard and fast rule as to when a more effective decrease in cholesterol becomes necessary. It is hardly ever justified to employ drug therapy other than bile-acid sequestrating agents in heterozygous children and even then these would only rarely be justified until the age of 10. In general the family history can be helpful in planning therapy. Thus in boys from families in whom the male members have developed coronary disease particularly early in their twenties or thirties, or female relatives before their menopause, HMG-CoA reductase therapy might be introduced in the middle to late teens. In women HMG-CoA reductase therapy should not be prescribed if there is a possibility of pregnancy and the personal risk of vascular disease would rarely justify their use before the mid-thirties and often not until considerably later or even at all, for example in some women who present late in life without any evidence of CHD. Clearly any woman with FH who does have CHD demands effective drug therapy, as do women whose family history is particularly adverse, for example whose mother developed CHD in her thirties or early forties. Where she has inherited the condition from her father an estimate of the age when she may develop CHD can be made by adding 9 years on to the age when he developed the symptoms. A small number of patients with heterozygous FH are genuinely resistant both to bile-acid sequestrating agents and to HMG-CoA reductase inhibitors[97]. These are rare. Presumably in them hepatic cholesterol biosynthesis must be occurring at such a low rate that boosting it by depleting the bile salt pool or inhibiting it produces insufficient decrease in the hepatocellular cholesterol concentration for any significant increase in hepatic LDL receptor expression to occur.

When bile-acid sequestrating agents are to be used it is essential that the physician explains fully the reasons for using such inconvenient drugs and does so with conviction. It is essential that they be introduced gradually, so that the bloating and dyspepsia that they often produce initially is overcome and that time is taken to explain how the ritual of taking them can easily be fitted into a busy life, as discussed in Chapter 10. A few patients can tolerate six or even eight sachets daily. As has been discussed it is becoming common to settle for two sachets in the morning and accept a rather limited therapeutic response in children and younger women and in other groups of patients to use this dose with HMG-CoA reductase inhibitor therapy. Many find they cannot manage six sachets daily, but will take a lower dose regularly. The serum cholesterol response is an excellent guide to compliance with bile-acid sequestrants. Some authors speak of patients whose hypercholesterolaemia is resistant to bile-acid sequestrating agents. True metabolic resistance is a rare event, as is testified by our experience of admitting patients who have not responded as outpatients to a metabolic ward where administration drug is supervised. The nicest and most plausible people, whose cholesterol has not fallen despite their assurance that they are taking the full dose of bile-acid sequestrant, often show a perfectly adequate response on the ward.

Another highly effective agent to combine with bile-acid sequestrants is nicotinic acid[43,98]. Again, it may be reasonably effective on its own. However, its use is severely limited by its side-effects which almost invariably occur (in patients who actually take it!). The worst of these is an unpleasant flushing. This is prostaglandin mediated and can be overcome to some extent by taking aspirin a short while before the nicotinic acid. Attempts have also been made to formulate nicotinic acid or to modify its structure in such a way that less variable plasma levels occur. These have led to a bewildering array of preparations. Unfortunately, the effect of many of these is simply to make the onset of the flushing more unpredictable than with the parent compound. At least if it occurs at a predictable time some patients can arrange to endure it privately in their own home. All too frequently the clinical circumstances in which nicotinic acid or its derivatives need to be considered is for the patient who has already found bile acid sequestrant therapy too much. That type of patient is thus unlikely to be tolerant of them and that unfortunately is the major practical obstacle to their use.

Other second-line agents are the fibrate drugs and probucol (Chapter 10). The fibrate drugs offer the potential advantage that clofibrate and bezafibrate often decrease, at least, serum fibrinogen (which is often raised in adult FH heterozygotes) and they all tend to increase serum HDL cholesterol. At one centre where serum fibrinogen is regularly measured, bezafibrate is given with cholestyramine for this reason[57]. On the other hand, fibrate drugs are much more effective at lowering triglycerides than cholesterol and may occasionally fail to have any effect on the serum cholesterol in FH. Perhaps the best type of FH patient to receive therapy with a fibrate is the unusual person who also has an increase in the triglycerides before treatment with a bile acid sequestrating agent or, more commonly, those whose triglycerides show a tendency to rise while on such treatment. In the occasional patient, particularly younger women, they may effectively lower cholesterol even when used alone. Uncertainties about the treatment's effect on the conceptus, however, limit their use in that group of patients. It should at all times be remembered that they must never be initiated in patients on anticoagulant therapy, except under the strictest supervision, or disastrous haemorrhage may result.

Probucol does sometimes effectively lower LDL cholesterol (Figure 5.4), although again this seems to be most often in younger women, in whom it should be regarded as contraindicated if there is any possibility of pregnancy, because not only are its effects on the conceptus unknown, but also it persists in the tissues for several months after it is discontinued. It is less well tolerated than the fibrate drugs, producing diarrhoea in a significant proportion of patients. Probucol also lowers serum HDL levels[99] and this is perhaps the major reason why its use has remained limited. However, this effect is less when it is used in combination with cholestyramine (Table 10.2). However, recently two (possibly linked) findings have emerged, which suggest that we should perhaps consider it more often in the management of FH. First, it decreased the size not only of xanthelasmata (Plate 6), but also tendon xanthomata[44] more impressively than other drugs. Secondly, LDL from patients receiving treatment with probucol has been shown to be resistant to oxidation, for example when incubated with copper or endothelial cells, so

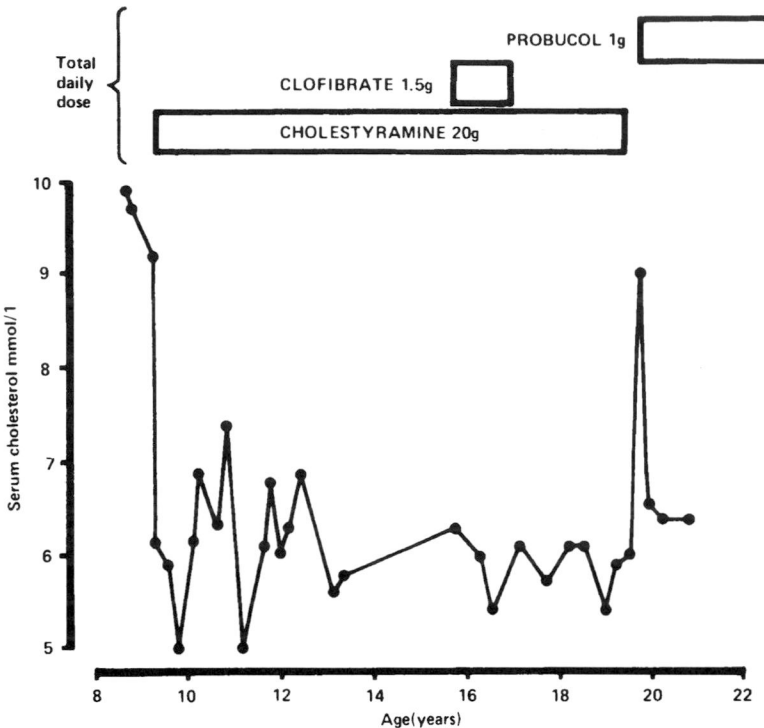

**Figure 5.4**   Miss K. B. was discovered to have hypercholesterolaemia at the age of 8 years. Her father had been discovered to have familial hypercholesterolaemia after a myocardial infarction when he was 28 years old. She was treated with cholestyramine 20 g daily in divided doses. At the age of 20, she took part in a placebo-control trial of probucol. The serum cholesterol rose while on placebo, but responded to probucol 500 mg b.d. (1 mmol/l = 39 mg/dl)

that it is not taken up by cultured macrophages to form foam cells, as is the case with LDL from patients not on probucol treated similarly[100]. In animal models it impedes the development of atherogenesis[101], but it has effects on reverse cholesterol transport in man which may be deleterious[102] (see Chapter 10).

In children who are heterozygotes for FH, long-term safety data do not really permit the use of any cholesterol-lowering medication other than cholestyramine or colestipol[103]. These agents effectively lower serum LDL cholesterol in children and do not appear to interfere with growth or development. There is some evidence to suggest that better compliance is achieved if treatment is instituted before the age of 10[103]. Parental attitudes are also important in that respect and the physician must ensure that adequate discussion has taken place with the surviving parent or parents before instituting bile-acid sequestrant therapy. Folate supplements should probably be given to children receiving such treatment[104].

Children who are homozygotes for FH do not usually respond well to bile-acid sequestrants or HMG-CoA reductase inhibitors (as would be expected if these agents act by increasing receptor expression[105]) or to fibrate drugs. There are reports that probucol may sometimes be useful[106]. Because of the diversity of mutations of the LDL receptor and because most homozygotes are actually mixed heterozygotes in the sense that they have different mutations affecting each of their LDL receptor genes, it is impossible to be certain of whether there will be any response and generally the whole range of cholesterol-lowering drugs should be systematically tried. Regular plasmapheresis or LDL apheresis will decrease the average serum LDL concentration (Figure 5.5)[25,107,108] and there is evidence that it may improve survival[53] (Figure 5.6). The most widely employed therapy is any drug therapy that helps to maintain a lower serum cholesterol in combination with LDL apheresis or plasmapheresis. In an 8-year-old patient, whose cardiac function was so compromised by ischaemia that she underwent cardiac transplantation, liver transplantation was also undertaken to provide her with an organ expressing LDL receptor[109]. This treatment was apparently effective and made possible an additional cholesterol reduction in response to an HMG-CoA reductase inhibitor[110]. This improvement has been maintained and liver transplantation has since been used in other patients. Portacaval anastomosis too has been used in the management of FH homozygotes[111–113], but a satisfactory response is not achieved sufficiently frequently to justify its regular use[18]. The hope is that familial hypercholesterolaemia will be one of the first diseases to be successfully treated by gene therapy.

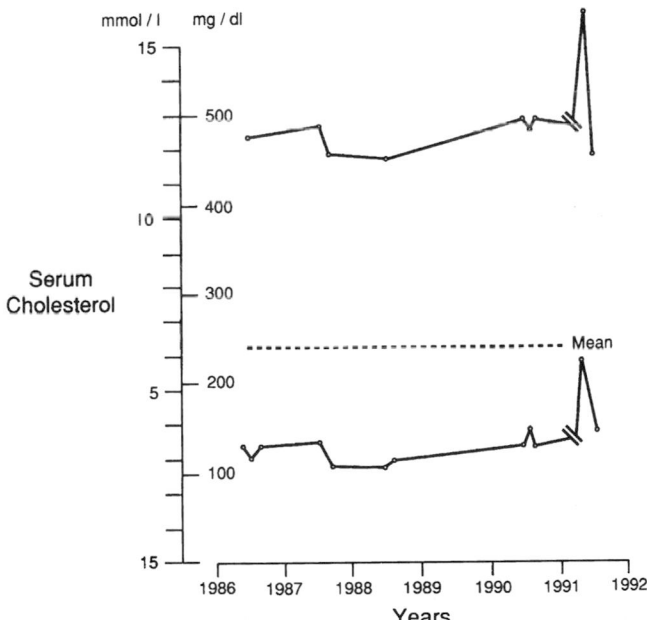

**Figure 5.5**   The effect of plasma pheresis (3.6 litre exchange every two weeks) on homozygote for familial hypercholesterolaemia. The upper continuous line in the serum cholesterol concentration immediately before plasmapheresis and the lower line the level at the end of the procedure. The broken line represents the mean serum cholesterol level on the treatment. In 1991 the patient discontinued plasmapheresis briefly and his cholesterol climbed to almost 20 mmol/l before treatment was recommenced

**Effects of plasma exchange on survival in 5 pairs
of siblings with homozygous FH**

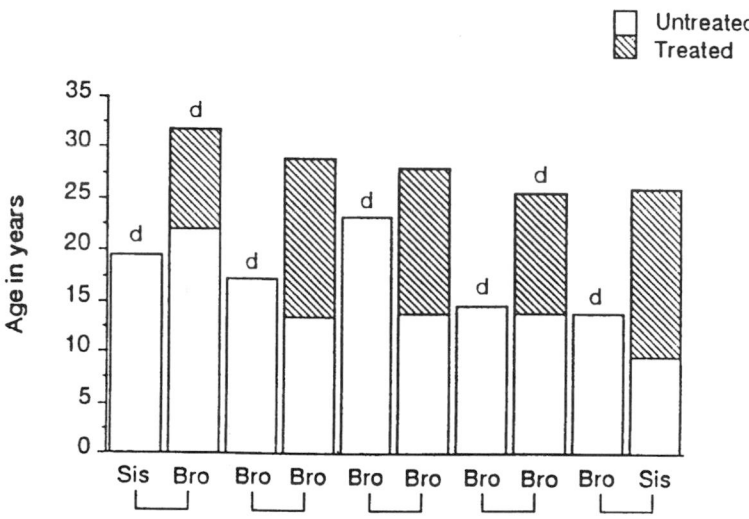

**Figure 5.6**  Comparison of the longevity of five pairs of siblings with homozygous familial hypercholesterolaemia. One of each pair were living when plasmapheresis or LDL apheresis became available (= treated). Their longevity has been compared with that of their sibling who did not receive this form of treatment (= untreated). In each case survival is prolonged by apheresis. **d** = dead. (Data from patients reported in reference [53] brought up to date in 1992 by Dr G.R. Thompson[108].)

The other surgical procedure which has been used in the management of FH is partial ileal bypass. This procedure is unsuitable for homozygotes. Like cholestyramine, it provides a means of interrupting the enterohepatic circulation of bile acids preventing their reabsorption through the terminal ileum[114]. The need for the operation has become much less since the introduction of the HMG-CoA reductase drugs. The operation bypasses the terminal third or 200 cm (whichever is the greater) of the small bowel[115]. The bowel is transected at that point and the proximal part anastomosed to the caecum. After closure of the cut end of the terminal ileum, it is left *in situ*. The operation is usually reserved for patients who are unwilling to take life-long medication. It is important not to undertake it because of failure to respond to cholestyramine, since this might indicate that the operation which relies on a similar diversion of bile acids would also be ineffective. A worthwhile reduction in serum cholesterol with cholestyramine should generally be demonstrated, for example by admission to hospital, in all patients in whom partial ileal bypass is contemplated (Figure 5.7). It is also essential to explain to patients that they will have diarrhoea following the operation. Generally the diarrhoea immediately after surgery abates and an acceptable bowel habit is possible, perhaps aided by codeine or other antidiarrhoeal agents. However, care must be taken in the choice of patient for the operation, otherwise the less stoical character, who has already been unprepared to accept the discomfiture or

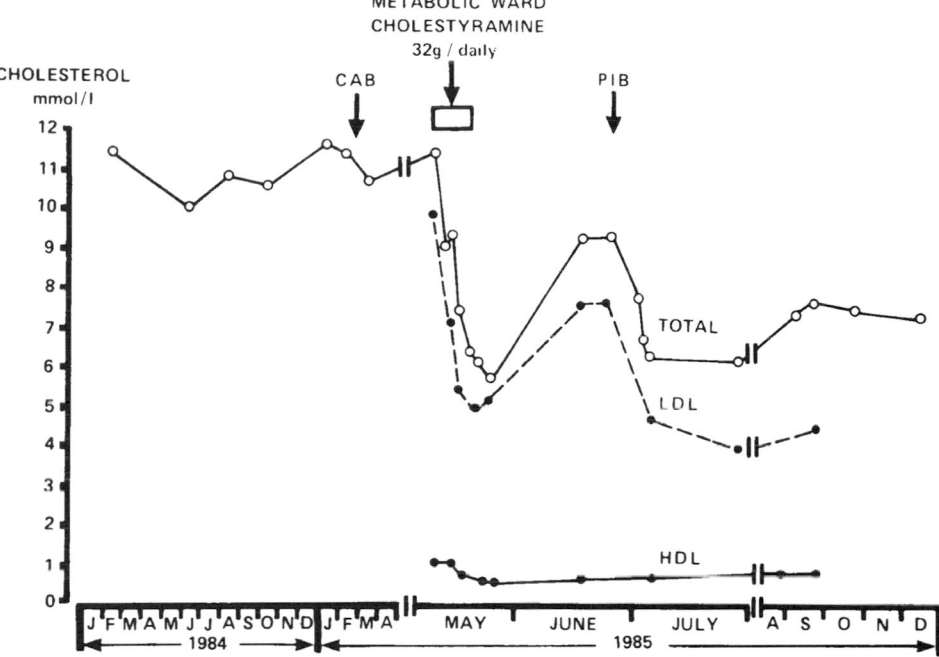

**Figure 5.7**   Mr D. W. presented with angina of effort at the age of 35. Treatment with bile acid sequestrating agents, fibrate drugs, probucol and nicotinic acid was unsuccessful because of non-compliance. Coronary artery bypass surgery (CAB) successfully relieved the angina. Later, it was shown that interruption of the enterohepatic circulation of bile acids would reduce the LDL cholesterol when cholestyramine was administered in hospital. Partial ileal bypass (PIB) surgery was therefore performed (1 mmol/l = 39 mg/dl)

routine imposed by medication, and who may be dissatisfied with the operation, may be offered it. The diarrhoea is of the cholorrhoeic type and may, of course, respond to cholestyramine, but this really defeats the purpose of the operation. Reversal of the surgery is possible. In a series of patients with CHD, but who mostly did not have FH partial ileal bypass produced a dramatic decrease in CHD morbidity and mortality and in the need for coronary artery bypass surgery[116].

Partial ileal bypass should not be confused with jejuno-ileal bypass, which has fallen into disrepute because of its frequent serious side-effects, including chronic liver disease. Partial ileal bypass does, however, create the need for vitamin $B_{12}$ injections and increases the likelihood of cholelithiasis. It may also produce enteropathic arthropathy. The latter should not be confused with tendinitis and periarthritis, which may follow the sudden decrease in LDL cholesterol and presumably mobilization of cholesterol deposits after the operation. A similar phenomenon is sometimes seen following the initiation of treatment with HMG-CoA reductase inhibitor therapy (page 126). A reduction in serum LDL cholesterol of about 30–40% occurs following the operation. There is, however, a tendency for the level to increase, usually over the space of a few years, and this increase is due to an increase in cholesterol biosynthesis. The ideal drugs for restoring lower serum cholesterol levels in these circumstances are the HMG-CoA reductase inhibitors[117]. The place of partial ileal bypass in the management of heterozygous FH is, however, very much dependent on the success of these and other newly developed drugs as primary therapy.

Because of the young average age of patients heterozygous for FH, questions about conception and pregnancy frequently occur. With regard to prevention of conception, my practice is to discourage oral contraception particularly strongly in the older women (Chapter 11). This is not because of its effects on serum lipids, but because it may exaggerate an already increased tendency to thrombosis which may cause myocardial infarction in patients who may have significant coronary atheroma. The absence of pre-existing angina is not likely to be an entirely reliable guide to this latter possibility. Obviously when a women with FH feels she has completed her family, there should be no discouragement to ligation of her uterine tubes (unless her coronary disease is so severe as to constitute a major anaesthetic risk) or to her husband's vasectomy.

Fortunately, genetic counselling in FH is fairly straightforward in countries such as Britain and the USA, where consanguineous marriages are unusual. It may be much more difficult, for example, in other societies. The great majority of heterozygotes will be married to a non-heterozygote and thus each child will have an even chance of being a heterozygote. This is no reason to discourage procreation, since the outlook for an affected child, even if male, is good with effective cholesterol-lowering treatment and with the various plasmacological and surgical advances in the management of coronary disease in recent years and hopefully future years. The worst outlook is for those patients whose physicians remain ignorant of their condition. In the unusual circumstances where a marriage between two heterozygotes has occurred, the risk of a child being a heterozygote is still even, but the risk that it might be a homozygote is 1 in 4. There is also, of course, a 1 in 4 chance that he or she will be normal. However, the risk that a child might be a homozygote is high and the miserable childhood and early demise of individuals so afflicted would argue against producing a large family. The possibility of prenatal diagnosis of homozygous FH does introduce the option of therapeutically aborting such conceptuses[79], so that children born will be either heterozygotes or normal.

## Familial defective apolipoprotein B

The great majority of patients identified clinically as having heterozygous FH have a mutation of one of their LDL receptor genes causing defective LDL catabolism. However, some 2% of patients indistinguishable clinically have impaired LDL catabolism due to a defective binding of their apo $B_{100}$ to normal LDL receptors[38,118], a condition first described by Vega and Grundy in 1986[119,120], although a similar case may have been reported as early as 1975[121]. This is most often due to a point mutation in codon 3500 in which adenine replaces guanine so that glutamine is coded for in place of arginine[122,123]. This condition is termed familial defective apolipoprotein $B_{100}$ 3500(FDB3500). A rarer mutation in codon 3531 has also been described associated with moderate hypercholesterolaemia [124]. This has not yet been reported in association with the full FH syndrome.

$FDB_{100}3500$ has been described in association with the heterozygous FH syndrome including accelerated CHD[118]. However, it has also been found in people and families with only moderate hypercholesterolaemia or with no elevation of serum cholesterol at all and with no clinical manifestations of premature CHD. The frequency of $FDB_{100}3500$ in the general population has been estimated from a survey of 5000 Californian bank employees to be 1 in 1300[125]. It is extremely difficult at the present time to be sure how frequently it is a cause of clinically significant hypercholesterolaemia. In some families it appears to be fully penetrant but in others serum cholesterol is not increased. Thus heterozygous $FDB_{100}3500$ is probably in general less severe in its clinical manifestations than heterozygous FH due defective LDL receptors. The same is also true of homozygous $FDB_{100}3500$. In the cases of this so far described only moderate hypercholesterolaemia has been evident[126,127]. Furthermore in the only case of $FDB_{100}3500$ and FH in the same individual FDB did not appear to make the FH more severe than in other members of the same family affected by FH without $FDB_{100}3500$[128]. In a series of 274 men with premature CHD none had $FDB_{100}3500$[129]. It must be a rare event for it to be sufficiently penetrant to cause CHD. Most of the patients with $FDB_{100}3500$ so far reported have come from screening Lipid Clinic populations and thus they are likely to represent the more severely affected end of the spectrum of $FDB_{100}3500$. The therapeutic response in their serum cholesterol has been similar to that of heterozygous FH so there is no immediate need to distinguish them from patients with FH or common hypercholesterolaemia. They do, however, have certain differences from FH which are of theoretical interest. All cases of $FDB_{100}3500$ have the same genetic mutation, whereas FH is produced by a variety of different LDL receptor mutations – almost 200 at the last count[130] and the number is growing. In FH therefore it is difficult to distinguish whether phenotypic variation is due to variation in the genetic mutation or to the milieu of other genes and acquired factors represented by the individual in whom it is expressed. $FDB_{100}3500$ tells us that even an identical genetic mutation affecting LDL catabolism expressed in different individuals can produce a range of manifestations from none to the complete FH clinical syndrome. Furthermore, it would appear that the clinical diagnosis of the syndrome is more closely associated with CHD risk than the genetic diagnosis. If this is confirmed, it will mean that the detection of genetic mutations associated with CHD itself will not itself be a very reliable guide as to individual risk – this will depend on other factors determining susceptibility to CHD in the individual possessing the mutation (a bit like the interpretation of the serum cholesterol!). Thus the identification of the genetic mutation in hyperlipidaemia will only be clinically relevant if the prognosis of the syndrome with which it is associated is judged to be so severe that gene therapy is contemplated.

FDP is also of theoretical interest in another context. In FH the LDL receptor is defective and this must interfere to some extent with LDL uptake of apo E-rich lipoproteins such as IDL. In many patients with FH therefore, in addition to the increased LDL, there is also some increase in IDL (obviously not to the same extent as in type III hyperlipoproteinaemia – because the remnant receptors for IDL are functioning and because apo E may still bind to mutant receptors better than apo $B_{100}$). In FDB only lipoproteins dependent on apo $B_{100}$ for receptor binding would be expected to accumulate in the circulation and thus serum LDL alone should be elevated if current theories about the clearance of apo E-containing lipoproteins are correct. Serum LDL does indeed appear to be the sole apolipoprotein which is increased in FDB[131].

# References

1. Fagge, C. H. General xanthelasma on vitiligoidea. *Trans. Path. Soc. Lond.*, **24**, 242–250 (1873)
2. Jensen, J. The story of xanthomatosis in England prior to the First World War. *Clio. Medica*, **2**, 289 305 (1967)

3. Ranking, W. H. Case of vitilogoidea with remarks. *Lancet*, **i**, 172–173 (1853)
4. Burns, F. S. A contribution to the study of the etiology of xanthoma. *Arch. Derm. Syph.*, **2**, 415–429 (1920)
5. Muller, C. Angina pectoris in hereditary xanthomatosis. *Arch. Int. Med.*, **64**, 675–700 (1939)
6. Thannhauser, S. J. and Magendanta, H. The different clinical groups of xanthomatous diseases: a clinical physiological study of 22 cases. *Ann. Intern. Med.*, **11**, 1662–1746 (1938)
7. Kachadurian, A. K. The inheritance of essential familial hypercholesterolaemia. *Am. J. Med.*, **37**, 402–407 (1964)
8. Gofman, J. W., De Lalla, O., Glazier, F., Freeman, N. K., Lindgren, F. T. *et al.* The serum lipoprotein transport system in health, metabolic diseases, atherosclerosis and coronary artery disease. *Plasma*, **2**, 413–484 (1954)
9. Langer, T., Strober, W. and Levy, R. I. The metabolism of low density lipoprotein in familial type II hyperlipoproteinaemia. *J. Clin. Invest.*, **51**, 1528–1536 (1972)
10. Goldstein, J. L. and Brown, M. S. Familial hypercholesterolaemia: identification of a defect in the regulation of 3-hydroxy-3-methylglutaryl coenzyme A reductase activity associated with overproduction of cholesterol. *Proc. Natl. Acad. Sci. USA*, **70**, 2804–2808 (1973)
11. Shepherd, J., Bicker, S., Lorimer, A. R. and Packard, C. J. Receptor-mediated low density lipoprotein catabolism in man. *J. Lipid Res.*, **20**, 999–1006 (1979)
12. Brown, M. S. and Goldstein, J. L. Receptor-mediated control of cholesterol metabolism. *Science*, **191**, 150–154 (1976)
13. Brown, M. S., Kovanen, P. T. and Goldstein, J. L. Evolution of the LDL receptor concept from cultured cells to intact animals. *Ann. NY Acad. Sci.*, **348**, 48–68 (1980)
14. Goldstein, J. L. and Brown, M. S. The LDL receptor locus and the genetics of familial hypercholesterolaemia. *Ann. Rev. Genet.*, **13**, 259–289 (1979)
15. Thompson, G. R. Familial hypercholesterolaemia: overcoming the metabolic defect. In *Atherosclerosis*, vol. VII (eds N. H. Fidge and P. J. Nestel), Elsevier, Amsterdam, pp. 177–180 (1986)
16. Goldstein, J. L. and Brown, M. S. Progress in understanding the LDL receptor and HMG-CoA reductase, two membrane proteins that regulate the plasma cholesterol. *J. Lipid Res.*, **25**, 1450–1461 (1985)
17. Lehrman, M. A., Schneider, W. J., Sudhof, T. C., Brown, M. S., Goldstein, J. L. and Russell, D. W. Mutation in LDL receptor: Alu-Alu recombination deletes eons encoding transmembrane and cytoplastmic domains. *Science*, **227**, 140–146 (1985)
18. Myant, N. B. Disorders of cholesterol metabolism: the hyperlipoproteinaemias. In *The Biology of Cholesterol and Related Steroids*, Heinemann Medical, London, pp. 689–772 (1981)
19. Simons, L. A., Reichl, D., Myant, N. B. and Mancini, M. The metabolism of the apoprotein of plasma low density lipoprotein in familial hyperbeta lipoproteinaemia in the homozygous form. *Atherosclerosis*, **21**, 283–298 (1975)
20. Packard, C. J., Third, J. L. H. C., Shepherd, J., Lorimer, A. R., Morgan, H. G. and Lawrie, T. D. V. Low density lipoprotein metabolism in a family of familial hypercholesterolaemic patients. *Metabolism*, **25**, 995–1006 (1976)
21. Kesaniemi, Y. A. and Grundy, S. M. Contribution of apoprotein B production rate in the regulation of lipoprotein levels in man. In *Atherosclerosis*, vol. VI (eds F. G. Schettler, A. M. Gotto, G. Middlehoff, A. J. R. Habenicht, and K. R. Jurutka), Springer-Verlag, Berlin, pp. 571–575 (1983)
22. Thompson, G. R., Soutar, A. K., Spengel, F. A., Jadhar, A., Gavigan, S. J. P. and Myant, N. B. Defects of receptor-mediated low density lipoprotein catabolism in homozygous familial hypercholesterolaemia and hypothyroidism *in vivo. Proc. Natl. Acad. Sci. USA*, **78**, 2591–2595 (1981)
23. Thompson, G. R., Spinks, T., Ranicar, A. and Myant, N. B. Non-steady-state studies of low density lipoprotein turnover in familial hypercholesterolaemia. *Clin. Sci. Mol. Med.*, **52**, 361–369 (1977)
24. Soutar, A. K., Myant, N. B. and Thompson, G. R. Simultaneous measurements of apolipoprotein B turnover in very-low and low-density lipoproteins in familial hypercholesterolaemia. *Atherosclerosis*, **28**, 247–256 (1977)
25. Soutar, A. K., Myant, N. B. and Thompson, G. R. Metabolism of apolipoprotein B-containing lipoproteins in familial hypercholesterolaemia. Effects of plasma exchange. *Atherosclerosis*, **32**, 315–325 (1979)

26. Janus, E. D., Nicoll, A., Wootton, R., Turner, P. R., Magill, P. J. and Lewis, B. Quantitative studies of very low density lipoprotein: conversion to low density lipoprotein in normal controls and primary hyperlipidaemic states and the role of direct secretion of low density lipoprotein in heterozygous familial hypercholesterolaemia. *Eur. J. Clin. Invest.*, **10**, 149–159 (1980)

27. Soutar, A. K., Myant, N. B. and Thompson, G. R. The metabolism of very-low-density and intermediate-density lipoproteins in patients with familial hypercholesterolaemia. *Atherosclerosis*, **43**, 217–231 (1982)

28. Myant, N. B. The metabolic basis of familial hypercholesterolaemia. *Klin. Wochenschr.*, **61**, 383–401 (1983)

29. Goldstein, J. L. and Brown, M. S. Familial hypercholesterolaemia. In *The Metabolic Basis of Inherited Disease*, 5th edn (eds J. B. Stanbury, J. B. Wyngaarden, D. S. Fredrickson, J. L. Goldstein and M. S. Brown), McGraw-Hill, New York, pp. 672–712 (1983)

30. Levy, R. A., Osthund, R. E., Goldberg, A. C. and Grundy, S. M. Long-term changes in cholesterol biosynthesis and the effect of plasma pheresis therapy in a hypercholesterolaemia homozygote. *Metabolism*, **35**, 415–418 (1986)

31. Mabuchi, H., Tatami, R., Veda, K., Veda, R., Haba, T. *et al.* Serum lipid and lipoprotein levels in Japanese patients with familial hypercholesterolaemia. *Atherosclerosis*, **32**, 435–444 (1979)

32. Myant, N. B. and Slack, J. Type II hyperlipoproteinaemia. *Clin. Endocrinol. Metabol.*, **2**, 81–109 (1973)

33. Torrington, M. and Botha, J. L. Familial hypercholesterolaemia and church affiliation. *Lancet*, **ii**, 1120 (1981)

34. Moorjani, S., Roy, M., Torres, A., Betard, C., Gagne, C. *et al.* Mutations of low-density-lipoprotein-receptor gene, variation in plasma cholesterol, and expression of coronary heart disease in homozygous familial hypercholesterolaemia. *Lancet*, **341**, 1303–1306 (1993)

35. Meiner, V., Landsberger, D., Berkman, N. *et al.* A common Lithuanian mutation causing familial hypercholesterolaemia in Ashkenazi Jews. *Am. J. Hum. Genet.*, **49**, 443–449 (1991)

36. Hayden, M.R., DeBraekeleer, M., Henderson, H.E. and Kastelein, J. Molecular geography of inherited disorders of lipoprotein metabolism: lipoprotein lipase deficiency and familial hypercholesterolaemia. In *Molecular Genetics of Coronary Artery Disease, Candidate Genes and Processes in Atherosclerosis.* (eds A. J. Lusis, J. I. Rotter and R. S. Sparkes), Karger, Basle, pp. 350–362 (1992)

37. Leitersdorf, E., Van der Westhuyzen, D.R., Coetzee, G.A. and Hobbs, H.H. Two common low density lipoprotein receptor gene mutations cause familial hypercholesterolaemia in Afrikaners. *J. Clin. Invest.*, **84**, 954–961 (1989)

38. Talmud, P., Tjbjaerg-Hansen, A., Bhatnagar, D., MBewu, A., Miller, J.P., Durrington, P. and Humphries, S. Rapid secreening for specific mutations in patients with a clinical diagnosis of familial hypercholesterolaemia. *Atherosclerosis*, **89**, 137–141 (1991)

39. Takahashi, W. and Naito, M. Lipid storage disease: Part 1. Ultrastructure of xanthoma cells in various xanthomatous diseases. *Acta Pathol. Jpn*, **33**, 959–977 (1983)

40. Salen, G., Shekr, S. and Berginer, V. M. Familial diseases with storage of sterols other than cholesterol: cerebrotendinous anthomatosis and sitosterolaemia with xanthomatosis. In *The Metabolic Basis of Inherited Disease*, 5th edn (eds J. B. Stanbury, J. B. Wyngaarden, D. S. Fredrickson, J. L. Goldstein and M. S. Brown), McGraw-Hill, New York, pp. 713–730 (1983)

41. Bhattacharyya, A. K. and Conner, W. E. β-sitosterolaemia and xanthomatosis. *J. Clin. Invest.*, **53**, 1033–1043 (1974)

42. Durrington, P. N., Adams, J. E. and Beastall, M. D. The assessment of Achilles tendon size in primary hypercholesterolaemia by computed tomography. *Atherosclerosis*, **45**, 345–358 (1982)

43. Kane, J. P., Malloy, M. J., Tun, P., Phillips, N. R., Freedman, D. D. *et al.* Normalization of LDL levels in heterozygous familial hypercholesterolaemia with a combined drug regimen. *N. Engl. J. Med.*, **304**, 251–257 (1981)

44. Yamamoto, A., Matsuzawa, Y., Yokoyama, S., Funahashi, T., Yamamura, T. and Kishino, B.-I. Effects of probucol on anthomata regression in familial hypercholeserolaemia. *Am. J. Cardiol.*, **57**, 29H–35H (1986)

45. Slack, J. Risks of ischaemic heart-disease in familial hyperlipoproteinaemia states. *Lancet*, **ii**, 1380–1382 (1969)

46. Bloch, A., Dinsmore, R. E. and Lees, R. S. Coronary arteriographic findings in type-II and type-IV hyperlipoproteinaemia. *Lancet*, **i**, 928–930 (1976)
47. Sugrue, D. D., Thompson, G. R., Oakley, C. M., Traynor, I. M. and Steiner, R. E. Contrasting patterns of coronary atherosclerosis in normocholesterolaemic smokers and patients with familial hypercholesterolaemia. *Br. Med. J.*, **283**, 1358–1360 (1981)
48. Heiberg, A. and Slack, J. Family similarities in the age at coronary death in familial hypercholesterolaemia. *Br. Med. J.*, **ii**, 493–495 (1977)
49. Miettinen, T. H. and Gytling, H. Mortality and cholesterol metabolism in familial hypercholesterolaemia. Long-term follow-up of 96 patients. *Arteriosclerosis*, **8**, 163–167 (1988)
50. Moorjani, S., Gagne, C., Lupien, P. J. and Brunn, D. Plasma triglyceride related decrease in high-density lipoprotein cholesterol and its association with myocardial infarction in heterozygous familial hypercholesterolaemia. *Metabolism*, **35**, 311–316 (1986)
51. Sprecher, D. L., Schaefer, E. J., Kent, K. M. *et al.* Cardiovascular features of homozygous familial hypercholesterolaemia: analysis of 16 patients. *Am. J. Cardiol.*, **54**, 20–30 (1984)
52. West, R., Gibson, P. and Lloyd, J. Treatment of homozygous familial hypercholesterolaemia: an informative sibship. *Br. Med. J.*, **291**, 1079–1080 (1985)
53. Thompson, G. R., Miller, J. P. and Breslow, J. L. Improved survival of patients with homozygous familial hypercholesterolaemia treated with plasma exchange. *Br. Med. J.*, **291**, 1671–1673 (1985)
54. Streja, D., Steiner, G. and Kwiterovich, P. O. Plasma high-density lipoproteins and ischaemic heart disease. Studies in a large kindred with familial hypercholesterolaemia. *Ann. Intern. Med.*, **89**, 871–880 (1978)
55. Hirobe, K., Matsuzawa, Y. and Ishikawa, K. Coronary artery disease in heterozygous familial hypercholesterolaemia. *Atherosclerosis*, **44**, 201–210 (1982)
56. Beaumont, V., Jacotot, B. and Beaumont, J.-L. Ischaemic disease in men and women with familial hypercholesterolaemia and xanthomatosis. A comparative study of genetic and environmental factors in 274 heterozygous cases. *Atherosclerosis*, **24**, 441–450 (1976)
57. Stone, M. C. Personal communication (1987)
58. Allen, J. M., Thompson, G. R., Myant, N. B., Steiner, R. and Oakley, C. M. Cardiovascular complications of homozygous familial hypercholesterolaemia. *Br. Heart J.*, **44**, 361–368 (1980)
59. Heiberg, A. The risk of atherosclerotic vascular disease in subjects with xanthomatosis. *Acta Med. Scand.*, **198**, 249–261 (1975)
60. Ribiero, P., Shapiro., L. M. Gonzalez, A., Thompson, G. R. and Oakley, C. M. Cross-sectional echocardiographic assessment of the aortic root and coronary osteal stenosis in familial hypercholesterolaemia. *Br. Heart J.*, **50**, 432–437 (1983)
61. Kachadurian, A. K. Migratory polyarthritis in familial hypercholesterolaemia (type II hyperlipoproteinaemia). *Arthr. Rheum.*, **11**, 385–393 (1968)
62. Frayha, R. A., Nasr, F. W. and Uthman, S. Synovial fluid findings in a case of familial hypercholesterolaemia. *Leb. Med. J.*, **25**, 435–439 (1972)
63. Glueck, C. J., Levy, R. I. and Fredrickson, D. S. Acute tendinitis and arthritis: a presenting symptom of familial type II hyperlipoproteinaemia. *J. Am. Med. Assoc.*, **206**, 2895–2897 (1968)
64. Rooney, P. J., Third, J., Madkour, M. M., Spencer, D. and Dick, W. C. Transient polyarthritis associated with familial hyperbetalipoproteinaemia. *Q. J. Med.*, **47**, 249–259 (1978)
65. Ott, J., Schrott, H. G., Goldstein, J. L., Hazzard, W. R., Allen, F. H. *et al.* Linkage studies in a large kindred with familial hypercholesterolaemia. *Am. J. Haem. Genet.*, **26**, 598–608 (1974)
66. Berg, K. and Heiberg, A. Linkage studies on familial hyperlipoproteinaemia with xanthomatosis: normal lipoprotein markers and the C3 polymorphism. *Cytogenet. Cell. Genet.*, **16**, 294–297 (1976)
67. Elston, R. C., Namboodini, K. W., Go, R. C. P., Siervogel, R. M. and Glueck, C. J. Probable linkage between essential familial hypercholesterolaemia and third complement component (C3). *Cytogenet. Cell. Genet.*, **16**, 294–297 (1976)
68. Quarfordt, S. H., de Vivo, J. C., Engel, W. K., Levy, R. I. and Fredrickson, D. S. Familial adult-onset proximal spinal muscular atrophy. Report of a family with type II hyperlipoproteinaemia. *Arch. Neurol.*, **22**, 541–549 (1970)
69. Thompson, G.R., Seed, M., Niththyananthan, S., McCarthy, S. and Thorogood, M. Genotypic and phenotypic variation in familial hypercholesterolaemia. *Arteriosclerosis*, **9**(Suppl.), I-76–I-80 (1989)

70. Luc, G., Chapman, M. J., De Gennes, J.-L. and Turpin, G. A study of the structural heterogeneity of low-density lipoproteins in two patients homozygous for familial hypercholesterolaemia, one of phenotype E2/2. *Eur. J. Clin. Invest.*, **16**, 329–337 (1986)

71. Seed, M., Hopplicher, F., Reaveley, D., McCarthy, S., Thompson, G. *et al*. Relation of serum lipoprotein (a) concentration and apolipoprotein (a) phenotype to coronary heart disease in patients with familial hypercholesterolaemia. *N. Engl. J. Med.*, **322**, 1494–1499 (1990)

72. Wiklund, O., Angelin, B., Oloffson, S., Eriksson, M., Fager, G. *et al*. Apolipoprotein (a) and ischaemic heart disease in familial hypercholesterolaemia. *Lancet*, **ii**, 1360–1363 (1990)

73. MBewu, A.D., Bhatnagar, D., Durrington, P.N., Hunt, L., Ishola, M. *et al*. Serum lipoprotein (a) in patients heterozygous for familial hypercholesterolaemia, their relatives and matched control populations. *Arteriosclerosis*, **11**, 940–946 (1991)

74. Kwiterovich, P. O., Levy, R. I. and Fredrickson, D. S. Neonatal diagnosis of familial type II hyperlipoproteinaemia. *Lancet*, **i**, 118–121 (1973)

75. Kwiterovich, P. O., Fredrickson, D. S. and Levy, R. I. Familial hypercholesterolaemia (one form of familial type II hyperlipoproteinaemia). A study of its biochemical, genetic and clinical presentation in childhood. *J. Clin. Invest.*, **53**, 1237–1249 (1974)

76. Leonard, J. V., Whitelaw, A. G., Wolff, O. H., Lloyd, J. K. and Slack, J. Diagnosing familial hypercholesterolaemia in childhood by measuring serum cholesterol. *Br. Med. J.*, **i**, 1566–1568 (1977)

77. Darmady, J. M., Fosbrooke, A. S. and Lloyd, J. K. Prospective study of serum cholesterol levels during first year of life. *Br. Med. J.*, **ii**, 685–688 (1972)

78. Tsang, R. C., Fallat, R. W. and Glueck, C. J. Cholesterol at birth and age 1: comparison of normal and hypercholesterolaemic neonates. *Pediatrics*, **53**, 458–470 (1974)

79. Brown, M. S., Kovanen, P. T., Goldstein, J. L., Eeckels, R., Vandenberghe, K. *et al*. Prenatal diagnosis of homozygous familial hypercholesterolaemia. Expression of a genetic receptor disease in utero. *Lancet*, **i**, 526–529 (1978)

80. Humphries, S. E., Kessling, A. M., Horsthemke, B., Donald, J. A., Seed, M. *et al*. A common DNA polymorphism of the low-density lipoprotein (LDL) receptor gene and its use in diagnosis. *Lancet*, **i**, 1003–1005 (1985)

81. Armston, A. E., Iverson, S. A. and Burke, J. F. Diagnosis of familial hypercholesterolaemia using DNA probes for the low-density lipoprotein (LDL) receptor gene. *Ann. Clin. Biochem.*, **25**, 142–149 (1988)

82. Schrott, H. G., Goldstein, J. L., Hazzard, W. R., McGoodwin, M. M. and Motulsky, A. G. Familial hypercholesterolaemia in a large kindred. Evidence for a monogenic mechanism. *Ann. Intern. Med.*, **76**, 711–720 (1972)

83. Scientific Steering Committee of the Simon Broome Register Group. Risk of fatal coronary heart disease in familial hypercholesterolaemia. *Br. Med. J.*, **303**, 893–896 (1991)

84. Zambon, A., Torres, A., Bijvoet, S., Gagne, C. Moorjani, S. *et al*. Prevention of raised low-density lipoprotein cholesterol in a patient with familial hypercholesterolaemia and lipoprotein lipase deficiency. *Lancet*, **341**, 1119–1121 (1993)

85. Mutsuri, E., Hegele, R.M., Hopkins, P.N. *et al*. Effects of three genetic loci in a pedigree with multiple lipoprotein phenotypes. *Arteriosclerosis*, **11**, 1349–1355 (1991)

86. Hobbs, H.H., Leitersdorf, E., Leffert, C., Cryer, D.R., Brown, M.S. and Goldstein, J.L. Evidence for a dominant gene that suppresses hypercholesterolaemia in a family with defective low density lipoprotein receptors. *J. Clin. Invest.*, **84**, 656–664 (1989)

87. Uauy, R., Vega, G.L. and Grundy, S.M. Coinheritance of two mild defects in low density lipoprotein receptor function produces severe hypercholesterolaemia. *J. Clin. Endocrinol. Metabol.* **72**, 179–187 (1991)

88. Utermann, G., Hopplicher, F., Dieplinger, H., Seed, M., Thompson, G. and Boerwinkle, E. Defects in the low density lipoprotein receptor gene affect lipoprotein (a) levels: multiplicative interactions of two gene loci associated with premature atherosclerosis. *Proc. Natl. Acad. Sci. USA*, **86**, 4171–4174 (1989)

89. Soutar, A.K., McCarthy, S.N., Seed, M. and Knight, B.L. Relationship between apolipoprotein(a) phenotype, lipoprotein (a) concentration in plasma, and low density lipoprotein receptor function in a large kindred with familial hypercholesterolaemia due to the $pro_{664}$-leu mutation in the LDL receptor gene. *J. Clin. Invest.*, **88**, 483– (1991)

90. Kane, J.P., Malloy, M.J., Ports, T.A., Phillips, N.R. *et al.* Regression of coronary atherosclerosis during treatment of familial hypercholesterolaemia with combined drug regimens. *J. Am. Med. Assoc.*, **264**, 3007–3012 (1990)

91. Mater, V.M.G. and Thompson, G.R. HMG CoA reductase inhibitors as lipid-lowering agents: five years' experience with lovastatin and an appraisal of simvastatin and pravastatin. *Q. J. Med.*, **74**, 165–175 (1990)

92. Illingworth, D.R. Mevinolin plus colestipol in therapy for severe heterozygous familial hypercholesterolaemia. *Ann. Intern. Med.*, **191**, 598 (1984)

93. Havel, R.J., Hunninglake, D.B., Illingworth, D.R. *et al.* Lovastatin (mevinolin) in the treatment of heterozygous familial hypercholesterolaemia. *Ann. Intern. Med.*, **107**, 609 (1987)

94. Mol, M.J.T.H., Erkelens, D.W., Leuvan, J.A.G., Schouten, J. A. and Stalenhoef, A.F.K. Effects of synvinolin (MK-733) on plasma lipids in familial hypercholesterolaemia. *Lancet*, **i**, 936–939 (1986)

95. Betteridge, D.J., Bhatnagar, D., Bing, D., Durrington, P.N., Evans, G. *et al.* Treatment of familial hypercholesterolaemia. The United Kingdom lipid clinics study of pravastatin and cholestyramine. *Br. Med. J.*, **304**, 1335–1338 (1992)

96. Bhatnagar, D., Durrington, P.N., Neary, R. and Miller, J.P. Elevation of skeletal muscle isoform of creatine kinase in heterozygous familial hypercholesterolaemia. *J. Intern. Med.*, **228**, 493–495 (1990)

97. Naoumora, R.P., Marais, D., Erkelens, W., Rendell, N.B., Taylor, G.W. and Thompson, G.R. Changes in plasma mevalonate predict responsiveness to HMG-CoA reductase inhibitors. *Atherosclerosis*, **103**, 297 (1993)

98. Illingworth, D. R. and Gowen, D. Management of lipoprotein abnormalities. In *Recent Advances in Cardiology*, vol. 10 (ed. D. J. Rowlands), Churchill Livingstone, Edinburgh, pp. 71–100 (1987)

99. Durrington, P.N. and Miller, J.P. Double-blind, placebo-controlled, cross-over trial of probucol in heterozygous familial hypercholesterolaemia. *Atherosclerosis*, **55**, 187–194 (1985)

100. Steinberg, D. Studies on the mechanism of action of probucol. *Am. J. Cardiol.*, **57**, 16H–21H (1986)

101. Witztum, J.L. Role of oxidised low density lipoprotein in atherogenesis. *Br. Heart J.*, **69** (Suppl.), S12–S18 (1993)

102. Franceschini, G., Sirtori, M., Vaccarino, V., Glanfranceschi, G., Rezzonico, L. *et al.* Mechanisms of HDL reduction after probucol: changes in HDL subfractions and increased cholesteryl ester transport. *Arteriosclerosis*, **9**, 462–468 (1989)

103. West, R. J., Lloyd, J. K. and Leonard, J. V. Long-term follow-up of children with familial hypercholesterolaemia treated with cholestyramine. *Lancet*, **ii**, 873–875 (1980)

104. West, R. J. and Lloyd, J. K. Effect of cholestyramine on intestinal absorption. *Gut*, **16**, 93–98 (1975)

105. Shepherd, J., Packard, C. J., Bicker, S., Lawrie, T. D. V. and Morgan, H. G. Cholestyramine promotes receptor-mediated low-density-lipoprotein catabolism. *N. Eng. J. Med.*, **302**, 1219–1222 (1980)

106. Baker, S.G., Joffe, B.I., Mendlesohn, D. and Seftel, H.C. Treatment of homozygous familial hypercholesterolaemia with probucol. *S. Afr. Med J.*, **62**, 7–11(1982)

107. Saal, S. D., Parker, T. S., Gordon, B. R., Studebaker, J., Hudgins, L. *et al.* Removal of low density lipoproteins in patients by extracorporeal immunoabsorption. *Am. J. Med.*, **80**, 583–589 (1986)

108. Thompson, G.R. Personal communication (1992)

109. Bilheimer, D. W., Goldstein, J. L., Grundy, S. M., Starzl, T. E. and Brown, M. S. Liver transplantation to provide low density lipoprotein receptors and lower plasma cholesterol in a child with homozygous familial hypercholesterolaemia. *N. Engl. J. Med.*, **311**, 1658–1662 (1984)

110. East, C., Grundy, S. M. and Bilheimer, D. W. Normal cholesterol levels with Lovastatin (mevinolin) therapy in a child with homozygous familial hypercholesterolaemia following liver transplantation. *J. Am. Med. Assoc.*, **256**, 2843–2848 (1986)

111. Starzl, T. E., Chase, H. P., Putnan, C. W. and Porter, K. A. Portacaval shunt in hyperlipoproteinaemia. *Lancet*, **ii**, 940–944 (1973)

112. Bilheimer, D. W., Goldstein, J. L., Grundy, S. M. and Brown, M. S. Reduction in cholesterol and low density lipoprotein synthesis after portacaval shunt surgery in a patient with homozygous familial hypercholesterolaemia. *J. Clin. Invest.*, **56**, 1420–1430 (1975)

113. Hoeg, J. M., Demosky, S. J., Schaefer, E. J., Starzl, T. E., Porter, K. A. and Brewer, H. B. The effects of portacaval shunt on hepatic lipoprotein metabolism in familial hypercholesterolaemia. *J. Surg. Res.*, **39**, 369–377 (1985)

114. Spengel, F. A., Jadhav, A., Duffield, R. G. M., Wood, C. B. and Thompson, G. R. Superiority of partial ileal bypass over cholestyramine in reducing cholesterol in familial hypercholesterolaemia. *Lancet*, **ii**, 768–771 (1981)

115. Buchwald, H. Moore, R. B. and Varco, R. L. Surgical treatment of hyperlipidaemia. *Circulation*, **49** (Suppl. I), I1–I37 (1974)

116. Buchwald, H., Varco, R.L., Matts, J.P., Long, J.M., Fitch, L.L. *et al.* and the POSCH Group. Effect of partial ileal bypass surgery on mortality and morbidity from coronary heart disease in patients with hypercholesterolaemia. *N. Engl. J. Med.*, **323**, 946–955 (1990)

117. Illingworth, D. R. and Connor, W. E. Hypercholesterolaemia persisting after distal ileal bypass: response to mevinolin. *Am. Intern. Med.*, **100**, 850–851 (1984)

118. Myant, N.B. Familial defective apolipoprotein B-100: a review, including some comparisons with familial hypercholesterolaemia. *Atherosclerosis*, **104**, 1–19 (1993)

119. Vega, G.L., Grundy, S.M. *In vivo* evidence for reduced binding of low density lipoprotein to receptors as a cause of primary moderate hypercholesterolaemia. *J. Clin. Invest.*, **78**, 1410–1414 (1986)

120. Innerarity, T. L., Weisgraber, K. H., Arnold, K. S, Mahley, R. W., Krauss, R. M. *et al.* Familial defective apolipoprotein B-100: low density lipoproteins with abnormal receptor binding. *Proc. Natl. Acad. Sci. USA*, **69**, 19–23 (1987)

121. Higgins, M.J.P., Lecamwasam, D.D. and Galton, D.J. A new type of familial hypercholesterolaemia. *Lancet*, **ii**, 737–740 (1975)

122. Soria, L.F., Ludwig, E.H., Clarke, H.R.G., Vega, G.L., Grundy, S.M. and McCarthy, B.J. Association between a specific apolipoprotein B mutation and familial defective apolipoprotein B-100. *Proc. Natl Acad. Sci. USA*, **86**, 587–591 (1989).

123. Lund-Katz, S., Innerarity, T.L., Arnold, K.S., Curtiss, L.K. and Phillips, M.C. [13]C NMR evidence that substitution of glutamine for arginine 3500 in familial defective apolipoprotein B-1 disrupts the conformation of the receptor-binding domain. *J. Biol. Chem.*, **266**, 2701–2704 (1991)

124. Pullinger, C.R., Hennessy, L.K., Love, J.A. *et al.* American Heart Association Meeting, Atlanta, November 1993 Abstracts, p.27

125. Bersot, T.P., Russell, S.J., Thatcher, S.R., Pomernacki, N.K., Mahley, R.W. *et al.* A unique hapotype of the apolipoprotein B-100 allele associated with familial giant defective apolipoprotein B-100 discovered during a study of the prevalence of this disorder. *J. Lipid Res.*, **34**, 1149–1154 (1993)

126. Marz, W., Baumstartk, M.W., Scharnagl, H. *et al.* Accumulation of small dense low dense lipoproteins in a homozygous patient with familial defective apolipoprotein B-100 results from heterozygous interaction of LDL-subfractions with the LDL receptor. *J. Clin. Invest.*, **92**, 2922–2933 (1993)

127. Funke, H., Rust, S., Seerdorf, U. *et al.* Homozygosity for familial defective apolipoprotein B-100 (FDB) is associated with lower plasma cholesterol concentration than homozygosity for familial hypercholesterolaemia. *Circulation*, **86** (Suppl. 1), I691 (1992)

128. Rauh, G., Schuster, H., Fischer, J., Keller, C.K., Wolfram, G. and Zollner, N. Identification of a heterozygous compound individual with familial hypercholesterolaemia and familial defective apolipoprotein B-100. *Klin. Wochenschr.* **69**, 320–324 (1991)

129. Deeb, S.S., Failor, R.A., Brown, B.G. *et al.* Association of apolipoprotein B gene variants with plasma apo B and low density lipoprotein cholesterol levels. *Hum. Genet.* **88**, 463–470 (1992)

130. Hobbs, H.H., Russell, D.W., Brown, M.S. and Goldstein, J.L. The LDL receptor locus in familial hypercholesterolaemia: mutational analysis of a membrane protein. *Ann. Rev. Genet.* **24**, 133–170 (1990)

131. Maher, V.M.G., Gallagher, J.J. and Myant, N.B. The binding of very-low-density lipoprotein remnants to the low-density lipoprotein receptor in familial defective apolipoprotein B-100. *Atherosclerosis*, **102**, 51–61 (1993)

# Chapter 6

# Common hypercholesterolaemia: polygenic hypercholesterolaemia and familial combined hyperlipidaemia

## Introduction

By now it will have become obvious that hypercholesterolaemia, however it is defined, is common (Chapter 3) and that, although an important cause of marked hypercholesterolaemia is heterozygous familial hypercholesterolaemia (FH), most hypercholesterolaemia is due to something else. Evidence that diet is a major cause of the commonly encountered hypercholesterolaemia is substantial. Nevertheless, not everybody consuming a Northern European or North American diet develops hypercholesterolaemia and evidence that individual dietary preferences is closely related to the serum cholesterol concentration is poor[1]. This argues strongly that other factors must determine the individual response to diet. Such factors are frequently considered to be substantially genetic. The frequency distribution of the serum cholesterol concentration is reasonably Gaussian, as it is, for example, for height. In the main, people at the top end of the cholesterol distribution are not there because of the influence of a single gene, as is the case for example in FH, but because of a combination of several genes. This type of hypercholesterolaemia is usually therefore referred to as polygenic hypercholesterolaemia.

In the UK, the cumulative death rate from ischaemic heart disease (IHD) for men up to the age of 60 is about 4%. The rates may be expected to be about two to four times greater in middle-aged men whose serum cholesterol exceeds 260 mg/dl (6.5 mmol/l) than in those in the lower part of the cholesterol distribution with levels around 200 mg/dl (5.2 mmol/l) (Figure 3.9). Most people with serum cholesterol levels over 260 mg/dl (6.5 mmol/l) have polygenic hypercholesterolaemia rather than FH (Chapter 5, page 118). Their risk is, of course, graded according to their serum cholesterol level (Figure 3.10). In middle-aged men with polygenic hypercholesterolaemia, whose cholesterol is around say 360–400 mg/dl (9.0–10 mmol/l), which is about the average in heterozygous FH (Chapter 5), the chance of dying from IHD is about eight times that of a man with a level of 200 mg/dl (5.20 mmol/l). It is generally assumed that the risk of premature death from IHD even then is less than in a man with a similar level of cholesterol due to FH, which is around 25 times higher. For the individual destined to die prematurely from IHD as a consequence of hypercholesterolaemia not due to FH, it is no comfort to know that he or she comes from a larger population who will generally not succumb similarly. For the physician it is less easy to pursue treatment of hypercholesterolaemia as rigorously, if the diagnosis of FH cannot be made. The essential question to ask is how evenly is the risk spread through the hypercholesterolaemic population left after those with clinical FH have been recognized? Is it possible to identify other individuals with a worse than average prognosis? It is known that the combination of hypercholesterolaemia with other risk factors for IHD, such as cigarette smoking, hypertension and diabetes mellitus, considerably increases the risk, often more than additively, and this is helpful in clinical practice (Fig. 3.12). However, there are still a large group of hypercholesterolaemic patients, with no other obvious risk factors, who are destined to develop IHD at an early age. Membership of this group may simply be the result of some random process, but a more attractive prospect is that they may either have disorders of lipoprotein metabolism, which are especially atherogenic, or that they have heightened susceptibility to IHD. Little is known about this latter possibility[2], which might involve anatomical variation in the coronary tree, differences in myocardial metabolism, in the response of tissue of the arterial wall to entry of lipoprotein (Chapter 2, page 60), in the chemical modification of lipoproteins making them more atherogenic, for example, due to the leakage of free radicals from oxidative pathways, or in the likelihood of thrombosis occurring on atheromatous plaques due possibly to variation in plasma levels of fibrinogen[3,4], factor 7[4], plasminogen activation[5], or apolipoprotein (a)[6].

The idea which has, however, received most attention is that among those hypercholesterolaemic individuals who do not have the FH syndrome, there may be some who have particular disorders of lipoprotein metabolism which are especially atherogenic. Familial hypercholesterolaemia and type III hyperlipoproteinaemia, with their substantially increased risk of atheroma, produce clinical syndromes which allow them to be clearly set apart from the broad mass of hypercholesterolaemia. Might there not be, within that mass, other disorders as risky, but which because they produce no clinical manifestations other than arterial disease are less easy to define? Analysis of survivors of early onset myocardial infarction should provide evidence for such disorders, if they exist, and investigation of their relatives should indicate whether they might have any genetic basis. If hyperlipidaemia is defined in terms of the 95th percentile, then studies show that about 30% of the survivors of myocardial infarction have either hypercholesterolaemia or hypertriglyceridaemia or both and that, of these, 30% or so will have a relative with some form of hyperlipidaemia[7-11]. Thus, overall about 10% of patients with premature myocardial infarction will have a type IIa, IIb or IV hyperlipoproteinaemia and come from families with hyperlipidaemia. Often, however, the affected relatives have a different lipoprotein phenotype. These patients were defined by one group of workers as having 'familial combined hyperlipidaemia' and it was further suggested that it represented a monogenic syndrome which led to early onset IHD[8,9,12]. There are many objections to this suggestion. For example, if one allows a variable phenotype, then one is increasing the likelihood of discovering affected family members on a purely sporadic basis. Also, the original study population appeared to include some patients with heterozygous FH (later definitions exclude patients with tendon xanthomata from the diagnosis of familial combined hyperlipidaemia). In addition, the evidence for monogenicity has been criticized because the genetic analysis must necessarily be biased, as the condition can only be identified in an individual if more than one family member is affected[7,13].

Furthermore, in the UK, for example, almost 10% of men have a heart attack before the age of 60, and we should have to allow that 10% of these had familial combined hyperlipidaemia (30% of 30%). If each of these had only one affected living relative, 1 in 50 of the population would have familial combined hyperlipidaemia. A similar prevalence of familial combined hyperlipidaemia has also been estimated in the USA[14]. To accept that such a condition was entirely genetic would be to accept impossibly large differences in gene frequencies between populations with high and low risks of IHD (Chapter 3, pages 73–84). Thus, whatever its mode of inheritance, environmental factors, probably nutritional, must have a considerable influence on its expression (penetrance).

Nevertheless there does appear to be an increased risk of premature IHD in families with multiple lipoprotein phenotypes and, accepting that the evidence for monogenicity is far from settled, the admittedly somewhat nebulous concept of familial combined hyperlipidaemia is of some practical clinical value in attempting to define the risk for an individual with hypercholesterolaemia.

## Familial combined hyperlipidaemia

In general even the larger case-control studies show only relatively small differences between the average serum cholesterol of myocardial infarction survivors and matched control populations and, indeed, this is to be expected from prospective studies. In Framingham, for example, the average serum cholesterol in men who developed coronary disease over 16 years was $244 \pm 51$ mg/dl ($6.3 \pm 1.3$ mmol/l) and in those who did not, $210 \pm 41$ mg/dl ($5.6 \pm 1.1$ mmol/l)[15]. As discussed in the previous section, hyperlipidaemic myocardial infarction survivors and presumably hyperlipidaemic individuals destined to develop IHD prematurely tend to come from families with hyperlipidaemia. Hypercholesterolaemia in myocardial infarction survivors, as in the community in general, is as prevalent as one cares to define it. Most of the studies which have attempted to define familial combined hyperlipidaemia (FCH) have relied on definitions of hyperlipidaemia considerably higher than those which are currently recommended[16–18], often the 95th percentile. The essential feature is that another family member is affected by type IIa, IIb or IV hyperlipoproteinaemia and that FH is excluded as a cause of type IIa or IIb. Of course, in clinical practice patients may present with one of these disorders without yet having any manifestation of coronary disease and, in order to entertain the diagnosis in them, a family history of premature IHD is required.

The finding of hyperlipidaemia in more than one member of a family does not necessarily confirm the diagnosis of FCH, since even using the 95th percentile to define hypercholesterolaemia and hypertriglyceridaemia the likelihood of finding hyperlipidaemia by chance is going to be about 1 in 10 with each family member screened. In families with FCH the chances of finding hyperlipidaemias should, however, be as high as 1 in 2. The finding of type IIb hyperlipoproteinaemia in a family does increase the likelihood that they have FCH, because this disorder affects only 3% of the general population[19], but occurs in more than 80% of families defined as having FCH[10]. Within affected family members the types IIa, IIb and IV phenotypes seem to be about evenly distributed [9–11].

Another supposed feature of FCH is the tendency for phenotypes to change readily with treatment, for example from IIb to IV with diet or from IIa to IIb or IV with cholestyramine or sometimes even without therapy[12]. This probably has more to do with the definition than with any unique metabolic defect, since many of the affected individuals cluster around the 95th percentile so that only small changes in either cholesterol or triglycerides will alter their phenotype[13].

Corneal arcus and xanthelasmata may occur in FCH, but their presence is not helpful in making the diagnosis. Other xanthomata do not occur in FCH. As in other hyperlipoproteinaemias, with the exception of FH, LDL receptor activity is normal in FCH. Unlike FH, obesity is over-represented in FCH.

Also unlike FH, the lipids in FCH, as is also the case in the other common hyperlipidaemias, are generally normal in childhood. The hyperlipidaemia does not become evident until the age of 25–30 years, with a tendency for hyper-triglyceridaemia to be apparent a little earlier than hypercholesterolaemia[9]. It has also been suggested that children with FCH who have one hypercholestero-laemic parent and one normal parent tend to develop hypertriglyceridaemia, whereas those with one hypertriglyceridaemic and one normal parent seem to manifest hypercholesterolaemia.

Since the previous edition of this book it has become more widely recognized that patients who exhibit the type IIb or IV phenotype, who will also generally have low serum HDL cholesterol levels (particularly $HDL_2$ cholesterol) and are frequently insulin-resistant. In most cases this may be as a result of their obesity, particularly if they have the male pattern of obesity. In this type of obesity there is greater tendency to put on weight around the waist and abdomen whilst retain-ing relatively lean thighs and buttocks whereas in the female type of obesity a relatively narrow waist may be retained, but fat is deposited in the thighs and buttocks (Chapter 11). In addition to the raised serum VLDL and LDL in this condition there is an increase in serum IDL and there is also an increase in the smaller particles in the LDL density range which are relatively depleted in lipids, particularly cholesteryl ester with triglycerides making up a greater proportion of their remaining lipid[20]. Both IDL and small dense LDL are atherogenic. IDL may behave like the $\beta$-VLDL of type III hyperlipoproteinaemia in atherogenesis and small LDL appears to be more susceptible to oxidative modification. This syndrome has attracted various names including syndrome X and plurimetabolic syndrome and there have been various claimants of eponymns, none of whom can be clearly shown to have first described it and some who have merely confused matters. I prefer to regard it as insulin-resistance syndrome because insulin resis-tance is frequently present. Often in practice Castelli's use of the term atherogenic profile provides the easiest description[21]. This seems appropriate because it was its prevalence in myocardial infarction survivors which first led to the suggestion that it should be regarded as a clinical syndrome[9] and this has been amply confirmed in a recent study of 6700 men and 1500 women with IHD[22]. Other components of the syndrome undoubtedly include glucose intolerance or frank diabetes and hyperuricaemia (Chapter 11). Hypertension is also frequently claimed as part of the syndrome, but whether the undoubted association of the syndrome with hypertension is the consequence of obesity or something more profound, perhaps related independently to insulin resistance, is uncertain (Chapter 12). It is undoubtedly the case that the use of $\beta$-blockers and/or thiazide diuretics in the management of hypertension, particularly in obese patients, will exacerbate the metabolic features of the condition often markedly (Chapter 11).

Insulin resistance syndrome is particularly common in migrant populations from India and Pakistan living in Britain in whom the incidence of IHD is higher than in the indigenous Europid population[23]. This is apparently due to the influence of the new culture because serum lipids, blood pressure and insulin resistance are greater in migrant siblings than those on the Indian subcontinent[24].

Whether FCH represents a specific disease or occurs merely as the result of factors which commonly underlie hyperlipidaemia, combining together in some families to produce more marked manifestations, is a matter of semantics. Kinetic studies have generally shown abnormally high production of VLDL apolipoprotein B[25–27]. This increase probably accounts for the increase in plasma LDL levels in FCH patients with the type IIa or IIb disorders, but the evidence for this notion is not conclusive[28]. An overproduction of VLDL apolipoprotein B is certainly not specific for FCH, since variations in VLDL apolipoprotein B production also account in substantial part for differences in plasma cholesterol within the population[29,30] and between populations[31], suggesting it is a more common cause of hyperlipidaemia than FCH. Increased VLDL apolipoprotein B production also appears to be the cause of type IV hyperlipoproteinaemia in many instances[32] and is a feature of obesity (Chapter 11, page 315). It would be possible to argue that this is because such type IV individuals come from FCH families, were it not that similar increases in production rate have been reported to be the metabolic basis of hyperapobetalipoproteinaemia[33] which, as discussed later in this chapter, appears to be more frequent in patients with premature coronary disease than FCH[34–36].

Whether a patient with overproduction of VLDL develops hypertriglyceridaemia will depend on how effectively VLDL is metabolized to LDL. This in turn will depend on the activity in particular of lipoprotein lipase, but also perhaps hepatic lipase. The report that heterozygotes for familial lipoprotein lipase deficiency have a lipoprotein profile which mimics that of the type IIb and IV phenotype in FCH[37] gives rise to the idea that mutations of the lipoprotein lipase gene or of apo CII, which activates it, might impair its activity, although not to the extent seen in severe hypertriglyceridaemia. If these mutations run in families with a tendency to overproduce VLDL either because of obesity or say some other independent genetic cause, type IV or IIb will occur only in those family members in whom both the gene defect affecting lipase activity and the overproduction of VLDL occur. Reports of linkage of FCH with an XmnI polymorphism in the apo AI-CIII-AIV gene cluster[38,39] might be explained, if this polymorphism was a marker for an increase in apo CIII levels which might decrease lipoprotein lipase activity and the hepatic clearance of remnants. Increased VLDL apolipoprotein B production has also been reported in patients developing IHD, even when they do not have any increase of VLDL and LDL[40], which poses the question as to whether people with normal lipids from FCH families are also at increased risk of IHD. This again brings us back to ask whether FCH families are really kindreds in which a susceptibility gene or other risk factors are running together with one or two genes predisposing to hyperlipidaemia. In purely practical terms, whatever FCH is or is not, hyperlipidaemic patients from families manifesting premature IHD or in which other family members have hyperlipidaemia appear to be at increased risk and presumably therefore more likely to benefit from lipid-lowering drugs should they fail to respond to dietary therapy.

Figure 6.1 shows how VLDL overproduction combined with acquired or genetic defects acting at different points in the conversion of VLDL to LDL can give rise to the different phenotypes associated with FCH, namely normal lipids, type IIa, type IIb or type IV or even V.

FCH, hyperapolipobetalipoproteinaemia and other hypertriglyceridaemic states are associated with small LDL. The larger LDL arising from large VLDL is thought to be actively cleared by the LDL receptor whereas a small dense LDL which is formed from smaller VLDL particles tends to accumulate in the circulation[41]. Why this small VLDL should be produced is not clear. An alternative perhaps complimentary view is that the enlarged triglyceride pool in these patients is responsible

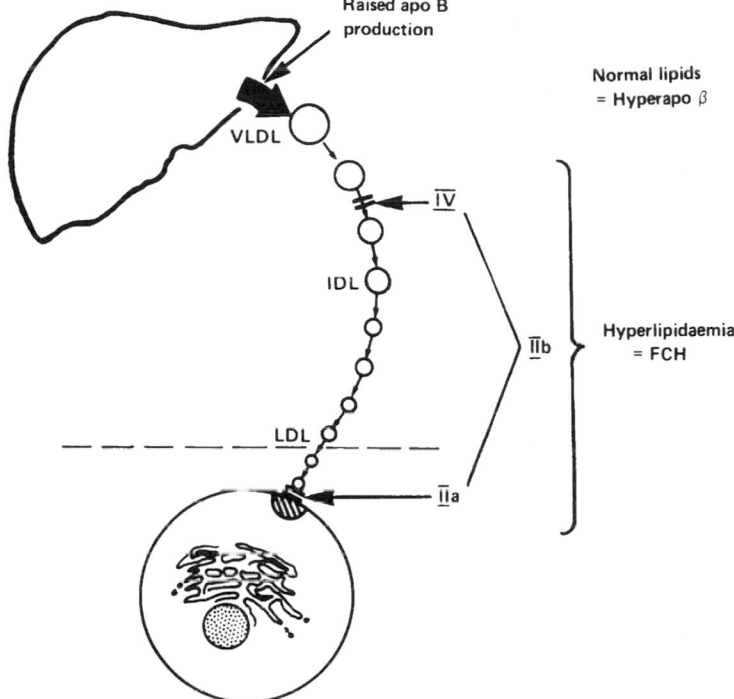

**Figure 6.1**   Increased production of apo $B_{100}$-containing lipoproteins characterizes familial combined hyperlipidaemia (FCH), hyperapobetalipoproteinaemia (hyperapo β) and many patients with polygenic hypercholesterolaemia and endogenous hypertriglyceridaemia. Individual variations in the rate of clearance of triglyceride-rich lipoprotein or LDL will determine whether type IIa, IIb or IV hyperlipoproteinaemia develop, or the patient remains normolipideamic. In both FCH and hyperapo β serum apolipoprotein B is raised. In FCH, there is hypercholesterolaemia or hypertriglyceridaemia but in hyperapo β, cholesterol is in the normal range

both for their low serum HDL cholesterol concentration and cholesteryl ester depleted small LDL. There is direct evidence that in patients with hypertriglyceridaemia the transfer of cholesteryl ester out of HDL to triglyceride-rich-lipoproteins is enhanced (see Cholesteryl ester transfer protein, Chapter 2, page 58)[42] and that this process is reversible when the triglyceride-rich lipoprotein levels are therapeutically lowered. Interestingly the quantity of free cholesterol in the triglyceride-rich lipoprotein pool may be a major determinant of the rate of cholesteryl ester transfer into it[43]. The transfer of cholesteryl ester from HDL to VLDL whence it may re-enter the IDL and LDL pool and of cholesteryl ester from LDL to VLDL in exchange for triglyceride could explain both the increase in IDL concentration and the cholesteryl ester-depleted small LDL associated with the syndrome.

## Other common hypercholesterolaemia

Hypercholesterolaemia is common and, as was discussed in the introduction, the term polygenic is frequently used to describe it. The case for the subdivision into

FCH is in parts dubious, as will be obvious from the previous section, and the argument in favour of further subdivision of common hypercholesterolaemia by the introduction of terms such as sporadic is even less strong. The absence of hyperlipidaemia in other members of a family does not rule out a genetic component in an affected individual any more than the presence of other affected members in the same kindred is necessarily genetic, since families frequently share a similar environment and habits[2].

In terms of its burden on society, polygenic hypercholesterolaemia should occupy a large part of this book. In fact most of the space it occupies is not so much concerned with its metabolic or clinical features as it is with the other primary hyperlipoproteinaemias, but by issues concerning whether it should be treated. The very great differences in the prevalence of polygenic hypercholesterolaemia between different communities (Chapter 3), usually closely related to their IHD rates, is thought to imply that it is largely nutritional in origin (Chapter 9) and that it is the root cause of most coronary disease. In general it appears due to an overproduction of VLDL apolipoprotein B[29–31], leading in turn to increased plasma LDL concentrations. Variation in the ability to catabolize LDL will also play some part in an individual's propensity to develop increased serum LDL levels[30,44].

Since the relationship between risk of IHD and the serum cholesterol concentration has no threshold, the definition of hypercholesterolaemia has provoked much discussion. The currently held view is that an appropriate target level for societies such as ours should be 200 mg/dl (5.2 mmol/l) and that levels exceeding this are potentially unhealthy[16–18]. The scale of polygenic hyperlipidaemia is enormous if it is defined in these terms (over 50% of middle-aged British men and women and almost as high a proportion of the middle-aged US population). Clearly this demands a public health approach aimed particularly at modifying national dietary preferences rather than a clinical approach on an individual basis. At what level of cholesterol clinical intervention is justified has been a matter of much debate, but most authorities have

**Table 6.1 Estimates of the proportion of men in the UK dying before the age of 60 years from CHD according to their serum cholesterol and whether they have the familial hypercholesterolaemia (FH) clinical syndrome***

| Serum cholesterol (mmol/l) | Risk of death before age of 60 yr (per 1000) | % UK male population with these cholesterol levels | % of UK male population dying before age of 60 from CHD with these cholesterol levels |
| --- | --- | --- | --- |
| <5 | 25 | 10 | 0.25 |
| 5–6 | 30 | 35 | 1.05 |
| 6–7 | 43 | 40 | 1.72 |
| 7–8 | 55 | 10 | 0.55 |
| 8–9 | 74 | 4 | 0.30 |
| >9 | 130 | 1 | 0.1 |
| Heterozygous FH | 500 | 0.2 | Total 4.1 |

* Death up to 60 in men is chosen because of limited data about cholesterol in older age groups, about morbidity and about women. Combined CHD death and non-fatal symptomatic CHD is probably 2–3 times that of CHD death

arrived at a figure of about 260 mg/dl (6.5 mmol/l). Even this constitutes a substantial burden, since in the UK and the USA around a quarter of the population have levels exceeding that. Furthermore it must be emphasized that a coronary disease prevention strategy purely confined to people whose cholesterol exceeds 260 mg/dl (6.5 mmol/l) will be relatively ineffective, since around 60% of early coronary deaths in men in the UK (Table 6.1) and the USA[45] occur in those whose serum cholesterol is less than that level. Thus a combined public health and clinical (or high risk) strategy is the only sensible means of coronary prevention.

The great difficulty with the clinical approach is the imprecise means we have available at present to determine an individual's risk of developing coronary disease. It is not possible to rely on cholesterol alone, except at the highest levels, to identify with certainty individuals likely to develop coronary disease prematurely. In the middle range of the cholesterol distribution, which encompasses the majority of people who will develop coronary disease, there is considerable overlap between cholesterol levels of people destined to have the disease and those who are not[15] (Figure 6.2). Even among men whose cholesterol exceeds 260 mg/dl(6.5 mmol/l), less than 10% are likely to die before the age of 60. A smaller proportion still will die of coronary disease in the range 220–260 mg/dl (5.2–6.5 mmol/l) (Table 6.1), but because this is a larger slice of the population a

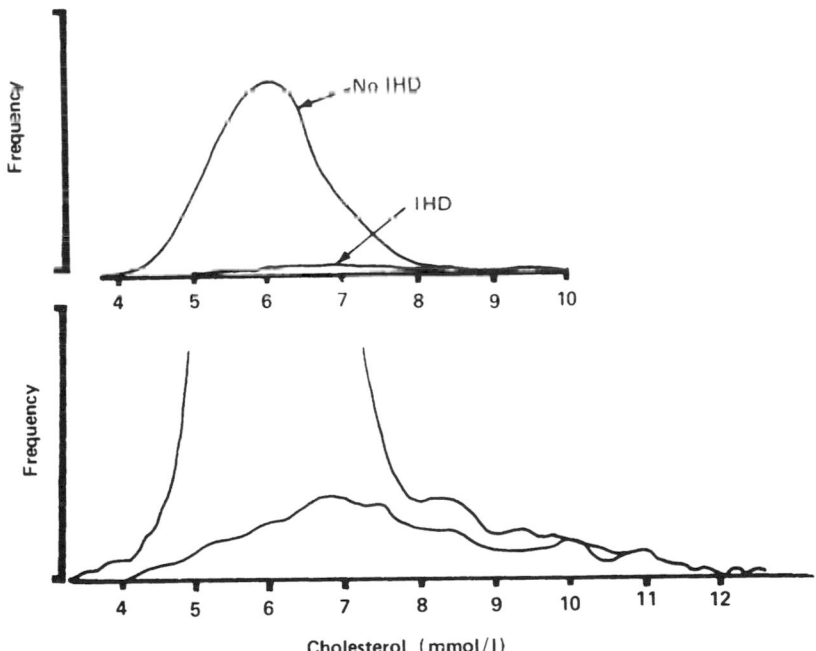

**Figure 6.2**  Except at the higher levels of serum cholesterol there is considerable overlap between the men who will die prematurely of coronary heart disease and those who will not. This poses an enormous problem for preventive cardiology, because those who will not are very much in the majority (Based loosely on Reference 15 and assuming a coronary death rate among men before the age of 60 years of 4% (1 mmol/l = 39 mg/dl)

substantial proportion (probably over half) of the total deaths will nevertheless come from this range.

Because the dietary approach to the management of hypercholesterolaemia (Chapter 10) is safe, efforts will need to be made to promote it to the community as a whole. A full discussion of this subject is beyond the scope of this book. An allied problem, however, is that if an individual approach is also to be applied, how are individuals with hypercholesterolaemia in the clinical range to be identified? Thus far, case finding has been largely restricted to the occasional screening of relatives of victims of heart attacks at an early age. It has now been reliably shown that attempts to identify hypercholesterolaemia by selective screening are little more efficient than unselective screening[46]. There is thus no justification for discouraging any individual who wishes to have his or her serum cholesterol measured, and this approach is actively advocated in the USA[47]. In Britain, the effectiveness of offering opportunistic screening to patients attending their general practitioners in detecting a substantial proportion of the hypercholesterolaemia present in the community has been demonstrated[46]. Confining such a strategy to men is probably not justified in terms of coronary prevention in the community as a whole, since the heightening of awareness among women, who are frequently more concerned about health issues than their spouses and who are generally more responsible for the family's nutrition, is also likely to reduce IHD risk more effectively in men and in children and adolescents, whose diet may imprint itself on their cholesterol metabolism in later life (Chapter 10).

# Evidence of benefit from cholesterol-lowering therapy

## Does spontaneously low cholesterol increase mortality *per se*?

This issue, which has now been reasonably satisfactorily resolved, is dealt with in Chapter 3.

## Benefit in patients with established atherosclerotic disease

### Clinical trials of IHD event rates

Many early trials of cholesterol-modification in patients with established coronary heart disease produced results which were hard to interpret. In retrospect this was to a large extent due to the relatively small size of the trials and the relative ineffectiveness of therapies used to lower cholesterol. None the less, for many years the view was prevalent that in patients who had already sustained a heart attack, lowering cholesterol was hopeless. This view was abetted by early reports that the serum cholesterol concentration in patients who had sustained a myocardial infarction was unrelated to the risk of having a second[48]. Since then there have been an overwhelming number of studies showing that both serum cholesterol[49–54] and HDL[53,55–58] cholesterol are related to the prognosis after myocardial infarction (Figure 6.3). It also appears that the long-term likelihood of occlusion of coronary artery bypass grafts is related to serum cholesterol levels[59–61]. The effect of serum cholesterol on the outcome of angioplasty is less

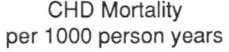

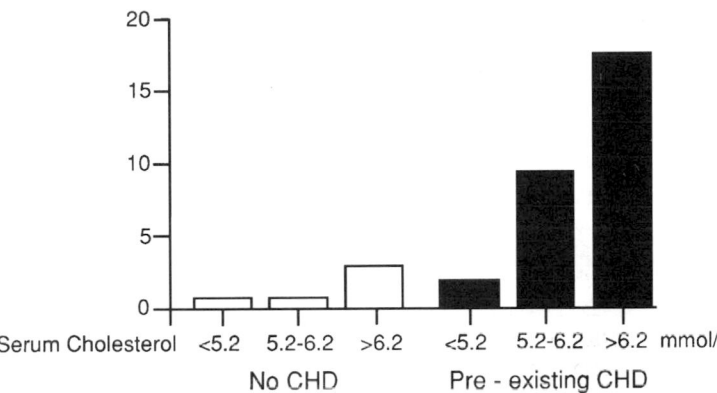

**Figure 6.3**   The increase in IHD risk with increments in serum cholesterol in men without evidence of pre-existing IHD and in men who have established IHD[53]

clear. This may be because the atheroma which recurs in arteries subjected to angioplasty results largely from fibrous tissue ('white' atheroma as opposed to 'yellow' atheroma). Serum HDL and lipoprotein (a) may none the less be relevant to restenosis[62,63].

Clearly if serum cholesterol is measured too close to the myocardial infarction its level may be falsely low and such a state could conceivably persist in patients with repeated episodes of angina following a heart attack (Chapter 3). The prognosis after myocardial infarction will be poor if it is complicated by ventricular dysrhythmia or significant heart failure, ventricular wall akinesis or aneurysm formation or mitral regurgitation. When these occur it would not be expected that determinants of the progression of coronary atheroma, such as cholesterol, would have a major impact on subsequent events, which may explain the early confusion surrounding cholesterol and risk after myocardial infarction.

Until recently, conclusive evidence that people with established IHD could benefit overall from cholesterol-lowering intervention was unavailable. In a recent meta-analysis, however, involving 21 trials and 2482 deaths in patients with IHD, there was a higher significant decrease in all-cause mortality ($P<0.008$) (Table 6.2). The decrease in IHD deaths was 6% in the first 2 years rising to 26% after 5 years (Table 6.3)[64,65]. There was a significant overall 26% decrease in IHD mortality in another meta-analysis of nine trials[66,67]. These meta-analyses include trials regarded as negative when published as well as those whose authors believed that lowering cholesterol had a beneficial outcome. Some of the trials relied on diet to lower cholesterol, others on lipid-lowering drugs as well and one on partial ileal bypass surgery. The greatest reduction in cholesterol was associated with greatest benefit[68]. In few, if any, of the trials were patients selected for hyperlipidaemia and thus their serum cholesterol at randomization was close to the population average. It is especially important to note that there was no adverse effect of cholesterol-lowering treatment on non-IHD mortality in trials in patients with established IHD[64-67].

**Table 6.2 Results of meta-analysis of 21 trials of cholesterol-lowering in patients with established ischaemic heart disease (IHD) involving 2482 deaths***

|                      | Odds ratio | % of all deaths |
|----------------------|-----------|-----------------|
| Non-IHD deaths       | 0.99†     | 14              |
| IHD deaths           | 0.89‡     | 86              |
| All causes of deaths | 0.90‡     | 100             |

* Many trials lasted less than 2 years and the average cholesterol decrease was only about 23 mg/dl (0.6 mmol/l).
Odds ratio is the rate in treatment group divided by rate in control group.
† NS; ‡ $P<0.01$.
Data from reference[65]

**Table 6.3 The decrease in IHD incidence in men aged 55–64 years for a 10% decrease in serum cholesterol***

| Type of trial        | Time since entry to trial |             |              |
|----------------------|---------------------------|-------------|--------------|
|                      | ≤2 years                  | 2.1–5 years | 5.1–12 years |
| Drug                 | 10%                       | 21%         | 22%          |
| Diet                 | 9%                        | 14%         | 37%          |
| Primary prevention   | 11%                       | 25%         | 24%          |
| Secondary prevention | 6%                        | 20%         | 26%          |
| All                  | 7%                        | 22%         | 25%          |

* Approximately 0.6 mmol/l or 23 mg/dl).
From a meta-analysis of clinical trials: reference[64]

**Table 6.4 The results of the Stockholm Secondary Prevention Study**

|                              | Total mortality | CHD mortality | Non-CHD mortality |
|------------------------------|-----------------|---------------|-------------------|
| Control ($n=276$)            | 82              | 73            | 9                 |
| Treatment ($n=279$)          | 61              | 47            | 14                |
| Odds ratio                   | 0.74            | 0.64          | 1.52              |
| % change in mortality        | −26             | −36           | +55               |
| Difference in number of patients dying | 21**  | 26***         | 5*                |

If the odds ratio or percentage change are quoted the misleading impression can be conveyed that there was an increase in non-CHD deaths, which more than counterbalanced favourable effect on CHD death rates. The actual numbers of people dying clearly, however, shows that as in the secondary prevention trials overall many more people survived in the treatment group than the control group.
*NS; **$P<0.05$; ***$P<0.01$
Data from reference[68]

Overall mortality has only been significantly decreased in one individual trial of cholesterol-lowering. Interestingly this was the only trial which combined highly effective lipid-lowering therapy with a group of myocardial infarction survivors who were at considerable risk of reinfarction[68].* This was the Stockholm

*Since going to print, the effectiveness of lipid-lowering therapy in decreasing all-cause mortality in pateints with angina of previous myocardial infarction has received powerful confirmation from the Scandinavian Simvastatin Survival Study [172].

Secondary Prevention Trial in which 555 men and women who had survived myocardial infarction were randomized to receive treatment with a combination of nicotinic acid (up to 1 g t.d.s) and clofibrate (1 g b.d.) or with placebo (Table 6.4). This led to a 13% decrease in cholesterol and a 19% decrease in triglycerides in the intervention group. Because of the flushing associated with nicotinic acid the trial was inevitably open. There was a 36% decrease in IHD mortality and a 26% decrease in all-cause mortality in the intervention group during the 5 years of the trial. In another trial, myocardial infarction survivors were treated with clofibrate or nicotinic acid[69]. The decrease in serum lipid concentrations was less than in the Stockholm Secondary Prevention study. There was a decrease in non-fatal IHD but not in fatal IHD in the 6 years of the study in the patients treated with nicotinic acid. However, the results of 15 years' observation showed that all-cause mortality was decreased by 11%[70]. This benefit persisting many years after discontinuing the drug suggests that the duration of observation of the participants in a trial is important and that the meta-analysis of results of multiple short trials will probably underestimate benefits.

The use of the odds ratio in assessing the outcome of clinical trials can cause confusion and lead to the misleading impression that the difficulty of influencing all cause mortality is due to an adverse effect of lipid-lowering therapy on non-coronary mortality. If such an effect does exist it is small in comparison with the beneficial effect of cholesterol reduction on IHD deaths. It can be seen in Table 6.4, which shows the results of the Stockholm Secondary Prevention Study[68], how this confusion can be created if no reference is made to the actual number of deaths in a trial. The apparently adverse effect on the odds ratio for non-cardiac deaths results from a tiny non-significant difference. The decrease in the total number of deaths in the intervention group greatly outweighed this probably chance difference in non-cardiac deaths. The meta-analysis of secondary prevention studies which subdivided cause of death strongly supports the same conclusion, there being, for example, only 11 more non-cardiovascular deaths in the intervention groups of the trials compared to their overall decrease of 217 deaths[66,67]. It is hard to believe that there are still people who have doubts about the wisdom of lowering cholesterol in patients with established IHD.

The POSCH trial[71] is a secondary prevention trial in which serum cholesterol was decreased by partial ileal bypass (Chapter 5, page 130). This resulted in a 23% decrease in serum cholesterol. Serum triglycerides, however, increased by 25% as a result of the operation. (Interestingly many of the more modern drugs lower cholesterol by more without the potentially adverse effects on triglycerides, see Chapter 10.) The result of the trial was a remarkable 34% decrease in further IHD events (fatal and non-fatal), a 39% decrease in IHD deaths in patients whose left ventricular function was not compromised and a decrease of 68% in the need for coronary artery surgery over a period of 10 years. Clearly the results should be regarded as of major importance in planning the management of myocardial infarction survivors. However, although the total mortality was decreased by 21%, this has not yet quite reached statistical significance. The reason for this illustrates the whole problem about the use of total mortality in clinical trials of cholesterol-lowering or indeed any other intervention when the prognosis of the condition being treated is not so disastrous as to cause staggeringly high death rates. The Stockholm Secondary Prevention Study was conducted in an era (recruitment 1972–76) before coronary angiography, angioplasty, bypass surgery and many pharmacological innovations to improve survival were available. The rate of IHD mortality in participants was 5.2% p.a. When POSCH was conducted (recruitment 1975–83) therapy had advanced. All patients considered for the trial had coronary angiograms. Those with severe left main stem coronary disease or triple-vessel disease were excluded. Other treatments were not withheld from the trial partici-pants including further coronary angiography and angioplasty and coronary surgery. As a result the mortality was 1.3% p.a. Even though the great majority of these deaths are due to IHD, such low rates in only 838 participants mean that it will either take a very long time to show a difference in total mortality (perhaps forever if the control group receive the newer cholesterol-lowering drugs) and that future trials will have to be in much larger numbers of patients.

The potential value of cholesterol-lowering therapy in people with established IHD must not be underestimated. Aspirin, β-adrenoreceptor blockers and angiostensin-converting enzymes inhibitors, which have been widely and rapidly introduced into clinical practice to improve prognosis in established IHD, benefit relatively small numbers of patients. Even if cholesterol-lowering treatment decreases mortality by as little as 10%, it is likely to be more beneficial than any of these.

*Regression trials*

The coronary angiographic atheroma regression studies are a remarkable series of investigations which in themselves probably do little to influence clinical manage-ment, but when considered alongside the results of the event trials previously reviewed provide further support for the conclusions previously discussed and have also led to some new insights into coronary disease and how its natural history might be modified. A summary of the results of the non-randomized coronary regression trials which have employed cholesterol-lowering treatment[71–79] is shown in Figure 6.4. It is always important not to exclude negative studies in forming a conclusion. However, the only randomized trial which is not included appears to be an early one of clofibrate in only 40 patients lasting only 1 year[80]: its inclusion would not alter the overall opinion. An overview would be that the likelihood of regression occurring in the intervention group is some three to four times that in the control group and the chances of progression are decreased by about half. The actual changes in the mean width of coronary arteries in these trials are minute fractions of a millimetre and attention has been drawn to the apparent rapid decrease in IHD event rates in the intervention groups[81], which is hard to attribute to the increased blood flow from such small changes in arterial diameter. Such changes in event rate could be dismissed as errors due to the relatively small size of the trials. However, in the regression trials there were much greater decreases in serum cholesterol than were achieved in many of the earlier trials employing event rates as their end-point. Furthermore, in another trial 1062 men and women with serum cholesterol averag-ing 265 mg/dl (6.8 mmol/l), who were at relatively high IHD risk because they also had two other risk factors (hypertension, family history, cigarette-smoking, estab-lished IHD), were randomized to receive pravastatin or placebo[82]. There was a large difference in IHD events within 6 months (13 events in the placebo group and one in the intervention group). Is it possible therefore that such profound decreases in serum cholesterol led to some relatively immediate benefit or was this simply an effect of chance? Various explanations have been advanced. The effect could be mediated through a rapid favourable effect of plasma lipid-lowering on blood coagu-lability due perhaps to changes in platelet aggregability and fibrinogen concentra-tion[83] and thus also in blood flow due to decreased plasma viscosity. However,

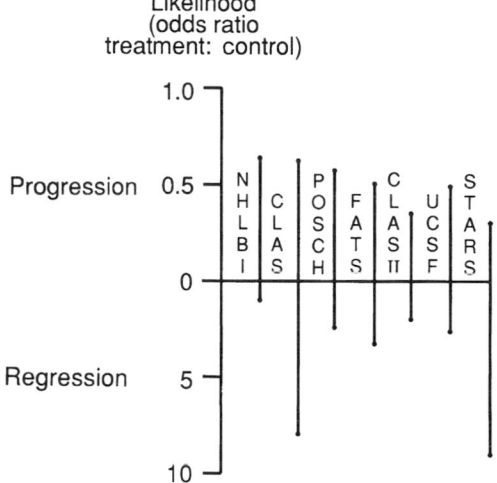

**Figure 6.4**   The likelihood of regression and progression of coronary artery disease in seven regression trials. The likelihood is expressed as the ratio of the proportion of treated to control patients in whom either regression or progression occurred[81]

not all of the lipid-lowering treatment employed in studies suggesting a rapid change in cardiac event rates has actually been shown to have very profound effects on these parameters which often relate more closely to triglyceride levels than to LDL effects. Endothelial dysfunction does occur in hypercholesterolaemia. One important function of endothelium which may be impaired is the release of endothelium-derived relaxing factor which might in its turn impair certain coronary vasodilatory responses[84]. In familial heterozygous hypercholesterolaemia, for example, femoral artery dilatation in response to reactive hyperaemia is impaired even in childhood before the development of atheromatous complications[85]. Lowering serum LDL in patients with established IHD might reduce the likelihood of coronary events by discouraging coronary artery spasm. The vascular endothelium when it has been damaged by oxidized LDL may also increase its procoagulant activity whilst its fibrinolytic activity is diminished[86]. The putative rapid-onset benefit of lipid-lowering therapy has, however, been shown in patients with IHD whose serum LDL is not as high as in patients shown to have endothelial dysfunction.

Another possible mechanism for the acute change in cardiac event rates with effective lipid-lowering therapy in IHD may be that a rapid change in the nature of the atheromatous lesions most vulnerable to rupture and subsequent thrombosis occurs (Chapter 2). In studies where attempts have been made to identify coronary lesions which have later led to coronary occlusion by studying earlier angiograms, the average degree of stenosis produced by the culprit lesions in the first angiogram was only around 50%[87,88]. Histologically such lesions are commonly the lipid-laden type of lesion. The overlying fibrous cap of such lesions is liable to rupture close to its junction with normal vessel wall where the circumferential shear stress is greatest[89] and where there is often an accumulation of lipid-laden foam cells[90]. Animal experiments show a marked reduction of lipid-laden foam cells in atheromatous lesions when hyperlipidaemia is treated. It is possible therefore that some critical phase for the rupture of an atheromatous plaque is rapidly reversed if cellular lipid-accumulation in actively progressing regions of the lesion is opposed by shutting down the supply of LDL from the circulation by lowering its concentration. It is also possible that there may be metabolic effects of some of the drugs such as the HMG-CoA reductase inhibitors within the lesion itself, which has been suggested as a possible mechanism by which simvastatin decreases accelerated graft vessel disease in transplanted rat hearts[91].

Trials showing regression of atherosclerosis are not confined to arteries of the coronary circulation. Favourable effects of lipid-lowering therapy on progression and regression of femoral atherosclerosis, at least in its early stages, have been reported[92,93].

## Benefit in people without clinically evident atherosclerotic disease

At least until recently, the case that treating hypercholesterolaemia was beneficial in the primary prevention of IHD was often considered inconclusive. There were several lines of evidence which, when considered as a whole, did, however, lead some expert committees to conclude that there was a case for encouraging cholesterol reduction as a means of coronary prevention and this was the origin of many of the longer running national coronary prevention programmes in countries such as Finland, Australia and more recently the USA. The evidence was as follows:

1. The effect of changes in the nutrition of certain populations on their ischaemic heart disease risk, such as the Japanese migrants to California and Hawaii in whom the prevalence of coronary disease increased, and the populations of countries such as the UK, whose IHD rates declined during the war years, when the national diet contained less fat and more carbohydrate (Chapter 3).
2. The presence of cholesterol in the atheromatous plaque that was derived from lipoproteins, which, with increasing understanding of the pathogenesis of atheroma, appeared to be present early in the process and to play an important role in the conversion of the fatty streak to a mature lesion (Chapter 2).
3. Evidence from animal experiments, particularly those involving primates, in which regression of atheroma occurred (these will not be considered further here)[94,95].
4. Evidence of regression of atheroma in man from post-mortem investigations (these will not be considered further here)[95].
5. Genetic disorders of lipoprotein metabolism associated with early onset atheroma (Chapter 12). (More recently gene manipulation in mice must also be considered)[96].
6. Evidence from clinical trials, which will now be discussed in detail.

Results of the three largest and longest primary trials are summarized in Table 6.5.

The publication of the first of these in 1978 – the WHO cooperative trial[98] was the first clear indication that modifying serum lipid levels could affect the likelihood of developing IHD. In the trial, 10 000 men with the highest cholesterol from about 30 000 screened in Edinburgh, Budapest and Prague were identified. Men with manifest IHD or other major disease were excluded from the trial. The study group were randomized to receive clofibrate 1.6 g daily or placebo capsules

**Table 6.5 Main findings of the WHO [98–100], LRC [102–105] and Helsinki [106–108] studies of primary prevention of ischaemic heart disease with lipid-modifying treatment**

| Trial | Number of men random-ized | Age (yr) | Treatment | Pretreatment lipid level (mg/dl; mmol/l) | | | Follow-up (yr) | Average difference in lipid levels (%) (active minus placebo) | | | Change in ischaemic heart disease rates | |
|---|---|---|---|---|---|---|---|---|---|---|---|---|
| | | | | Cholesterol | Triglycerides | HDL cholesterol | | Cholesterol | Triglycerides | HDL cholesterol | Overall | Non-fatal myocardial infarction |
| WHO | 10 627 | 30–59 | Clofibrate 800 mg b.d. | 248 (6.4) | – | – | 5.3 | – 9 | – | – | – 20 | – 25 |
| LRC | 3 806 | 35–59 | Cholestyramine 8 g t.d.s. | 280 (7.2) | 155 (1.7) | 44 (1.1) | 7.4 | – 8.5 | +3 | +3 | – 19 | – 19 |
| Helsinki | 4 081 | 40–55 | Gemfibrozil 600 mg b.d. | 270 (6.9) | 176 (2.0) | 47 (1.2) | 5.4 | – 10 | – 35 | +10 | – 34 | – 37 |

containing a similar quantity of olive oil. These men, and another control group of 5000 men from the lowest third of the cholesterol distribution, were observed for an average of 5.3 years. The men receiving clofibrate during the study had on average reduced their serum cholesterol level by 9% and this resulted in an overall decrease in IHD events of 20%. This decrease was mainly due to a 25% fall in non-fatal myocardial infarction, whereas the incidence of fatal myocardial infarction was not significantly different. Since, however, the incidence of fatal myocardial infarction was only 0.7% throughout the study, even with 10 000 participants, it is doubtful that a significant decrease could have been expected. The age-standardized mortality rates did not differ significantly between the three groups during the trial, but 4 years after its completion they were reported to be significantly increased in the men who had received clofibrate[99]. Unfortunately this conclusion was not based on an intention-to-treat analysis, which has only recently been reported, and reveals no excess mortality in the men treated with clofibrate even 4 years after completion of the trial[100].

The causes of mortality in the WHO trial are discussed elsewhere (Chapter 10, pages 269). The main criticism of the WHO trial is not that it failed to show any benefit, but rather that its design meant that any benefits, against which side-effects could be set, could only be minimal and it thus has little relevance to clinical practice. In a group of patients whose serum cholesterol averaged only 6.4 mmol/l (248 mg/dl) (Table 6.2), only a few would be at sufficiently high cardiovascular risk for drug treatment to produce overall benefit. The truth of this was demonstrated in the WHO trial itself, since patients with serum cholesterol levels above the median got the most benefit from clofibrate, especially when other risk factors were present, whereas the side-effects were unrelated to cholesterol lowering. In clinical practice, a lipid-lowering drug would be discontinued if it failed to produce a reduction in cholesterol and with hindsight would not be used at all unless the IHD risk was much greater than in most of the men in the WHO trial. In fact the 20% reduction in IHD for a 9% reduction in cholesterol is close to what would have been predicted from prospective epidemiological studies. This was also a feature of the LRC trial and even more potently of the Helsinki Heart Study, which are reviewed next. At the time of the publication of the WHO trial there was considerable misunderstanding of its findings and many patients at considerable risk of IHD, even those with FH, refused cholesterol-lowering treatment of any type in the mistaken belief that it has been shown to cause cancer (which it had not) and that it was of no benefit in the treatment even of specific hyperlipidaemias (which it was). Obviously no single drug is likely to be the answer to the prevention of IHD in the population as a whole. Before using a lipid-lowering drug we have to define the levels of cholesterol and IHD risk above which benefit will accrue. In the words of Oliver: 'The results of this [the WHO] trial will be debated in many places. What is clear, at least, is that reduction of serum cholesterol concentration is relevant to the prevention of coronary heart disease'[101].

The Lipid Research Clinics (LRC) trial was begun in the early 1970s from several centres in Northern America, created by the US National Heart, Lung and Blood Institute for the purposes of the trial and the Prevalence Program (Chapter 3)[102–105]. Almost 4000 middle-aged men, with no evidence of IHD and whose serum cholesterol persisted above the 95th percentile for the US population after the introduction of a fairly unrestrictive lipid-lowering diet, participated. Their average cholesterol was 280 mg/dl (7.2 mmol/l). Men whose serum triglycerides exceeded 300 mg/dl (3.4 mmol/l) were not included. They were randomized to receive either cholestyramine (Questran) six sachets daily or placebo. After an average of just over 7 years' treatment the trial was analysed on an 'intention-to-treat' basis. This means that participants allocated to a particular group were analysed as part of that group, even if they did not comply with the medication. This was thus a more rigorous assessment of therapy than is applicable to clinical practice, but it minimizes the possibility of bias. There was thus only a small difference in cholesterol between the placebo and active treatment groups of 8.5%. Nevertheless, the effect on coronary morbidity was dramatic, there being approximately a 20% decrease in all coronary heart disease, fatal myocardial infarction, non-fatal myocardial infarction, development of positive exercise ECG, new angina and coronary bypass surgery. The consistent change in all these end-points is important, because some authorities argued that the result lacked statistical significance because a one-tailed test had been used to analyse the results rather than a two-tailed test (disallowing the hypothesis that lowering cholesterol might increase the risk of IHD). The consistency of the effect on so many end-points makes it only remotely possible that their improvement occurred by chance and also strongly in support of that conclusion was the almost 50% decrease in coronary morbidity and mortality in men who took the full dose of cholestyramine, achieving a 25% decrease in their cholesterol.

The Helsinki Heart Study[106–108] was conducted in several clinics in Finland, beginning in 1981. In many respects it was of similar design to the LRC trial and also involved about 4000 middle-aged men. They were asked to participate if the cholesterol in their serum after subtraction of that in HDL exceeded 200 mg/dl (5.2 mmol/l). Patients with hypertriglyceridaemia were included. The average total serum cholesterol was 289 mg/dl (7.4 mmol/l) and the fasting triglycerides 176 mg/dl (2.0 mmol/l). The men were randomly assigned to receive placebo or gemfibrozil 600 mg b.d. Both groups received similar counselling about a lipid-lowering diet. Their serum cholesterol before the introduction of drug or placebo was 270 mg/dl (6.9 mmol/l). After 5 years the study was analysed on an 'intention-to-treat' basis, but as the compliance with therapy was high the lipid responses were much closer to those which might be encountered in clinical practice. There was a clear 34% decrease in cardiac events in the drug-treated group, a 37% difference in non-fatal myocardial infarction and a 28% decline in total cardiac deaths. The decrease in serum cholesterol to achieve this was 10%.

The Helsinki Heart Study raises an important question about whether modification of serum levels of lipoproteins other than LDL cholesterol is important. In the LRC study and the WHO study, the 2% decrease in IHD for every 1% decrease in cholesterol was exactly in accord with the prediction from the relationship between serum cholesterol and IHD in prospective studies[105]. In the Helsinki study, the decrease in IHD was closer to 3% for a 1% cholesterol reduction. Was this due to the additional effect of decreasing triglycerides or of increasing HDL? One analysis suggests that the HDL effect was most important[108]. This is considered further in the context of the rationale for treating hypertriglyceridaemia (Chapter 7).

One feature common to both the LRC and Helsinki trials was that the difference in IHD between drug- and placebo-treated men was evident after 2 years. This rather seems to support the idea that IHD risk can change quite quickly, gleaned from the rather rapid shift in IHD mortality in the UK during the war years and more recently from other clinical trials (see Benefit in patients with established atherosclerotic disease, page 148), and is encouraging for patients whose hyperlipidaemia is not discovered until middle age or later. At the same time it must call into question conclusions drawn from trials which have lasted less than 2 years and in which the reduction in cholesterol has been 10% or less (Table 6.3).

Neither the LRC nor the Helsinki Heart Study nor the WHO trial demonstrated a decrease in all-cause mortality between drug- and placebo-treated men. Much has been made of this by the traditional detractors of the 'cholesterol hypothesis'. Their argument is somewhat specious. The men in these studies, because they had been specifically selected for their lack of evidence of pre-existing IHD, were probably fitter in cardiovascular terms than middle-aged men in general. The studies were therefore not equipped to show an effect on all-cause mortality, since cardiovascular mortality would be under-represented. Any unfavourable or favourable effect on total mortality could only arise by chance. Evidence that cholesterol-lowering does reduce total mortality can only come from studies that are so large as to be impossible on grounds of cost, or studies involving men whose coronary risk is substantially increased above normal, but which, with the present knowledge that their cardiovascular morbidity can be reduced, may be considered unethical in some countries. Despite this, it is important to realize that evidence that cholesterol reduction will reduce all-cause mortality is not an essential prerequisite to getting on with treating hypercholesterolaemia in patients at substantially increased IHD risk, because of more importance is the very secure evidence that cholesterol reduction decreases morbidity. If IHD were to be abolished altogether, it would extend the life expectancy of the average man or woman by only 3–4 years[109]. Although, as doctors, we tend to regard ourselves as saving lives, medicine has had in reality very little impact on the life expectancy of the average person once he or she has survived childhood, which remains little more than 'three score and ten' as it was in the Psalms[110].

If our *raison d'être* as doctors were to reduce mortality, society need have little use for our humble efforts, a fact which has not gone unnoticed by health economists. Fortunately, we are much better at reducing morbidity, which is the traditional role of medicine, and the scale of morbidity from IHD is enormous. In the UK, 20 million working days are lost each year due to IHD, more than influenza or arthritis and rheumatism[111], making not only an impressive economic case for reducing serum cholesterol levels as a means of prevention but, when translated into terms of human suffering, a persuasive moral case as well. Further extrapolation beyond the working population to an even slightly older age group amplifies the impact of preventable coronary morbidity even more. In the USA in 1980 it was estimated that the annual cost of IHD was $80 billion, with direct health costs of $30 billion[112]. These figures must be higher today.

The issue of whether there is evidence that lowering cholesterol decreases total mortality does, however, remain an important one. First this is because it has been widely publicized not only amongst physicians but also amongst the lay public. It is not sufficiently widely appreciated that similar questions remain unanswered about the treatment of other common medical conditions, for example hypertension, non-insulin-dependent diabetes mellitus, arthritis and dyspepsia. Nonetheless in many doctors' minds it has acted as a disincentive to detect or to treat hypercholesterolaemia appropriately, often even in patients with established IHD or familial hypercholesterolaemia. Secondly, the issue is an important one if we are to adopt rational strategies for the use of lipid-lowering diets and drugs and to design relevant future trials, which will permit the development and adoption of effective newer approaches to IHD prevention.

There are really three aspects of the issue to consider. First, is either a low level of serum cholesterol or lowering the serum cholesterol concentration harmful in any way, and secondly, as corollary to this are any of the diets or drugs in use for the treatment of hypercholesterolaemia harmful? Thirdly, can we draw from current evidence reliable conclusions about which groups of patients will benefit overall from cholesterol-lowering?

## IHD mortality and non-IHD mortality in cholesterol-lowering trials

All of the cholesterol-lowering trials have had too few clinical events in them to individually provide any reliable conclusions about any end-point other than that for which they have been designed, namely to demonstrate a reduction in all IHD events (IHD mortality and morbidity). Few would dispute their success in that respect, particularly that of the larger and longer ones. In order, however, to get any idea of what effect cholesterol-lowering has on IHD mortality, overall mortality and any specific causes of mortality, meta-analysis, a technique for pooling the results of several trials, must be used. This has led to considerable disagreement and a lot of silly speculation in the press. Reporters, who are not as a group by nature abstemious, delight in any story that alcohol, cigarette smoking or high cholesterol is good for them. From a purely scientific standpoint the controversy is not so much about the technique of meta-analysis, but which trials should be included and whether there are sufficient numbers of participants in the trials even when pooled to draw any reliable conclusions. This does not, of course, mean that the conclusion that lowering cholesterol decreases combined IHD mortality and morbidity, arrived at without the aid of meta-analysis, is in any way diminished. The major published meta-analyses are those of Holme[113,114], Davey Smith and colleagues[115], Ravnskov[116] and Law and co-workers[64,65]. Holme's meta-analysis included 19 trials with follow-up greater than 2 years in which it was intended to lower cholesterol including trials in which other coronary risk factors were also modified. He had a total of 135 000 patients. Ravnskov included 22 trials regardless of duration. Davey Smith and colleagues included trials of more than 6 months duration with at least one death. In all, 35 trials were included with 57 000 participants. Law et al. analysed 28 trials giving a total of 52 000 patients. They exclude trials of oestrogen and D-thyroxine but inclusion of these makes no difference to results of meta-analysis[68,115].

The results of one meta-analysis[116] are inconsistent with those of the other three in several respects. First, the author of the trial disputes that cholesterol-lowering in meta-analysis is associated with significant decrease in IHD mortality whereas this has been a consistent finding in the other meta-analyses. The explanation is that included in this meta-analysis were trials in which virtually no difference between the cholesterol levels in the intervention and control groups had been achieved. His decrease in fatal IHD ($P<0.06$) is consistent with the overall decrease in cholesterol of only 15 mg/dl (0.4 mmol/l) in the treated patients which has generally been around 23 mg/dl (0.6 mmol/l) in the other meta-analyses. Secondly, he disputed any relationship between the degree of reduction in serum cholesterol and the extent to which coronary risk was decreased. This is inexplicable, because it was not only evident in the other meta-analyses in which it was sought[64,65,113–115 ] but is also seen in the larger of the primary prevention trials themselves[98,105,108]. Thirdly, Ravnskov disputed the relationship between the duration of a trial and the degree of decrease in IHD incidence. Again this is inexplicable and runs counter with the other meta-analyses (Table 6.3) and with individual trials[117].

If we consider the other three meta-analyses we are really considering patient populations which differ according to whether trials involving multiple interventions besides cholesterol-lowering were included. Holme's meta-analysis has the largest population by virtue of including multiple risk factor intervention trials[113,114]. Unfortunately, some of these trials produced the most disappointing reduction in serum cholesterol. His analysis provides strong evidence that lowering cholesterol in addition to reducing IHD morbidity also decreases IHD mortality. It shows a trend towards a reduction in all-cause mortality and shows that this like the decrease in IHD morbidity and mortality is related to the degree to which serum cholesterol is decreased.

The other two meta-analyses[64,65,115] include only trials in which it was intended primarily to reduce cholesterol. Although the inclusion in one of these[115] of trials using D-thyroxine and oestrogen in men, both treatments abandoned due to their obvious adverse effects in causing dysrhythmias and thromboembolic complications, has been criticized, these trials considered together did actually show overall benefit of cholesterol-lowering[118], although, of course, that benefit would be expected to be diminished by these side-effects. The advantage of this meta-analysis is that it included 35 trials and that this was a sufficient number to allow stratification of the trials according to the IHD risk of their participants. It was then evident that there was a decrease in all-cause mortality in those trials which have been in patients at high risk of death from IHD. The decrease in all-cause mortality occurred when the risk of IHD death exceeded 30 per 1000 per annum (Table 6.6). There was a significant relationship between the extent of cholesterol lowering and the reduction in IHD deaths. Conversely, deaths from other causes were not significantly related to the reduction in the cholesterol level and, if anything, mortality from other causes was lower when cholesterol reduction was greater, confirming that cholesterol reduction itself was unlikely to produce an increased risk of death from non-IHD causes. There was, however, an adverse effect on the odds ratio for deaths from non-IHD risk which hardly dented the benefit in terms of reduction of IHD risk which was 0.78 compared to 0.81 for all-cause mortality. This means that the excess non-IHD deaths were few in number compared to the lives saved (see also page 151 for discussion of odds ratio). No adverse effect of cholesterol-lowering was seen with non-pharmacological treatment.

**Table 6.6 The ratio of death rates in the intervention to those in the control groups in clinical trials of cholesterol-lowering**

| | No. of trials | No. of participants | Odds ratio | | |
|---|---|---|---|---|---|
| | | | IHD deaths | Non-IHD deaths | All deaths |
| *Drugs Trials* | | | | | |
| IHD deaths ≥ 3% p.a. | 11 | 11 106 | 0.78 | 1.14 | 0.81 |
| IHD deaths < 3% p.a. | 13 | 31 165 | 0.97 | 1.27 | 1.08 |
| *Non-drug trials* | | | | | |
| IHD deaths ≥ 3% p.a. | 6 | 4 009 | 0.79 | 0.98 | 0.80 |
| IHD deaths < 3% p.a. | 6 | 10 874 | 1.09 | 1.05 | 1.07 |

Data from reference [115]

The meta-analysis of Law *et al.*[64,65] was smaller than that of Davey Smith *et al.* largely because of the exclusion of trials of oestrogen and D-thyroxine. They did not stratify the trials according to IHD risk. There was a clear reduction in IHD deaths with intervention to decrease cholesterol ($P<0.004$). This was related to the duration of the trials (Table 6.3) and to the degree of reduction in cholesterol[65]. There was no significant decrease in all-cause mortality in the primary prevention trials. There was, however, a decrease in all-cause mortality in patients with established IHD ($P<0.008$). In these patients there was no change in mortality rates from causes of death other than IHD.

Neither the meta-analysis of Law and colleagues nor that of Davey-Smith and colleagues demonstrated any adverse effect of cholesterol-lowering by diet in the primary prevention trials. However, in the primary prevention trials which employed medication there was a significant ($P<0.02$) increase in deaths due to causes other than IHD. This increase stemmed from a slightly greater death rate in the intervention group, roughly in the region of one to two deaths per 1000 per year. It is important to realize that the apparent small increase in non-IHD deaths was not the reason for a failure of the primary prevention trials to show a significant reduction in total mortality despite their success in decreasing IHD deaths. The explanation was because there were too few IHD deaths in the relatively low risk populations studied for their decrease to influence overall mortality significantly. This is not a criticism of the individual trials because the end-point for which they were designed was the combined end-point of IHD morbidity and mortality. Many of the trials were relatively short and it is therefore reasonable to assume that the expected decrease in IHD mortality from a 10% decrease in cholesterol in the trials would be between 6 and 20% (Table 6.3), say 10%. Even if we combine the data from primary prevention trials together with that of the secondary prevention trials (in which there was a decrease in all-cause mortality and in which over 80% of deaths were due to IHD) so that IHD deaths comprise 65% of the total deaths from any cause would be only 6.5% fewer in the intervention groups. Well over 100 000 patients would be required for it to be detected with any degree of certainty[119]. In the meta-analysis of Law *et al.*[65] the observed difference from a 10% reduction in cholesterol was 4% (95% confidence intervals, 10% reduction to 2% increase) so that the actual trial results are quite compatible with this line of reasoning.

As to the question of whether there is an increase in non-IHD mortality with lipid-lowering drugs, albeit small, most statisticians have argued that the size of the trials is still too small to be sure of this. There is no doubt that the hazard of dying from gall bladder surgery in, for example, the WHO trial can be laid at the door of clofibrate (although, of course, the risk may be more to do with surgeons)[98]. Apart from this, no other individual cause of non-IHD death is plausibly or significantly increased. One small 'meta-analysis' did claim to show a significant increase in non-medical deaths (accidents, suicide or violence)[120]. The biological plausibility of the results of such a subset analysis are questionable when plainly the antecedents of taking one's own life and being the passenger in an airliner which crashes are very different. The result was obtained by including in the meta-analysis only six trials, two of which lasted less than 2 years, two of which were in people in long-term residential care because they were mentally ill or elderly and only four of which involved lipid-lowering drugs.

Despite its implausibility, despite the fact that larger meta-analyses have discounted its findings, despite the fact that it has been clearly shown that non-IHD deaths in trials are unrelated to the extent of cholesterol-lowering and despite a careful analysis of the non-medical deaths in the two most recent large primary prevention trials, which has shown that the deaths were unrelated even to medication (many of the deaths being in non-compliant patients)[121], the idea that cholesterol-lowering drugs cause aggressive behaviour or depression persists and continues to surface in newspapers. Research has been funded on a grand scale to investigate the effect of cholesterol-lowering on the psyche and the various theories linking a decrease in cholesterol in CNS cell membranes to mental changes. The CNS generally makes its own cholesterol and patients with hypobetalipoproteinaemia live happily into old age (page 370). I feel the issue of whether cholesterol-lowering drugs are in any way harmful is something of a red herring, because the trials have already told me that there are *no* substantial benefits of cholesterol-lowering medication in patients whose risk was as low as most included in the primary prevention trials. There is thus no purpose in exposing such people to possible adverse effects of drug therapy in clinical practice no matter how remote the possibility. The overall balance of evidence is, however, strongly in favour of introducing lipid-lowering drugs, if diet is inadequate to control hyperlipidaemia in patients at high risk of IHD. The outstanding question is how high is high? It is also, of course, the case that newly introduced lipid modifying drugs should undergo trials to establish their long-term safety, but in that respect they do not differ from any other medication for chronic medical conditions.

## When to introduce medication?

This section will discuss at what level of IHD risk it is reasonable to go beyond dietary therapy and introduce medication.

### Management of FCH and polygenic hypercholesterolaemia

In purely practical terms it can be extremely difficult to allocate the diagnosis of FCH as opposed to polygenic hypercholesterolaemia to a particular patient. Indeed the diagnosis of familial hypercholesterolaemia (FH) itself can be elusive in, for example, patients in their twenties or thirties who do not have tendon xanthomata and when none of their first-degree relatives is available for examination. The great majority of patients will present therefore with an undifferentiated hypercholesterolaemia. Guidelines for their management have been suggested by several groups[16–18,50,122–126].

The first set were published by the National Institutes of Health Consensus Conference in 1985[16]. Since then there have been a plethora of guidelines from numerous international and national bodies. It would be pointless to discuss all of these here, particularly because they embody similar principles and a few sets suffice to illustrate the difficulties of writing such guidelines. Guidelines in any area of clinical medicine are difficult to write and easy to criticize. They will always epitomize Herman Melville's aphorism 'Truth uncompromisingly told will always have its ragged edges'. Three sets of guidelines will be considered, all of which have been recently revised: those of the National Cholesterol Education Program (NCEP)[50,126], the European Atherosclerosis Society (EAS)[17,123] and the British Hyperlipidaemia Association (BHA)[18,124,125] (Tables 6.7–6.9).

**Table 6.7 The guidelines of the Second Adult Treatment Panel (ATPII) of the US National Cholesterol Education Panel who state that 'these general principles may not always pertain to individual patients, and clinical judgment is required for shaping the best therapy for individuals' [126]**

**Case detection**

A. *Non-fasting total serum cholesterol and HDL cholesterol should be measured in all adults ≥ 20 years old without IHD or other atherosclerotic diseases.* Repeat at 5-yearly intervals if cholesterol desirable, i.e. ≤200 mg/dl (≤5.2 mmol/l) and HDL cholesterol >35 mg/dl (>0.91 mmol/l). More often if cholesterol 200–239 mg/dl (5.17–6.21 mmol/l) and/or other risk factors

B. *Fasting serum triglycerides, total cholesterol, HDL cholesterol and LDL cholesterol* should be measured in:
1. All patients with established IHD or other atherosclerotic disease
2. People discovered in A to have high cholesterol, i.e. ≥240 mg/dl (≥6.21 mmol/l)
3. People discovered in A to have borderline high cholesterol, i.e. 200–239 mg/dl (5.17–6.21 mmol/l) who in addition have two risk factors or who in addition have HDL cholesterol ≤35 mg/dl (≤0.91 mmol/l)

*Risk factors:*
(i) Male ≥45 years old
(ii) Female ≥55 years old or premature menopause without oestrogen replacement therapy
(iii) Family history of premature IHD
(iv) Cigarette smoking
(v) Hypertension
(vi) Diabetes mellitus
(vii) Low HDL (≤35 mg/dl; ≤0.91 mmol/l)
(viii) HDL ≥60 mg/dl (>1.55 mmol/l) is a negative risk factor. Subtract one of (i)–(vi)

**Action limits** are based on LDL cholesterol
*Primary prevention*
(i) *Definitions*
Desirable LDL cholesterol <130 mg/dl (<3.36 mmol/l)
Borderline LDL cholesterol 130–159 mg/dl (3.36–4.11 mmol/l)
High LDL cholesterol >160 mg/dl (≥4.14 mmol/l)
(ii) *Indications for dietary therapy*
Institute dietary therapy if LDL cholesterol >160 mg/dl (4.14 mmol/l) or is 130–159 mg/dl (3.36–4.11 mmol/l) with two or more additional risk factors
(iii) *Dietary therapy*
Total fat restricted to 30% of dietary energy, saturated fat restricted to 8–10% dietary energy and dietary cholesterol to <300 mg/day. If LDL cholesterol still ≥160 mg/dl (≥4.11 mmol/l) or ≥130 mg/dl (≥3.36 mmol/l) when two or more additional risk factors present intensify diet so that saturated fat is <7% dietary energy and dietary cholesterol <200 mg/day.
(iv) *Indications for drug therapy*
Institute lipid-lowering drug therapy if despite dietary therapy LDL cholesterol ≥190 mg/dl(≥4.91 mmol/l) or ≥160 mg/dl(≥4.14 mmol/l) in the presence of two or more additional risk factors. Goal is LDL cholesterol <160 mg/dl (<4.14 mmol/l) if one or no other risk factors or <130 mg/dl (<3.36 mmol/l) if two or more additional risk factors are present

Exceptions are young men (≤35 years old) and premenopausal women in whom drug therapy should generally be restricted to those with LDL cholesterol ≥220 mg/dl (≥5.69 mmol/l), 'unless multiple risk factors are present'. On the other hand, the cut-points may be decreased for some patients with single additional risk factors such as diabetes mellitus or family history of premature IHD

*Secondary prevention*
Lipid-lowering therapy should be initiated in all patients with established IHD or other atherosclerotic disease whose LDL >100 mg/dl (>2.59 mmol/l) on dietary treatment

**Table 6.8 Recommendation of the International Task Force of the European Atherosclerosis Society, who state 'Since most risk factors are continuous variables, e.g. plasma cholesterol, specific action limits are no more than a guide to therapy. Global risk must therefore be judged on the basis of the doctor's knowledge of the patient as a whole'[123]**

**Case detection**
A. *Serum cholesterol is measured in all adults as part of screening for global coronary risk offered opportunistically when patient attends doctor for some other purpose.* Genetic hyperlipidaemia should be diagnosed before the age of 40 years. Diagnosis of hyperlipidaemia requires a minimum of two consistent analyses

B. *Fasting cholesterol, triglycerides and HDL cholesterol*
    (i)    in all patients with cardiovascular disease
    (ii)   in people with serum cholesterol >250 mg/dl (>6.5 mmol/l)
    (iii)  in people with serum cholesterol >200 mg/dl (>5.2 mmol/l) plus non-lipid risk factors, and in diabetes and hypertension
    (iv)  mandatory if drug treatment is being considered, but need not be repeated on each occasion when therapy is being monitored, serum cholesterol measurement often sufficing

*Risk factors*
    (i)    Age. Risk factor reduction necessary at all ages except where life expectancy limited. Not stated how age should be used in determination of global risk
    (ii)   Sex. After menopause women require same management as men. Not stated how male sex should be used in determination of global risk
    (iii)  Family history of premature IHD
    (iv)  Cigarette smoking
    (v)   Hypertension
    (vi)  HDL cholesterol <35 mg/dl (<0.9 mmol/l) in men
    (vii)  HDL cholesterol <42 mg/dl (<1.1mmol/l) in women (high risk in women if serum total cholesterol : HDL cholesterol >5)
  (viii)  High serum fibrinogen (level not stated)
    (ix)  Obesity, especially if truncal distribution

**Action limits**
*Primary prevention*
    (i)    *Definitions based on total serum cholesterol*
         Desirable <200 mg/dl(<5.2 mmol/l)
         Mildly increased risk 200–300 mg/dl (5.2–7.8 mmol/l) + no non-lipid risk factors or HDL <39 mg/dl (<1.0 mmol/l). Higher risk >300 mg/dl (>7.8 mmol/l) or familial hypercholesterolaemia or 200–300 mg/dl (5.2–7.8 mmol/l) + two non-lipid factors or one severe non-lipid risk factor
    (ii)   *Indication for dietary therapy*
         Cholesterol >200 mg/dl (>5.2 mmol/l) or LDL cholesterol >135 mg/dl(>3.5 mmol/l)
    (iii)  *Dietary therapy*
         Correction of overweight. Restrict saturated fats and replace (if diet not primarily intended to be reducing) with unsaturated fats and foods providing complex carbohydrate and soluble fibre. Restrict dietary cholesterol
         Specific dietary items which may be eaten freely, in moderation or avoided are tabulated.
    (iv)  *Indications for drug therapy should be based on LDL cholesterol*
      (a) Consider in those with serum cholesterol >300 mg/dl (>7.8 mmol/l) or LDL cholesterol >215 mg/dl (>5.5 mmol/l). Commonly needed for major genetic hyperlipidaemias, e.g. familial hypercholesterolaemia, after a 3 months trial of conservative measures
      (b) Consider in those with serum cholesterol 250–300 mg/dl (6.5–7.8 mmol/l) or LDL cholesterol 175–215 mg/dl (4.5–5.5 mmol/l) at high risk after 3–6 month trial of conservative measures
      (c) Required uncommonly even for patients at high risk of coronary disease with serum cholesterol 200–250 mg/dl (5.2–6.5 mmol/l) or LDL cholesterol 135–175 mg/dl (3.5–4.5 mmol/l) after prolonged trial of conservative measures. NB: This recommendation does not apply to patients with established IHD – see Secondary prevention

**Table 6.8 continued**
   (d) The guidelines differentiate between hypercholesterolaemia in the absence and in the presence of hypertriglyceridaemia (>200 mg/dl; >2.3 mmol/l). In the latter recommendations for patients with serum cholesterol 200–250 mg/dl (5.2–6.5 mmol/l) are the same as for those with serum cholesterol 250–300 mg/dl (6.5–7.8 mmol/l) without hypertriglyceridaemia
   (e) Goal of therapy is to reduce LDL cholesterol to 115–135 mg/dl (3.0–3.5 mmol/l) in those at high risk, to 135–155 mg/dl(3.5–4.0 mmol/l) in those at moderately increased risk and to 155–175 mg/dl (4.0–4.5 mmol/l) in those at mildly increased risk

*Secondary prevention*
Unclear in the desk-top summary, but it does appear to be the intention of the authors that diet and drugs should be used in patients with established coronary disease with LDL cholesterol >135 mg/dl (3.5 mmol/l) with the aim of reducing it to 115–135 mg/dl (3.0–3.5 mmol/l), some of the committee opting for a LDL target of 95–115 mg/dl (2.5–3.0 mmol/l).

*All of the guidelines to be reviewed make the overall IHD risk rather than the absolute level of serum cholesterol the most important indication for lipid-lowering drug therapy.*

The NCEP guidelines were first published in 1988 and were revised recently to take account of (a) stronger evidence of benefit from cholesterol-lowering in patients with established IHD, (b) concerns about whether the earlier guidelines might not lead to the use of lipid-lowering drugs in patients not at sufficiently high IHD risk for benefit with possible adverse consequences[127] and inconsistencies in the degree of IHD risk in different categories for which drug treatment was recommended[128] and (c) to include HDL cholesterol in the assessment of risk.

## Detection of hyperlipidaemia

The NCEP guidelines are most strongly in favour of population screening and make clear recommendations that screening should begin at the age of 20 in both men and women and continue at 5-yearly intervals. Both random serum cholesterol and HDL cholesterol are recommended for screening. The EAS is also in favour of population screening, but is less prescriptive and considers that the best approach is an opportunistic one, in which patients are invited to be screened for cardiovascular risk when they attend their family practitioner for some other purpose. It is known that 80–90% of patients visit their family medical practice for some purpose every 2 years. Both the EAS and the BHA recommend random total serum cholesterol as the screening test. There is, however, controversy in Britain about whether there should be population screening or whether cholesterol should only be measured in patients with established atherosclerosis or in whom cardiovascular risk is already sufficiently high that the discovery of a high cholesterol level might justify treatment on the basis of clinical trial evidence. In terms of the cost of the actual screening there is not likely to be great economic advantages in the selective approach, because it is known that the prevalence of risk factors in the middle-aged population would mean that perhaps as many as 50% would still require cholesterol testing[129] and there would be no saving on the cost of the initial screening process, which must involve enquiring about risk factors, examination for stigmata of hyperlipidaemia and blood pressure measurement to determine who qualifies for cholesterol measurement. Furthermore a

**Table 6.9 Guidelines for the management of hypercholesterolaemia from the British Hyperlipidaemia Association, who state that 'Drug therapy should be reserved for those patients at high risk where life style measures have failed to result in acceptable plasma lipid levels'[124]**

**Case detection**
A. *Non-fasting serum cholesterol: minimum standard of medical practice should be to measure cholesterol in patients with overt atherosclerotic disease, clinical stigmata of hyperlipidaemia, a strong family history of premature IHD and those with other risk factors for IHD such as hypertension, diabetes mellitus and obesity.* In children of parents with FH the diagnosis should be made by the age of 5 years. No specific policy possible at present about whether there should be mass-screening

B. *Fasting serum cholesterol, triglycerides, HDL cholesterol and LDL cholesterol*
   (i)    Patients with serum cholesterol >200 mg/dl (>5.2 mmol/l) + established IHD or other clinically significant vascular disease
   (ii)   people with serum cholesterol 250–300 mg/dl (6.5–7.8 mmol/l) + another significant risk factor
   (iii)  people with serum cholesterol >300 mg/dl (>7.8 mmol/l) regardless of presence of other risk factors

*Risk factors*
Cigarette-smoking, hypertension, diabetes mellitus, strong family history of premature IHD, renal disease

**Action limits**
*Primary and secondary prevention*
   (i)   *Definitions*
        Terms such as high risk etc. attaching to particular cholesterol levels are avoided. Instead treatment is prioritized according to the strength of the evidence favouring intervention with lipid-lowering drug therapy and the ease of identifying patients whose IHD risk justifies intervention. See Indications for drug therapy
   (ii)  *Indications for dietary therapy*
        Serum cholesterol ≥200 mg/dl (≥5.2 mmol/l) or LDL cholesterol 160 mg/dl (≥4.1 mmol/l) in primary prevention and LDL ≥130 mg/dl (≥3.4 mmol/l) in secondary. Dietary treatment in children with heterozygous FH should begin at the age of 5 years
   (iii) *Dietary therapy*
        Total fat ≤ 30% with saturated fat <10% total dietary energy and cholesterol <300 mg/day. The extent to which any intensification of this dietary advice is possible is a matter for individual counselling. Failure of the achievement of some arbitrary target is not in itself an indication for lipid-lowering drug therapy
   (iv) *Indications for drug therapy*

| Degree of priority | Clinical features | Cholesterol* mg/dl (mmol/l) (Total) | (LDL) |
|---|---|---|---|
| First (highest) | Established IHD, coronary artery bypass surgery or angioplasty, cardiac transplant, other significant atherosclerosis | >200 (>5.2) | >130 (>3.4) |
| Second | Genetic hyperlipidaemia, e.g. FH or multiple major risk factors | >250 (>6.5) | >190 (>5.0) |
| Third | Men without overt atherosclerosis or risk factors | >300 (>7.8) | >230 (>6.0) |
| Fourth (lowest) | Postmenopausal women† without overt atherosclerosis or risk factors | >300 (>7.8) + total cholesterol : HDL cholesterol >5.0 | >230 (>6.0) |

* Generally after dietary measures, preferably individual counselling for 3–6 months.
† Consider use of HRT before lipid-lowering drug therapy.

significant population of people, in whom severely elevated serum cholesterol constitutes their only known coronary risk factor, will be missed by such an approach. For example, a large proportion of men with heterozygous familial hypercholesterolaemia inherited from their mother may develop clinical IHD without any adverse family history or other risk factors[130].

The real fear of those opposed to population screening for hypercholesterolaemia is that the medical profession will misinterpret the result and otherwise healthy people at modest risk of premature IHD will be worried unduly and, worse, may be given unnecessarily restrictive dietary advice and perhaps pharmacotherapy. The widespread use of lipid-lowering drugs without hope of any substantial benefit would, of course, be extremely costly and a misuse of resources which at least in a state health care system might be more effectively directed elsewhere. Support for this view has been rallied by the huge publicity which has been given to reports that cholesterol-lowering medication may have adverse effects on non-cardiovascular mortality. This fear is largely unjustified (pages 159–162). In the author's view, a better argument against wholesale cholesterol screening is the lack of evidence of any substantial beneficial effect of treatment in people with relatively modest elevations of serum cholesterol in the absence of other major risk factors or heightened susceptibility to IHD. The prescription of therapy from which the patient does not stand to benefit is, therefore, quite simply poor medical practice and is to be decried.

There is thus a strong case for ensuring that any guidelines about the management of hypercholesterolaemia are not couched in such terms that they may lead to the unnecessary administration of lipid-lowering drugs, but of considerably greater importance is the education of doctors and medical students about how to assess cardiovascular risk and to interpret lipoprotein levels and diagnose dyslipoproteinaemia. The NCEP, EAS and BHA are quite clear in their recommendations that cholesterol screening should be part of a programme of overall cardiovascular risk factor management. Implicit in this must be that the doctors and nurses administering such a programme should be sufficiently knowledgeable to interpret the information sensibly and without causing undue anxiety. A physician's first duty is, in the case of the great majority of people who consult him or her, to improve the health of that individual and whether society, as a whole, benefits from the therapy advised for that patient is generally of lesser importance. It should, however, be the responsibility of any health service in any state in which IHD is a major health problem to introduce a universal system of risk factor screening including the management of serum cholesterol as soon as there is adequate reassurance that this will not lead to the misuse of pharmacotherapy or encourage excessive phobia about one risk factor. An education programme for the medical and nursing profession in advance of or in parallel with the introduction of population screening is thus essential. There has been widespread use of antihypertensive medication (Chapter 11) in most prosperous countries with probably the majority of the recipients unlikely to receive any benefit[131]. A more selective approach is now beginning to be advocated in the management of hypertension[132] so it seems unreasonable to use this as an argument against detecting and treating significant hyperlipidaemia when current recommendations for the management of hypercholesterolaemia already appear to be more rational than those for hypertension.

There probably has been an inappropriate use of lipid-lowering drugs. Even in the USA and many European countries where the consumption of cholesterol-lowering medication is high, there has probably been a failure to institute treatment in many high risk patients, a failure which cannot be laid at the door of those responsible for the guidelines. On the other hand, there may be significant numbers of people receiving lipid-lowering drugs from which there is little evidence that they will benefit[128] and who regard themselves as unhealthy as a result of the knowledge that their cholesterol is high. This could have been aggravated by some of the guidelines. At the present time in Britain the debate about the overall benefit to society of cholesterol screening continues and is unfortunately one factor which has led to a low rate of cholesterol testing even in people who are clearly at high IHD risk, such as those who have developed the disease prematurely, and a rate of cholesterol testing lower than most other countries even with less IHD and smaller health care budgets. In Britain at present therefore the effective introduction of a selective programme for cholesterol measurement must be viewed as a stage in the development of a universal screening programme linked with an education programme allowing rational interpretation of the results. In the USA where a universal screening programme was launched *ab initio* a re-evaluation of the indications for lipid-lowering medication has been necessary[126].

The NCEP, EAS and BHA agree that a proportion of people with undesirable cholesterol levels should have a fasting lipoprotein profile (cholesterol, triglycerides, HDL cholesterol and LDL cholesterol calculated from the Friedewald formula, page 98). There is agreement that cholesterol levels above 200 mg/dl (5.2 mmol/l) are undesirable. There is agreement that all patients with established IHD should have a fasting lipoprotein profile, certainly if their cholesterol level exceeds 200 mg/dl (5.2 mmol/l). The NCEP advises a full profile if the serum cholesterol exceeds 240 mg/dl (6.2 mmol/l) or 200 mg/dl (5.2 mmol/l) if two or more risk factors are also present or if the HDL cholesterol is also less than 35 mg/dl (0.91 mmol/l). The EAS recommends levels above 250 mg/dl (6.5 mmol/l), if no other risk factor is present, but above 200 mg/dl (5.2 mmol/l) even in the presence of only one risk factor. However, given that the NCEP regard being a man aged 45 or more or female of 55 or more years of age as a risk factor, the EAS and NCEP guidelines are probably little different in their advocacy of measuring fasting lipoprotein profiles. The BHA is more conservative and regards 250 mg/dl (6.5 mmol/l) as a suitable cut-off above which the fasting lipoproteins should be measured when other risk factors are present and 300 mg/dl (7.8 mmol/l) if there are none.

## Intervention

### Primary prevention

All of the sets of guidelines recommend dietary modification if serum cholesterol exceeds 200 mg/dl (5.2 mmol/l). All would wish people who are obese to adopt a weight-reducing diet and all people whose cholesterol exceeds 200 mg/dl (5.2 mmol/l) to reduce their consumption of fat to no more than 30% of their total dietary energy intake, saturated fat to 10% or less and cholesterol to under 300 mg/day (this is the American Heart Association Step 1 diet). Ramsay, who comes from a clinical pharmacology background, has criticized this fat-modified diet recommendation on the grounds that an overview of controlled clinical trials of this diet reveals it to produce on average a less than 2% decrease in cholesterol[133]. Experimental data suggest a bigger decrease in serum cholesterol[134], but this is not a counter-argument to Ramsay's, because in practice results are likely to be closer to those suggested by Ramsay's analysis. Those patients who are obese and actually achieve weight loss frequently show much larger decreases in cholesterol (Chapter 11) and the guidelines certainly advise weight reduction. Furthermore they all advocate a more stringent decrease in saturated fat and cholesterol consumption, if serum cholesterol does not decrease with the Step 1 diet. More stringent diets do appear to decrease cholesterol but there is a great variation in by how much[134–136]. Clearly the effectiveness of weight reduction and of stricter fat modification will depend on how acceptable they are to patients and for how long they are maintained. It is probable that weight reduction is always going to be difficult to maintain. Modification of dietary fat intake need not, however, lead to an unpalatable diet. No one can convince me that the average Italian workman's diet is less enjoyable than that of the British workman: the unpalatability of a low saturated fat diet lies simply in inadequate culinary skills, prejudice and the lack of availability of cheap healthy food because of misguided and inappropriate nutritional policies. Ramsay is, however, largely correct in his case, because many people in practice in North America and North-ern Europe will not lower their serum cholesterol concentration by following dietary advice.

There is, however, a much more important point stemming from Ramsay's work which has not been challenged. This is that people who fall into the categories defined in the guidelines as being at insufficient IHD risk to warrant the use of lipid-lowering drugs are unlikely to achieve the target cholesterol levels set for them by diet alone. In other words, an asymptomatic man with a serum choles-terol of 240 mg/dl (6.2 mmol/l) in the USA or of 250 mg/dl (6.5 mmol/l) in France or of 300 mg/dl (7.8 mmol/l) in Britain is extraordinarily unlikely to achieve levels of less than 5.2 mmol/l by dietary means. Patients could, however, have been set such unrealistic targets and, furthermore, because terms such as 'high risk' may have been used initially based simply on cholesterol values, people in these categories will be alarmed at their inability to lower their cholesterol to 'safer' levels. It should be clearly stated in the guidelines that the failure of serum choles-terol to fall below some set level by dietary intervention is not an indication for lipid-lowering medication. If the patient was not at genuinely high IHD risk at the outset so that drug therapy was never a possible outcome of inadequate dietary response, explanation and reassurance should have been provided rather than exhortation to achieve the impossible. Otherwise the outcome may be that patients will be given lipid-lowering drugs for the wrong indications or will believe themselves to have a disease which cannot be treated and for which they are to blame.

Although the latest NCEP and BHA guidelines are still open to this type of misinterpretation by robotic practitioners, this is clearly not the intention of their authors. Of more concern are the latest EAC guidelines which, although they now currently state that the decision to introduce lipid-lowering medication must be based on a global assessment of coronary risk rather than the absolute cholesterol level, nevertheless repeatedly also state that diet is effective in lowering choles-terol and that there are categories of patients in whom only a minority will not respond to diet and require lipid-lowering medication. Authors of guidelines must be more careful not to classify patients as at high enough IHD risk to justify lipid-lowering medication in the expectation that the serum cholesterol in the great majority will respond adequately to diet.

## Indications for drug therapy

All three sets of guidelines are in agreement that major therapeutic decisions should only be made after at least two determinations of fasting serum cholesterol, triglycerides and HDL cholesterol which are in close agreement. This is necessary for the following reasons:

1 Measurement of triglycerides and HDL are necessary for the calculation of the LDL cholesterol (using the Friedewald equation) upon which the guidelines at least for drug therapy are based. In prospective epidemiological studies LDL cholesterol has not been more closely associated with IHD risk than total cholesterol. This may, however, be due to the greater error in estimating LDL cholesterol on a single occasion (which is generally the case in a prospective study in contrast to the clinic) compared to total serum cholesterol, because the LDL cholesterol calculation combines errors from the measurement of total serum cholesterol, triglycerides and HDL cholesterol. Furthermore in deciding the risk attaching to a particular cholesterol level in an individual as opposed to a segment of the population it is necessary to remove the effect of the cholesterol in HDL, which is inversely rather than positively related to risk. Some cholesterol too will be contained within VLDL. It is, however, somewhat debatable whether the quantity is particularly important clinically at levels of serum triglycerides up to 400 mg/dl (4.5 mmol/l), when the Friedwald formula becomes inaccurate. If VLDL cholesterol does contribute to IHD risk then, of course, the non-HDL cholesterol (i.e. total serum cholesterol – HDL cholesterol) may be a better indicator of risk than the calculated LDL cholesterol; it is certainly more accurately measured because of the additional analytical error posed by triglyceride measurement in the Friedwald formula. It is a mistake, however, to believe that the total cholesterol : HDL cholesterol ratio which has been widely advocated is more accurately measured than the LDL cholesterol calculated by the Friedwald formula because division of the triglyceride concentration by a fixed number (5 in mg/dl or 2.19 in mmol/l) reduces the impact on the overall error due to its analytical variation and the error in the HDL cholesterol measurement is subtracted from the total cholesterol rather than being its divisor which amplifies the influence of error in its measurement. Nonetheless certainly in the middle range of the serum cholesterol distribution the cholesterol: HDL cholesterol ratio may be the most accurate determination of risk, particularly if based on repeated measurements [21,137,138].

2 The LDL cholesterol is necessary to assess accurately the response to therapy, particularly in combined hyperlipidaemia. For example, administration of a fibrate drug in a patient whose cholesterol is 350 mg/dl (9.0 mmol/l), triglycerides 400 mg/dl (4.5 mmol/l) and HDL cholesterol 35 mg/dl (0.9 mmol/l) might lead to a serum cholesterol of 300 mg/dl (7.8 mmol/l), triglycerides of 200 mg/dl (2.3 mmol/l) and an HDL cholesterol value of 47 mg/dl (1.2 mmol/l), whereas on a statin (HMG-CoA reductase inhibitor) the cholesterol, triglyceride and HDL cholesterol levels might be 250 mg/dl (6.5 mmol/l), 300 mg/dl (3.5 mmol/l) and 35 mg/dl (0.8 mmol/l) respectively. Total serum cholesterol : HDL cholesterol is thus 10.0 on no drug therapy, 6.6 on fibrate therapy and 7.1 on the statin. The LDL cholesterol response is, however, dramatically different, the LDL cholesterol being 235 mg/dl (6.2 mmol/l) on no drug therapy, 213 mg/dl (5.5 mmol/l) on the fibrate and 155 mg/dl (4.0 mmol/l) on the statin.

3 A knowledge of the HDL cholesterol is important because it gives additional information about risk: there is no clinical trial evidence that raising its level *per se* will decrease IHD risk, but a low level can make it much more important to reduce the LDL cholesterol and, of course, to treat hypertension and stop smoking[21,137]. In the NCEP guidelines serum HDL cholesterol of 35 mg/dl (0.91 mmol/l) is regarded as low. The EAS makes <35 mg/dl <0.91 mmol/l) low for men, but 42 mg/dl (<1.1 mmol/l) low for women. This has been justifiably criticized because there is no evidence that the absolute risk of IHD is increased by more in a woman with an HDL cholesterol of 42 mg/dl (1.1 mmol/l) than in a man with an HDL cholesterol value of 35 mg/dl (0.91 mmol/l) whose lipoprotein levels are otherwise similar even though the levels of 42 and 35 mg/dl (1.1 and 0.9 mmol/l) may represent similar percentiles in the two sexes [139]. The measurement of HDL cholesterol is, however, particularly critical in a woman with a high cholesterol regardless of whether she is pre- or post-menopausal. This is because, unlike LDL cholesterol which generally rises at the menopause, HDL cholesterol frequently remains unchanged (Figures 3.3 and 3.8). Thus many women with a high total serum cholesterol even after the menopause, because of their preserved high HDL cholesterol, may not be at great IHD risk[140].

4 The presence of hypertriglyceridaemia may alert the clinician to the possibility that the patient has type III hyperlipoproteinaemia (Chapter 8), is at risk of pancreatitis (Chapter 7), has a high ethanol consumption (perhaps hitherto not revealed) (Chapter 11), and also reveals that the patient has an additional risk factor for IHD namely hypertriglyceridaemia which increases the risk from the raised LDL cholesterol or more accurately raised LDL:HDL cholesterol ratio[141–143].

The latest NCEP guidelines also make high levels of HDL a negative risk factor allowing the subtraction of another positive factor from the overall assessment of risk. This is an attractive concept, although the clinician should be aware that some patients at high IHD risk may have raised HDL cholesterol, for example those with insulin-treated diabetes mellitus. Given the inclusion of male gender over the age of 45 and female gender over the age of 55 years as positive risk factors subtracting one for an HDL value in excess of 60 mg/dl (1.55 mmol/l) probably restores a reasonable balance in the overall risk assessment.

5 Knowledge of the HDL and triglycerides may be helpful in determining the choice of lipid-lowering drug and occasionally diet.

All the guidelines make high global coronary risk the main indication for introducing lipid-lowering medication. None of them states the level of absolute IHD risk at which its authors believe benefit from such treatment occurs. The NCEP guidelines give the most precise advice about numbers of risk factors and levels of LDL cholesterol at which drug therapy should be introduced. They have been criticized previously for appearing to favour the introduction of lipid-lowering medication in women at lower levels of risk than in men despite the greater degree of uncertainty about benefit in women[128]. Risk factors are generally continuous variables, the degree of risk they confer depending on their severity. With the exception of cholesterol, all of the guidelines treat them as all-or-none phenomena. The BHA use the term 'major risk factors', implying that mild hypertension or trivial smoking does not count, but even it is not more specific. The EAS raises the issue, but in many ways is the least clear about how the clinician should use such information. Thus in all the guidelines there is a large element of clinical acumen required. This is of course precisely what health economists and epidemiologists most mistrust. In theory it should be possible to write a mathematical equation which would allow an estimate of an individual's absolute risk to be calculated. In practice this is not easy, largely because no prospective epidemiological study has included all the IHD risk factors which the clinician routinely has at his or her disposal when making an assessment of cardiovascular risk. These would be:

1. A clinician's history of chest pain currently and in the past and relevant cardiological investigations.
2. Physical examination to identify tendon xanthomata, tuberoeruptive xanthomata, striate palmar xanthomata.
3. Family history.
4. Age.
5. Gender.
6. Age of menopause.
7. Use of hormone replacement therapy.
8. Blood pressure and history of hypertension.
9. Diabetes mellitus, especially if proteinuria present (and glucose intolerance). Loss of female protection in diabetes.
10. Current and previous smoking habit.
11. Serum cholesterol level.
12. Fasting serum triglyceride level.
13. Serum HDL cholesterol level.

If we were to devise a risk equation therefore, we should have to pool the results from studies that had omitted to measure many of these, had not assessed the participants as rigorously as in the clinic and had not made as accurate assessments of the true mean values of variables such as lipids and blood pressure as can be made by repeated clinical measurement. Furthermore, it would be difficult to assess how much of the apparent risk conferred by a factor measured in a trial would be diminished by taking into account another risk factor not measured, e.g. if triglycerides were measured, but not HDL, then triglycerides would explain a larger proportion of the variation in risk than if HDL were also included in multivariate analysis, because the two are inversely related. Furthermore, such observational studies would contain very few people at the extremes of risk such as those with familial hypercholesterolaemia and the relative importance of serum cholesterol and other risk factors determined at lower points in their frequency distribution may be misleading.

Nevertheless, clinicians must have some concept of the absolute levels of IHD risk that they are seeking in deciding which of their patients can benefit from lipid-lowering intervention. The meta-analysis of cholesterol-lowering trials in which they were stratified according to the IHD risk of the control patients[115] provides some point of reference in this respect. Evidence of a decrease in all-cause mortality was not observed until the IHD risk had reached 3% per annum mortality[115]. As we have discussed previously (page 159), this comparatively high figure is not due to a high incidence of adverse events associated with cholesterol lowering, but to the large numbers of people who will not die of IHD during relatively short trials relative to those who will. We have also rehearsed the argument that the true benefit of lipid-lowering treatment must really include the decrease in IHD morbidity as well as mortality (page 158). Nevertheless, we should not adopt clinical practices, which may mean that unacceptably large numbers of people are exposed to long-term medication when only a handful can benefit. Let us therefore take the figure of 3% p.a. risk of IHD death obtained in the meta-analysis of clinical trials, accepting it may be an overestimate of the level at which benefit from lipid-lowering occurs and see how this can make clinical practice more objective.

First, it is important to remember that a direct translation of meta-analyses into clinical practice is not going to be possible. This is because:

1 Many of the trials included in meta-analyses have been short-term, lasting less than 2 years. It was evident in the meta-analysis of Law et al.[64] (Table 6.3) that the decrease in coronary incidence in trials lasting under 2 years was 7% whereas that in trials lasting longer was 25%.

2 Many, if not all, of the trials included in meta-analyses were analysed on an intention-to-treat basis. That means that patients not complying with medication were included in the intervention group. In the Lipid Research Clinic Trial it was evident that the decrease in cholesterol in the intervention group as a whole was 8% and the decrease in coronary incidence 19%[105]. It was estimated that in the patients fully compliant with medication the decrease in cholesterol was 25% and the decrease in coronary incidence 49%. Intention-to-treat analysis is the only unbiased way to analyse a trial, but the result it gives is qualitative and a quantitatively greater benefit is likely to accrue in clinical practice. This is because in clinical practice patients are not expected to persist with medication which is either ineffective in lowering cholesterol or not well tolerated. A more effective medication is selected, if the first drug proves inadequate. This argument could be challenged if the incidence of adverse side-effects was related to cholesterol-lowering, but it is known that non-cardiovascular deaths are unrelated to cholesterol reduction[98,115] or even to compliance with medication[121].

3 In clinical practice we identify particular patterns of hyperlipidaemia for which certain lipid-lowering drugs are particularly suited: in clinical trials only one choice of agent is available.

4 Included in some of the meta-analyses were trials involving medications such as high dose oestrogen and dextrothyroxine, both of which have been abandoned in clinical practice because of their adverse effects. The effect of this might be to overestimate the disadvantages of medication[65].

The clinical trial evidence would thus suggest that in clinical practice an overall benefit in terms of mortality will occur at an IHD mortality rate closer to 1.5% rather than the 3% in clinical trials.

Secondly, if one attempts to use prospective studies to assess the levels of coronary risk in patients identified by the guidelines the risk may be underestimated for three reasons:

The first is regression dilution bias. In a prospective study one measurement of cholesterol made at the outset is related to the subsequent incidence of events. No matter how large the study is, this procedure is going to give an underestimate of risk associated with factors like cholesterol[144] or blood pressure[145]. This is because of biological and analytical variation in the measurement. A participant in a prospective study categorized in the upper range for cholesterol on the basis of one measurement is more likely to have a true mean value (which can only be estimated as the mean of several measurements) which is lower than the initial value rather than higher. At the lower end of the scale the opposite is the case. The effect of this is that the true relationship between mean cholesterol and risk is steeper than that reported in studies employing single measurements which are frequently used to establish risk in prospective trials. It has been calculated that the 17% difference in IHD mortality associated with a difference in serum cholesterol of 2.3 mg/dl (0.6 mmol/l) is increased to 24% if this effect is taken into account (4) (Figure 6.5). Thus, a man of 55 years of age with a cholesterol of 300 mg/dl (7.8 mmol/l), normal triglycerides and an LDL cholesterol of 235 mg/dl (6 mmol/l) and no other risk factors would have an annual risk of IHD death of 1% predicted from Framingham data. If the value of 300 mg/dl (7.8 mmol/l) had been established after a series of measurements as recommended by the NCEP, EAS and BHA guidelines this risk is probably closer to 1.5%.

Secondly, the risk attaching to a particular cholesterol level when it has been achieved from a previously higher value as the result of dietary modification will almost certainly be greater than for a spontaneously occurring similar cholesterol concentration.

Thirdly, there is a tendency in prospective studies to recruit a cohort, who are more healthy than the general population, so that in the first years of the study there is a tendency to underestimate the true effect of a risk factor, the incidence of IHD being less than that in the general population. It is difficult to quantitate the extent to which this would underestimate the true impact of a risk factor such as cholesterol when compared with people who are clinically evaluated for the presence of IHD; it will mean that the risk of a particular cholesterol level is likely to be underestimated from epidemiological trials.

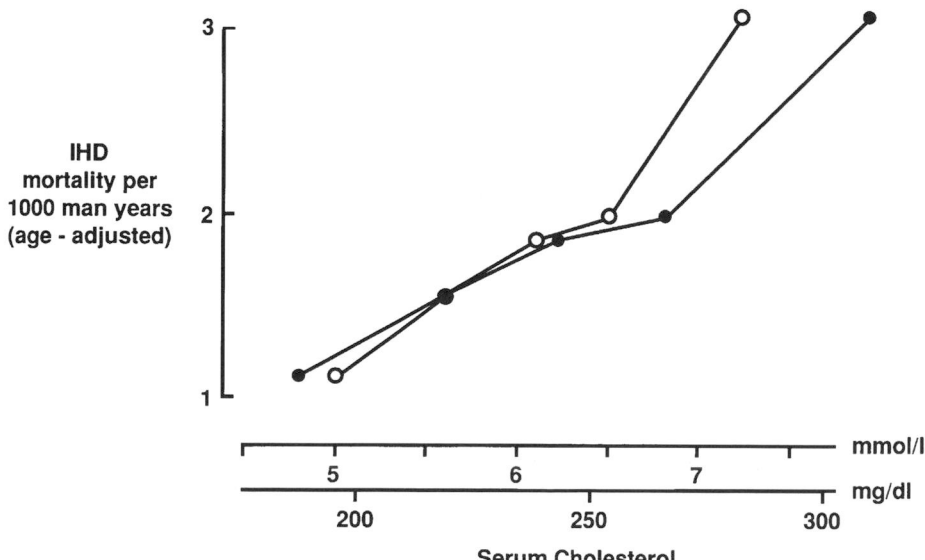

**Figure 6.5**   The difference in the relationship between serum cholesterol and IHD risk before (●) and after adjustment for the effect of regression dilution bias (○)[144]

Taking these points into consideration, an even stronger argument that the rate of 3% per annum for CHD death where all-cause mortality is decreased in clinical trials established by Davey Smith *et al.*[115] can certainly be at least halved in clinical practice. Thus priorities as low as the third category in the British Hyperlipidaemia Association guidelines fit with present evidence. The lowest priority (women with cholesterol >7.8 mmol/l and no other risk) would certainly include some patients in whom evidence of benefit was dubious, but if serum high density lipoprotein cholesterol was low or the level of cholesterol was substantially greater than 7.8 mmol/l coronary risk could be high enough to justify lipid-lowering drug therapy, if diet was insufficiently effective. The relatively low priority in women is because of the limited trial data in women, the uncertainty about optimum cholesterol levels in women and the necessity that lipoprotein levels with which many clinicians, who have not specialized in this area will be unfamiliar, must be taken into account. It must be emphasized that this argument is not intended to apply to women with established genetic hyperlipidaemia, atherosclerosis or multiple risk factors, particularly diabetes. Furthermore age at the menopause is important in assessing cardiovascular risk and hormone replacement therapy should frequently be considered before lipid-lowering drug treatment as a means of decreasing cardiovascular risk.

Therefore if both the underestimation of benefit from meta-analyses of clinical trials of intervention and the underestimation of risk from data obtained in prospective cohort studies are taken into account, the guidelines for primary prevention of IHD may not have strayed so far from epidemiological and clinical trial evidence as has been suggested by some of their critics.

## Secondary prevention

It is now well established that patients who have established IHD will benefit from lipid-lowering therapy both in terms of decreased IHD morbidity and overall death rate (pages 148–154). The guidelines are unanimous on this point, all set a cholesterol level below that considered desirable in the general population as the target. The BHA sets an LDL cholesterol level of <130 mg/dl (<3.4 mmol/l), the EAS 115–135 mg/dl (3.0–3.5 mmol/l) and the NCEP <100 mg/dl (<2.59 mmol/l). Some of the EAS committee also wanted to go as low as the NCEP. The justification for aiming to reduce LDL to these low levels is three-fold.

First, the patients entered into the secondary prevention trials were generally not selected for their cholesterol levels and as such the average cholesterol concentration at randomization was about average for the population, around 230 mg/dl (6.0 mmol/l). Thus probably about half had levels below this. The benefit did not seem to be confined to those with the highest levels, but, if anything, was most closely correlated with the percentage reduction in LDL cholesterol (pages 159–162).

Secondly, presumably those people who develop IHD with a below average level of serum LDL cholesterol are more susceptible to its effect in producing coronary atheroma. Hence the slope of relationship between serum cholesterol and IHD risk is steeper in people who have revealed themselves to be susceptible to the disease by already having had a heart attack (Figure 6.3). This would be supported by epidemiological studies which do not show any clear threshold for LDL cholesterol below which IHD ceases to occur. There appears to be a straight-line relationship between serum cholesterol and log to the base 2 of IHD risk which continues in populations such as the Japanese and Chinese in whom the frequency of low cholesterol levels is much higher than in countries such as Britain and the USA[146]. Cholesterol at low levels continues to be a risk factor, but only in those few people who are the most susceptible. On the other hand, the atheroma that does develop in susceptible individuals with low cholesterol, although less frequent is histologically no different from that in people with higher levels. Thus it is reasonable to conclude that individuals who develop IHD despite low cholesterol levels have arteries that respond to LDL cholesterol by producing atheroma in the same way as those who are less susceptible but do so at lower levels. Any LDL cholesterol concentration in an individual with IHD should therefore be regarded as too high for that person and there may be benefit from lowering it.

Thirdly, the regression studies using cholesterol reduction as the intervention in both animals[147] and humans[148] (pages 152–154) suggest LDL cholesterol levels of 100 mg/dl (2.5 mmol/l) or less may be associated with the best results in terms of the regression or arrest of progression of coronary lesions.

It is not widely enough appreciated that whereas recurrence of IHD events can be decreased by aspirin, beta-blockers and ACE inhibitors, LDL cholesterol reduction can produce results of at least a similar magnitude. It should be remembered that the 25% reduction in IHD deaths in trials of 3 years or more was achieved with only a 10% decrease in serum cholesterol (Table 6.3). Greater reductions which are now possible with newer drugs would be expected to produce an even greater benefit. Furthermore, LDL cholesterol-lowering is the only intervention which has been shown to arrest progression or even to induce regression. Even in the USA this conclusion has been slow to enter clinical practice[149]. Half of coronary events occur in patients who can be identified by the presence of existing IHD[66,150]. There should therefore be no difficulty in identifying and intervening in a substantial proportion of the population otherwise destined to die from the disease. This is why all the guidelines make this group of patients the first priority.

## Should treatment guidelines be based on current IHD risk or on future IHD risk?

The risk of death in patients with established IHD, certainly in the earlier cholesterol-lowering trials, was around 6% per annum[66]. We have seen that one meta-analysis which has examined this in cholesterol-lowering trials as a whole finds evidence of benefit in terms of reduction of all-cause mortality when the incidence of IHD death is around 3% per annum[115]. We have further argued that even in these terms (ignoring benefits in terms of reduced morbidity, less need for coronary surgery etc.) a conservative extrapolation to clinical practice would be to group with a 1.5% per annum risk of IHD death (pages 172–175). The important question is should we wait until that risk is achieved or should we start treatment at an earlier stage, if it is known with reasonable certainty that a risk as high as this is likely to occur before old age. To take the example of a man with heterozygous FH aged 20: his current risk is likely to be less than 1.5% per annum (unless he has a particularly adverse family history). However, on average, by the age of 50 he will have comfortably reached an even higher risk than 1.5% per annum. It seems reasonable not to wait, but to try to avert this happening by commencing lipid-lowering treatment earlier. A similar argument must apply to the patients whose risk might be predicted with similar certainty such as patients with clear features of FCH, type III hyperlipoproteinaemia or diabetic patients, particularly if their dyslipidaemia is marked or it is occurring in association with hypertension, proteinuria or an adverse family history.

# The elderly

Table 6.10 shows the benefit calculated from epidemiological data by Law and colleagues[64] from decreasing cholesterol by 10% at different ages. Gordon and Rifkind obtained a similar, but somewhat higher decrease in all age groups, using data from the MRFIT study and Framingham assuming a 33% decrease in cholesterol[151]. In percentage terms there appears to be a progressive attenuation of the benefits of cholesterol lowering with advancing age. However, this is because the slope of the relationship between IHD and serum cholesterol becomes progressively less with advancing age (Figure 3.9). A similar effect is seen with blood pressure. However, trials of blood pressure-lowering showed that the benefit of anti-hypertensives in the elderly is greater than in younger age groups. This is at least partly because the incidence of myocardial and cerebral infarction is much higher in the elderly than in the young so that even a reduced percentage decrease results in a substantially greater number of such events being prevented. In the study of Gordon and Rifkind it was calculated that 1.8 per 1000 IHD deaths might be prevented in people aged 35–44 years from a 77% decrease in CHD death resulting from a decrease in serum cholesterol from 285 to 200 mg/dl (7.4 to 5.2 mmol/l)[151], whereas in people aged 75–84 a 23% decrease in CHD risk from a similar cholesterol reduction would prevent 12.7 per 1000 deaths. Morbidity from acute myocardial infarction is also much greater in the elderly than in the young, because it is much more likely to lead to chronic ill-health due to persistent ventricular dysfunction. The case for a trial of cholesterol reduction in the elderly is strong. In the meantime it is my practice to treat hyperlipidaemia in elderly people, who have had coronary artery bypass surgery. I do not advocate screening the elderly for hypercholesterolaemia on present evidence, but from time to time elderly people are referred to me with high cholesterol levels and then it is

**Table 6.10 Effect of a 10% decrease in serum cholesterol***

| Men aged | Decrease in IHD incidence |
|---|---|
| 40 years | 54% |
| 50 years | 39% |
| 60 years | 27% (25%†) |
| 70 years | 20% |
| 80 years | 19% |

* The expected decrease in IHD incidence from a 10% decrease in serum cholesterol (approximately 0.6 mmol/l or 23 mg/dl) for men of different ages and (†) the decrease in IHD incidence in men aged 55–64 years from meta-analysis of clinical trials of cholesterol-lowering lasting longer than 5 years
Data from reference[64]

often a matter of great tact and frankness to decide the most appropriate action, taking into account any other co-existent diseases or factors which are likely to lead to death before IHD, always bearing in mind that harm rather than good may follow. A higher level of cholesterol should be set both for intervention and as a goal. It should also be remembered that many elderly women continue to have relatively high HDL cholesterol (Figure 3.8). It is also the case that a lipid-lowering diet may remove the only pleasure in life from a great many elderly people and may thus be a greater imposition than medication. It is probably not true to say that if one postpones IHD death the patient will die of something worse, such as cancer. They will probably still die of IHD if they have one or more major risk factors or established disease, but perhaps a little later. In terms of cost, the duration of treatment will be shorter than in a young person. This together with the high absolute risk makes the cost per year of life gained potentially substantially cheaper than that of a younger person. There may also be the potential to prevent stroke in the elderly which probably because of its relative rarity in the younger populations in clinical trials, has not so far been prevented by lipid-lowering therapy despite evidence that cholesterol is a risk factor for occlusive stroke[152]. I can offer the reader no more adequate guidance than these few thoughts.

## Monitoring of patients borderline for lipid-lowering drugs

By now it will be obvious that the decision to introduce lipid-lowering medication should not be lightly undertaken and is generally for life. Often patients will not quite fulfil the indications for lipid-lowering drug treatment. The decision not to prescribe such medication should not be regarded as a once-and-for-all decision. The serum lipids should be monitored thereafter, perhaps annually. This is because:

1. The serum cholesterol may rise with age or the serum HDL cholesterol diminish.
2. Another risk factor may become evident with age. Diabetes may develop (particularly if the serum triglycerides are also raised), blood pressure may rise, a positive family history may declare itself. Most regrettably, of course, the patient may develop symptoms of IHD. Where there is any doubt about whether a patient with a normal resting ECG does have IHD, I consider exercise stress testing perfectly justified.

   On the other hand, risk can be favourably altered if a patient stops smoking, removing the patient from a category borderline for lipid-lowering medication.

3. Advancing age itself may add to the risk. The clinician is often on the horns of dilemma. When it is obvious that a patient will move into a high risk category in only a few years, it may be unreasonable to withhold lipid-lowering drug therapy. On the other hand, if that high risk is not achieved until the patient is comparatively elderly one is dealing, at least on present evidence, with those imponderables previously discussed (pages 177–178).
4. The patient's dietary compliance (? response to diet) may decline with time.

# Hyperapobetalipoproteinaemia

Apolipoprotein $B_{100}$ is the main component of the protein moiety of VLDL and LDL. Since one molecule of apo B is present in each VLDL or LDL molecule, the apo B concentration of each reflects their molar concentration. LDL particles generally predominate over VLDL particles even in the postprandial state, and more than 90% of the circulating apo B is normally present in LDL[153].

Most investigations have relied on measurements of cholesterol to assess the concentration of LDL. However, it has become increasingly apparent that the loading of LDL with cholesterol may vary considerably between individuals and that measurement of serum apolipoprotein B levels is a better means of assessing the concentration of LDL particles. It may therefore give a more precise indication of coronary risk. The first suggestion that this might be the case was from a study in which apo B was measured in serum and lipoproteins in various hyperlipoproteinaemias[153]. It was discovered that some of the patients with type IV hyperlipoproteinaemia, who by definition had LDL cholesterol levels in the normal range, nevertheless had LDL apo B levels and total serum apo B levels quite as high as many patients with type II hyperlipoproteinaemia and therefore acknowledged increases in LDL cholesterol. The implication was that it was possible to have high molar concentrations of LDL not revealed by cholesterol testing.

Soon afterwards, Avogaro and colleagues showed that apo B discriminated between survivors of myocardial infarction and controls better than cholesterol[154], and Sniderman and co-workers reported an association between serum apo B and coronary atherosclerosis in people whose serum LDL concentration was in the normal range[34]. They coined the term hyperapobetalipoproteinaemia (HABL) for this condition. They confirmed that some people with HABL had type IV hyperlipoproteinaemia, although many had a normal lipoprotein phenotype. Only a proportion of patients with type IV hyperlipoproteinaemia have HABL, and these tend to be those whose serum cholesterol, although by definition in the normal range, is at the upper end of that range. It is in this group of patients with type IV hyperlipoproteinaemia that coronary atherosclerosis is particularly evident[155]. The incidence of HABL in type IV hyperlipoproteinaemia in general does not, however, appear to be greatly increased[36]. As will be evident from the previous discussion of FCH, patients with IHD and type IV hyperlipoproteinaemia are likely to fall within the group labelled FCH. Since we now know that most of these will have HABL, the question arises as to whether FCH and HABL are really the same syndrome[14,156]. Both are characterized by raised levels of serum apo B and in both there is overproduction of apo B-containing lipoproteins[33] (Figure 6.1). Furthermore, in both FCH and HABL the circulating LDL is dense and its apo B is less saturated with cholesteryl ester than normal or than in FH[156,157]. This has also been reported in hypertriglyceridaemia in general, but appears to be even more pronounced in patients with hypertriglyceridaemia and HABL[157].

The major difference between FCH and HABL is thus one of definition. Serum apo B levels are elevated in both. In FCH, however, either the serum cholesterol or triglycerides must also be elevated, whereas in HABL the LDL cholesterol must be within the normal range. There is also the implication in FCH that it is an inherited condition and thus that other members of the family should be affected and that premature IHD should also run in the family. This is not required in the definition of HABL, but higher than average serum apo B levels were found in the children of patients with early onset coronary atheroma[158]. On the other hand, a family history of myocardial infarction in early life is not a major determinant of serum apo B concentration in adults[36], in whom nutritional influences may swamp the genetic influence[159,160]. The combination of high levels of apo B and apo (a) also seems to be particularly associated with premature IHD[6,161]. Apo (a) is strongly genetically determined and people with HABL from families in which high levels of apo (a) are running may be particularly at risk[6].

Another question which arises in this context is what is the coronary risk of the normolipidaemic members of FCH families? Do they have HABL? One is frequently referred patients with a poor family history of IHD, but with normal cholesterol and triglycerides and no other conventional risk factors, so this is an important clinical consideration. The explanation for HABL must inevitably be that LDL which is relatively depleted in cholesteryl ester must exist in the circulation of patients with the condition. Such LDL particles must be similar, if not identical, with the small LDL found in type IV and IIb hyperlipoproteinaemia. Increasingly, genetic polymorphisms of apo B or the DNA sequences flanking its gene are being reported in association with variations in serum apo B levels and in LDL composition and metabolism (Chapter 12, page 374). None of these satisfactorily explains the occurrence of HABL. There may thus be a metabolic explanation. There does appear to be an association between HABL and hypertriglyceridaemia and patients with HABL who do not have fasting hypertriglyceridaemia commonly have delayed postprandial triglyceride clearance[162,163]. Throughout much of the day, therefore, most if not all patients with HABL will have an expanded circulating triglyceride-rich lipoprotein pool. Sniderman and his colleagues believe that there is a protein they term acylation stimulating protein, which stimulates triglyceride synthesis from circulating NEFA in peripheral tissues[164]. Tissues in HABL may be less responsive to this, perhaps delaying triglyceride clearance peripherally and causing more NEFA to be cleared by the liver which may increase hepatic triglyceride synthesis and thence increase hepatic secretion of apo B. The expanded VLDL pool, regardless of its explanation, would be expected to accelerate the transfer of cholesteryl ester from LDL to it under the agency of CETP, which could explain the small apo B-rich, cholesteryl ester depleted LDL in HABL.

Another feature of HABL which might make this process more likely is that the free cholesterol content of VLDL is increased in HABL. This is a factor known to enhance cholesteryl ester transfer into VLDL. Free cholesterol in the triglyceride-rich lipoprotein pool must largely arise from newly secreted hepatic VLDL rather than gut triglyceride-rich lipoproteins, because the liver unlike the gut exports cholesterol unesterified. Thus it is conceivable that in HABL (and perhaps in FCH or indeed any condition associated with small LDL) the rate of hepatic secretion of VLDL is high enough to exceed the capacity of LCAT to esterify it without there being a rise in the free cholesterol content of VLDL[43]. It has also been proposed that small LDL may arise from a smaller VLDL secreted in this condition as has been proposed in frank hypertriglyceridaemia[41]. This explanation and the explanation based on accelerated cholesteryl ester transfer out of LDL are not necessarily incompatible. Further studies will be of considerable interest.

Whatever the underlying cause of HABL and FCH, more immediate practical implications arise, because in case-control studies apo B is often more discriminating than any other lipoprotein variable in identifying individuals with premature

IHD[6,35,36,154]. Some case-control studies will undoubtedly have underestimated the strength of the association between apo B and risk of coronary disease in favour of apo AI and triglycerides, because they include patients on beta-blockers which depress apo AI (Chapter 11) and they neglect the effect of myocardial ischaemia itself, which is to reduce apo B while increasing triglycerides and decreasing apo AI[165,166].

There have been two prospective studies in which serum apo B has been measured. One of these did not reveal apo B to be superior to the total cholesterol : HDL ratio in predicting IHD risk and combining apo B with HDL or apo AI was no better than the ratio using total cholesterol[143]. In the other prospective study apo B did perform better than any other parameter in predicting IHD incidence[167] and the results were compatible with previously published case-control studies. It was also the case that in a trial of angiographic coronary atheroma regression in which an elevated serum apo B was an entry requirement, the decrease in apo B and the increase in HDL cholesterol were the two factors that best predicted regression and favourable clinical outcome[76].

Whether any of this actually has any clinical utility depends on attitudes to population screening, certainly even the combination of apo B or cholesterol with HDL cholesterol would not allow the identification of all people destined to sustain heart attacks without the inclusion of large numbers who would not. As always a knowledge of other coronary risk factors is critical in the assessment of risk. In a recent debate it was proposed that apolipoprotein B could already be of value in identifying people at high IHD risk[168]. The opponents of this viewpoint argued that apo B would not provide more information than the serum cholesterol level after subtraction of HDL cholesterol which is already measured by most routine laboratories[169]. It is perfectly true that there is a good correlation between serum apo B and the non-HDL cholesterol level. However, this is only the case if the full range of non-HDL cholesterol encountered in the population is plotted against apo B giving a range of say 100–300 mg/dl (2.5–7.8 mmol/l). The potential value of apo B would be over a much narrower range where IHD risk was in doubt, perhaps 150–200 mg/dl (3.8–5.2 mmol/l) equivalent to a group of people with total serum cholesterol levels in the range 200–250 mg/dl (5.2–6.5 mmol/l). There is nowhere near such a good correlation between serum apo B and non-HDL cholesterol in this segment of the population as opposed to the whole population and this is the segment of the population from which most ischaemic heart disease deaths will come (greatest attributable risk). Knowledge of the serum apo B level may also be helpful in assessing the IHD risk posed by hypertriglyceridaemia[170,171].

There is a need for an agreed definition of the level of apo B which constitutes the upper limit of normal. At present, this latter requirement is difficult to fulfil, because of the range of different immunoassays for apo B and the lack of an agreed standard. The antiserum may well be critical in view of the growing evidence that serum apo B is itself heterogeneous (Chapter 12, page 374), and an antiserum which has a higher affinity for isoforms of apo B particularly associated with atherosclerosis may provide a better assay for the identification of individuals at risk than one which is perhaps more accurate in purely analytical terms.

There is also a need to have more precise information about the effects of lipid-modifying therapy on serum apo B levels. Dietary treatment, at least in normal individuals, lowers serum apo B in parallel with cholesterol[159,160]. The same, however, may not be true of all drug therapy.

# References

1. Shekelle, R. B., Shryock, A. M., Paul, O., Lepper, M., Stamler, J. *et al.* Diet, serum cholesterol and death from coronary heart disease – the Western Electric Study. *N. Engl. J. Med.*, **304**, 65–70 (1981)
2. Burn, J., Durrington, P. and Harris, R. Genetics and cardiovascular disease. In *Recent Advances in Cardiology* (ed. D. J. Rowlands), Churchill Livingstone, Edinburgh, pp. 27–47 (1987)
3. Stone, M. C. and Thorp, J. M. Plasma fibrinogen – a major coronary risk factor. *J. R. Coll. Gen. Pract.*, **35**, 565–569 (1985)
4. Meade, T. W., Mellows, S., Brosovic, M., Miiler, G. J., Chakrabarti, R. R. *et al.* Haemostatic function and ischaemic heart disease: principal results of the Northwick Park heart study. *Lancet*, **ii**, 533–537 (1986)
5. Hamsten, A., de Faire, U., Walldius, G., Dahlen, G., Szamos, A. *et al.* Plasminogen activator inhibitor in plasma: risk factor for recurrent myocardial infarction. *Lancet*, **ii**, 3–9 (1987)
6. Durrington, P. N., Ishola, M., Hunt, L., Arrol, S. and Bhatnagar, D. Apolipoproteins (a), AI and B and parental history in men with early onset ischaemic heart disease. *Lancet*, **i**, 1070–1073 (1988)
7. Slack, J. The genetic contribution to coronary heart disease through lipoprotein concentrations. *Postgrad. Med. J.*, **51** (Suppl. 8), 27–32 (1975)
8. Goldstein, J. L., Hazzard, W. R., Schrott, A. G., Bierman, E. L. and Motulsky, A. G. Hyperlipidaemia in coronary heart disease I. Lipid levels in 500 survivors of myocardial infarction. *J. Clin. Invest.*, **52**, 1533–1534 (1973)
9. Goldstein, J. L., Schrott, H. G., Hazzard, W. R., Bierman, E. L. and Motulsky, A. G. Hyperlipidaemia in coronary heart disease II. Genetic analysis of lipid levels in 176 families and delineation of a new inherited disorder, combined hyperlipidaemia. *J. Clin. Invest.*, **52**, 1544–1568 (1973)
10. Nikkila, E. A. and Aro, A. Family study of serum lipids and lipoproteins in coronary heart disease. *Lancet*, **i**, 954–958 (1973)
11. Rose, H. G., Kranz, P., Winstock, H., Juliano, J. and Haft, J. I. Combined hyperlipoproteinaemia: evidence for a new lipoprotein phenotype. *Atherosclerosis*, **20**, 51–64 (1974)
12. Hazzard, W. R., Goldstein, J. L., Schrott, H. G., Motulsky, A. G. and Bierman, E. L. Hyperlipidaemia in coronary heart disease III. Evaluation of lipoprotein phenotypes of 156 genetically defined survivors of myocardial infarction. *J. Clin. Invest.*, **52**, 1569–1577 (1973)
13. Havel, R. J., Goldstein, J. L. and Brown, M. S. Lipoproteins and lipid transport. In *Metabolic Control and Disease* (eds P. K. Bondy and L. E. Rosenberg), W. B. Saunders, Philadelphia, pp. 393–494 (1980)
14. Grundy, S. M., Chait, A. and Brunzell, J. D. Familial combined hyperlipidaemia workshop. *Arteriosclerosis*, **7**, 203–207 (1987)
15. Kannel, W. B., Castelli, W. P., Gordon, T. and McNamara, P. Serum cholesterol lipoproteins and risk of coronary heart disease: the Framingham Study. *Ann. Intern. Med.*, **74**, 1–12 (1971)
16. Consensus Conference. Lowering blood cholesterol to prevent heart disease: National Institutes of Health. *J. Am. Med. Assoc.*, **253**, 2080–2086 (1985)
17. European Atherosclerosis Society Study Group. Strategies for the prevention of coronary heart disease: a policy statement of the European Atherosclemis Society. *Eur. Heart J.*, **8**, 77–88 (1987)
18. Shepherd, J., Betteridge, D. J., Durrington, P., Laker, M., Lewis, B. *et al.* Strategies for reducing coronary heart disease and desirable limits for blood lipid concentrations: guidelines of the British Hyperlipidaemia Association. *Br. Med. J.*, **295**, 1245–1246 (1987)
19. Lewis, B., Chait, A., Oakley, C. M., Wooton, I. D. P., Krikler, D. M. *et al.* Serum lipoprotein abnormalities in patients with ischaemic heart disease. Comparisons with a control population. *Br. Med. J.*, **iii**, 489–493 (1974)
20. Austin, M.A., King, M.C., Vranizan, K.M. and Krauss, R.M. Atherogenic lipoprotein phenotype: a proposed genetic marker for coronary heart disease risk. *Circulation*, **82**, 492–506 (1990)
21. Castelli, W.P. The fact and fiction of lowering cholesterol concentrations in the primary prevention of coronary heart disease. *Br. Heart J.*, **69** (Suppl.), S70–S73 (1993)
22. Bezafibrate Infarction Prevention (BIP) Study Group, Israel. Lipids and lipoproteins in symptomatic coronary heart disease. Distribution, intercorrelations, and significance for risk classification in 6,700 men and 1,500 women. *Circulation*, **86**, 839–848 (1992)

23. McKeigue, P.M. and Keen, H. Diabetes, insulin, ethnicity, and coronary heart disease. In *Coronary Heart Disease Epidemiology. From Aetiology to Public Health.* (eds M. Marmot and P. Elliott), Oxford University Press, Oxford (1992)
24. Bhatnagar, D., Mackness, M.I., Britt, R., Anand, I.S. and Durrington, P.N. Serum lipids and apolipoproteins in South Asians living in the UK and their siblings in India. *Atherosclerosis*, **103**, 296 (1993)
25. Berman, M., Hall, M., Levy, R. I., Eisenberg, S., Bilheimer, D. W. *et al.* Metabolism of apo B and apo C lipoproteins in man: kinetic studies in normal and hyperlipoproteinaemic subjects. *J. Lipid Res.*, **19**, 38–56 (1978)
26. Janus, E. D., Nicoll, A. M., Turner, P. R., Magill, P. and Lewis, B. Kinetic bases of the primary hyperlipidaemias: studies of apolipoprotein B turnover in genetically defined subjects. *Eur. J. Clin. Invest.*, **10**, 161–172 (1980)
27. Kissebah, A. H., Alfarsi, S. and Evans, D. C. Low density lipoprotein metabolism in familial combined hyperlipidaemia: mechanisms of the multiple lipoprotein phenotypic expression. *Arteriosclerosis*, **4**, 614–624 (1984)
28. Chait, A., Foster, D. B., Albers, J. J., Failor, A. and Brunzell, J. D. Low density lipoprotein metabolism in familial combined hyperlipidaemia and familial hypercholesterolaemia: kinetic analysis using an integrated model. *Metabolism*, **35**, 697–704 (1986)
29. Kesaniemi, Y. A. and Grundy, S. M. The significance of low density lipoprotein production in the regulation of plasma cholesterol level in man. *J. Clin. Invest.*, **70**, 13–22 (1982)
30. Turner, P. R., Konarska, R., Revill, J., Masana, L. I., LaVille, A. *et al.* Metabolic study of variations in plasma cholesterol level in normal men. *Lancet*, **ii**, 663–665 (1984)
31. International Collaborative Study Group. Metabolic epidemiology of plasma cholesterol. Mechanisms of variation of plasma cholesterol within populations and between populations. *Lancet*, **ii**, 991–995 (1986)
32. Sigurdsson, G., Nicoll, A. and Lewis, B. Metabolism of VLDL in hyperlipidaemia. Studies of VLDL-apo B kinetics in men. *Eur. J. Clin. Invest.*, **6**, 167–177 (1976)
33. Teng, B., Sniderman, A. D., Soutar, A. K. and Thompson, G. R. Metabolic basis of hyperapobetalipoproteinaemia. Turnover of apolipoprotein B in low density lipoprotein and its precursors and subfractions compared with normal and familial hypercholesterolaemia. *J. Clin. Invest.*, **77**, 663–672 (1986)
34. Sniderman, A. D., Shapiro, S., Marpole, D., Skinner, B., Teng, B. and Kwiterovich, P. O. Association of coronary atherosclerosis with hyperapobetalipoproteinaemia (increased protein, but normal cholesterol levels in human plasma, low density (o lipoproteins)). *Proc. Natl Acad. Sci. USA*, **77**, 604–608 (1980)
35. Brunzell, J. D., Sniderman, A. D., Albers, J. J. and Kwiterovich, P. O. Apoprotein B and AI and coronary artery disease in humans. *Arteriosclerosis*, **4**, 79–83 (1984)
36. Durrington, P. N., Hunt, L., Ishola, M., Kane, J. and Stephens, W. P. Serum apolipoproteins AI and B and lipoproteins in middle-aged men with and without previous myocardial infarction. *Br. Heart J.*, **56**, 206–212 (1986)
37. Babirak, S.P., Iverius, P-H., Fujimoto, W.Y., Brunzell, J.D. Detection and characterisation of the heterozygote state for lipoprotien lipase deficiency. *Arteriosclerosis*, **9**, 326–334 (1989)
38. Wojciechowski, A.P., Farrall, M., Cullen, P., Wilson, T.E.M., Bayliss, J.D. *et al.* Familial combined hyperlipidaemia linked to the apolipoprotein AI-CII-AIV gene cluster on chromosome 11q 23-q24. *Nature*, **349**, 161–164 (1991)
39. Hayden, J., Rabkin, S., McLeod, R. and Hewitt, J. DNA polymorphisms in and around the apo-AI-CIII genes and genetic hyperlipidaemias. *Am. J. Hum. Genet.*, **40**, 421–430 (1987)
40. Kesaniemi, Y. A. and Grundy, S. M. Overproduction of low density lipoproteins associated with coronary heart disease. *Arteriosclerosis*, **3**, 40–46 (1983)
41. Shepherd, J., Caslake, M., Gaw, A., Griffin, B., Lindsay, G. and Packard, C. Atherogenicity of triglyceride-rich lipoproteins: clinical aspects. In *Drugs Affecting Lipid Metabolism.* (eds A. L. Catapano, L. C. Smith and R. Paoletti), Kluwer Academic Publishers, Dordrecht, pp. 453–466 (1993)
42. Bhatnagar, D., Durrington, P.N., Mackness, M.I., Arrol, S., Winocour, P.H. and Prais, H. Effects of treatment of hypertriglyceridaemia with gemfibrozil on serum lipoproteins and the transfer of

cholesteryl ester from high density lipoproteins to low density lipoproteins. *Atherosclerosis*, **92**, 49–57 (1992)

43. Bhatnagar, D., Durrington, P.N., Channon, K.M., Prais, H. and Mackness, M.I. Increased transfer of cholesteryl esters from high density lipoproteins to low density and very low density lipoproteins in patients with angiographic evidence of coronary artery disease. *Atherosclerosis*, **98**, 25–32 (1992)

44. Mistry, P., Miller, N. E., Laker, M., Hazzard, W. R. and Lewis, B. Individual variation in the effects of dietary cholesterol on plasma lipoproteins and cellular homeostasis in man. *J. Clin. Invest.*, **87**, 493–502 (1981)

45. Stamler, J., Wentworth, D. and Neaton, J. D. Is relationship between serum cholesterol and risk of premature death from coronary heart disease continuous and graded? Findings in 356 222 primary screens of the Multiple Risk Factor Intervention Trial (MRFIT). *J. Am. Med. Assoc.*, **256**, 2823–2828 (1986)

46. Mann, J. I., Lewis, B., Shepherd, J., Winder, A. F., Fenster, S. *et al.* Blood lipid concentrations and other cardiovascular risk factors: distribution, prevalence and detection in Britain. *Br. Med. J.*, **296**, 1702–1706 (1988)

47. Report on the National Cholesterol Education Program Expert Panel on Detection, Evaluation and Treatment of High Blood Cholesterol in Adults. *Arch. Intern. Med.*, **148**, 36–39 (1988)

48. Shanoff, H.M. and Little, J.A. C sima A studies of male survivors of myocardial infarction XII. Relation of serum lipids and lipoproteins to survival over a 10-year period. *Canad. Med. Assoc. J.*, **103**, 927–931 (1970)

49. Jenkins, C.D., Zyzanski, S.J. and Rosenman, R.H. Risk of new myocardial infarction in middle-aged men with manifest coronary heart disease. *Circulation*, **53**, 342–347 (1976)

50. Schlant, R.C., Forman, S., Stamler, J. and Canner, P.L. The natural history of coronary heart disease: prognostic factors after recovery from myocardial infarction in 2,789 men. The 5-year findings of the coronary drug project. *Circulation*, **66**, 401–414 (1982)

51. Heliövaara, M., Karronen, M.J., Punsar, S. and Haapakoski, J. Importance of coronary risk factors in the presence or absence of myocardial ischaemia. *Am. J. Cardiol.*, **50**, 1248–1252 (1982)

52. Frost, P.H., Verter, J. and Miller, D. Serum lipids and lipoproteins after myocardial infarction: associations with cardiovascular mortality and experience in the Aspirin Myocardial Infarction Study. *Am. Heart J.*, **113**, 1356–1364 (1987)

53. Pekkanen, J., Linn, S., Heiss, G., Suchindran, C.M., Leon, A. *et al.* Ten-year mortality from cardiovascular disease in relation to cholesterol level among men with and without pre-exisiting cardiovascular disease. *N. Engl. J. Med.*, **322**, 1700–1707 (1990)

54. Wong, N.D., Wilson, P.W.F. and Kannel, W.B. Serum cholesterol as a prognostic factor after myocardial infarction: the Framingham Study. *Ann. Intern. Med.*, **115**, 687–693 (1991)

55. Berge, K.G., Canner, P.L. and Hainline A. High-density lipoprotein cholesterol and prognosis after myocardial infarction. *Circulation*, **66**, 1176–1178 (1982)

56. Franzer, J., Johansson, B.W. and Gustafson, A. Reduced high density lipoproteins as a risk factor after myocardial infarction. *Acta Med. Scand.*, **221**, 357–362 (1987)

57. Goldbort, U., Cohen, L. and Neufeld, H.N. High density lipoprotein cholesterol: prognosis after myocardial infarction: the Israeli Ischaemic Heart Disease Study. *Int. J. Epidemiol.*, **15**, 51–55 (1986)

58. Shah, P.K. and Amin, J. Low high density lipoprotein level is associated with increased restenosis rate after coronary angioplasty. *Circulation*, **85**, 1279–1285 (1992)

59. Palac, R. T., Meadows, W. R., Hwang, M. H., Loeb, H. S., Pifarre, R. and Gunnar, R. M. Risk factors related to progressive narrowing in aortocoronary vein graft studies 1 and 5 years after surgery. *Circulation*, **66** (Suppl. I), I-40–61 (1982)

60. Campau, L., Enjalbert, M., Lesprance, J., Bourassa, M. G., Kwiterovich, P. O. *et al.* The relation of risk factors to the development of atherosclerosis in saphenous-vein bypass grafts and the progression of disease in the native circulation. *N. Engl. J. Med.*, **311**, 1329–1332 (1984)

61. Fox, M. H., Gruchow, H. W., Barboriak, J. J., Anderson, A. J., Hoffmann, R. G. *et al.* Risk factors among patients undergoing repeat aorto-coronary bypass procedures. *J. Thorac. Cardiovasc. Surg.*, **93** 56–61 (1987)

62. Shah, P.K. and Amin, J. Low high density lipoprotein level is associated with increased restenosis rate after coronary angioplasty. *Circulation*, **85**, 1279–1285 (1992)

63. Hearn, J.A. Donohue, B.C., Ba'albaki H. *et al.* Usefulness of serum lipoprotein (a) as a predictor of restenosis after precutaneous transluminal coronary angioplasty. *Am. J. Cardiol.*, **69**, 736–739 (1992)

64. Law, M.R., Wald, N.J. and Thompson, S.G. By how much and how quickly does reduction in serum cholesterol concentration lower risk of ischaemic heart disease? *Br. Med. J.*, **308**, 367–373 (1994)

65. Law, M.R., Thompson, S.G. and Wald, N.J. Assessing possible hazards of reducing cholesterol. *Br. Med. J.*, **308**, 373–379 (1994)

66. Rossouw, J.E., Lewis, B. and Rifkind, B.M. The value of lowering cholesterol after myocardial infarction. *N. Engl. J. Med.*, **323**, 1112–1119 (1990)

67. Rossouw, J.E., Canner, P.L. and Hulley, S.B. Deaths from injury, violence and suicide in secondary prevention trials of cholesterol lowering. *N. Engl. J. Med.*, **325**, 1813 (1991)

68. Carlson, L. A. and Rosenhamer, G. Reduction of mortality in the Stockholm Ischaemic Heart Disease Secondary Prevention Study by combined treatment with clofibrate and nicotinic acid. *Acta Med. Scand.*, **223**, 405–418 (1988)

69. Coronary Drug Project Research Group. Clofibrate and niacin in coronary heart disease. *J. Am. Med. Assoc.*, **231**, 360–381(1975)

70. Canner, P. I., Berge, K. G., Wenger, N. K., Stamler, J., Friedman, L. *et al.* Fifteen year mortality in Coronary Drug Project patients: long term benefit with niacin. *J. Am. Coll. Cardiol.*, **8**, 1245–1255 (1986)

71. Buchwald, H., Varco, R.L., Matts, J.P., Long, J.M., Fitch, L.L. *et al.* Effect of partial ileal bypass surgery on mortality and morbidity from coronary heart disease in patients with hypercholesterolaemia. Report of the Program on the Surgical Control of Hyperlipidaemia (POSCH). *N. Engl. J. Med.*, **323**, 946–955 (1990)

72. Brensike, J.F., Levy, R.I., Kelsey, S.F. *et al.* Effects of therapy with cholestyraine on progressions of coronary arteriosclerosis. Results of NHLBI Type II Coronary Intervention Study. *Circulation*, **69**, 313–324 (1984)

73. Levy, R.I. Brenskie, J.F., Epstein, S.E., Kelsey, S.F., Passamoni, E.R. *et al.* The influence of changes in lipid values induced by cholestyramine and diet on progression of coronary artery disease. Results of the NHLBI type II Coronary Intervention Study. *Circulation*, **69**, 325–337 (1984)

74. Blankenhorn, D.H., Nessim, S.A., Johnson, R.I., Sanmarco, M.E., Azen, S.P. and Cachin-Hamphill, L. Beneficial effects of combined colestipol-niacin therapy on coronary atherosclerosis and coronary venous bypass grafts. *J. Am. Med. Assoc.*, **257**, 3233–3240 (1987)

75. Cachin-Hemphill, L., Mack, W.J., Pogoda, M.J., Sanmorco, M.E., Azen, S.P. and Blankenhorn, D.H. Beneficial effects of colestipol-niacin on coronary atherosclerosis. *J. Am. Med. Assoc.*, **264**, 3013–3017 (1990)

76. Brown, B.G., Albers, J.J., Fisher, L.D., Schaefer, S.M., Lin, J-T. *et al.* Regression of coronary artery disease as a result of intensive lipid-lowering therapy in men with high levels of apolipoprotein B. *N. Engl. J. Med.*, **323**, 1289–1298 (1990)

77. Kane, J.P., Malloy, M.J., Prots, T.A., Phillips, N.R., Dietil, J.C. and Havel, R.J. Regression of coronary atherosclerosis during treatment of familial hypercholesterolaemia with combined drug regimens. *J. Am. Med. Assoc.*, **264**, 3007–3012 (1990)

78. Ornish, D., Brown, S.E., Scherwitz, L.W., Billings, J.H., Armstrong, W.T. *et al.* Can lifestyle changes reverse coronary heart disease? *Lancet*, **336**, 129–133 (1990)

79. Watts, G.F., Lewis, B., Brunt, J.N.H., Lewis, E.S., Coltart, D.J. *et al.* Effects on coronary artery disease of lipid-lowering diet, or diet plus cholestyramine, in the St Thomas' Atherosclerosis Regression Study (STARS). *Lancet*, **339**, 563–569 (1992)

80. Cohn, K., Sakai, F.J. and Langston, M.F. Effect of clofibrate on progression of coronary disease: a prospective angiographic study in man. *Am. Heart J.*, **89**, 591–598 (1975)

81. Brown, B.G., Zhao X-Q., Sacco, D.E. and Albers, J.J. Arteriographic view of treatment to achieve regression of coronary atherosclerosis and to prevent plaque disruption and clinical cardiovascular events. *Br. Heart J.*, **69** (Suppl.), S48–S53 (1993)

82. The Pravastatin Multinational Study Group for Cardiac Risk Patients. Effects of pravastatin in patients with serum total cholesterol levels from 5.2 to 7.8 mmol/l (200–300 mg/dl) plus two additional atherosclerotic risk factors. *Am. J. Cardiol.*, **72**, 1031–1037 (1993)

83. Sirtori, C.R. and Colli, S. Drugs affecting thrombosis and atherosclerosis. In *Drugs Affecting Lipid Metabolism*. (eds A. L. Catapano, A. M. Gotto, L. C. Smith and R. Paoletti), Kluwer Academic Publishers, Dordrecht, pp. 215–229 (1993)

84. Flavalian N.A. Atherosclerosis or lipid-induced endothelial dysfunction. Potential mechanism underlying reduction EDRF/nitric oxide activity. *Circulation*, **85**, 1927–1938 (1992)

85. Celermajer, D.S., Sorensen, K.E., Gooch, V.M., Spiegelhalter, D.J., Miller, O.I. *et al.* Non-invasive detection of endothelial dysfunction in children and adults at risk of atherosclerosis. *Lancet*, **340**, 111–1115 (1992)

86. Tremoli, E., Camera, M., Colli, S., Sironi, L., Prati, L., Banfi, C. and Mussoni, L. Influence of atherogenic lipoproteins on the thrombotic potential of endothelial cells. In *Drugs Affecting Lipid Metabolism*. (eds A. L. Catapano, A. M. Gotto, L. C. Smith. and R. Paoletti), Kluwer Academic Publishers, Dordrecht, pp. 15–22 (1993)

87. Brown, B.G., Gallery, C.A., Badger, R.S., Kennedy, J.W., Mathey, D. *et al.* Incomplete lysis of thrombus in the moderate underlying atherosclerotic lesion during intracoronary infusion of strep-tokinase for acute myocardial infarction: quantitative angiographic observations. *Circulation*, **73**, 653–661 (1986)

88. Little, W.C., Constantinescu, M., Applegate, R.M., Kutcher, M.A., Burrows, M.T. *et al.* Can coronary angiography predict the site of a subsequent myocardial infarction in patients with mild-to-moderate coronary artery disease? *Circulation*, **78**, 1157–1166 (1988)

89. Richardson, P.D., Davies, M.J. and Born, G.V.R. Influence of plaque configuration and stress distribution on fissuring of coronary atherosclerotic plaques. *Lancet*, **ii**, 941–944 (1989)

90. Lendon, C.L., Davies, M.J., Born, G.V.R. and Richardson, P.D. Atherosclerotic plaque caps are locally weakened when macrophage density is increased. *Atherosclerosis*, **87**, 87–90 (1991)

91. Meiser, B.M., Wenke, K., Thiery, J., Wolf, S., Devens, Ch. *et al.* Simvastatin decreases acceler-ated graft vessel disease after heart transplantation in an animal model. *Trans Proc*, **25**, 2077–2079 (1993)

92. Barndt, R., Blakenhorn, D.H., Crawford, D.W. and Brooks, S.H. Regression and progression of early femoral atherosclerosis in treated hyperlipoproteinaemic patients. *Ann. Intern. Med.*, **86**, 139–146 (1977)

93. Duffield, R.G.M., Lewis, B., Miller, N.E., Jamieson, C.W., Brunt, J.N.H. and Colchester, A.C.F. Treatment of hyperlipidaemia retards progression of symptomatic femoral atherosclerosis. *Lancet*, **ii**, 639–643 (1983)

94. Wissler, R.W. and Vesselinovitch, D. Atherosclerosis in non human primates. *Adv. Vet. Med. Sci. Comp. Med.*, **21**, 351–420 (1977)

95. Berliner, J.A. and Gerrity, R.G. Pathology of atherosclerosis. In *Molecular Genetics of Coronary Artery Disease. Candidate Genes and Processes in Atherosclerosis* (eds A. J. Lusio, J. J. Rotter, and R. S. Sparkes), Karger, Basle, pp. 1–17 (1992)

96. Wilens, S.L. The resorption of arterial atheromatous deposits in wasting disease. *Arch. Intern. Med.*, **79**, 793–804 (1947)

97. Brown, M.S. and Goldstein, J.L. Koch's postulates for cholesterol. *Cell*, **71**, 187–188 (1992)

98. Committee of Principal Investigators. Report on a cooperative trial in the primary prevention of ischaemic heart disease using clofibrate. *Br. Heart J.*, **40**, 1069–1118 (1978)

99. Report of the Committee of Principal Investigators. WHO cooperative trial on primary preven-tion of ischaemic heart disease using clofibrate to lower serum cholesterol: mortality follow-up. *Lancet*, **ii**, 379–385 (1980)

100. Heady, J.A., Morris, J.N. and Oliver, M.F. WHO clofibrate/cholesterol trial: clarifications. *Lancet*, **340**, 1405–1406 (1992)

101. Oliver, M. F. Cholesterol, coronaries, clofibrate and death. *N. Engl. J. Med.*, **299**, 1360–1361 (1978)

102. The Lipid Research Clinics Program. Participant recruitment to the coronary primary prevention trial. *J. Chron. Dis.*, **36**, 451–465 (1983)

103. The Lipid Research Clinics Program. Pre-entry characteristics of participants in the Lipid Research Clinics Coronary Primary Prevention Trial. *J. Chron. Dis.*, **36**, 467–479 (1983)

104. Lipid Research Clinics Program. The Lipid Research Clinics Coronary Primary Prevention Trial results 1. Reduction in incidence of coronary heart disease. *J. Am. Med. Assoc.*, **251**, 351–364 (1984)

105. Lipid Research Clinics Program. The Lipid Research Clinics Coronary Primary Prevention Trial results. II The relationship of reduction in incidence of coronary heart disease to cholesterol lowering. *J. Am. Med. Assoc.*, **251**, 365–374 (1984)
106. Manttari, M., Elo, O., Frick, M. H., Haapa, K., Heinonen, O. P. *et al.* The Helsinki Heart Study: basic design and randomisation procedure. *Eur. Heart J.*, **8** (Suppl. I), 1–29 (1987)
107. Frick, M. H., Elo, O., Haapa, K., Heinonen, O. P., Heinsalmi, P. *et al.* The Helsinki Heart Study: primary prevention trial with gemfibrozil in middle-aged men with dyslipidaemia. Safety of treatment, changes in risk factors, and incidence of coronary heart disease. *N. Engl. J. Med.*, **317**, 1237–1245 (1987)
108. Manninen, V., Elo, O., Frick, H., Haapa, K., Heinonen, O. P. *et al.* Lipid alterations and decline in the incidence of coronary heart disease in the Helsinki Heart Study. *J. Am. Med. Assoc.*, **260**, 641–651 (1988)
109. Tsevat, J., Weinstein, M.C., Williams, L.W., Tosteson, A.N.A. and Goldman, L. Expected gains in life expectancy from various coronary heart disease risk factor modifications. *Circulation*, **83**, 1194–1201 (1991)
110. McManus, I. Life expectation of Italian renaissance artists. *Lancet*, **i**, 266–267 (1975)
111. Silman, A. J. Routinely collected data and ischaemic heart disease in the United Kingdom. *Health Trends*, **13**, 3s–n (1981)
112. Rice, D.P., Hodgson, T.A. and Kopstein, A.N. The economic cost of illness: a replication and update. *Health Care Finance. Rev.*, **7**, 61–80 (1985)
113. Holme, I. An analysis of randomised trials evaluating the effect of cholesterol reduction on total mortality and coronary heart disease incidence. *Circulation*, **82**, 1916–1924
114. Holme, I. Relationship of cholesterol lowering to outcome in randomised clinical trials. Chapter 5 in *Cholesterol Lowering Trials. Advice for the British Physician* (eds M. Laker, A. Neil, and C. Wood), Royal College of Physicians, London, 59–69 (1993)
115. Davey Smith, G., Song, F. and Sheldon, T.A. Cholesterol lowering and mortality: the importance of considering initial level of risk. *Br. Med. J.*, **306**, 1367–1373 (1993)
116. Ravnskov, U. Cholesterol lowering trials in coronary heart disease: frequency of citation and outcome. *Br. Med. J.*, **305**, 15–19
117. Durrington, P.N. Hyperlipidaemia: Should we treat patients? Should we treat populations? What treatment should we use? Chapter 3 in *Recent Advances in Cardiology*, vol. 11 (ed. D. J. Rowlands), Churchill Livingstone, Edinburgh, pp. 47–71 (1992)
118. Sheldon, T.A. and Davey Smith, G. Personal communication (1994)
119. Collins, R., Keech, A., Peto, R., Sleight, P., Kjekshus, J. *et al.* Cholesterol and total mortality: need for larger trials. *Br. Med. J.*, **304**, 1689 (1992)
120. Muldoon, M.F., Manuck, S.B. and Matthews, K.A. Lowering cholesterol concentrations and mortality: a quantitative review of primary prevention trials. *Br. Med. J.*, **301**, 309–314 (1990)
121. Wysowski, D.K. and Gross, T.P. Deaths due to accidents and violence in two recent trials of cholesterol-lowering drugs. *Arch. Intern. Med.*, **150**, 2169–2172 (1990)
122. The British Cardiac Society Working Group on Coronary Prevention. Conclusions and recommendations. *Br. Heart J.*, **57**, 188–189 (1987)
123. European Atherosclerosis Society International Task Force for Prevention of Coronary Heart Disease. Prevention of coronary heart disease: scientific background and new clinical guidelines. *Nutr. Metabol. Cardiovasc. Dis.*, **2**, 113–156 (1992)
124. Betteridge, D.J., Dodson, P.M., Durrington, P.N., Hughes, E.A. *et al.* Management of hyperlipidaemia: guidelines of the British Hyperlipidaemia Association. *Postgrad. Med. J.*, **69**, 359–369 (1993)
125. Durrington, P.N. Summary and BHA guidelines. Chapter 9 in *Cholesterol Lowering Trials. Advice for the British Physician* (eds M. Laker, A. Neil, and C. Wood), Royal College of Physicians, London, pp. 105–113 (1993)
126. NCEP (National Cholesterol Education Program). *J. Am. Med. Assoc.*, **269**, 3015–3023 (1993)
127. Hulley, S.B., Walsh, J.M.B. and Newman, T.B. Health policy on blood cholesterol. Time to change directions. *Circulation*, **86**, 1026–1029 (1992)
128. McIsaac, W.J., Naylor, C.D. and Basinski, A. Mismatch coronary risk and treatment intensity under the National Cholesterol Education Program Guidelines. *J. Genet. Intern. Med.*, **6**, 518–523 (1991)

129. Imperial Cancer Research Fund Oxcheck Study Group. Prevalence of risk factors for heart disease in OXCHECK trial: implication for screening in primary care. *Br. Med. J.*, **302**, 1057–1060 (1991)
130. The Scientific Steering Committee on behalf of the Simon Broome Register Group. The risk of fatal coronary heart disease in familial hypercholesterolaemia. *Br. Med. J.*, **303**, 893–896 (1991)
131. Collins, R., Peto, R., MacMahone, S., Hebert, P., Fiebach, N.H. *et al.* Blood pressure, stroke and coronary heart disease. Part 2 Short-term reductions in blood pressure: overview of randomised drug trials in their epidemiological context. *Lancet*, **335**, 827–838 (1990)
132. Subcommittee of WHO/ISH Mild Hypertension Liaison Committee. Summary of 1993 World Health Organisation–International Society of Hypertension guidelines for the management of mild hypertension. *Br. Med. J.*, **307**, 1541–1546 (1993)
133. Ramsay, L.E., Yeo, W.W. and Jackson, P.R. Dietary reduction of serum cholesterol concentration: time to think again. *Br. Med. J.*, **303**, 953–957 (1991)
134. Hegsted, D.M., Augman, L.M., Johnson, J.A. and Dallal, G.E. Dietary fat and serum lipids: an evaluation of the experimental data. *Am. J. Clin. Nutr.*, **57**, 875–883 (1993)
135. Thompson, G.R. Dietary reduction of serum cholesterol concentration. *Br. Med. J.*, **303**, 1332 (1991)
136. Hunninghake, D.B., Stein, E.A., Dujovne, C.A., Harns, W.S., Feldman, E.B. *et al.* The efficacy of intensive dietary therapy alone or combined with lovastatin in outpatients with hypercholesterolaemia. *N. Engl. J. Med.*, **328**, 121–1219 (1993)
137. Assman, G. Identification of patients at high-risk for myocardial infarction: screening procedures and their implementation. In *Current Views of Prevention, Diagnosis and Treatment of Hyperlipidaemia* (eds B. Lewis, and G. Assman), Royal Society of Medicine, London, pp. 17–23 (1987)
138. Kovanen, P. The cholesterol ratio: simplifying clinical management. In *HDL: Where Should the Clinician Stand?* (ed. P. N. Durrington), Mark Allen Publishing, London, pp. 17–20 (1992)
139. Silva, J.M. and Silva, P.S. Sexless HDL. *Lancet*, **343**, 129–130 (1994)
140. Neil, H.A.W., Mant, D., Jones, L., Morgan, B. and Mann. J.I. Lipid screening: is it enough to measure total cholesterol concentration? *Br. Med. J.*, **301**, 584–587 (1990)
141. Assmann, G. and Schulte, H. Relation of high-density lipoprotein cholesterol and triglycerides to incidence of atherosclerotic coronary artery disease (the PROCAM experience) *Am. J. Cardiol.*, **70**, 733–737 (1992)
142. Manninen, V., Tenkanen, L., Koskinen, P., Huttunen, J.K., Manttari, M. *et al.* Joint effects of serum triglyceride and LDL cholesterol and HDL cholesterol concentrations on coronary heart disease risk in the Helsinki Heart Study. Implications for treatment. *Circulation*, **85**, 37–45 (1992)
143. Stampfer, M.J., Sacks, F.M., Salvini, S., Willet, W.C. and Hennekens, C.H. A prospective study of cholesterol, apolipoproteins, and the risk of myocardial infarction. *N. Engl. J. Med.*, **325**, 373–381 (1991)
144. Law, M.R., Wald, N.J., Wu, T., Hackshaw, A. and Bailey, A. Systematic underestimation of association between serum cholesterol concentration and ischaemic heart disease in observational studies: data from the BUPA study. *Br. Med. J.*, **308**, 363–366 (1994)
145. MacMahone, S., Peto, R., Cutter, J., Collins, R., Sorlie, P. *et al.* Blood pressure, stroke and coronary heart disease. Part 1 Prolonged differences in blood pressure: prospective observational studies corrected for the regression dilution bias. *Lancet*, **335**, 765–774 (1990)
146. Chen, Z., Peto, R., Collins, R., MacMahon, S., Lu, J. and Li, W. Serum cholesterol concentration and coronary heart disease in population with low cholesterol concentrations. *Br. Med. J.*, **303**, 276–282 (1991)
147. St Clair, R.S.W. Atherosclerosis regression in animal models: current concepts of cellular and biochemical mechanisms. *Progr. Cardiovasc. Dis.*, **26**, 109–132 (1983)
148. La Rosa, J.C. and Cleeman, J.I. Cholesterol lowering as a treatment for established coronary heart disease. *Circulation*, **85**, 1229–1233 (1992)
149. Cohn, M.V., Byrne, M-J., Levine, B., Gutowski, T. and Adelson R. Low rate of treatment of hypercholesterolaemia by cardiologists in patients with suspected and proven coronary artery disease. *Circulation*, **83**, 1294–1304 (1991)
150. Shaper, A.G., Pocock, S.J., Phillips, A.N. and Walker, M. Identifying men at high risk of heart attacks: strategy for use in general practice. *Br. Med. J.*, **293**, 474–479 (1986)

151. Gordon, D.J. and Rifkind, B.M. Treating high blood cholesterol in the older patient. *Am. J. Cardiol.*, **63**, 4811–? (1989)
152. Qizilbash, N., Duffy, S.W., Warlow, C. and Mann, J. Lipids are risk factors for ischaemic stroke: overview and review. *Cerebrovasc. Dis.*, **2**, 127–136 (1992)
153. Durrington, P. N., Bolton, C. H. and Hartog, M. Serum and lipoprotein apolipoprotein B levels in normal subjects and patients with hyperlipoproteinaemia. *Clin. Chim. Acta*, **82**, 151–160 (1978)
154. Avogaro, P., Bittolo Bon, G., Cazzolato, G. and Quinci, G. B. Are apolipoproteins better discriminators than lipids for atherosclemis? *Lancet*, **i**, 901–903 (1979)
155. Sniderman, A. D., Wolfson, C., Teng, B., Franklin, F. A., Bachorik, P. S. and Kwiterovich, P. O. Association of hyperapobetalipoproteinaemia with endogenous hypertriglyceridemia and atherosclerosis. *Ann. Intern. Med.*, **97**, 833–839 (1982)
156. Lippl, K., Gianturco, S., Fogelman, A., Nestel, P., Grundy, S. M. *et al.* Lipoprotein heterogeneity workshop. *Arteriosclerosis*, **7**, 315–323 (1987)
157. Teng, B., Thompson, G. R., Sniderman, A. D., Forte, T. M., Krauss, R. M. and Kwiterovich, P. O. Composition and distribution of low density lipoprotein fractions in hyprapobetalipoproteinaemia, normolipidaemia and familial hypercholesterolaemia. *Proc. Natl Acad. Sci, USA*, **80**, 6662–6666 (1983)
158. Sniderman, A. D., Teng, B., Genest, J., Cianflore, K., Wacholder, S. and Kwiterovich, P. Familial aggregation and early expression of hyerapobetalipoproteinaemia. *Am. J. Cardiol.*, **55**, 291–295 (1985)
159. Durrington, P. N., Bolton, C. H., Hartog, M., Angelinetta, R., Emmett, P. and Furniss, S. The effect of a low-cholesterol high-polyunsaturate diet on serum lipid levels, apolipoprotein B levels and triglyceride fatty acid composition. *Atherosclerosis*, **27**, 465–475 (1977)
160. Vega, G. L., Groszek, E., Wolf, R. and Grundy, S. M. Influence of polyunsaturated fat on composition of plasma lipoproteins and apolipoproteins. *J. Lipid Res.*, **23**, 811–822 (1982)
161. Armstrong, V. W., Cremer, P., Eberle, E., Marke, A., Schulze, F. *et al.* The association between serum Lp(a) concentrations and angiographically assessed coronary atherosclerosis. Dependence on serum LDL levels. *Atherosclerosis*, **C2**, 249–257 (1986)
162. Genest, J., Sniderman, A.D., Cianflone, K., Teng, B., Wacholders, S. *et al.* Hyperapobetalipoproteinaemia: plasma lipoprotein responses to oral fat load. *Arteriosclerosis*, **6**, 297–304 (1986)
163. Bhatnagar, D., Durrington, P.N. and Arrol, S. Postprandial plasma lipoprotein responses to a mixed meal in subjects with hyperapobetalipoproteinaemia. *Clin. Biochem..*, **25**, 341–343 (1992)
164. Sniderman, A., Baldo, A. and Cianflone, K. The potential role of acylation stimulating protein as a determinant of plasma triglyceride clearance and intracellular triglyceride synthesis. *Curr. Opin. Lipidol.*, **3**, 202–207 (1992)
165. Avogaro, P., Bittolo Bon, G., Cazzolato, G., Quinci, G. B., Sanson, A. *et al.* Variations in apolipoproteins B and Al during the course of myocardial infarction. *Eur. J. Clin. Invest.*, **8**, 121–129 (1978)
166. MBewu, A.D., Durrington, P.N., Bulleid, S. and Mackness, M.I. The immediate effect of streptokinase on serum lipoprotein (a) concentration and the effect of myocardial infarction on serum lipoprotein (a), apolipoprotein AI and B, lipids and C-reactive protein. *Atherosclerosis*, **103**, 65–71 (1993)
167. Wald, N.J., Law, M., Watt, H., Wu, T., Bailey, A. *et al.* Apolipoproteins and ischaemic heart disease, implications for screening. *Lancet*, **343**, 75–79 (1994)
168. Sniderman, A.D. and Silberberg, J. Is it time to measure apolipoprotein B? *Arteriosclerosis*, **10**, 665–667 (1990)
169. Vega, G.L. and Grundy, S.M. Does measurement of apolipoprotein B have a place in cholesterol management? *Arteriosclerosis*, **10**, 668–671 (1990)
170. Durrington, P.N. and Bhatnagar, D. Does measurement of apolipoproteins add to the clinical diagnosis and management of dyslipidaemias? *Curr. Opin. Lipidol.*, **4**, 299–304 (1993)
171. Bhatnagar, D. and Durrington, P.N. Clinical value of apolipoprotein measurements. *Ann. Clin. Biochem.*, **28**, 427–437 (1991)
172. Scandinavian Simvastatin Survival Study Group. Randomized trial of cholesterol lowering in 4444 patients with coronary heart disease: The Scandinavian Simvastatin Survival Study (4S). *Lancet*, **344**, 1383–1389 (1994).

Chapter 7

# Hypertriglyceridaemia

In its extreme form there seems little doubt that treatment of hypertriglyceri-daemia is justified by the risk of acute pancreatitis. Even in severe hypertriglyc-eridaemia, however, the association with coronary disease is as complex as in the milder forms of hypertriglyceridaemia. This chapter, therefore, will discuss patients with moderate fasting hypertriglyceridaemia of less than 450 mg/dl (5 mmol/l) and those with higher levels separately. There is, of course, no sharp division and a few people with only modestly raised triglycerides have the capacity, under certain circumstances, to develop gross hypertriglyceridaemia leading to acute pancreati-tis, whereas others who habitually run serum triglycerides of even 2500 mg/dl (30 mmol/l) or more can live to a ripe old age without complications.

## Moderate hypertriglyceridaemia

For some years we have tended to regard the upper limit of normal for serum triglycerides as being 200 mg/dl (2.3 mmol/l), although the NIH consensus group have tried to increase this to the 95th percentile (around 300 mg/dl or 3.4 mmol/l in middle-aged men) (Chapter 3). Their reasoning would seem to be largely on the basis of the lack of evidence for an association between triglycerides and IHD risk in prospective studies analysed by multivariate analysis[1], although the present author knows of no substantial evidence that multivariate analysis reveals any stronger association at the higher levels of serum triglycerides.

It is important to correct the commonly held misconception that triglycerides are poor indicators of coronary risk. This is quite untrue. In the great majority of case-control studies and prospective studies, univariate analysis shows a relation-ship between coronary atheroma and triglycerides, which may in some be even stronger than for cholesterol (see references [2] and [3] for a list of publications on the subject). Hypertriglyceridaemia is often the most common hyperlipidaemia found in myocardial infarction survivors. Triglycerides are, however, themselves positively correlated with other cardiovascular risk factors such as cholesterol, obesity, glucose intolerance, cigarette smoking and hyperuricaemia and, negatively, with HDL cholesterol. When all or some of these are included in multi-variate analysis the element of risk attributable to triglycerides *per se* becomes much less and is often statistically insignificant[1,4]. Those studies which have claimed to show an independent triglyceride effect have often not included HDL measurements in their multivariate analysis. On the other hand, the way that multivariate analysis treats variables which are highly intercorrelated can be criti-cized[5]. Furthermore, it must be remembered that multivariate analysis estab-lishes only a mathematical probability that the variation in one factor (in this case coronary risk) is related to variation in another. It does not establish a causal relationship. A variable, such as the triglyceride concentration, which is subject to enormous biological variation (Chapter 3, page 88), will fare badly in most mathematical models beside, say, cholesterol or HDL cholesterol.

In a number of important areas triglycerides do survive statistical analysis as risk factors for ischaemic heart disease and that makes one wary of entirely dismissing them. In women over the age of 50, triglycerides were a significant risk factor in Framingham even using conventional multivariate analysis, which included HDL. Indeed, they were ahead of LDL[4]. An independent risk from triglycerides was present in Framingham men over 50, using a technique which compensated for their association with other risk factors such as HDL[5]. Of clinical importance too are the apparent interactions between triglycerides and other risk factors in determining cardiovascular risk. These are discussed in the following sections.

## HDL

In the Framingham study, hypertriglyceridaemia is more likely to lead to ischaemic heart disease when it is associated with levels of HDL cholesterol less than 40 mg/dl (1 mmol/l)[4]. Castelli has suggested that people in whom this association is most likely to occur are usually overweight, have twice the likelihood of developing non-insulin-dependent diabetes and often have hyperuricaemia.

## LDL

There have been a number of studies, the most famous of which is the Stockholm Prospective study, that have suggested that the risk from an elevated cholesterol is greater when the triglycerides are also raised[6]. A review of prospective trials involving triglyceride measurements lends further support to this view[3]. Although it could be argued that in many studies HDL was not measured and that the apparent association between triglycerides and IHD risk was, at least in part, the result of a high LDL in the presence of a low HDL cholesterol for which a high triglyceride concentration was a surrogate, a stronger metabolic basis than this is suggested by the relatively common clinical disorder of familial combined hyperlipidaemia (FCH) (Chapter 6). Type IIb hyperlipoproteinaemia is a frequent manifestation of FCH and is more closely associated with premature IHD than other even commoner forms of hypercholesterolaemia. Since one phenotypic expression of FCH is type IV hyperlipoproteinaemia, this also suggests that at least some patients with type IV hyperlipoproteinaemia are at increased risk of coronary disease. The extent to which FCH overlaps with hyperapobetalipoproteinaemia (HABL) is discussed in Chapter 6, but in that condition hypertriglyceridaemia, when it occurs, is invariably associated with increased LDL apo B and this type of hypertriglyceridaemia is a frequent accompaniment of coronary atherosclerosis (Chapter 6, page 179). It should be emphasized, however, that the evidence for FCH and HABL is at present based largely on case-control studies. One prospective investigation which does lend support for an independent effect of triglycerides on IHD risk is the Helsinki Heart Study in which the risk in men in the placebo group was even greater in those with raised triglycerides and low HDL than in those with low HDL and normal levels of serum triglycerides[7]. In that study all the men had moderate hypercholesterolaemia and this respect resembled those in the earlier Stockholm study[6].

In heterozygotes for familial hypercholesterolaemia, who present with type IIb hyperlipoproteinaemia rather than the usual IIa phenotype, the prognosis has been reported to be poorer (Chapter 5, page 115), which again indicates that LDL may be more atherogenic when hypertriglyceridaemia is also present.

The reason for the increased risk of atheroma attaching to a particular LDL level when hypertriglyceridaemia is also present may be:

1. Intermediate density lipoproteins are frequently elevated in type IIb hyperlipoproteinaemia as opposed to IIa (page 143).
2. Reverse cholesterol transport may operate unfavourable (page 145). There is increased transfer of cholesteryl ester out of HDL into the increased pool of triglyceride-rich lipoproteins where in the case of VLDL it can re-enter the LDL pool and thus contribute to atheroma risk. The effect may be compounded because it will decrease the concentration of circulating HDL cholesterol and thus the quantity which can be transferred directly to the liver during the passage of HDL through the hepatic microcirculation. This will be further compromised if HDL competes unfavourably with triglyceride-rich lipoproteins for hepatic lipase which is though to be important in this process. Thus the transfer of cholesteryl ester will be shifted away from hepatic disposal towards re-entry in the LDL pool.
3. Small readily oxidizable LDL readily cleared from the circulation through non-receptor mediated pathways is present, perhaps as the result of increased transfer of cholesteryl ester out of LDL into the VLDL in exchange for triglyceride (page 59).
4. Raised triglycerides are frequently associated with glucose intolerance and insulin resistance. Even if this does not amount to frank diabetes mellitus, it increases IHD risk.
5. Raised triglycerides are frequently associated with an increased tendency to thrombosis.

### Diabetes mellitus

In the WHO multinational study of diabetes mellitus, triglycerides were more strongly associated with IHD than cholesterol on multiple regression analysis[8]. This is generally considered to indicate that triglycerides are an independent risk factor in diabetes, but it must be pointed out that HDL was not measured. However, the stronger relationship between IHD and triglycerides was present in insulin-dependent diabetes, which, unlike non-insulin-dependent diabetes, is not noted for low serum HDL concentrations (Chapter 11, page 293).

### Type III hyperlipoproteinaemia

Clearly, type III hyperlipoproteinaemia, in which both hypertriglyceridaemia and hypercholesterolaemia are present, is associated with premature arterial disease (Chapter 8, page 216). This relationship does not occur via an increase in LDL apo B or LDL cholesterol, which are decreased. There is, however, an increase in β-VLDL, which is a cholesterol-carrying lipoprotein arising as a result of the accumulation within the circulation of IDL and chylomicron remnants (Chapter 8, page 217). The condition does hint that perhaps analogous lipoprotein particles occurring in other hypertriglyceridaemic patients, for example postprandially, might be atherogenic[9].

In diabetes, in which hypertriglyceridaemia frequently occurs, there is some evidence for the existence of such particles, even in the fasting state[10–12]. In some people, hypertriglyceridaemia may occur in association with insulin resistance without glycaemia, if their increased insulin secretion is increased sufficiently to overcome their resistance. This may be the phenomenon identified in those epidemiological studies which identify serum insulin as a risk factor for atherosclerosis in non-diabetic people (Chapter 11, page 293).

### Hypercoagulability

There is growing evidence that fibrinogen is an independent risk factor for coronary heart disease[13,14]. Patients with hypertriglyceridaemia have increased levels of plasma fibrinogen, decreased fibrinolytic activity and increases in activated clotting factors such as factor VIIc[15–19]. Interestingly patients with familial lipoprotein lipase deficiency although usually manifesting extremely high levels of circulating triglycerides do not have an increase, in for example, plasma fibrinogen and factor VIIc. The combination of a high serum triglyceride level and lipolytic activity seems to be important for the activation of factor VII, probably via factor XII activation[20].

## Clinical features of patients with moderate hypertriglyceridaemia

As with the great majority of hypercholesterolaemic patients, those with hyper-triglyceridaemia do not conform to any readily definable clinical syndrome. Some patients have relatives who also have hyperlipidaemia. Frequently, however, the condition is sporadic[21] When other relatives are affected they most frequently display multiple lipoprotein phenotypes (i.e. types IIa and IIb, in addition to type IV) indicating the presence of familial combined hyperlipidaemia (Chapter 6, page 142). More rarely when the kindred is sufficiently large, it has been possible to demonstrate pure hypertriglyceridaemia of a similar degree in several other relatives and this condition has been termed familial endogenous hypertriglyceridaemia and may perhaps be inherited as an autosomal dominant[22–25]. Occasionally some members of such families have more marked hypertriglyceridaemia with fasting chylomicron-aemia (exogenous hypertriglyceridaemia). Variation in the severity of hypertriglyc-eridaemia in different members of the same family can also occur because some other primary defect in triglyceride metabolism is also running in the family, thus in some members a minor defect in catabolism may combine with another causing overpro-duction to produce spectacular results, whereas their relatives having only a single defect have only minor hypertriglyceridaemia. One way this can arise is if the members of the family are heterozygotes for familial lipoprotein deficiency[26,27].

It is not known how commonly mutations in one lipoprotein lipase gene contribute to familial endogenous hypertriglyceridaemia or to familial combined hyperlipidaemia or hyperapobetalipoproteinaemia. More commonly, some acquired additional precipitant of hypertriglyceridaemia such as alcohol, diabetes mellitus or beta-adrenoreceptor blockade is involved. Occasionally, too, relatives of patients with type III hyperlipoproteinaemia (Chapter 8, page 218) prove to have type IV hyperlipoproteinaemia and this is often taken to indicate that the coincidence of familial endogenous hypertriglyceridaemia with apolipoprotein E2 homozygosity in the patient has been the additional perturbation provoking the accumulation of remnant lipoproteins in the circulation of the patient.

Primary endogenous hypertriglyceridaemia is rare before the age of 20 years and this seems also to be the case even in the familial form unless it is the rare homozygous familial lipoprotein lipase deficiency (see Severe hypertriglyceridaemia)[22].

Hypertriglyceridaemia much more commonly occurs in secondary hyperlipoproteinaemia than does hypercholesterolaemia. Obesity is a leading cause of hypertriglyceridaemia, and alcohol abuse and diabetes mellitus are also often present in patients presenting with hypertriglyceridaemia. Beta-adrenoreceptor blocking drugs are also very commonly a major contributing factor to hypertriglyceridaemia in patients referred to the lipid clinic. Secondary causes of hypertriglyceridaemia are discussed in Chapter 11. A minority of patients with type IV hyperlipoproteinaemia are, however, lean and have no obvious explanation other than presumably a strong genetic tendency.

Another cause of increased serum triglycerides which is frequently overlooked is physical stress. Although it is widely recognized that myocardial infarction may provoke hypertriglyceridaemia, it is often not realized that the same may be true of severe angina or of procedures such as coronary angioplasty, coronary artery bypass or indeed any surgical operation. If serum lipids are estimated close to such events, a type IV phenotype is often found. Later, however, the true picture emerges as the triglycerides fall and the cholesterol rises (Chapter 3, page 87), which may well be a type IIa or IIb hyperlipoproteinaemia.

Hyperuricaemia and gout are strikingly associated with all forms of hypertriglyceridaemia, except the rare lipoprotein lipase deficiency (page 198; gout is discussed in Chapter 11, page 337).

## Metabolic basis of type IV hyperlipoproteinaemia

It will be obvious from the foregoing that type IV hyperlipoproteinaemia is heterogeneous and that it is unlikely therefore to have any single metabolic cause. Despite methodological difficulties associated with the interpretation of the results of experiments in which triglyceride turnover or VLDL apo B turnover have been investigated[28,29], it is evident that in the majority of patients with type IV hyperlipoproteinaemia the cause is an increased input of hepatic VLDL into the circulation[25,30–41]. Since the triglyceride removal mechanism is readily saturable, its capacity becomes a more significant factor in those patients in whom increases in production are extreme. Often, too, some partial defect in catabolism or a catabolic rate towards the lower end of the normal distribution seems to be present[42–45], which in the absence of any increase in production would be insufficient to take the serum triglyceride concentration out of the normal range. The so-called familial endogenous hypertriglyceridaemia may be an expression of a more marked catabolic defect[37] and it is in this type of patient that some additional stimulus to triglyceride production such as alcohol, oestrogen administration or diabetes mellitus or some further slowing of catabolism such as β-blockade, hypothyroidism or diabetes mellitus may lead to the progression of relatively mild type IV hyperlipoproteinaemia to the type V phenotype with its attendant risk of acute pancreatitis[46].

The fraction of the VLDL apo B which enters the LDL apo B is decreased in hypertriglyceridaemia[29,34,39–41]. The LDL present in hypertriglyceridaemia is characterized by several features, all of which are more marked when the hypertriglyceridaemia is severe. It is smaller and denser than normal LDL and is composed of relatively more apo B and triglycerides and less cholesteryl ester[47]. It has been suggested that the increased triglyceride and decreased cholesteryl ester content of LDL might be due to the greatly expanded pool of triglyceride-rich lipoproteins (page 59). CETP activity in hypertriglyceridaemia is increased[47,48]. In at least some patients with more severe hypertriglyceridaemia there is an increased fractional catabolism of LDL[29,33,37,39]. There is a reduced affinity of LDL from hypertriglyceridaemic patients for its receptor[47] which is consistent with the view that the increased LDL catabolism in hypertriglyceridaemia does not proceed via the receptor-mediated pathway, but is non-receptor mediated[48]. Possibly increased LDL catabolism, together with an increased fraction of VLDL being removed before its conversion to LDL, which has been observed in type IV hyperlipoproteinaemia[29], might account for the even lower levels of LDL in type V hyperlipoproteinaemia.

In some patients with type IV hypertriglyceridaemia typical lipid values might be triglycerides 350 mg/dl (4 mmol/l) and cholesterol 200 mg/dl (5 mmol/l) or even less. The treatment of such patients, for example with fibrate drugs, often causes an increase in the LDL cholesterol level as the hypertriglyceridaemia subsides (Chapter 10, page 266). The LDL composition changes towards normal[49] and its non-receptor mediated catabolic rate, which was previously high, declines, which is the reason for the increase in serum LDL levels[50]. In another type of patient, the LDL cholesterol levels are higher and the distinction between this phenotype and type IIb hyperlipoproteinaemia is somewhat arbitrary depending on what is considered the upper limit of normal for LDL cholesterol. This type of patient often responds to fibrate drugs by lowering their triglycerides, whilst their LDL cholesterol level remains relatively constant, although in them too there will be an increase in receptor-mediated LDL clearance and a decrease in non-receptor mediated clearance[50]. The kinetic mechanism underlying type IV hyperlipoproteinaemia thus has much in common with familial combined hyperlipidaemia or hyperapobetalipoproteinaemia (Chapter 6, page 144).

Much of the early literature about hypertriglyceridaemia concerned the hypothesis that it resulted from dietary carbohydrate. Diets high in carbohydrate can undoubtedly induce a rise in serum triglyceride levels not only in patients with pre-existing hypertriglyceridaemia, but also in normal people. However, the evidence that patients with hypertriglyceridaemia are more susceptible to carbohydrate induction is not convincing[51], and even on very low carbohydrate diets the great majority of patients with hypertriglyceridaemia do not revert to normal[52]. Certainly in normal people carbohydrate induction is not sustained (Chapter 9, page 234): it is not known whether it is in patients with pre-existing hypertriglyceridaemias. In purely practical terms the withdrawal of saturated fat from the diet is more effective therapy (Chapter 9, page 226).

The concentration of serum HDL tends to be decreased in primary and most secondary hypertriglyceridaemias. As outlined in Chapter 2, the metabolism of triglyceride-rich lipoproteins and HDL is intimately linked. The decrease in HDL in hypertriglyceridaemia is principally in $HDL_2$. The $HDL_3$ particles present are frequently denser than those of normal $HDL_3$ and contain less cholesteryl ester and more triglyceride relative to protein[47].

Low concentrations of HDL may be explained in those hypertriglyceridaemic states which are associated with decreased or absent lipoprotein lipase activity, since the conversion of HDL3 to HDL2 and the acquisition of many components of HDL is dependent on lipolysis of triglyceride-rich lipoproteins[53].

Increased activity of cholesteryl ester transfer protein (see Chapter 2, page 58) also characterizes many hypertriglyceridaemic states[48,54–57] and this might have some bearing on the decreased proportion of cholesteryl ester in HDL.

A further observation has been that the rate of catabolism of apolipoproteins AI and AII is increased in hypertriglyceridaemia[58–60]. The explanation for this is at present uncertain[61], but it too might contribute to the low levels of HDL.

## Treatment of moderate hypertriglyceridaemia

The presence of triglyceride levels in excess of 200 mg/dl (2.3 mmol/l) when they occur in association with a raised cholesterol are an additional factor favouring therapy aimed at reducing the LDL cholesterol level if it persists above 250 mg/dl (6.5 mmol/l) despite dietary treatment, particularly if an additional risk factor such as diabetes mellitus or hypertension is present (Chapter 6). In this section the possible indications for therapy in patients with primary type IV hyperlipoproteinaemia, whose serum cholesterol levels are less than this, will be considered. Generally, hypertriglyceridaemic patients will have serum cholesterol levels in excess of 200 mg/dl (5.2 mmol/l) and dietary advice will as usual be the starting point of therapy. Many will be obese (Chapter 11, page 315) and so the saturated fat withdrawn from the diet will not need to be replaced (Chapter 9). In patients who remain hypertriglyceridaemic despite such a diet, it is important to review the possibility that their hyperlipoproteinaemia may be secondary. If secret high alcohol consumption is suspected, then investigations such as a blood ethanol level or mean red cell volume should be considered. Results of γ-glutamyl transpeptidase should be interpreted with caution in this context, since one report suggests that its serum activity may be increased in hypertriglyceridaemia from causes other than alcohol[62]. The possibility that the patient has not been truly fasting is also important in a borderline decision as to whether to introduce lipid-lowering drug therapy.

A Consensus Conference of the US National Institutes of Health concluded that for patients whose triglycerides were in the range 250–500 mg/dl (2.8–5.6 mmol/l), 'In the absence of elevated serum cholesterol levels (in the person or family members), other risk factors for heart disease, or premature cardiovascular disease in other family members, there is no evidence for increased cardiovascular risk; specific triglyceride-lowering therapy seems unnecessary. If the person has other major risk factors, such as hypertension, smoking, or obesity, vigorous attempts to modify these factors should be undertaken'[63]. The statement that 'there is no evidence for increased cardiovascular risk' would appear to run counter to the findings of the Framingham study discussed previously (page 191). Also, since such patients frequently have low HDL levels this would be an additional hazard. Nevertheless the rest of the statement is fair, since even if we recognize that such individuals are at increased risk we have no evidence that pharmacological intervention will affect this. As is discussed earlier and in Chapter 10, therapy such as fibrates or fish oil in hypertriglyceridaemic patients with low LDL cholesterol may actually raise its concentration. It might be argued that some benefit might accrue from raising HDL cholesterol with a fibrate such as gemfibrozil. In the Helsinki Heart Study[64], however, in which the participants with the type IV phenotype were of the type whose cholesterol was at the upper end of the normal range and who might thus have been expected to benefit more than patients with lower cholesterol levels, there was no significant effects of therapy on coronary disease.

It must, however, be said that there were too few men with type IV hyper-lipoproteinaemia for this to be regarded as a conclusive finding and a future study designed to answer this question would be important.

As has been previously pointed out, hypertriglyceridaemia is a relatively common finding in patients presenting with ischaemic heart disease even after recovery from the immediate effects of physical illness and the elimination of effects of therapy. In an open trial of nicotinic acid combined with clofibrate in the survivors of myocardial infarction, a significant reduction in subsequent mortality was observed in the treated group compared with controls[65]. The apparently beneficial effect of the therapy occurred only in patients with an initial triglyceride of >135 mg/dl (>1.5 mmol/l) and was greatest when the decrease in triglycerides was marked. It was not related to changes in serum cholesterol. Clofibrate is more active in lowering plasma fibrinogen than gemfibrozil and this may have had some bearing on the success of this study.

Additional evidence for the treatment of patients with moderate hypertriglyceridaemia when they have some manifestation of cardiovascular disease comes from investigations of patients who have undergone coronary bypass surgery. Three studies indicate that hyperlipidaemia is a major risk factor to graft occlusion and for progression of disease in mature vessels[66–68]. In this respect, triglyceride levels seem as important as cholesterol, although in the one study in which it was measured, apolipoprotein B was more important than either[67]. Certainly in our present state of knowledge it seems reasonable to treat both hypercholesterolaemia and hypertriglyceridaemia in such patients. Evidence for this comes from coronary angiographic studies showing similar benefit in patients treated with combinations of drugs which lowered LDL predominantly compared to drug combinations producing a less pronounced LDL reduction but which was accompanied by decreased serum triglyceride levels[69,70] (Chapter 6, page 152). If there is a strong indication that a man with moderate hypertriglyceridaemia is predisposed to myocardial infarction, perhaps by virtue of a strong family history, it seems reasonable to extrapolate from the present evidence and prescribe triglyceride-lowering drug therapy, if his response to diet is unsatisfactory, rather than wait for a myocardial infarction to occur.

## Marked hypertriglyceridaemia

Fasting serum triglyceride levels in excess of 450 mg/dl (5 mmol/l) are not commonly encountered in population surveys (Chapter 3, page 78) and levels exceeding 1000 mg/dl (11 mmol/l) occur with a frequency of probably no more than 1 in 5000. Up to 1000 mg/dl (11 mmol/l), the triglyceride-rich lipoproteins responsible for the hypertriglyceridaemia are largely VLDL of hepatic origin (endogenous hypertriglyceridaemia) and the serum appears opalescent. As the levels approach 1000 mg/dl (11 mmol/l), however, chylomicrons from the gut become increasingly prominent (exogenous hypertriglyceridaemia) and the plasma becomes milky in appearance. This is not surprising since milk, of course, consists of chylomicrons. When the plasma triglycerides reach 4000 mg/dl (45 mmol/l), its fat content is the same as that of whole milk. The particular clinical importance of this type of hypertriglyceridaemia is that as the triglyceride levels climb above 20 mmol/l there is in many patients a likelihood of acute pancreatitis. Some individuals left to their own devices seem to run levels of triglycerides persistently above this level, whereas others can fluctuate between levels almost into the normal range at times, but at others (usually because of some provoking factor) produce very high levels. Up to 13 000 mg/dl (150 mmol/l) has been recorded in our lipid clinic. The great majority of patients with this type of severe hyper-triglyceridaemia due to chylomicronaemia have a type V phenotype, the VLDL concentration also being grossly elevated. In a small number (generally young people with a familial lipoprotein lipase deficiency), the chylomicrons alone are elevated giving the type I phenotype. When this is the case the chylomicrons, which float to the top to form a creamy layer (just as they do in milk) when plasma is allowed to stand or centrifuged at low speed, leave behind a clear plasma. In type V hyperlipoproteinaemia, the plasma remains opalescent or turbid, indicating the presence of VLDL.

Milky serum was well described in the seventeenth century when blood-letting was still common practice[71] and many of its associations including diabetes mellitus, alcohol abuse, nephrotic syndrome, abdominal pain, eruptive xanthomata and splenomegaly, had been reported. Hewson (1771)[72] and Christison (1830)[73] established that the appearance was due to fat particles of splanchnic origin. However, the first clear descriptions of the full clinical syndrome associated with the inherited form were those of Burger and Grutz (1932)[74] and of Holt and colleagues (1939)[75]. The initial demonstration that it was due to lipoprotein lipase deficiency was by Havel and Gordon (1960)[76].

The most common cause of type V hyperlipoproteinaemia is, however, not a profound defect in lipoprotein lipase inherited as an autosomal recessive, but a combination of genetic and acquired factors often combining tendencies for overproduction and delayed clearance of triglyceride-rich lipoproteins. The clinical manifestations of hyperchylomicronaemia are, however, similar regardless of causation. Therefore we shall consider causes first, before considering the clinical consequences common to all.

## Metabolic basis of gross hypertriglyceridaemia (Figure 7.1)

### Familial lipoprotein lipase deficiency

Familial lipoprotein lipase deficiency probably occurs in no more than one person in 1 million[77]. In some populations it is more frequent, such as the French Canadians and some immigrant populations from the Indian subcontinent due to a founder gene effect[78]. A growing number of mutations of the lipoprotein lipase gene associated with the clinical syndrome are being reported, the affected patients being true homozygotes for one of them or compound heterozygotes. A recent review listed 27 mutations in familial lipoprotein lipase deficiency[79]. Familial lipoprotein lipase deficiency produces hyperchylomicronaemia in all affected individuals from childhood onwards. This distinguishes it from the much greater number of patients presenting as a consequence of hyperchylomicronaemia developing in adult life. Lipoprotein lipase deficiency is not, however, the only cause of severe hypertriglyceridaemia in childhood and occasionally children in families with a strong predisposition to type IV or type V hyperlipoproteinaemia are found to have hyperchylomicronaemia[80,81].

The term lipoprotein lipase deficiency implies a virtually complete lack of enzyme activity. Its inheritance is usually considered to be autosomal recessive, although it is now realized that in some families that at least one of the mutations

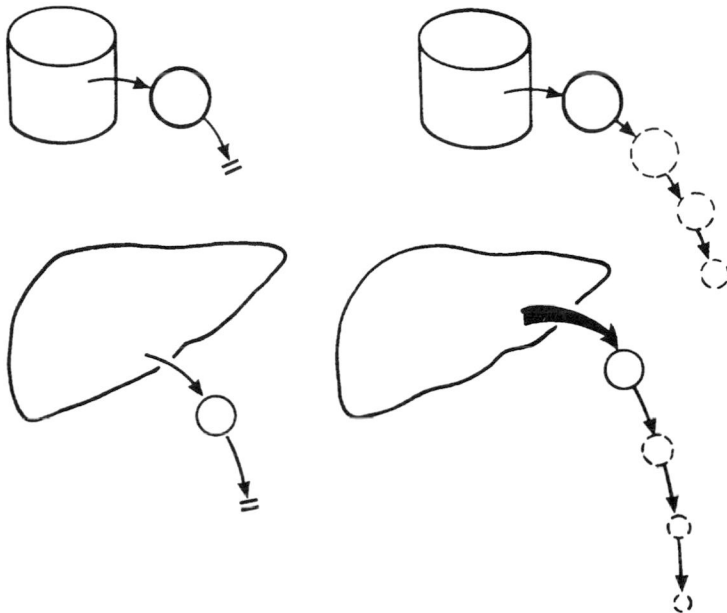

**Figure 7.1**  Metabolic defects leading to severe hypertriglyceridaemia. On the left is shown the effect of familial lipoprotein lipase deficiency, whereas on the right is the more common cause: an increase in hepatic VLDL production combined with partially defective clearance of triglyceride-rich lipoproteins

in the lipoprotein lipase gene can be expressed in heterozygotes as a comparatively mild type IV or IIb phenotype[82]. Until recently it was considered due to a failure of expression of the enzyme because of a true failure of synthesis or a structural abnormality. Recently, however, some cases have been shown to be due to failure to produce apo CII, the apolipoprotein which activates lipoprotein lipase[83–86] (Chapter 2, page 50). Another suggestion that the sialylation of apo CIII might influence the efficiency of triglyceride-rich lipoproteins as lipolytic substrates awaits further confirmation[87].

Although present in childhood, the presenting features are often not recognized nor appropriate therapy instituted until adult life or, sometimes with disastrous results, not at all. Thus, an adult may give a history of recurrent abdominal pain throughout childhood and perhaps eruptive xanthomata in adolescence, the significance of which has escaped medical attention, possibly even after more typical attacks of acute pancreatitis have occurred in adult life.

If identified in childhood, the majority, if not all, patients with lipoprotein lipase deficiency will have type I hyperlipoproteinaemia rather than type V hyperlipoproteinaemia. The impression gained from the literature is that some of these patients do occasionally have the type V phenotype even in childhood. It is a great problem to explain why they all do not, since the same enzyme is responsible for the catabolism of both chylomicrons and VLDL and thus the concentration of both might be expected to increase[88]. It seems that with the progression into adult life, the effect of advancing age is to convert the type I phenotype to the expected type V. It must be extraordinarily rare, if not unknown, for the type I patterns to exist after the age of 30 years. One suggestion to explain the type I phenotype has been that the liver may produce larger triglyceride-rich particles indistinguishable from chylomicrons, but direct evidence for this hypothesis is lacking[89]. Another hypothesis might be that children have a greater capacity than adults to switch off the production of hepatic VLDL when high levels of exogenous triglyceride-rich lipoproteins are circulating. Evidence that such a mechanism might exist at all is at present insubstantial, although a possible mechanism involving insulin has been suggested[90] and its decreased sensitivity in adulthood might relate to increasing insulin resistance. Another explanation might be that in childhood at least one of the other lipases, such as hepatic lipase, may have the capacity to hydrolyse triglycerides on VLDL[91,92]. Lipoprotein lipase itself appears to show a preference for triglycerides in larger particles[93]. Hepatic lipase may, however, show preference for smaller VLDL particles. Recently this hypothesis has received substantial confirmation as the result of kinetic studies in patients with lipoprotein lipase deficiency[94]. By injecting large and small VLDL labelled with different isotopes of iodine it was shown that whereas the clearance of chylomicrons and big VLDL was considerably delayed the clearance of small VLDL was relatively normal (Figure 7.2). Thus expression of the type I phenotype is dependent on the capacity of this alternative pathway (presumably hepatic lipase) to clear small VLDL. Once its capacity is exceeded type V ensues. The type I phenotype does not persist when a low fat diet is instituted and dietary

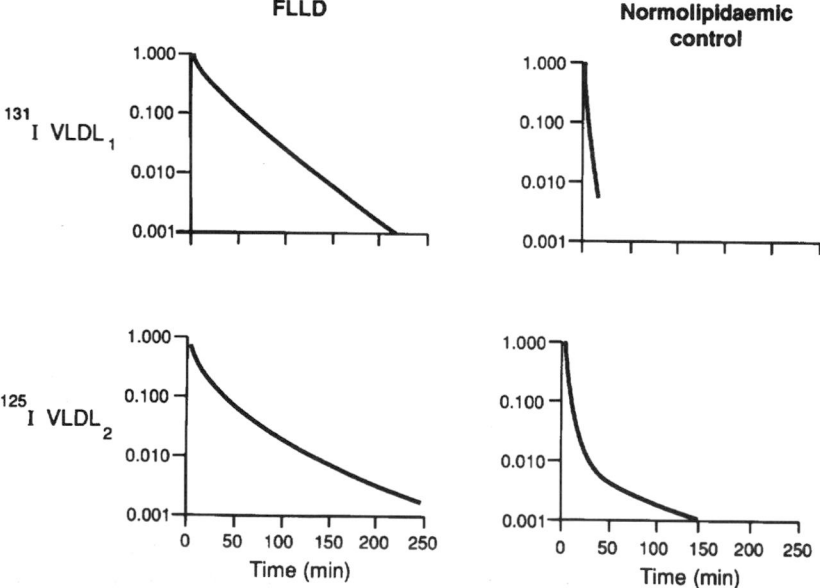

**Figure 7.2**    The disappearance of radiolabelled large VLDL (VLDL₁, sf 60–400) and small VLDL (VLDL₂, sf 20–60) from the circulation of a patient with familial lipoprotein lipase deficiency (FLLD) and in a normolipidaemic control. The more profound difference is in the disappearance rate of large VLDL, probably because hepatic lipase can in the absence of lipoprotein lipase be recruited to hydrolyse triglycerides on the smaller VLDL particles. (Data from reference[94])

energy replaced by carbohydrates: it is converted to a type IV or V pattern. Many patients by the time they reach specialized lipid clinics may be in this partially treated state.

Unlike most other hypertriglyceridaemias, hyperuricaemia and glucose intolerance do not feature in familial lipoprotein lipase deficiency. In patients in whom glucose intolerance does occur there is usually ample evidence that it is secondary to recurrent acute pancreatitis occurring as a consequence of the hyperchylomicronaemia[77,83].

## Commoner forms of hyperchylomicronaemia

Type I hyperlipoproteinaemia seems only exceptionally to result from any cause other than familial lipoprotein lipase deficiency or apo CII deficiency[77]. Type V hyperlipoproteinaemia, although uncommon, is by no means as rare as type I and probably affects at least 1 in 10 000 people at some time. Only exceptionally are patients presenting with type V hyperlipoproteinaemia found to have familial lipoprotein lipase deficiency. It may be familial, but even then it is only occasionally manifest before the third decade. Type IV hyperlipoproteinaemia is found more commonly than type V in other family members, implying that in the proband the familial tendency to endogenous hypertriglyceridaemia has perhaps coincided with some partial defect in lipoprotein lipase or some additional stimulus to overproduction. This probably accounts for why type V hyperlipoproteinaemia occurs at least as frequently as a secondary hyperlipoproteinaemia as it does in its primary form. Thus diabetes mellitus or alcohol abuse, which commonly lead to a type IV hyperlipoproteinaemia, may in an individual who already has an underlying tendency to primary hypertriglyceridaemia combine to produce a severe type V disorder[77,95,96]. The conditions which are known to contribute to the development of chylomicronaemia in susceptible individuals are as follows:

1. Obesity (Chapter 11, pages 315–322).
2. Alcohol abuse[97] (Chapter 11, pages 322–325).
3. Diabetes mellitus[98] (Chapter 11, pages 293–314).
4. Pregnancy[99] (Chapter 3, page 89).
5. Oestrogen[100] (Chapter 11, pages 334–335).
6. Beta-adrenoreceptor blockade[101,102] (Chapter 11, pages 333–334).
7. Bile acid-sequestrating agent inappropriately prescribed (Chapter 10, page 263).
8. Hypothyroidism (Chapter 11, pages 314–315).
9. Renal disease (Chapter 11, pages 328–331).

## Laboratory diagnosis

The detection of hyperchylomicronaemia does not usually present any problem, since it is revealed by the milky appearance of the serum or plasma and by the appearance of a creamier layer on the surface of the plasma when left to stand (Plate 7). It may be confirmed by routine paper or agarose gel electrophoresis or by nephelometry[103]. The serum triglyceride concentration is invariably greater than that of cholesterol, but also in type V hyperlipoproteinaemia marked increases in cholesterol are frequently found.

The diagnostic problem is to identify the small number of patients with familial lipoprotein lipase deficiency. From the previous discussion it will be obvious that the finding of some secondary cause or of hyperuricaemia makes familial lipoprotein lipase deficiency unlikely. Type III hyperlipoproteinaemia which occasionally causes some accumulation of chylomicrons should be excluded (Chapter 8, page 221). A low fat diet should be instituted to clear chylomicron-aemia before isolation of VLDL in the ultracentrifuge for cholesterol determination to detect the presence of β-VLDL. The diagnosis of familial lipoprotein lipase deficiency is more likely if the patient presents in childhood. It is also helpful if the clinical history extends back to childhood. Lipoprotein lipase deficiency is more certain if VLDL is absent (type I phenotype), as revealed by clear plasma after the chylomicrons have floated to the surface either on standing or low speed centrifugation or by lipoprotein electrophoresis or by nephelometry. In practice, these tests are not always easy to interpret, since when the triglyceride levels are several thousand mg/dl chylomicrons are not always easily cleared from plasma on standing, and on electrophoresis they may smear the area usually occupied by VLDL. Stone and Thorp nephelometry[103] is potentially the best means of distinguishing type I from type V hyperlipoproteinaemia, but this has not been tested in the largest series of patients studied[22].

Confirmation of the diagnosis of lipoprotein lipase deficiency requires the demonstration of a profound decrease in its activity. Methods to do this are available in only a few centres and, even then, the interpretation of results is not always easy. When the diagnosis is suspected, a number of more generally available tests can, however, be performed before resorting to assay of the lipase. First, polyacrylamide gel electrophoresis and isoelectric focusing is widely available and the presence or absence of apo CII can thus be easily determined. Secondly, the intravenous fat tolerance test, in which 10% Intralipid (1 ml/kg body weight) is injected intravenously as a bolus and its disappearance followed by nephelometry for 45 min[104], will demonstrate whether any significant triglyceride clearance is taking place. This test should be done after the patient's plasma has been largely cleared following institution of a low fat diet (page 245). Another simple test for lipoprotein lipase is to compare the results of lipoprotein electrophoresis before and 10 min after the intravenous injection of heparin (20 U/kg body weight). If lipoprotein lipase is present, it will be released from the vascular endothelium and the ensuing intravascular lipolysis will release non-esterified fatty acids which are absorbed by all the lipoproteins, altering their charge and markedly accelerating their electrophoretic mobility[22,105].

The difficulty in measuring lipoprotein lipase activity largely relates to its site on the vascular endothelium of skeletal muscle and adipose tissue. It is released into the circulation within minutes of the intravenous administration of heparin, but so also is hepatic lipase. Although hepatic lipase does not appear to function effectively as a triglyceride lipase *in vivo*, in post-heparin plasma, its hydrolytic activity against the radioactive triolein emulsion used in the assay is quantitatively similar to that of lipoprotein lipase. Total post-heparin lipolytic activity is therefore of no diagnostic value. There have been two approaches to overcome this difficulty. One is to inactivate one of the enzymes in post-heparin plasma. This has been accomplished by inactivating lipoprotein lipase with protamine[106]. Lipoprotein lipase is then calculated as the difference between the lipolytic activity of post-heparin plasma in the presence and absence of protamine. A more direct method in which the hepatic lipase in post-heparin plasma is inactivated with a specific antiserum has also been used[107,108]. Another approach to the problem has been to avoid post-heparin plasma altogether and measure the enzyme in extracts of adipose tissue obtained by biopsy, either in terms of its activity against an artificial triglyceride emulsion[109–111] or by immunoassay[112]. Adipose tissue can fairly easily be aspirated subcutaneously from the anterior abdominal wall with a syringe and needle. Direct assay of tissue lipoprotein lipase is probably the diagnostic method of choice.

In purely practical terms, the only value of knowing with certainty that lipoprotein lipase is inactive is that it largely rules out the possibility of drug therapy. However, where uncertainty remains or the method is unavailable, the question of therapeutic responsiveness can in any case be settled by a trial of a fibrate drug.

## Clinical features of severe hypertriglyceridaemia

### Acute pancreatitis

Abdominal pain occurs fairly commonly in patients with hyperchylomicronaemia. Some individuals appear to be resistant and only rarely or perhaps never experience any symptoms even as a consequence of serum triglyceride levels exceeding 10 000 mg/dl (110 mmol/l). In others, it is difficult to say what the threshold is, particularly when theirs is the more evanescent form of the disorder and during intervals between episodes of pancreatitis serum triglycerides may be less than 480 mg/dl (5 mmol/l)[46]. This has undoubtedly led some authors to suggest that hyperchylomicronaemia was a consequence rather than a cause of acute pancreatitis[113,114]. The demonstration that acute pancreatitis occurs in patients with persistently elevated triglycerides, that in those in whom the hypertriglyceridaemia is transient the rise precedes the development of pancreatitis, and that recurrent episodes of pancreatitis are abolished by treatment of the hypertriglyceridaemia, are convincing evidence that the hypertriglyceridaemia is the cause of the pancreatitis[75,77,97,100,115–119].

In my view, acute pancreatitis is unlikely to be caused by hyperchylomicronaemia when triglyceride concentrations are less than 2000 mg/dl (22 mmol/l). Often, however, when a patient is admitted with severe abdominal pain, no serum is kept for serum triglyceride determination. By the time such a test is considered, the patient has been on intravenous fluid and gastric aspiration for several days and the triglyceride levels may have fallen even to within the normal range. This has certainly led to a failure to appreciate that 10% or more of acute pancreatitis is due to hypertriglyceridaemia[46,113,116,117].

The presentation of acute pancreatitis probably varies little from that of other causes of the disorder. It may occur as a relatively isolated episode of abdominal pain or as a more severe attack in the type of patient who has been having recurring less severe pains. The patient is generally seen as an emergency and the usual differential diagnosis is a perforated peptic ulcer. All too frequently the decision as to whether to subject the patient to laparotomy turns on the serum amylase level. Unfortunately it is not widely appreciated that the serum amylase may be within normal limits or only marginally elevated in patients with hyperchylomicronaemia, even at the height of an episode of acute pancreatitis[95,96,117,120–122]. The reasons for this are probably that in some instances the high level of lipoprotein particles interferes with the assay of amylase[120]. Diluting serum or measuring the urinary amylase may sometimes reveal the true hyperamylasaemia[95], but this does not seem invariably to be the case. A laparotomy during acute pancreatitis increases the likelihood of mortality at least ten-fold. In my view, the emergency biochemist should never report an amylase value in a patient whose serum is grossly lipaemic without informing the admitting doctor of its limitations. The presence of milky serum in a patient with severe abdominal pain should almost invariably be taken as confirmation of the diagnosis of acute pancreatitis regardless of the amylase value, and appropriate conservative measures instituted, when the great majority of patients recover surprisingly quickly.

The reason that hyperchylomicronaemia provokes pancreatitis is not known with certainty, but a very plausible theory has been proposed by Havel[118]. It is known that the normal pancreas releases small amounts of lipase into the circulation. It is also likely (see later) that in severe hyperchylomicronaemia the microcirculation of many organs is sluggish, because of the difficult passage of the large lipoprotein particles through their capillaries. Any lipase entering the pancreatic capillaries would encounter an abundance of slowly moving substrate there, and large quantities of non-esterified fatty acids might thus be generated locally. These are irritants and the resulting local inflammation might increase the tendency for amylase to leak into the blood stream and so create a vicious circle, eventually producing clinical pancreatitis. The triglyceride sluggishly circulating through the pancreatic microcirculation would also be very vulnerable to attack by free radicals and thus the generation of lipid peroxides, ketones, aldehydes and lyso-phospholipids all of which could cause cytotoxicity and inflammation. The risk of free radical attack may be high in the pancreas because of their high level in bile[123]. Acute pancreatitis in hypertriglyceridaemia can give rise to complications including pseudocyst, and recurring episodes may occasionally cause pancreatic exocrine or endocrine insufficiency. One oddity from my own experience has been how infrequently patients with primary diabetes seem to develop acute pancreatitis, even in the presence of grossly elevated triglycerides. The same is not true of alcohol abusers, in whom gross chylomicronaemia is quite frequently a precipitant of acute pancreatitis. Alcohol *per se* can, of course, in susceptible individuals, cause acute pancreatitis without the agency of hypertriglyceridaemia.

### *Hepatosplenomegaly*

Hepatosplenomegaly is fairly common in patients with marked hypertriglyceridaemia and it is sometimes difficult to know whether disturbances of serum liver enzymes and the appearance of fatty infiltration on liver scanning are due to the hypertriglyceridaemia or to alcohol abuse or both. However, hepatomegaly and occasionally splenomegaly undoubtedly occur in patients with hyperchylomicronaemia, and marked defects in triglyceride catabolism when alcohol plays no part. The reason is that, in the absence of the lipolytic clearance pathway or when it is overloaded, the reticulo-endothelial system clears the triglyceride-rich lipoproteins from the circulation. Bone marrow biopsy in such patients reveals the presence of numerous foam-laden macrophages (Plate 8), which are also the cause of the fatty enlargement of the liver and spleen. In patients with splenomegaly, splenic infarction is a possible cause of abdominal pain and it is also said that sudden increases in size of the liver and spleen due to over-indulgence in fat may also be a cause.

It has sometimes been said that hypersplenism does not result from the splenomegaly. However, we have reported an undoubted case of pancytopenia due to this cause in an adult[111] and have subsequently discovered two others.

Whatever Zieve's syndrome is[96], it was not present in our patients. Similar cases have also occurred in infancy[124,125].

## Other abdominal pain in hypertriglyceridaemia

Some patients with hyperchylomicronaemia have recurrent abdominal pain, which is neither severe enough to be typical of acute pancreatitis nor is it related to hepatosplenomegaly. Abdominal pain is, of course, a common reason for medical consultation and thus unrelated abdominal pain may then lead to the discovery of milky plasma when the blood is taken for some other purpose. Clinical impression is, however, that recurring abdominal pain is more common than can be accounted for in this way. Patients may frequently have previously been diagnosed as having irritable bowel syndrome, functional abdominal pain or even as malingerers or possibly having Munchausen's syndrome[96,126]. It should furthermore be remembered that cholelithiasis is also prevalent in hypertriglyceridaemia[127].

## Eruptive xanthomata

Cutaneous xanthomata consisting of papules with raised yellow centres (1–5 mm diameter) or an erythematous base appear on the extensor surfaces especially of the arms, back, buttocks and legs (Plate 9). They show less tendency to coalesce and to cluster over tuberosities than the tuberoeruptive xanthomata of type III hyperlipoproteinaemia (Chapter 8, page 216). The presence of tuberoeruptive xanthomata together with eruptive xanthomata suggests that a type III disorder is the underlying cause of the hyperchylomicronaemia. Occasionally, eruptive xanthomata are itchy, particularly during resolution. In extreme cases almost any skin surface and even mucous membranes can be affected. Histologically, eruptive xanthomata consist of fat-filled macrophages and, unlike other xanthomata, they contain substantial amounts of triglycerides in addition to cholesteryl esters, particularly when they first appear[128]. They usually disappear within a few weeks of commencing treatment. Eruptive xanthomata are not encountered in patients whose triglycerides do not exceed at least 2000 mg/dl (22 mmol/l) and thus their presence in association with lower levels implies that a more severe hypertriglyceridaemia has recently resolved or some other diagnosis such as acne, seborrhoea, xanthoma disseminatum[129] or juvenile xanthogranuloma[130] should be considered (Plates 10a–c).

## Spurious laboratory results

Pseudohyponatraemia is a feature of severe hypertriglyceridaemia of any cause. It occurs when the triglyceride-rich lipoproteins occupy a volume sufficiently great to reduce the volume of water in a sample so that the sodium concentration appears low when expressed in terms of the total rather than the aqueous volume. A formula has been devised for the calculation of the true serum sodium concentration[131]. However, this requires the determination of the serum triglyceride concentration and assumes that the average size of the lipoproteins at a given level of triglycerides is the same in every patient. If it is considered necessary to know the serum sodium level, centrifugation to reduce the level of the chylomicrons is an alternative approach. Also the plasma osmolality may be measured.

Pseudohyponatraemia can lead to serious complications if it is not appreciated by the medical attendants. This applies frequently to patients admitted to intensive treatment units with acute pancreatitis, but also occasionally to patients with diabetic ketoacidosis, who erroneously receive large quantities of intravenous saline, sometimes even hypertonic saline. Sometimes such management results in true serum sodium concentrations of 160 mmol/l or more. In any case, one cannot but marvel at the ignorance of doctors who equate a low serum sodium level with sodium deficiency; perhaps it is precisely such people who would be unable to grasp the concept of pseudohypernatraemia. On one occasion the author has even seen it develop following persistent and wholly pointless infusions of Intralipid in a severely ill patient who was then subjected to infusions of hypertonic saline.

Almost any biochemical test performed on the plasma or serum, including the liver enzymes, can give spurious results when lipaemia is extreme. This need not be due to any chemical interference but can be mechanical, for example due to clogging of the sampler of an autoanalyser, especially if the sample pot stands for a while in the carriage allowing chylomicrons to build up on the surface. This latter factor, too, may make calculations of the true sodium level based on triglyceride levels erroneous if the sodium analyser has sampled plasma enriched in chylomicrons.

### Glucose intolerance and insulin

Diabetes mellitus frequently accompanies type V hyperlipoproteinaemia (Chapter 11, page 295)[77]. In addition, a substantial proportion of patients with type V hyperlipoproteinaemia who do not have diabetes mellitus have oral or intravenous glucose responses in the upper part of the normal range[22,132]. This is apparently due to insulin resistance, since insulin levels are also increased[132]. Obesity and/or a family history of diabetes are often present in such patients. These observations raise important, but unresolved, questions about whether insulin resistance influences the expression of hypertriglyceridaemia or whether hypertriglyceridaemia contributes to insulin resistance.

### Accelerated atheroma

As discussed in connection with less severe forms of hypertriglyceridaemia, the evidence for a substantially increased risk of atheroma overall does not exist. Clearly, however, in the presence of glucose intolerance, a poor family history or some other risk factor such as hypertension, risk may be increased. Many patients are, of course, discovered because their serum lipids are checked when they present with vascular disease and the clinical impression of an association may thus be gained from the population of patients seen at lipid clinics.

Increased risk of atherosclerosis might be expected on the basis of the low plasma HDL levels typical of both type V and type I hyperlipoproteinaemia. However, the LDL cholesterol concentration in both these disorders is also typically low and this applies equally to LDL apo B. In fact, the total serum and LDL apo B levels in many patients with moderate type IV hyperlipoproteinaemia are much higher than in patients with marked type V hyperlipoproteinaemia[133].

## Lipaemia retinalis

In hyperchylomicronaemia the blood may appear paler ('melted strawberry ice cream')[134]. This paleness can be observed in the retina as a whole. Also, within the microcirculation of the retina the presumably slower movement of the chylomicrons compared with the red cells can actually be observed as a white central streak along the veins which thus appear to have the same white line along their centre as the normal arteries. These appearances are known as 'lipaemia retinalis'[75] (Plate 11). Presumably a similar phenomenon is present in the microcirculation of all organs and this may give rise to some of the transient apparently ischaemic complications (see later).

## Hyperuricaemia

See Chapter 11, page 337.

## Polyarthritis

Musculoskeletal symptoms and polyarthralgias are reported to occur more commonly in hypertriglyceridaemia than by chance[135,136].

## Sicca syndrome

Sicca syndrome is also believed to be associated with type V hyperlipoproteinaemia[137].

## Polyneuropathy

Paraesthesiae and altered sensation in various parts of the body occur in severe hypertriglyceridaemia. It is often difficult to eliminate associated diabetes as the cause, but there probably is a specific peripheral neuropathy due to the hyperlipidaemia itself[138–140].

## Other neurological features

Occasionally, transient focal neurological complications of chylomicronaemia have been reported, including hemiparesis, but it is difficult to attribute them to the hyperchylomicronaemia with confidence. Mild confusion and recent memory loss has also been reported when triglycerides are at their height, with improvement as their level subsides[98]. It has also been suggested that severe hypertriglyceridaemia might play a part in depression and dementia[141,142].

## Miscellaneous features

Earlier reports that hypertriglyceridaemia might contribute to ischaemia by inducing hypoxaemia, abnormal haemoglobin oxygen affinity and decreased pulmonary diffusing capacity have not been confirmed when techniques have been employed which allow for artefacts due to the lipaemia[98].

## Management of severe hypertriglyceridaemia

In both types I and V hyperlipoproteinaemia the essential part of management is a diet low in total fat to limit the formation of chylomicrons (Chapter 9, page 245). Secondary factors should be treated or regulated as far as possible, including of course alcohol abuse and obesity. Diets as low as 10 g of fat may occasionally be necessary, but the response to diets in the range 20–40 g daily should be carefully assessed before resorting to such extremes. Considerable resolution of the hypertriglyceridaemia within a few days of instituting such a diet on the ward is the rule, although responses are more variable in outpatients. Dietary energy replacement presents a problem in some patients who may require large quantities of carbohydrate. Medium chain triglycerides as energy supplements have not in the author's experience proved particularly helpful and the place of fish oils needs to be more fully explored. At present they should be used with caution as they must contribute to chylomicron formation. In many patients, normal levels of triglyceride cannot be a realizable aim of therapy. Average levels of less than 2000 mg/dl (22 mmol/l) are generally sufficient to prevent the clinical features developing and some patients tolerate much higher levels without apparent ill-effect.

Drug therapy does not appear to be of any value in familial lipoprotein lipase deficiency. Fibrate drugs may be useful in the majority of patients whose hypertriglyceridaemia is not due to that cause and who are able to express lipoprotein lipase. Other drugs such as nicotinic acid may occasionally be used. Bile acid-sequestrating agents are contraindicated, since they may further exacerbate hypertriglyceridaemia.

## References

1. Hulley, S.B., Rosenman, R.H., Bawol, R.D. and Brand, R.J. Epidemiology as a guide to clinical decisions. The association between triglyceride and coronary heart disease. *N. Engl. J. Med.*, **302**, 1383–1389 (1980)
2. Cambien, F., Jacqueson, A., Richard, J.L., Warnet, J.M., Ducimetiere, P. and Claude, J.R. Is the level of serum triglyceride a significant predictor of coronary death in 'normocholesterolemic' subjects? *Am. J. Epidemiol*, **124**, 624–632 (1986)
3. Austin, M. Plasma triglyceride and coronary heart disease. *Arteriosclerosis*, **11**, 2–14 (1991)
4. Castelli, W.P. The triglyceride issue: a view from Framingham. *Am. Heart J.*, **112**, 432–437 (1986)
5. Abbott, R.D. and Carroll, R.J. Interpreting multiple logistic regression coefficients in prospective observational studies. *Am. J. Epidemiol.*, **119**, 830–836 (1984)
6. Carlson, L.A. and Bottiger, L.E. Ischaemic heart disease in relation to fasting values of plasma triglycerides and cholesterol. Stockholm Prospective Study. *Lancet*, **i**, 865–868 (1972)
7. Manninen, V., Huttunen, J.K., Tenkanen, L., Heinonen, O.P., Manttari, M. and Frick, M.H. High density lipoprotein cholesterol as a risk factor for coronary disease in the Helsinki Heart Study. In *High Density Lipoprotein and Atherosclerosis II*, Amsterdam, Excerpta Medica, pp. 35–42 (1989)
8. West, K.M., Ahuja, M.M.S., Bennett, P.H., Czyzyk, A., de Acosta, O.M. *et al.* The role of circulating glucose and triglyceride concentrations and their interactions with other 'risk factors' as determinants of arterial disease in nine diabetic population samples from the WHO Multinational Study. *Diabetes Care*, **6**, 361–369 (1983)
9. Zilversmit, D.B. Atherogenesis: a postprandial phenomenon. *Circulation*, **60**, 473–485 (1979)
10. Winocour, P.H., Durrington, P.N., Ishola, M. and Anderson, D.C. Lipoprotein abnormalities in insulin-dependent diabetes mellitus. *Lancet*, **i**, 1176–1178 (1986)
11. Winocour, P.H., Bhatnagar, D. Durrington, P.N., Ishola, M., Arrol, S. and Mackness, M.I. Abnormalities of VLDL, IDL and LDL characterise insulin-dependent diabetes mellitus. *Arteriosclerosis*, **12**, 920–928 (1992)

12. Steiner, G. Hypertriglyceridemia and carbohydrate intolerance: interrelations and therapeutic implications. *Am. J. Cardiol.*, **57**, 279–309 (1986)
13. Stone, M.C. and Thorp, J.M. Plasma fibrinogen – a major coronary risk factor. *J. R. Coll. Gen. Pract.*, **35**, 565–569 (1985)
14. Meade, T.W., Mellows, S.M., Brozovic, M., Miller, G.J., Chakrabarti, R.R. *et al.* Haemostatic function and ischaemic heart disease: principal results of the Northwick Park heart study. *Lancet*, **ii**, 533–537 (1986)
15. Simpson, H. C. R., Man, J. I., Meade, T. W., Chakrabarti, R., Stirling, Y. and Woolf, L. Hypertriglyceridaemia and hypercoagulability. *Lancet*, **i**, 786–790 (1983)
16. Mitropoulos, K.A., Miller, G.J., Reeves, B.E.A., Wilkes, H.C. and Cruickshank, J.K. Factor VII coagulant activity is strongly associated with the plasma concentration of large lipoprotein particles in middle-aged men. *Atherosclerosis*, **76**, 203 (1989)
17. Miller, G.J., Martin, J.C., Mitropoulos, K.A., Reeves, B.E.A., Thompson, R.L. *et al.* Plasma factor VII is activated by postprandial triglyceridaemia irrespective of dietary fat composition. *Atherosclerosis*, **86**, 163 (1991)
18. Hamsten, A., Wiman, B., deFaire, U. and Blomback, M. Increased plasma levels of a rapid inhibitor of tissue plasminogen activator in young survivors of myocardial infarction. *N. Engl. J. Med.*, **313**, 1557–1563 (1985)
19. Sirtori, C.R. and Lovati, M.R. Triglyceride-rich lipoproteins: role in atherogenesis and thrombogenesis. In *Drugs Affecting Lipid Metabolism* (eds A.L. Catapani, A.M. Gotto, L.C. Smith, and R. Pasletti), Kluwer Academic Publishers, Dordrecht, pp. 215–229 (1993)
20. Mitropoulos, K.A., Miller, G.J., Watts, G.F. and Durrington, P.N. Lipolysis of triglyceride-rich lipoproteins activates coagulant factor XII: a study in familial lipoprotein lipase deficiency. *Atherosclerosis*, **95**, 119–125 (1992)
21. Nikkila, E. A. and Aro, A. Inheritance of endogenous hypertriglyceridaemia type IIb or IV. *Postgrad. Med. J.*, **51**, (Suppl. 8), 32–35 (1975)
22. Fredrickson, D. S. and Levy, R. I. Familial hyperlipoproteinaemia. In *The Metabolic Basis of Inherited Disease*, 3rd edn (eds J.B. Stanbury, J.B. Wyngaarden and D.S. Fredrickson), McGraw-Hill, New York (1972)
23. Glueck, C. J., Tsang, R., Fallat, R., Buncher, C. R., Evans, G. and Steiner, P. Familial hypertriglyceridaemia: studies in 130 children and 45 siblings of 36 index cases. *Metabolism*, **22**, 1287–1309 (1973)
24. Goldstein, J. L., Schrott, H. G., Hazzard, W. R., Bierman, E. L. and Motulsky, A. G. Hyperlipidaemia in coronary heart disease II. Genetic analysis of lipid levels in 176 families and delineation of a new inherited disorder, combined hyperlipidaemia. *J. Clin. Invest.*, **52**, 1544–1568 (1973)
25. Brunzell, J. D., Albers, J. J., Chait, A. I., Grundy, S. M., Groszek, E. and McDonald, G. B. Plasma lipoproteins in familial combined hyperlipidaemia and monogenic familial hypertriglyceridaemia. *J. Lipid Res.*, **24**, 147–155 (1983)
26. Babirak, S.P., Iverius, P-H., Fjimoto, W.Y. and Brunzell, J.D. Detection and characterisation of the heterozygous state for lipoprotein lipase deficiency. *Arteriosclerosis*, **9**, 326–334 (1989)
27. Auwerx, J.H., Barbirak, S.P., Hopkanson, J.E., Stahnke, G., Will, H. *et al.* Co-existance of abnormalities of hepatic lipase and lipoprotein lipase in a large family. *Am. J. Hum. Genet.*, **46**, 470–477 (1990)
28. Carlson, L. A. Regulation of endogenous plasma triglyceride concentration. Can we measure the rate of production or removal of endogenous triglycerides in man? *Eur. J. Clin. Invest.*, **10**, 5–7 (1980)
29. Beltz, W. F., Kesaniemi, A., Howard, B. V. and Grundy, S. M. Development of an integrated model for analysis of the kinetics of apolipoprotein B in plasma very low density lipoproteins, intermediate density lipoproteins, and low density lipoproteins. *J. Clin. Invest.*, **76**, 575–585 (1985)
30. Reaven, G. M., Hill, D. B., Gross, R. C. and Farquhar, J. W. Kinetics of triglyceride turnover of very low density lipoproteins of human plasma. *J. Clin. Invest.*, **44**, 1826–1833 (1969)
31. Nikkila, E. A. and Kekki, M. Polymorphism of plasma triglyceride kinetics in normal human adult subjects. *Acta Med. Scand*, **190**, 49–59 (1971)
32. Adams, P. W., Kissebah, A. H., Harrigan, P., Stokes, T. and Wynn, V. The kinetics of plasma free fatty acid and triglyceride transport in patients with ideopathic hypertriglyceridaemia and their relation to carbohydrate metabolism. *Eur. J. Clin. Invest.*, **4**, 149–161 (1974)

33. Sigurdsson, G., Nicoll, A. and Lewis, B. The metabolism of low density lipoprotein in endoge-nous hypertriglyceridaemia. *Eur. J. Clin. Invest.*, **6**, 151–158 (1976)
34. Berman, M., Hall, M., Levy, R. I., Eisenberg, S., Bilheimer, D. W. *et al*. Metabolism of apo B and apo C apolipoproteins in man: kinetic studies in normal and hyperlipoproteinaemic subjects. *J. Lipid Res.*, **19**, 38–56 (1978)
35. Grundy, S. M., Mok, H. Y. I., Zech, L., Steinberg, D. and Berman, M. Transport of very low density lipoprotein triglycerides in varying degrees of obesity and hypertriglyceridaemia. *J. Clin. Invest.*, **63**, 1274–1283 (1979)
36. Kekki, M. Plasma triglyceride turnover in ninety-two adult normolipidaemic and thirty hyper-triglyceridaemic subjects. The effect of age, synthesis rate and removal capacity on plasma triglyc-eride concentration. *Ann. Clin. Res.*, **12**, 64–76 (1980)
37. Janus, E. D., Nicoll, A. M., Turner, P. R., Magill, P. and Lewis, B. Kinetic bases of the primary hyperlipidaemias. Studies of apolipoprotein B turnover in genetically defined subjects. *Eur. J. Clin. Invest.*, **10**, 161–172 (1980)
38. Chait, A., Albers, J. J. and Brunzell, J. D. Very low density lipoprotein overproduction in genetic forms of hypertriglyceridaemia. *Eur. J. Clin. Invest.*, **10**, 17–22 (1980)
39. Packard, C. J., Shepherd, J., Jeorns, S., Goko, A. M. and Taunton, O. D. Apolipoprotein B metab-olism in normal, type IV, and type V hyperlipoproteinaemic subjects. *Metabolism*, **29**, 213–221 (1980)
40. Shepherd, J., Packard, C. J., Stewart, J. M., Almeh, R. F., Clark, R. S. *et al*. Apolipoprotein A and B (sf 100–400) metabolism during bezafibrate therapy in hypertriglyceridaemic subjects. *J. Clin. Invest.*, **74**, 2164–2177 (1984)
41. Reardon, M. F., Fidge, N. H. and Nestel, P. J. Catabolism of very low density lipoprotein B apolipoprotein in man. *J. Clin. Invest.*, **61**, 850–860 (1978)
42. Krauss, R. H., Levy, R. I. and Fredrickson, D. S. Selective measurement of two lipase activities in postheparin plasma from normal subjects and patients with hyperlipoproteinaemia. *J. Clin. Invest.*, **54**, 1107–1124 (1974)
43. Huttunen, J. K., Ehnholm, C., Kekki, M. and Nikkila, E. A. Post heparin plasma lipoprotein lipase and hepatic lipase in normal subjects and in patients with hypertriglyceridaemia. Correlations to sex, age and various parameters of triglyceride metabolism. *Clin. Sci. Mol. Med.*, **50**, 249–260 (1976)
44. Rossner, S. Further methodological studies on the intravenous fat intolerance with intralipid emulsion. *Scand. J. Clin. Lab. Invest.*, **36**, 155–159 (1976)
45. Liwel, K., Tyroler, H., Eder, H., Gotto, A. and Vahouny, G. Relationship of hypertriglyceridaemia to atherosclerosis. *Arteriosclerosis*, **i**, 406–417 (1981)
46. Durrington, P. N., Twentyman, O. P., Braganza, J. M. and Miller, J. P. Hypertriglyceridaemia and abnormalities of triglyceride metabolism persisting after pancreatitis. *Int. J. Pancreatol.*, **1**, 195–203 (1986)
47. Eisenberg, S. Lipoprotein abnormalities in hypertriglyceridaemia. Significance in atherosclerosis. *Am. Heart J.*, **113**, 555–561 (1987)
48. Bhatnagar, D., Durrington, P.N., Mackness, M.I., Arrol, S. and Winocour, P.H. Effects of treat-ment of hypertriglyceridaemia with gemfibrozil on serum lipoproteins and the transfer of choles-teryl ester from high density lipoproteins to low density lipoproteins. *Atherosclerosis*, **92**, 49–57 (1992)
49. Eisenberg, S., Gavish, D., Oschry, Y., Fainaru, M. and Deckekbaum, R. J. Abnormalities in very low, low, and high density lipoproteins in hypertriglyceridaemia. Reversal toward normal with bezifibrate treatment. *J. Clin. Invest.*, **74**, 470–482 (1984)
50. Shepherd, J., Caslake, M., Gaw, A., Griffin, B., Lindsay, G. and Packard, C. Atherogenicity of triglyceride-rich lipoproteins: clinical aspects. In *Drugs Affecting Metabolism* (eds A.L. Catapani, A.M. Gotto, L.C. Smith and R. Pasletti), Kluwer Academic Publishers, Dordrecht, pp. 215–229 (1993)
51. Bierman, E. L. and Porte, D. Carbohydrate tolerance and lipemia. *Ann. Intern. Med.*, **68**, 926–933 (1968)
52. Schonfeld, G. and Kudzma, D. J. Type IV hyperlipoproteinaemia. A critical appraisal. *Arch. Intern. Med.*, **132**, 55–62 (1973)

53. Nikkila, E. A. HDL in relation to the metabolism of triglyceride-rich lipoproteins. In *Clinical and Metabolic Aspects of High-Density Lipoproteins* (eds N. E. Miller and G. J. Miller), Elsevier, Amsterdam, pp. 217–245 (1984)

54. Fielding, P. E., Fielding, C. J., Havel, R.J., Kane, P. J. and Tun, P. Cholesterol net transport, esterification, and transfer in human hyperlipidemic plasma. *J. Clin. Invest.*, **71**, 449–460 (1983)

55. Tall, A., Granot, E., Brocia, R., Tabas, I., Hester, C. *et al.* Accelerated transfer of cholesteryl ester in dyslipidaemic plasma. Role of cholesterol ester transfer protein. *J. Clin. Invest.*, **79**, 1217–1225 (1987)

56. Barter, P. J., Hopkins, G. J. and Ying, C. The role of lipid transfer proteins in plasma lipoprotein metabolism. *Am. Heart J.*, **113**, 538–542 (1987)

57. Patsch, J. R., Karlin, J. B., Scott, L. W., Smith, L. C. and Gotto, A. M. Inverse relationship between blood levels of high density lipoprotein subfraction 2 and magnitude of postprandial lipemia. *Proc. Natl Acad. Sci. USA*, **80**, 1449–1453 (1983)

58. Furman, R. H., Sanbar, S. S., Alaupovic, P., Brandford, R.H. and Howard, R. P. Studies of the metabolism of radioiodinated human serum alpha lipoprotein in normal and hyperlipidaemic subjects. *J. Lab. Clin. Med.*, **63**, 193–204 (1964)

59. Schaefer, E. J., Zech, L. A., Jenkins, L. L., Bronzert, T. J., Rubalcaba, E. A. *et al.* Human apolipoprotein AI and AII metabolism. *J. Lipid Res.*, **23**, 850–862 (1982)

60. Magill, P., Rao, S. N., Miller, N. E., Nicoll, A., Brunzell, J. *et al.* Relationships between the metabolism of high-density and very-low-density lipoproteins in man. Studies of apolipoprotein kinetics and adipose tissue lipoprotein lipase activity. *Eur. J. Clin. Invest.*, **12**, 113–120 (1982)

61. Nikkila, E. A. and Taskinen, M. R. Plasma high-density lipoprotein concentration and subfraction distribution in relation to triglyceride metabolism. *Am. Heart J.*, **113**, 543–548 (1987)

62. Martin, P. J., Martin, J. V. and Goldberg, D. M. γ-Glutamyl transpeptidase, triglycerides and enzyme induction. *Br. Med. J.*, **i**, 17–18 (1975)

63. Consensus Development Panel. Consensus Conference. Treatment of hypertriglyceridaemia. *J. Am. Med. Assoc.*, **251**, 1196–1200 (1984)

64. Manninen, V., Elo, O., Frick, H., Haapa, W., Heinonen, O. P. *et al.* Lipid alterations and decline in the incidence of coronary heart disease in the Helsinki Heart Study. *J. Am. Med. Assoc.*, **260**, 641–651 (1988)

65. Carlson, L. A. and Rosenhamer, G. Reduction of mortality in the Stockholm Ischaemic Heart Disease Secondary Preventive Study by combined treatment with clofibrate and nicotinic acid. *Acta Med. Scand.*, **223**, 405–418 (1988)

66. Palac, R. T., Meadows, W. R., Hwang, M. H., Loeb, H. S., Pifarre, R. and Gunnar, R. M. Risk factors related to progressive narrowing in aortocoronay vein grafts studied 1 and 5 years after surgery. *Circulation*, **66**, (Suppl. I), I40–I44 (1982)

67. Campeau, L., Engjalbert, M., Lesperance, J., Bourassa, M. G., Kwiterovich, P. *et al.* The relation of risk factors to the development of atherosclerosis in saphenous-vein bypass grafts and the progression of disease in the native circulation. A study 10 years after aortocoronary bypass surgery. *N. Engl. J. Med.*, **311**, 1329–1332 (1984)

68. Fox, M. H., Gruchow, H. W., Barboriak, J. J., Anderson, A. J., Hoffman, R. G. *et al.* Risk factors among patients undergoing repeat aorto-coronary bypass procedures. *J. Thorac. Cardiovasc. Surg.*, **93**, 56–61(1987)

69. Blankenhorn, D. M., Nessim, S. A., Johnson, R. L., Sanmarco, M. E., Azen, S. P. and Cashin-Hemphill, L. Beneficial effects of combined colestipol–niacin therapy on coronary atherosclerosis and coronary venous bypass grafts. *J. Am. Med. Assoc.*, **257**, 3233–3240 (1987)

70. Brown, B.G., Albers, J.J., Fisher, L.D., Schaefer, S.M., Lin, J-T. *et al.* Regression of coronary artery disease as a result of intensive lipid-lowering therapy in men with high levels of apoprotein B. *N. Engl. J. Med.*, **323**, 1289–1298 (1990)

71. Fischer, B. Uber lipamie und cholesteremie, sowie uber veranderungen des pankrea und der leber bei diabetes mellitus. *Virchow's Archiv.*, **172**, 30–71(1903)

72. Hewson, W. *An experimental enquiry into the properties of the blood with remarks on some of its morbid appearances and an appendix relating to the discovery of the lymphatic system in birds, fish and the animals called amphibious.* T. Cadell, London (1771)

73. Christison, R. On the cause of the milky and whey-like appearances sometimes observed in the blood. *Edinb. Med. Surg. J.*, **33**, 274–280 (1830)

74. Burger, M. and Grutz, O. Uber hepatosplenomegale lipoidose mit xanthomatosen veranderungen in haut und schleimhaut. *Arch. Dermatol. Syph.*, **166**, 542–575 (1932)

75. Holt, L. E., Aylward, F. X. and Timbres, H. G. Idiopathic familial lipaemia. *Johns Hopkins Hosp. Bull.*, **64**, 279–314 (1939)

76. Havel, R. J. and Gordon, R. J. Idiopathic hyperlipidaemia. Metabolic studies in an affected family. *J. Clin. Invest.*, **39**, 1777–1790 (1960)

77. Nikkila, E. A. Familial lipoprotein lipase deficiency and related disorders of chylomicron metabolism. In *The Metabolic Basis of Inherited Disease*, 5th edn (eds J. B. Stanbury, J. B. Wyngaarden, D. S. Fredrickson, J. L. Goldstein and M. S. Brown), McGraw-Hill, New York (1983)

78. Hayden, M., DeBraekeleer, M., Henderson, H.E. and Kastelein, J. Molecular geography of inherited disorders of lipoprotein metabolism: lipoprotein lipase deficiency and familial hypercholesterolaemia. In *Molecular Genetics of Coronary Artery Disease. Candidate Genes and Processes in Atherosclerosis* (eds A. J. Lewis, J. I. Rotter and R.D. Sparkes), no. 14 in Monographs in Human Genetics series, Karger, Basle, pp. 350–362 (1992)

79. Lalonel, J-M., Wilson, D.E. and Iverius, P-H. Lipoprotein lipase and hepatic triglyceride lipase: molecular and genetic aspects. *Curr. Opin. Lipidol.*, **3**, 86–95 (1992)

80. Kwiterovich, P.O., Farah, J.R., Brown, W.V., Bachorik, P.S., Baylin, S.B. and Neill, C.A. The clinical biochemical and familial presentation of type V hyperlipoproteinaemia in childhood. *Pediatrics*, **59**, 513–525 (1977)

81. Yeshuran, D., Chung, H., Gotto, A. M. and Taunton, D. O. Primary type V hyperlipoproteinaemia in childhood. *J. Am. Med. Assoc.*, **238**, 2518–2520 (1977)

82. Babirak, S.P., Iverius, P-H, Fujimoto, W.Y. and Brunzell, J.D. Detection and characterisation of the heterozygote state for lipoprotein lipase deficiency. *Arteriosclerosis*, **9**, 326–334 (1989)

83. Breckenridge, W. C., Little, J. A., Steiner, G., Chow, A. and Poapst, M. Hypertriglyceridaemia associated with deficiency of apolipoprotein C-II. *N. Engl. J. Med.*, **298**, 1265–1273 (1978)

84. Yamamura, T., Sudo, H., Ishikawa, K. and Yamamoto, A. Familial type I hyperlipoproteinaemia caused by apolipoprotein CII deficiency. *Atherosclerosis*, **34**, 53–65 (1979)

85. Cox, D. W., Breckenridge, W. C. and Little, J. A. Inheritance of apolipoprotein CII deficiency with hypertriglyceridaemia and pancreatitis. *N. Engl. J. Med.*, **29**, 1421–1424 (1978)

86. Quinn, D., Shiraai, W. and Jackson, R. L. Lipoprotein lipase. Mechanism of action and role in lipoprotein metabolism. *Prog. Lipid Res.*, **22**, 35–78 (1982)

87. Holdsworth, G., Stocks, J., Dodson, P. and Galton, D. J. An abnormal triglyceride-rich lipoprotein containing excess sialylated apolipoprotein C-III. *J. Clin. Invest.*, **69**, 932–939 (1982)

88. Durrington, P.N. Lipoprotein lipase activity in the pathological metabolism of lipoproteins. *In Esterases Lipases, and Phospholipases. From Structure to Clinical Significance.* (eds M. I. Mackness and M. Clerc) NATO Advanced Science Institution Series Vol. 266. Plenum Press, New York, pp. 129–138 (1994)

89. Berger, G. M. Why very low density lipoprotein levels are normal in familial hyperchylomicronaemma. *Atherosclerosis*, **34**, 83–86 (1979)

90. Durrington, P. N., Newton, R. S., Weinstein, D. B. and Steinberg, D. Effects of insulin and glucose on very low density lipoprotein triglyceride secretion by cultured rat hepatocytes. *J. Clin. Invest.*, **70**, 63–73 (1982)

91. Nicoll, A. and Lewis, B. Evaluation of the roles of lipoprotein and hepatic lipase in lipoprotein metabolism: *in vivo* and *in vitro* studies in man. *Eur. J. Clin. Invest.*, **10**, 487–495 (1980)

92. Fielding, P.E. and Fielding, C.J. Dynamics of lipoprotein transport in the circulatory system. Chapter 15 in *Biochemistry of Lipids, Lipoproteins and Membrane* (eds D.E. Vance and J. Vance), Elsevier, Amsterdam, pp. 427–459 (1991)

93. Musliner, T. A., Herbert, P. N. and Kingston, J. J. Lipoprotein substrates of lipoprotein lipase and hepatic triglycerol lipase from human post-heparin plasma. *Biochim. Biophys. Acta*, **575**, 277–288 (1979)

94. Demant, T., Gaw., A., Watts, G.F., Durrington, P., Buckley, B. *et al.* Metabolism of apo B-100-containing lipoproteins in familial hyperchylomicronaemia. *J. Lipid Res.*, **34**, 147–156 (1993)

95. Brunzell, J. D. and Schrott, H. G. The interaction of familial and secondary causes of hypertriglyceridaemia. Role in pancreatitis. *Trans. Assoc. Am. Phys.*, **86**, 245–254 (1973)

96. Brunzell, J. D. and Bierman, E. L. Chylomicronaemia syndrome. Interaction of genetic and acquired hypertriglyceridaemia. *Med. Clin. North Am.*, **66**, 455–468 (1982)

97. Chait, A., Mancini, M., February, A. W. and Lewis, B. Clinical and metabolic study of alcoholic hyperlipidaemia. *Lancet*, **ii**, 62–64 (1972)

98. Chait, A., Robenson, H. T. and Brunzell, J. D. Chylomicronaemia syndrome in diabetes mellitus. *Diabetes Care*, **4**, 343–348 (1981)

99. Glueck, C. J., Christopher, C., Mishkel, M., Tsang, R. C. and Mellies, M. J. Pancreatitis, familial hypertriglyceridaemia, and pregnancy. *Am. J. Obstet. Gynaecol.*, **136**, 755–761 (1980)

100. Glueck, C. J., Scheel, D., Fishbank, J. and Steiner, P. Oestrogen-induced pancreatitis in patients with previously covert familial type V hyperlipoproteinaemia. *Metabolism*, **21**, 657–665 (1972)

101. Durrington, P. N. and Cairns, S. A. Acute pancreatitis. A complication of beta-blockade. *Br. Med. J.*, **284**, 1016 (1982)

102. Durrington, P. N., Brownlee, W. C. and Large, D. M. Short-term effects of β-adrenoreceptor blocking drugs with and without cardioselectivity and intrinsic sympathomimetic activity on lipoprotein metabolism in hypertriglyceridaemic patients and in normal men. *Clin. Sci.*, **69**, 713–719 (1985)

103. Stone, M. C. and Thorp, J. M. A new technique for the investigation of the low density lipoprotein in health and disease. *Clin. Chim. Acta*, **14**, 812–830 (1966)

104. Rossner, S. Studies on an intravenous fat tolerance test. Methodological experimental and clinical experiences with intralipid. *Acta Med. Scand. (Suppl.)*, **564**, 1–24 (1974)

105. Gotto, A. M. Type V hyperlipoproteinaemia. *Clin. Endocrinol. Metabol.*, **2**, 11–39 (1973)

106. Krauss, R. M., Levy, R.I. and Fredrickson, D. S. Selective measurement of two lipase activities in postheparin plasma from normal subjects and patients with hyperlipoproteinaemia. *J. Clin. Invest.*, **54**, 1107–1124 (1974)

107. Greten, M., De Grella, R., Klose, G., Rashcer, W. *et al.* Measurement of two plasma triglyceride lipases by an immunochemical method. Studies in patients with hypertriglyceridaemia. *J. Lipid Res.*, **17**, 203–210 (1976)

108. Huttunen, J. K., Ehnholm, C., Kekki, M. and Nikkila, E. A. Post-heparin plasma lipoprotein lipase and hepatic lipase in normal subjects and in patients with hypertriglyceridaemia. Correlations to sex, age and various parameters of triglyceride metabolism. *Clin. Sci. Mol. Med.*, **50**, 249–260 (1976)

109. Harlan, W. R., Winesett, P. S. and Wasserman, A. J. Tissue lipoprotein lipase in normal individuals and in individuals with exogenous hypertridyceridaemia and the relationship of this enzyme to assimilation of fat. *J. Clin. Invest.*, **46**, 239–247 (1967)

110. Taylor, K. G., Holdsworth, G. and Galton, D. J. Lipoprotein lipase in adipose tissue and plasma triglyceride clearance in patients with primary hypertriglyceridaemia. *Eur. J. Clin. Invest.*, **10**, 133–138 (1980)

111. Durrington, P. N., MacIver, J. E., Holdsworth, G. and Galton, D. J. Severe hypertriglyceridaemia associated with pancytopenia and lipoprotein lipase deficiency. *Ann. Intern. Med.*, **94**, 211–212 (1981)

112. Pykalisto, O. J., Smith, P. H. and Brunzell, J. D. Human adipose tissue lipoprotein lipase: comparison of assay methods and expressions of activity. *Proc. Soc. Exp. Biol. Med.*, **148**, 297–300 (1975)

113. Greenberger, N. J., Hatch, F. T., Drummery, G. D. and Kselbacher, K. J. Pancreatitis and hyperlipemia. A study of serum lipid alterations in 25 patients with acute pancreatitis. *Medicine*, **48**, 161–174 (1966)

114. Stackhouse, K. L., Glass, D. D. and Zimmerman, B. Relationships of lipoprotein lipase and hyperlipidaemia in pancreatitis. *Surg. Forum*, **17**, 343–444 (1966)

115. Klatskin, G. and Gordon, M. Relationship between relapsing pancreatitis and essential hyperlipemia. *Am. J. Med.*, **12**, 3–23 (1952)

116. Farmer, R. G., Winkelman, E. I., Brown, H. B. and Lewis, L. A. Hyperlipoproteinaemia and pancreatitis. *Am. J. Med.*, **54**, 161–165 (1973)

117. Cameron, J.L., Capuzzi, D.M., Zuidema, G.D and Margolis, S. Acute pancreatitis with hyperlipaemia. The incidence of lipid abnormalities in acute pancreatitis. *Ann. Surg.*, **177**, 483–489 (1973)

118. Havel, R.J. Pathogenesis, differentiation and management of hypertriglyceridaemia. *Adv. Intern. Med.*, **15**, 117–154 (1969)

119. Cameron, J. L., Capuzzi, D. M., Zuidema, G. D. and Margolis, S. Acute pancreatitis with hyper-lipemia. Evidence for a persistent defect in lipid metabolism. *Am. J. Med.*, **56**, 482–487 (1974)

120. Fallat, R. W., Vestor, J. W. and Glueck, C. J. Suppression of amylase activity by hypertriglyceri-daemia. *J. Am. Med. Assoc.*, **225**, 1331–1334 (1973)

121. Lesser, P. B. and Warshaw, A. L. Diagnosis of pancreatitis masked by hyperlipidemia. *Am. Intern. Med.*, **82**, 795–798 (1975)

122. Warshaw, A. L., Bellini, C. A. and Lesser, P. B. Inhibition of serum and urine amylase activity in pancreatitis with hyperlipaemia. *Ann. Surg.*, **182**, 72–75 (1975)

123. Braganza, J.M., Pancreatic disease: a casualty of hepatic 'detoxification'? *Lancet*, **ii**, 1002 (1993)

124. Hagberg, B., Hultquist, G., Svennerholm, L. and Voss, H. Malignant hyperlipemia in infancy. *Am. J. Dis. Child.*, **107**, 267–276 (1964)

125. Jacken, J., Casteels-van Dacke, M., Harvengt, L., Corbeel, L., Brokaert-Van Orshoven, A. *et al..* A hyperlipemia syndrome in infancy with rapidly fatal evolution. *Helv. Paediat. Acta*, **28**, 67–71 (1973)

126. Himsworth, R. L., Bangham, C., Mason, A. M. S. and Nixon, J. Has anyone else seen Betty? *Lancet*, **i**, 796–797 (1974)

127. Einarsson, K., Hellstrom, K. and Kallner, M. Gallbladder disease in hyperlipoproteinaemia. *Lancet*, **i**, 484–487 (1975)

128. Parker, F., Bagdade, J. D., Odland, G. F. and Bierman, E. L. Evidence for the chylomicron origin of lipids accumulating in diabetic eruptive xanthomas. A correlative lipid biochemical, histo-chemical and electron microscopic study. *J. Clin. Invest.*, **49**, 2172–2187 (1970)

129. Altman, J. and Winkelmann, R. K. Xanthoma disseminatum. *Arch. Dermatol.*, **86**, 582–596 (1962)

130. Gianotti, F. and Zina, G. *Xanthogranulomatoses Juveniles*. XIII Congres de l'Assocation des Dermatologistes et Syphilgraphes de Langue Francais., Masson et Cie, Paris, p. 103 (1971)

131. Steffes, M. W. and Freier, E. F. A simple and precise method of determining true sodium, potas-sium and chloride concentrations in hyperlipemia. *J. Lab. Clin. Med.*, **88**, 683–688 (1976)

132. Glueck, C. J., Levy, R. I. and Fredrickson, D. S. Immunoreactive insulin, glucose tolerance, and carbohydrate inducibility in types II, III, IV and V hyperlipoproteinaemia. *Diabetes*, **18**, 739–747 (1969)

133. Durrington, P. N., Bolton, C. H. and Hartog, M. Serum and lipoprotein apolipoprotein B levels in normal subjects and patients with hyperlipoproteinaemia. *Clin. Chim. Acta*, **82**, 151–160 (1978)

134. Brown, W. V. and Greten, H. Type I hyperlipoproteinaemia. *Clin. Endocrinol. Metabol.*, **2**, 73–80 (1973)

135. Golman, J. A., Abrams, N. R., Glueck, C. J., Steiner, P. and Herman, J. H. Musculoskeletal disor-ders associated with type IV hyperlipoproteinaemia. *Lancet*, **ii**, 449–452 (1972)

136. Buckingham, R. B., Bole, G. G. and Bassett, D. R. Polyarthritis associated with type IV hyper-lipoproteinaemia. *Arch. Intern. Med.*, **135**, 286–290 (1975)

137. Reinertsen, J. L., Schaefer, E. J., Brewer, H. B. and Moutsopoulos, H. M. Sicca-like syndrome in type V hyperlipoproteinaemia. *Arth. Rheum.*, **23**, 114–118 (1980)

138. Fessel, W. J. Fat disorders and peripheral neuropathy. *Brain*, **94**, 531–540 (1971)

139. Sandbank, U., Bechar, M. and Bornstein, B. Hyperlipemic neuropathy. *Acta Neuropathol.*, **19**, 290–300 (1971)

140. Nausieda, P. A. Hyperlipemic neuropathy. In *Handbook of Clinical Neurology*, vol. 29 (eds P. J. Vinken and G. W. Bruyn), Elsevier, Amsterdam (1977)

141. Heilman, K. M. and Fisher, W. D. Hyperlipidemic dementia. *Arch. Neurol.*, **31**, 67–68 (1974)

142. Mathew, N. T., Meyer, J. S., Archari, A. N. and Dodson, R. F. Hyperlipidaemic neuropathy and dementia. *Eur. Neurol.*, **14**, 370–382 (1976)

# Chapter 8

# Type III hyperlipoproteinaemia

## Introduction

Type III hyperlipoproteinaemia has several synonyms: broad beta disease, floating beta disease, dysbetalipoproteinaemia and remnant removal disease. The earliest description of the clinical syndrome was by Addison and Gull (1851)[1] in a young man with diabetes from Kingsbridge in Devon, UK, who had the typical xanthomata of type III hyperlipoproteinaemia, which they termed vitiligoidea plana and vitiligoidea tuberosa. The terminology changed in subsequent years to xanthoma striatum palmaris (striate palmar xanthoma) and xanthoma tuberosum (tuberose xanthomata). Gofman and colleagues first demonstrated the essential abnormality of the lipoproteins associated with these skin lesions[2]. Using analytical ultracentrifugation they reported an unusual increase in the Sf 10–50 lipoproteins (small VLDL and IDL) and a decrease in the Sf 0–10 range (LDL)[2]. Later, with the introduction of paper electrophoresis, it was reported by Fredrickson and his group that these same patients, instead of having the prebeta and beta bands commonly associated with increased serum cholesterol and triglycerides (type IIb hyperlipoproteinaemia), had a broad band stretching across prebeta and beta ranges[3]. Isolation of the VLDL from such patients revealed that it contained much more cholesteryl ester than normal or than in any of the other primary hyperlipoproteinaemias[4]. This abnormal VLDL possessed beta rather than prebeta mobility on electrophoresis[5]. Later it was shown that these lipoproteins were abnormally rich in apolipoprotein E[6] and even more recently that the majority of individuals with type III hyperlipoproteinaemia are homozygotes for its $E_2$ isoform[7].

## Clinical features

### General

The definition of type III hyperlipoproteinaemia is difficult, because it cannot simply rely on the presence of the cholesterol-rich β-VLDL (page 220), since this can be detected in some apparently healthy people with normal levels or even low levels of serum cholesterol and triglycerides. For clinical purposes, type III will therefore be considered as the presence of cholesterol-rich β-VLDL together with hyperlipidaemia. On the basis of this definition, type III hyperlipoproteinaemia is a rare disorder affecting no more than one person in 10 000. It is exceptionally unusual to encounter it until the end of the second decade. It tends to be present in men earlier than in women, in whom it frequently does not produce signs until after the menopause. Many patients will have some other disorder predisposing them to hyperlipidaemia, such as obesity, diabetes or hypothyroidism, before the clinical syndrome of type III hyperlipoproteinaemia develops. In others, it must be presumed that some other genetic cause of hyperlipidaemia has led to its expression (page 217).

## Xanthomata

The characteristic xanthomata of type III hyperlipoproteinaemia are striate palmar xanthomata (Plates 12a–c), which are yellow–orange discoloration of the skin creases of the palms of the hands and sometimes the creases of the palmar surfaces of the fingers and wrists[8]. Sometimes these may be quite flat and can be missed, unless sought with care. In other patients, more well-defined seed-like raised areas appear within the areas of discoloration and the xanthomata are more obvious. Occasionally, additional larger subcutaneous raised xanthomata are deposited over the pulp of the fingers and the pressure areas of the palms. Tuberose xanthomata (Plates 13a, b), which are the other common skin manifestation of type III hyperlipoproteinaemia, occur over the tuberosities of the elbows and knees in particular. They usually appear as a cluster of yellowish papules, which coalesce to form a single cauliflower-like lesion often 2 cm or more in diameter, which itself becomes raised up further. They are not uncommon on the parts of the foot subjected to pressure by shoes (especially when the pressure is excessive due to obesity). They may thus occur over the heels (Plate 14), where they can usually be differentiated from Achilles tendon xanthomata because of their yellowish appearance and subcutaneous location. The presence of genuine tendon xanthomata in a patient with striate palmar and/or tuberose xanthomata strongly suggests that the patient has the combination of familial hypercholesterolaemia and type III hyperlipoproteinaemia, which is occasionally encountered. Tuberose xanthomata are also found over the knuckles and dorsum of finger joints, particularly in manual workers (Plates 15a, b), and occasionally in other sites including internally such as in the bone marrow or thorax, where they may be encountered by radiologists. Often tuberose xanthomata appear inflamed and those on the foot, particularly if there is associated diabetes, may become infected.

The term tuberoeruptive is often used to describe tuberose xanthomata when they have small satellite xanthomata similar to eruptive xanthomata, which have not been amalgamated into the main lesion. Occasionally patients have more widespread eruptive xanthomata over the extensor surfaces and soft-tissue pressure areas, as described in chylomicronaemia (Chapter 7, page 205). These are patients in whom chylomicronaemia has recently been or still is present in association with the accumulation of chylomicron remnants.

Tuberose xanthomata and striate palmar xanthomata generally occur together. Some patients, however, have tuberose xanthomata only and a smaller number have only the striate palmar ones. This makes tuberose xanthomata the more common of the two, occurring in 57% of one collected series compared with a prevalence of 47% for the striate palmar xanthomata[9].

Similar xanthomata to those of type III hyperlipoproteinaemia may occur in secondary lipoprotein disorders such as obstructive liver disease, paraproteinaemia and systemic lupus erythematosus (Chapter 11).

## Arterial disease

Patients with type III hyperlipoproteinaemia are certainly at increased risk of atherosclerosis. In one series, about one-third had premature ischaemic heart disease (mean age of onset in men 38 years) and a similar proportion had peripheral arterial disease[10]. Since a proportion of patients will present by virtue of their ischaemic symptoms, this may overestimate the overall risk. However, the precise risk is difficult to gauge because not only is the condition uncommon, so that few presymptomatic individuals are found on screening the general population, but, even within the family of affected probands, it is uncommon to find a similarly affected individual. The only presymptomatic people available for study will be those presenting because of xanthomata and such patients do prove to have fewer atheromatous complications[11]. Even if one assumed that lipid clinic statistics double the apparent risk, overall the likelihood of premature coronary disease is probably of the same order as heterozygous FH, but there is in addition a very much greater chance of intermittent claudication and other manifestations of peripheral arterial disease.

**Other features**

The most frequent association of type III hyperlipoproteinaemia is obesity[9,10,12] and this probably accounts for the frequency of mild glucose intolerance[10,13]. There does, however, appear to be a genuinely increased incidence of diabetes mellitus, which probably occurs in at least 4% of patients with type III hyperlipoproteinaemia[9]. Type III hyperlipoproteinaemia is also encountered with greater than expected frequency in diabetic populations[14].

Hypothyroidism also provokes the type III syndrome in susceptible individuals[15], perhaps because of its effect on lipoprotein catabolism[16]. The menopause, too, seems to be important, because of the relative infrequency of type III in premenopausal women[9,12]. The marked reduction in the hyperlipidaemia in some patients with type III hyperlipoproteinaemia, when oestrogen is administered, suggests that the decrease in oestrogen secretion associated with the menopause may account for the development of type III in many women[17–19]. Since the effect of oestrogen is to increase the production of hepatic VLDL, it is likely that in type III, as opposed to other hypertriglyceridaemic states, which are exacerbated, enhanced catabolism of chylomicron remnants and IDL outstrips this effect[17]. Pharmacological doses of oestrogen do induce an apo E receptor on rat liver[20]. Direct evidence that naturally occurring levels of oestrogen regulate such a receptor in women is lacking at present.

Gout certainly occurs in type III hyperlipoproteinaemia[9,12], but whether it does so more or less frequently than in other conditions associated with hypertriglyceridaemia is uncertain.

# Genetics and metabolic basis of type III hyperlipoproteinaemia (Figure 8.1)

The genetic basis of type III hyperlipoproteinaemia has become much clearer following the discovery of the apolipoprotein E polymorphisms. It had previously been realized from screening the families of probands[10,21–23] that quite commonly there was no other relative affected. Sometimes affected relatives were found, but there was no evidence of vertical transmission. It was also noted that in families where type III hyperlipoproteinaemia did run, up to half of the

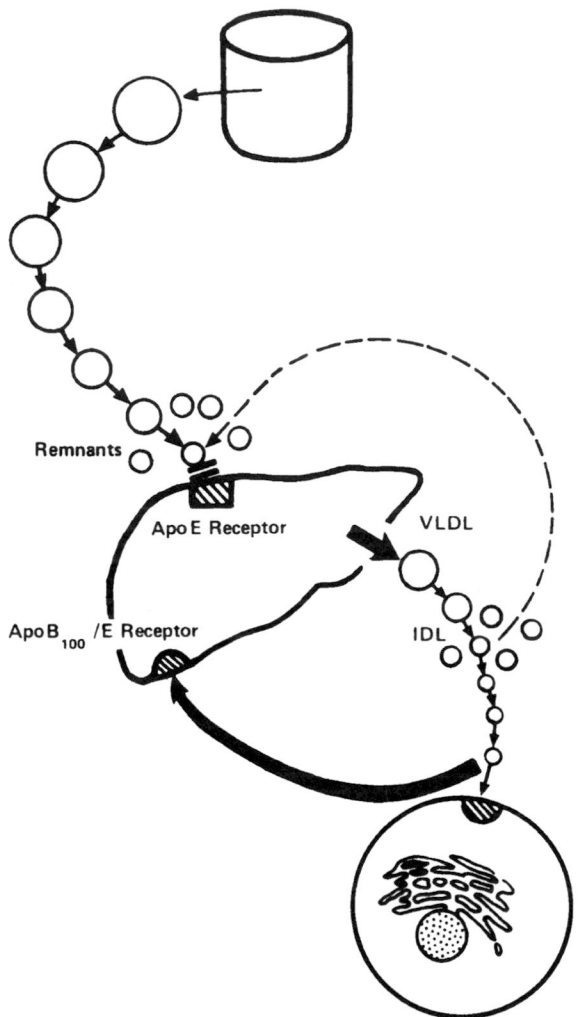

**Figure 8.1** Lipoprotein metabolism in type III hyperlipoproteinaemia. There is an accumulation of chylomicron remnants and intermediate density lipoprotein (IDL) (known collectively as β-VLDL) due to their defective clearance, usually because of apo $E_2$ homozygosity. High concentrations result from a coincidental overproduction of very low density lipoproteins (VLDL). Low density lipoprotein catabolism is increased probably because of increased hepatic LDL (apo $B_{100}$/E) receptor activity in response to diminished entry of cholesterol via the apo E receptor

first-degree relatives had hyperlipidaemia, but that only half of these had type III hyperlipoproteinaemia.

Other hyperlipidaemias such as type IV hyperlipoproteinaemia or occasionally type IIb or IIa hyperlipoproteinaemia, were equally frequent. It was concluded therefore that the gene or genes permitting the development of the β-VLDL had to coincide with some other genetic hyperlipoproteinaemia such as familial hypertriglyceridaemia (Chapter 7, page 193) or familial combined hyper-lipidaemia (Chapter 6, page 142), before sufficient β-VLDL was produced to cause the hyperlipidaemia and often the clinical syndrome associated with type III hyperlipoproteinaemia.

The discovery of the association of type III hyperlipoproteinaemia and apo $E_2$ homozygosity[24,25] has done much to explain the basis of its mode of transmission. Apolipoprotein E has three common genetically determined isoforms which may be detected by isoelectric focusing on polyacrylamide gel[24,25] (Chapter 2, page 51 and Chapter 12, page 375). Genetic studies showed that these were alleles operating at a single genetic locus on each chromosome and that the phenotype expression might thus be $E_{2/2}$, $E_{2/3}$, $E_{3/3}$, $E_{3/4}$, $E_{4/4}$ and $E_{2/4}$. The commonest are $E_{3/3}$ and $E_{3/2}$. The $E_{2/2}$ phenotype occurs in between 0.2 and 1.6% of the unselected populations studied in various countries, but more than 90% of patients with type III hyperlipoproteinaemia have it[24]. It has been shown that the affinity of apo $E_2$ for both fibroblast[25,26] and hepatic receptors[27] is less than that of apo $E_3$, which, in turn, is less than that of apo $E_4$. The binding affinity relates to the arginine content of the apo E isoforms, specifically to amino acid substitution of cysteine for arginine[26,28]. Thus apo $E_4$ has arginine at both amino acid positions 112 and 158 (Figure 2.14), whereas in the more common apo $E_3$ amino acid 112 is cysteine and in apo $E_2$ both 112 and 158 are cysteine[28]. The apo $E_2$ and $E_4$ polymorphisms have probably arisen from mutations of apo $E_3$. Probably 90% or more of patients with type III hyperlipoproteinaemia prove to be homozygotes for apo $E_2$ using isoelectric focusing. The majority of the rest are apo $E_{2/3}$ heterozygotes or exceptionally $E_{3/3}$ homozygotes. Properly performed isoelectric focusing is accurate in identifying the $E_{2/2}$ phenotype when the method is compared with genotyping[29], which has become widely available using PCR and RFLP[30] or allele-specific oligonucleotides[31] since the first edition of this book.

In addition to the three apo E polymorphisms already discussed at least 18 other rarer variants of apo E have been described[29], which explain some of the cases of type III hyperlipoproteinaemia not associated with $E_{2/2}$ phenotype. Some have the same isoelectric point as apo $E_2$ such as $Arg_{145} \rightarrow Cys$ (25,26) and $Lys_{146} \rightarrow Gln$[32]. Others have similar isoelectric points to apo $E_3$[33], such as $Arg_{142} \rightarrow Cys$[34] and apo $E_{Leiden}$ (duplication of amino acid residues 121–127)[35]. In yet others the amino acid substitution has the effect of creating a variant with an isoelectric point dissimilar from apo $E_2$, $E_3$ or $E_4$, such as $E_1$ or $E_5$.

If a patient develops type III hyperlipoproteinaemia with an $E_2$ gene and a mutant $E_3$ gene decreasing the receptor binding of the apo $E_3$ then inheritance is recessive, as in the case of the $E_{2/2}$ phenotype generally associated with the type III hyperlipoproteinaemia. However, occasionally patients with type III hyper-lipoproteinaemia have been described with the $E_{2/3}$ or $E_{3/3}$ phenotype in whom one $E_3$ gene has proved normal. The mutation in the other gene ($E_2$ in the case of such $E_{2/3}$ heterozygotes and the other $E_3$ gene in the case of $E_{3/3}$ homozygotes) must therefore be acting in a dominant fashion. Examples in the case of $E_2$ would be $Lys_{146} \rightarrow Gln$ and the case of $E_3$ $Arg_{142} \rightarrow Cys$ and $E_{3\ Leiden}$. One of the $E_1$ variants, $Lys_{146} \rightarrow Gln$, also produces type III hyperlipoproteinaemia dominantly[36]. Since these patient will have VLDL and chylomicron remnants with normal apo $E_3$ as well as apo $E_2$ or $E_3$ with decreased receptor binding, they should have no more tendency to type III hyperlipoproteinaemia than the common $E_{2/3}$ heterozygote. Yet they have severe type III hyperlipoproteinaemia with no other predisposing cause (in the case of $E_3$ $Arg_{142}$ → Cys type III occurs in childhood[34]). The most likely explanation is that this dominantly expressed apo E mutation interferes with the receptor binding of the normal apo $E_3$.

In addition to apo E variants type III hyperlipoproteinaemia has also been described in apo E deficiency[37] (due to a splice defect in intron (30)[38].

In $E_{2/2}$ homozygotes who have not developed type III hyperlipoproteinaemia (i.e. do not have hyperlipidaemia), an increase in the VLDL cholesterol content is detectable, probably because of slower clearance of their apo $E_2$-containing lipoproteins. It is assumed therefore that some other stimulus to hyperlipidaemia must be present before type III hyperlipoproteinaemia will develop (Figure 8.1). This would be compatible with earlier studies in which both genetic (e.g. familial hypertriglyceridaemia or familial combined hyperlipidaemia) or acquired hyper- lipidaemia (e.g. diabetes mellitus, hypothyroidism, obesity, menopause) were criti- cal to its development. Of wider interest still is the finding that, in the absence of type III hyperlipoproteinaemia, possession of the apo $E_2$ gene is associated with low levels of LDL cholesterol and serum apo B, whereas the $E_4$ gene tends to produce high levels and $E_3$ intermediate levels[24] (Chapter 2, page 51, and Chapter 12, page 375). It has been suggested that increased hepatic uptake of apo $E_4$-containing lipoproteins will lead to higher intracellular cholesterol levels and down-regulation of the LDL receptor (apo $B_{100}$/E receptor) and that this will lead to higher LDL levels[24].

In type III hyperlipoproteinaemia, kinetic studies employing radiolabelled lipoproteins gave results which were difficult to interpret until recently. There was agreement that delayed remnant and IDL clearance occurred in all patients[17,39,40]. This is, of course, compatible with their decreased receptor binding of apo E. In many patients, however, an increase in the production of IDL was also found[41–43] which we would now interpret as due to a second coinci- dental defect unrelated to the apo E genotype, but which was acting as the stimu- lus to hyperlipidaemia. Furthermore, the ready exchange of apo E between lipoproteins would explain why the residence time of VLDL from a patient with type IV hyperlipoproteinaemia when injected into a patient with type III hyper- lipoproteinaemia was found to be just as delayed as was their own VLDL and did not indicate a defect in the clearance mechanism itself[39]. Thus far, type III hyperlipoproteinaemia has not been reported due to a defect in the remnant (apo E) receptor. The increased catabolic rate of LDL observed in turnover studies, which accounts for the low serum LDL concentrations in most patients with type III hyperlipoproteinaemia, would also be explicable on the basis of their $E_{2/2}$ phenotype, as discussed previously.

## Laboratory diagnosis

The clinical syndrome associated with type III hyperlipoproteinaemia may make the diagnosis inescapable. In other patients, suspicion of the diagnosis may be raised simply by the finding of a combined increase in both serum cholesterol and triglyceride concentrations. Usually, in type IIb hyperlipoproteinaemia, the increase in the cholesterol level is greater than the triglycerides and in type V it is the converse. In type III the serum cholesterol concentration in mmol/l is frequently very similar to that of the triglycerides (in mg/dl it is about half that of the triglycerides). On paper or agarose gel electrophoresis, a broad beta band is helpful, but similar electrophoretic appearances can sometimes be produced by other hyperlipoproteinaemias such as type V. Now that apo E phenotyping is more generally available, the detection of the apo $E_{2/2}$ phenotype in the presence of hyperlipidaemia can probably be regarded as diagnostic. The finding of a different apo E phenotype does not, of course, exclude the diagnosis, because a small number of patients with type III will be $E_{2/3}$ or even $E_{3/3}$.

The only way to make the diagnosis with certainty is by ultracentrifugation. Very low density lipoproteins may be easily isolated in the preparative ultracentrifuge in a fixed angle or swing-out rotor. For example, using a 6.5 ml capacity tube, 5 ml of EDTA plasma may be overlayered with 1 ml of 1.006 g/ml saline and then be centrifuged for 24 h at 100 000 $\times$ g. The VLDL is next isolated by tube-slicing and transferred to a 5 ml volumetric flask, where it can be combined with washings from the upper part of the ultracentrifuge tube to restore it to a volume of 5 ml. The VLDL cholesterol concentration is then measured and expressed as a ratio of the total serum triglycerides[44]. In most other hyperlipoproteinaemias, the ratio is less than 0.15 (calculated from mg/dl) or 0.3 (from mmol/l). In type III, ratios exceeding 0.3 (from mg/dl) or 0.68 (from mmol/l) are commonly found and are regarded as diagnostic. Ratios exceeding 0.25 (from mg/dl) or 0.57 (from mmol/l) are highly suspicious. This procedure should not be applied unless there is a hyperlipidaemia present, as some normal people have similar ratios. Falsely low ratios, on the other hand, can be found in the occasional type III patient who also has marked chylomicronaemia. Under these circumstances, the test should be repeated after several days on a 20 g fat diet.

It is, of course, essential to exclude secondary causes of hyperlipoproteinaemia, as discussed previously. Myeloma, paraproteinaemia and systemic lupus erythematosus can mimic the syndrome too, without there necessarily being any genetic cause for decreased apo E receptor binding (Chapter 11, page 336).

## Treatment

Fortunately, the therapy for type III hyperlipoproteinaemia does not usually require to be so radical that a definite diagnosis is mandatory. Centres without access to ultracentrifugation or apo E phenotyping need rarely therefore be at any disadvantage in instituting therapy.

Weight reduction should be strongly encouraged in the obese type III patient. Calories derived from fat, particularly saturated fat, should most strenuously be avoided. In the lean patient the question arises as to what should be substituted. As usual the easiest compromise is probably a combination of carbohydrate and unsaturated fat, although particularly in the patient with associated chylomicronaemia a generalized fat restriction may be better[12].

Most patients will show a good response to diet. In those in whom both cholesterol and triglycerides remain elevated, the decision to introduce drug therapy in addition to diet is easy. However, in many the serum cholesterol will decline into the normal range, but they will nevertheless continue to have a raised serum triglyceride value. The decision to introduce drug therapy may then be more difficult. Clearly, close monitoring of all patients in the long term is desirable in order that decisions about drug therapy may be reviewed as the patient gets older and to maintain dietary compliance.

Type III hyperlipoproteinaemia is often remarkably responsive to fibric acid derivatives (Chapter 10, page 266). The newer ones (gemfibrozil, bezafibrate, fenofibrate, ciprofibrate) should be used as first-line agents in preference to clofibrate. Some authorities, however, regard clofibrate as the most active[45], and in the occasional patient who does not show a satisfactory response to one of the other fibrates, it may be tried. Such therapy will cause a resolution of xanthomata in virtually all patients and lipid levels will fall to normal in the majority. Some, however, can be remarkably resistant to treatment.

Type III hyperlipoproteinaemia can also respond to nicotinic acid (niacin), but this is not an easy medication for the patient (Chapter 10, page 264). Rarely, if ever, is therapeutic use made of the responsiveness of type III hyperlipoproteinaemia to oestrogens[17–19]. In theory hormone replacement therapy might be appropriate to use when the type III syndrome presents soon after the menopause. Since, however, oestrogen will exacerbate the hypertriglyceridaemia which is the driving force for the type III hyperlipoproteinaemia, this may outweigh favourable effects on remnant receptors and careful monitoring is required to decide whether in an individual patient HRT is beneficial.

HMG-CoA reductase inhibitors are effective therapy in the management of type III hyperlipoproteinaemia[45,46]. Whether they offer any advantage over fibrate drugs is not clear. I suspect that they are most often currently being used in patients with type III hyperlipoproteinaemia who have proved unresponsive to fibrates. How often they prove efficacious in this context will only become apparent with increasing clinical experience.

# References

1. Addison, T. and Gull, W. On a certain affection of the skin. *Guy's Hosp. Rep.*, ser. II, **7**, 265–270 (1851)
2. Gofman, I. W., Rubin, L., McGinley, J. P. and Jones, H. B. Hyperlipoproteinaemia. *Am. J. Med.*, **17**, 514–520 (1954)
3. Fredrickson, D. S., Levy, R. I. and Lees, R. S. Fat transport in lipoproteins. An integrated approach to mechanisms and disorders. *N. Engl. J. Med.*, **276**, 32–44, 94–103, 148–156, 215–226, 273–281 (1967)
4. Hazzard, W. R., Porte, D. and Bierman, E. L. Abnormal lipid composition of chylomicrons in broad-beta disease (type III hyperlipoproteinaemia). *J. Clin. Invest.*, **49**, 1853–1858 (1970)
5. Sata, T., Havel, R. J. and Jones, A. L. Characterization of subfraction of triglyceride-rich lipoproteins separated by gel chromatography from blood serum of normolipemic and hyerlipemic humans. *J. Lipid Res.*, **13**, 757–768 (1972)
6. Havel, R. J. and Kane, J. P. Primary dysbetalipoproteinaemia a predominance of a specific apoprotein species in triglyceride-rich lipoproteins. *Proc. Natl Acad. Sci., USA.*, **70**, 2015–2019 (1973)
7. Utermann, G., Jaeschke, M. and Menzel, J. Familial hyperlipoproteinaemia type III. Deficiency of a specific apolipoprotein (apo E-III) in the very low density lipoproteins. *FEBS Lett.*, **56**, 352–355 (1975)
8. Polano, M. K. Xanthomatosis and hyperlipoproteinaemia. *Dermatologica*, **149**, 1–9 (1974)
9. Brown, M. S., Goldstein, J. L. and Fredrickson, D. S. Familial type 3 hyperlipoproteinaemia (dysbetalipoproteinaemia). In *The Metabolic Basis of Inherited Disease*, 5th edn (eds J. B. Stanbury, J. B. Wyngaarden, D. S. Fredrickson, J. L. Goldstein and M. S. Brown), McGraw-Hill, New York, pp. 655–671 (1973)
10. Morganroth, J., Levy, R. I. and Fredrickson, D. S. The biochemical, clinical and genetic features of type III hyperlipoproteinaemia. *Ann. Intern. Med.*, **82**, 158–174 (1975)

11. Borrie, P. Type III hyperlipoproteinaemia. *Br. Med. J.*, **ii**, 665–667 (1969)
12. Brewer, H. B., Zech, L. A., Gregg, R. E., Schwartz, D. and Schefer, E. J. Type III hyperlipoproteinaemia. Diagnosis, molecular defects, pathology and treatment. *Ann. Intern. Med.*, **98**, 623–640 (1983)
13. Glueck, C. J., Levy, R. I. and Fredrickson, D. S. Immunoreactive insulin, glucose tolerance and carbohydrate inducibility in types II, III, IV and V hyperlipoproteinaemia. *Diabetes*, **18**, 739–747 (1969)
14. Winocour, P. H., Tetlow, L., Durrington, P. N., Ishola, M., Hillier, V. and Anderson, D. C. Apolipoprotein E polymorphism and lipoproteins in insulin-treated diabetes mellitus. *Atherosclerosis*, **75**, 161–173 (1989)
15. Hazzard, W. R. and Bierman, E. L. Aggravation of broad-beta disease (type 3 hyperlipoproteinaemia) by hypothroidism. *Arch. Intern. Med.*, **130**, 822–828 (1972)
16. Thompson, G. R., Soutar, A. K., Spengel, F. A., Jadhav, A., Gavigan, S. J. and Myant, N. B. Defects of receptor-mediated low density lipoprotein catabolism in homozygous familial hyper-cholesterolaemia and hypothyroidism *in vivo*. *Proc. Natl Acad. Sci., USA.*, **78**, 2591–2595 (1981)
17. Chait, A., Brunzell, J. D., Albers, J. J. and Hazzard, W. R. Type III hyperlipoproteinaemia ('remnant removal disease'). *Lancet*, **ii**, 1176–1178 (1977)
18. Kushwaha, R. S., Hazzard, W. R., Gagne, C., Chait, A. and Albers, J. J. Type III hyperlipoproteinaemia: paradoxical hypolipidaemic response to estrogen. *Ann. Intern. Med.*, **87**, 517–525 (1977)
19. Falko, J. M., Schonfeld, G., Witztum, J. L., Kolar, J. and Weidman, S. W. Effect of estrogen therapy on apolipoprotein E in type III hyperlipoproteinaemia. *Metabolism*, **28**, 1171–1177 (1979)
20. Windler, E. E., Kovanen, P. T., Chao, Y.-S., Brown, M. S., Havel, R. J. and Goldstein, J. L. The estradiol-stimulated lipoprotein receptor of rat liver. A binding site that mediates the uptake of rat lipoproteins containing apoproteins B and E. *J. Biol. Chem.*, **225**, 10464–10471 (1980)
21. Hazzard, W. R., O'Donell, T. F. and Lee, Y. L. Broad β disease (type III hyperlipoproteinaemia) in a large kindred: evidence for a monogenic mechanism. *Ann. Intern. Med.*, **82**, 141–149 (1975)
22. Vessby, B., Hedstrand, H., Lundin, L.-G. and Olsson, U. Inheritance of type III hyperlipoproteinaemia. Lipoprotein patterns in first-degree relatives. *Metabolism*, **26**, 225–254 (1977)
23. Moser, H., Slack, J. and Borrie, P. Type III hyperlipoproteinaemia. A genetic study with an account of the risks of coronary deaths in first degree relatives. In *Atherosclerosis*, vol. III (eds G. Schettler and A. Weizel), Springer-Verlag, Berlin, pp. 845–871
24. Utermann, G. Apolipoprotein E polymorphisms in health and disease. *Am. Heart J.*, **113**, 433–440 (1987)
25. Mahley, R. W. and Angelin, B. Type III hyperlipoproteinaemia. Recent insights into the genetic defect of familial dysbetalipoproteinaemia. *Adv. Int. Med.*, **29**, 385–441 (1984)
26. Rall, S. C., Weisgraber, K. H., Innerarity, T. L. and Mahley, R. W. Structural basis for receptor-binding heterogeneity of apolipoprotein E from type III hyperlipoproteinaemic subjects. *Proc. Natl Acad. Sci., USA.*, **79**, 4696–4700 (1982)
27. Hui, D. Y., Innerarity, T. L. and Mahley, R. W. Defective hepatic lipoprotein receptor binding of β-very low density lipoproteins from type III hyperlipoproteinaemic patients. *J. Biol. Chem.*, **259**, 860–869 (1984)
28. Weisgraber, K. H., Rall, S. C. and Mahley, R. W. Human E apoproteins heterogeneity. Cysteine-arginine interchanges in the amino acid sequence of apo-E isoforms. *J. Biol. Chem.*, **256**, 9077–9083 (1981)
29. Talmud, P. Detection and physiological relevance of mutations in the apolipoprotein E, C-II and B genes. Chapter 5 in *Structure and Function of Apolipoproteins* (ed. M. Rosseneu), CRC Press Inc., Boca Raton, pp. 123–158 (1992)
30. Emi, M., Wu, L.L., Robertson, M.A., Muers, R.L., Hegele, R.A. *et al*. Gentoyping and sequence analysis of apolipoprotein E isoforms. *Genomics*, **3**, 373–379 (1988)
31. Hixson, J.E. and Vernier, D.T. Restriction isotyping of human apolipoprotein E by gene amplification and cleavage with HhaI. *J. Lipid Res.*, **31**, 545–548 (1990)
32. Rall, S.C. Jr., Weisgraber, K.H., Innerarity, T.L., Bersot, T.P., Mahley, R.W. and Blum, C.B. Identification of a new structural variant of human apolipoprotein E, E2 (Lys146 leads to Gln), in a type III hyperlipoproteinaemic subject with the E3/2 phenotype. *J. Clin. Invest.*, **72**, 1288 (1993)

33. Havel, R. J., Kotite, L., Kane, J. P., Tun, P. and Bersot, T. Atypical familial dysbetalipopro-teinaemia associated with apolipoprotein phenotype E3/3. *J. Clin. Invest.*, **72**, 379–387 (1983)
34. Rall, S.C. Jr., Newhouse, Y.M., Clarke, H.R.G., Weisgraber, K.H., McCarthy, B.J. *et al.* Type III hyperlipoproteinaemia associated with apolipoprotein phenotype E3/3. Structure and genetics of an apolipoprotein E3 variant. *J. Clin. Invest.*, **83**, 1095–1101 (1989)
35. Wardell, M.R., Weisgraber, K.H., Havekes, L.M. and Rall, S.C. Jr. Apolipoprotein E3-Leiden contains a seven-amino acid insertion that is a random repeat of residues 121–127. *J. Biol. Chem.*, **264**, 21205–21210 (1989)
36. Mann, W.A., Gregg, R.E., Sprecher, D.L. and Brewer, H.B. Jr. Apolipoprotein E-I Harrisburg: a new variant of apolipoprotein E dominantly associated with type III hyperlipoproteinaemia. *Biochim. Biophys. Acta*, **1005**, 239–244 (1989)
37. Ghiselli, G., Schefer, E. J., Garscon, P. and Brewer, H. B. Type III hyperlipoproteinaemia associ-ated with apolipoprotein E deficiency. *Science*, **214**, 1239–1241 (1981)
38. Cladaras, C., Hadzopoulou-Cladaras, M., Felber, B.K., Pavlakis, B. and Zannis, V.I. The molecu-lar basis of a familial apo E deficiency. An acceptor splice site mutation in the third intron of the deficient apo E gene. *J. Biol. Chem.*, **262**, 2310–2315 (1987)
39. Chait, A., Hazard, W. R., Albers, J. J., Kushwaha, R. P. and Brunzell, J. D. Impaired very low density lipoprotein and triglyceride removal in broad beta disease. Comparison with endogenous hypertriglyceridaemia. *Metabolism*, **27**, 1055–1066 (1978)
40. Janus, E. D., Nicoll, A. M., Turner, P. R., Magill, P. and Lewis, B. Kinetic bases of the primary hyperlipidaemias. Studies of apolipoprotein B turnover in genetically defined subjects. *Eur. J. Clin. Invest.*, **10**, 161–172 (1980)
41. Berman, M., Hall, M., Levy, R. I., Eisenberg, S., Bilheimer, D. W. *et al.* Metabolism of apo B and apo C lipoproteins in man. Kinetic studies in normal and hyperlipoproteinaemic subjects. *J. Lipid Res.*, **19**, 38–56 (1978)
42. Reardon, M. F., Poapst M. E. and Steiner, G. The independent synthesis of intermediate density lipoproteins in type III hyperlipoproteinaemia. *Metabolism*, **31**, 421–427 (1982)
43. Packard, C. J., Clegg, R. J., Dominiczak, M. H., Lorimer, A. R. and Shepherd, J. Effects of bezafi-brate on apolipoprotein B metabolism in type III hyperlipoproteinaemic subjects. *J. Lipid Res.*, **27**, 930–938 (1986)
44. Fredrickson, D. S., Morganroth, J. and Levy, R. I. Type III hyperlipoproteinaemia. An analysis of two contemporary definitions. *Ann. Intern. Med.*, **82**, 150–157 (1975)
45. Illingworth, D.R. and O'Malley, J.P. The hypolipidaemia effects of lovastatin and clofibrate alone and in combination in patients with type III hyperlipoproteinaemia. *Metabolism*, **39**, 403–409 (1990)
46. Feussner, G., Eichinger, M. and Ziegler, R. The influence of simvastatin alone or in combination with gemfibrozil on plasma lipids and lipoproteins in patients with type III hyperlipoproteinaemia. *Clin. Invest.*, **70**, 1027–1235 (1992)

# Chapter 9

# Diet

## Introduction

Diet is widely regarded as the major reason for the enormous variation in the serum cholesterol concentration and hence the coronary death rate in different parts of the world[1]. The observation that populations with low intake of fat, particularly saturated fat, and in whom a greater portion of dietary energy is derived from carbohydrate, tend to have lower serum cholesterol levels and lower mortality rates from ischaemic heart disease when compared to populations whose dietary energy is substantially derived from fat is scarcely old[2]. The incidence of diabetes, too, seems to follow a similar pattern[3]. Despite the virtually certain involvement of nutrition in these diseases, which are a major cause of morbidity and premature mortality in nations with a Northern European diet, which includes the USA, Canada, Australia, New Zealand and white South Africa, very few well-designed experiments have been done to support the enormous quantity of frequently ill-informed, if not merely capricious, writing on the subject. What is known for certain has often been buried beneath a deluge of trivial and insubstantial observations. The sadness of this has been in the sage words of one journal editorial[4] that, in the UK for example, 'conflict has bred inactivity in strategies to improve the nation's diet'. In the management of patients, all too frequently failure to see the wood for the trees has produced dietetic advice which is more appropriate to an evangelical crusade than to medicine. Impossible demands made on patients are, of course, ineffective therapy.

In this chapter some of the harder facts about soft fats will be reviewed before outlining some of the policies advocated for altering the diet of whole populations and then discussing specific therapeutic diets for individuals with hyperlipidaemia and some of the practical problems associated with them.

## Obesity

Obesity has a major influence on serum lipid and lipoprotein levels. There is no hyperlipidaemia which, when associated with obesity, is not improved by weight reduction. Confusion seems to exist in the minds of many because of the conclusion of some investigators[5–7] that obesity is not an independent risk factor for ischaemic heart disease. That conclusion may be perfectly valid, but it is based on multivariate analysis, in which the effects of, for example, serum cholesterol and blood pressure are removed mathematically before an effect of obesity is sought. Body weight is directly related to coronary risk on univariate analysis (Chapter 11, page 315). It is thus a useful means by which the clinician may identify an individual at risk of coronary disease. Multivariate analysis, however, demonstrates that much of its effect is through other risk factors.

Obesity is associated with an increase in serum triglycerides and, in susceptible individuals, raised serum cholesterol, whereas serum HDL cholesterol levels tend to be low (Chapter 11, page 319). Correction of obesity in patients with hyperlipidaemia leads to a decrease in both serum cholesterol and triglycerides[8,9], although its effect on serum HDL cholesterol remains less certain[10].

## Saturated fatty acids

These undoubtedly have a greater effect on the concentrations of serum cholesterol and triglycerides than any other dietary constituent. They are frequently lumped together as if they were a single substance when, in fact, those occurring in the diet represent a diverse collection of fatty acids of chain lengths from 6 to more than 20. Those seeking to oversimplify matters and thus inadvertently nullify their advice, refer to them as animal fats. This is an horrific misnomer since many plant oils are rich in saturated fats and, with the exception of mammals adapted to warm or temperate environments, many animal species contain considerable quantities of polyunsaturates, inappropriately referred to by the same people as plant or vegetable fats.

The commonest dietary saturated fatty acids are C12 : 0 (lauric acid), C14 : 0 (myristic acid), C16 : 0 (palmitic acid) and C18 : 0 (stearic acid). Of these, palmitic acid is the most abundant in the Northern European style diet because of its great reliance on dairy, beef, pork and lamb products. Milk products and coconut also contain substantial amounts of myristic acid, and beef, pork and mutton are rich in stearate. The importance of the saturated fats lies in the fact that in rigorously conducted metabolic studies, in which saturated fat was added or subtracted from isocaloric diets, consistent changes in serum cholesterol occurred of sufficient magnitude to be of therapeutic value[11–13]. An isocaloric substitution of one dietary component for another, of course, leaves open the question of whether the component substituted has an effect in its own right. Generally speaking, monounsaturated fats, such as oleic acid, or carbohydrate have been assumed to have little effect on serum cholesterol in the interpretation of experiments. Set against this yardstick, saturated fats such as C12 : 0, C14 : 0 and C16 : 0 increase cholesterol by about 2.6 mg/dl (0.07 mmol/l) for each 1% they contribute (as calories) to the total diet. Clearly, of course, this is a considerable generalization and there will be some individuals who show more marked response than others.

Myristic acid may be more potent than palmitic acid in raising cholesterol[12]. Stearic acid, on the other hand, may not do so at all[14–16]. On this rating, butter fat, palm oil and coconut oil are even more potent in raising cholesterol than beef, mutton and pork fat. The benefit from the knowledge that stearic acid does not raise cholesterol is not likely to be great because in practice foods rich in stearic acid, but not in other saturated fats or cholesterol, are not available[17] and stearic acid is the most potent fatty acid in raising factor VII coagulant activity[18]. The effects of saturated fatty acids with 20 or more carbon atoms, such as those present in peanut (arachis) oil is uncertain. Medium-chain saturated fatty acids (C < 10) do not appear to influence serum cholesterol levels[19], although this may not be the case in patients with major defects in triglyceride catabolism (page 208).

In addition to the effect of replacing dietary saturated fats with polyunsaturated fats on serum cholesterol levels, most investigations have also shown that there is a decrease in the fasting concentration of serum triglycerides[20–26]. Diets in which carbohydrate or mono-unsaturated fat replaces saturated fat are generally less effective in reducing serum triglycerides. Stearate (C18 : 0) and medium-chain fatty acids (C < 10)[27,28], too, seem at least as effective as other saturated fats in raising serum triglycerides (unlike serum cholesterol). There may, however, be considerable individual variation in the relative importance of nutritional and constitutional factors in determining the serum triglyceride level. Thus, for example, in patients with a defect in triglyceride clearance (Chapter 7, page 208) a decrease in total fat consumption, since it reduces exogenous hypertriglyceridaemia, may produce a marked decrease in serum triglycerides, despite the increase in dietary carbohydrate necessitated if the diet is to provide sufficient calories.

## Mono-unsaturated fatty acids

The main mono-unsaturated fatty acid in the diet is oleic acid (C18 : 1). It is the principal fat in olive oil and in rapeseed oil, but is also a major component of fats in other vegetable oils, dairy products and meat, since both plants and animals can create a double bond in the $\omega 9$ position. Because it is so ubiquitous in the European diet, it is often the predominant fatty acid in the circulating triglycerides[26]. The independent effect of oleic acid on serum cholesterol in isocaloric feeding experiments was initially thought to be similar to $\omega 6$ polyunsaturated fatty acids which decrease serum cholesterol concentration by more than would be expected if they are 'inertly' replacing saturated fat[26]. However, many later reports were that mono-unsaturated fatty acids had no significant effect on serum cholesterol levels[12,30–33]. The whole question has recently been reopened by experiments in which there was a similar reduction in serum cholesterol regardless of whether oleic acid (C18 : 1) or linoleic acid (C18 : 2) were substituted for palmitic acid (C16 : 0)[17, 34–36].

## Polyunsaturated fatty acids

There are two major types of polyunsaturated fatty acids in the diet: the $\omega 6$ and the $\omega 3$ series.

### Omega 6 fatty acids

Those from the safflower, sunflower, maize and other higher plants are characterized by a double bond six carbon atoms from the methyl (omega) end and are know as omega 6 ($\omega 6$) fatty acids (Chapter 1, page 6). The predominant one in the diet is linoleic acid (C18 : 2). Their major role, like that of any fatty acid, is, of course, as an energy source and a component of structural lipids, but in addition they are essential for the synthesis of arachidonic acid and thence essential humoral substances such as prostaglandins and leukotrienes (Chapter 1, page 22). They are thus essential fatty acids.

In the experiments of Keys[13,30] and Hegsted[12,33], linoleic acid appeared to have a specific cholesterol-lowering effect. Thus, there was an additional decrease in serum cholesterol when linoleic acid rather than oleic acid or carbohydrate was substituted for C12–C16 saturated fatty acids. Implicit in these conclusions, too, was that an alteration in the ratio of saturated fat to polyunsaturated fat would alter the serum cholesterol level even without any change in the total fat energy in the diet[33]. This was the rationale for the use of the P : S ratio, in which the calories derived from polyunsaturated fats (P) are expressed as the ratio of those obtained from saturates (S). Mono-unsaturated fats are disregarded in this ratio. It is frequently used today, but account has never been taken of the apparent neutrality of stearate, which is included in S, nor that the $\omega 6$ fatty acids, principally linoleic, were what was meant by P. Frequently now, $\omega 3$ fatty acids are included as P. Furthermore the neutrality of mono-unsaturated fatty acids is no longer acceptable[37]. It also appears that *trans* isomers of unsaturated fats behave like saturated fat in raising cholesterol[38].

Formulae to predict the change in serum cholesterol have been developed from a large number of dietary experiences by three groups. These have in common an insignificant effect of mono-unsaturated fatty acids and an independent cholesterol-lowering effect of polyunsaturated fats at least half as great as the removal of a similar quantity of saturated fat energy from the diet[12,13,32]. Two of these which also take into account changes in dietary cholesterol are as follows:

$$\text{Serum cholesterol} = 1.3 \ (2S - P) + 1.5\sqrt{C} \qquad \qquad \text{[Ref. 12]}$$
$$= 2.16S - 1.65P + 6.77C - 0.53 \qquad \text{[Ref. 13]}$$

where S is the percentage of change in dietary energy from saturated fat; P is the percentage of change in dietary energy from polyunsaturated fat; and C is the change in dietary cholesterol in multiples of 100 mg/day.

Although these must now be considered inaccurate, they do serve to illustrate that a 10% reduction in calories from saturated fat, if accompanied by a similar increase in polyunsaturated fat, and no change in mono-unsaturated fat will lower serum cholesterol by 38–39 mg/dl (1.0 mmol/l), whereas substitution of the saturated fat energy by carbohydrate would produce only a 22–26 mg/dl (0.6–0.7 mmol/l) reduction. This assumes that no change in the cholesterol intake was made. In practice, because foods rich in saturated fat contain more cholesterol than carbohydrate-rich or linoleic acid-rich foods, there would on average be an even greater decrease in serum cholesterol with both diets.

## Omega 3 fatty acids

Omega 3 fatty acids have a double bond at the third carbon from the methyl end (Chapter 1, page 6). The creation of a double bond at this site is typical of lower plants, such as the algae present in plankton, which are rich in $\omega 3$, C18 polyunsaturates, such as linolenic acid (C18 : 3)[39]. Fish, which graze on plankton, and their predators thus have a ready source of $\omega 3$ fatty acids and many species, particularly those adapted to a cold environment, elongate these and create further double bonds to form other fatty acids in the omega 3 series, in particular eicosapentaenoic (C20 : 5), eicosahexaenoic (C20 : 6) and docosahexaenoic (C22 : 6) acids. These are also, of course, present in the blubber of fish-eating mammals, such as seals, whales, etc. The importance of fatty acids with a low melting point in a cold environment is discussed elsewhere (Chapter 1, page 9).

The highly polyunsaturated fish oils have a peculiar significance, because of their presence in substantial amounts in the traditional Eskimo diet. As such they constitute as important a component of the 'red herring' as they do of the herring.

Although it is widely accepted that Eskimos have low rates of ischaemic heart disease. One-third of deaths in Eskimos are due to accidents[40], such as drowning or hypothermia. Critical epidemiological or post-mortem evaluation of the evidence that Eskimos are unusual with regard to coronary heart disease frequency is scanty. Few primitive Eskimos survive to the age when coronary heart disease is most common[1]. In any case, the primitive diet of the Eskimo was fatty only during the sealing season, but quite low in fat during the fishing season. In both seasons it was relatively unsaturated and the low intake of saturated fats may have more to do the low serum cholesterol of the Greenland Eskimos than their ω3 polyunsaturated fatty acid intake although this would undoubtedly contribute to changes in coagulation such as prolonged bleeding time which could help to prevent IHD.

The main effect on plasma lipids of marine fish oils is a decrease in serum triglycerides[41–46]. There may be a small effect in lowering cholesterol, but this is due to a decrease in VLDL cholesterol, and LDL cholesterol may actually increase[47]. When they are substituted for saturated fat, the anticipated decrease in serum cholesterol due to the decrease in saturated fat does, however, occur[48]. Fish liver oils do contain cholesterol and also saturated fats (20% or so in the case of herring and even more in salmon)[39]. In the Eskimo, who may have few other dietary sources of saturated fat, this will still result in low consumption of saturates, but this may not be so when added to a typical Western diet. In experiments, fish oil supplements of the order of 20 g/day (equivalent to 200 g/day of, say, mackerel) have generally been given. At this level of consumption, antithrombotic and anti-inflammatory effects are also observed[43]. The former effect results from an inhibition of platelet aggregation[44,49,50]. Such an effect might be beneficial in decreasing the likelihood of thrombosis. There are also reports of reductions in blood pressure by a fish-oil diet[45]. Whether these effects are sufficiently beneficial to outweigh any disadvantages in other aspects of health (Eskimos were generally considered susceptible to infections) has never been the subject of any proper clinical trial. In myocardial infarction survivors, however, a diet including fatty fish or fish oil supplements, was more effective in reducing deaths in a large clinical trial than either a diet enriched in linoleic acid or in fibre[51]. Marine fish oil supplements should be regarded as medicaments rather than nutrients and are included in Chapter 10 (page 277).

## Mechanisms by which dietary fats influence serum lipoproteins

The decrease in serum cholesterol in response to reduction in dietary energy derived from saturated fat results from a decrease in LDL[52]. A small contribution is also made by the decrease in VLDL, although of course the major result of the decreased concentration of that lipoprotein is a reduction in serum triglycerides[25,26]. A more profound decrease in LDL is likely when linoleic acid or oleic acid, rather than carbohydrate, is substituted for the saturated fat. No enhancement of the LDL-lowering effect of saturated fat withdrawal has been reported with ω3 polyunsaturates.

It was suggested that the decrease in LDL cholesterol occurring during linoleic acid feeding might not be due to a decrease in the concentration of LDL particles, but result from a reduction in the quantity of cholesterol, which could be accommodated in each particle when it was esterified with the bulkier linoleic acid[53], with its kinked hydrocarbon chain, compared with, say, palmitate, with its straight flexible structure (Chapter 1, page 6). Although difficulty in accommodating polyunsaturated fatty acids on enzymes involved in triglyceride synthesis or in packaging them during lipoprotein synthesis may be important, it does not explain their action on LDL cholesterol, since the decrease in LDL cholesterol is matched by a parallel decrease in apolipoprotein B, its principal protein component[26,54]. Also LCAT on HDL (Chapter 2, page 57) has a preference for esterifying cholesterol to linoleic acid[55], so that difficulty in transferring that ester of cholesterol back to LDL would seem unlikely.

There is no single consistently reported and entirely convincing explanation for the effect of dietary fatty acids on serum LDL cholesterol. They do not appear to alter the rate of cholesterol biosynthesis[56]. The balance of evidence does favour an increase in the output of faecal neutral sterols[57–59], and of faecal bile acids[58–62]. This would be consistent with an effect on cholesterol absorption and on conversion of cholesterol to bile salts. By whatever mechanism a low saturated fat diet lowers serum cholesterol, the results of studies using the external sterol balance technique do refute the fear that the effect is due to movement of cholesterol out of the plasma into the tissues. The effect of saturated fat does appear to be enhanced by dietary cholesterol (see later), which it has been suggested may influence hepatic LDL receptor expression by its effect on the intrahepatic cholesterol pool.

The effect of low saturated fat, polyunsaturated fat substituted diets on serum triglycerides is probably mediated through a decrease in hepatic VLDL production[25,63–65]. Since VLDL is the precursor of much of the circulating LDL, this might also explain the decrease in LDL with such a diet. In the International Collaborative Study, saturated fat intake was directly correlated with LDL production rate[66]. However, this cannot be the whole explanation for the decrease in LDL, because stearic acid (page 227) and medium-chain fatty acids[27,28] increase serum triglycerides without affecting serum cholesterol. Also, ω3 fatty acids lower serum triglycerides by decreasing VLDL production[67], but they do not reduce serum LDL cholesterol levels[44].

The additional explanation for the LDL lowering effect of unsaturated fatty acids may be that they oppose the down-regulation of hepatic LDL receptors due to cholesterol in the diet[68–70] (presumably secondary to chylomicron remnant uptake, Chapter 2 page 41). Interestingly, however, ω3 polyunsaturates which have no LDL-lowering effect in man are more active than ω6 polyunsaturated fatty acids in this respect[68]. There is a dearth of human information. Mediterranean populations are reported to have enhanced LDL catabolism[66]. Their olive oil (oleic acid) intake is high, but so also is their intake of linoleic acid high and their saturated fat intake low.

One effect of substitution of saturated fat with linoleic acid is a decrease in the serum concentration of HDL cholesterol[10,34,71,72]. This effect is due to a decrease in the production of apolipoproteins AI[71] and occurs when the intake of linoleic acid exceeds 10% of the dietary energy. This decrease in HDL cholesterol did not occur in experiments in which mono-unsaturated fat was substituted for saturated fat[34,73], but it does occur when carbohydrate is substituted for a saturated fat[73,74]. Since most of the world's population, particularly those with a low prevalence of coronary disease, have a diet which is low in fat and rich in carbohydrate, it is hard to imagine that these changes in HDL concentration actually increase the risk of coronary atheroma. In Chapter 3 (page 83) it was pointed out that many populations with a low prevalence of ischaemic

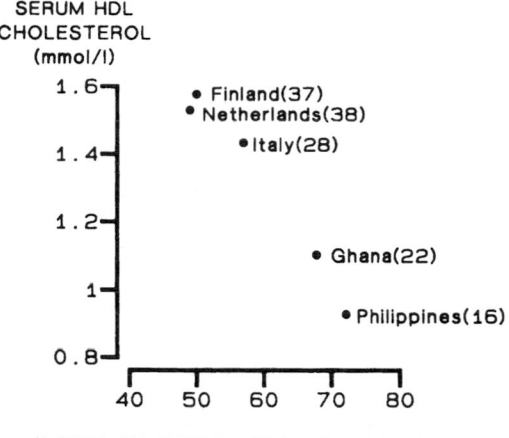

**Figure 9.1**   Mean serum high density lipoprotein cholesterol concentration of boys living in different countries plotted against the proportion of dietary energy they derive from carbohydrate (After Kruiman *et al*.[75])

heart disease subsisting on low saturated fat, high carbohydrate diets have low HDL cholesterol values in comparison with populations with a high fat intake[75] (Figure 9.1). While not denying the inverse relationship between ischaemic heart disease risk and HDL cholesterol within single populations, it does nevertheless appear that decreases of HDL due to diet are not necessarily harmful. The concentration of cholesterol in serum HDL may, for example, be a poor guide to the flux of cholesterol through HDL. Also, it should not be forgotten that dietary saturated fats are obtained from organisms further up the food chain than plant polyunsaturates. There is thus the possibility that a high intake of saturated fat leads to exposure to lipid-soluble chemicals, such as pesticides, concentrated there. A wide variety of chemicals, which induce hepatic microsomal enzymes, including pesticides, increase serum HDL cholesterol levels[76–78]. Marked differences in enzyme induction exist between populations with a high saturated fat intake and rural Africans subsisting on a high carbohydrate diet[79].

Marine fish oils generally tend to increase HDL cholesterol levels[45] unless substantial quantities are present in the diet when, as with linoleic acid, serum HDL decreases[70].

## *Trans* polyunsaturated fatty acids and other unusual dietary fatty acids

The *trans* fatty acids are present in the UK diet in amounts averaging about 7 g/day. They are isomers of the *cis* polyunsaturated fatty acids in which the hydrogen atoms on carbon atoms linked by double bonds are on opposite sides (Chapter 1, page 5). There is thus no kink in the hydrocarbon chain at the double bond as in the *cis* forms. Because of the straight chain which results, the properties of the resulting fatty acid may more closely resemble those of a saturated fatty acid. The commonest dietary *trans* fatty acid is elaidic acid. The melting point of elaidic acid (*trans* ω9, C18 : 1) is, for example, 44 °C compared with its *cis* isomer, oleic acid (*cis* ω9, C18 : 1), which has a melting point of 11 °C.

*Trans* fatty acids are often included with saturated fat in the calculation of the P : S ratio and it is sometimes assumed that they will raise serum cholesterol. There is now experimental evidence for this[38], but it is difficult to be sure at present how great an effect *trans* fatty acids have and it should be remembered that stearate (C18 : 0), the saturated fatty acid with a similar length to elaidic acid, has no effect on serum cholesterol. It is generally considered advisable to keep their production in the food industry to a minimum[80].

*Trans* fatty acids arise in the diet as a result of partial hydrogenation of, for example, linoleic acid (*cis, cis*, ω6, C18 : 2) when the ω6 double bond becomes saturated, but the one at ω9 is rearranged to a *trans* bond. This occurs naturally to some extent in the rumen of ruminant animals whence they may enter depot fat. Industrially they are produced when polyunsaturated fatty acids are hydrogenated in order to raise their melting points and thus produce margarine or other spreads. Depending on the catalyst and conditions used, up to 30–50% of hydrogenated vegetable oil may be *trans* isomerized. The extent of hydrogenation both partial and complete in the production of margarine should be considered in recommending its use, both because *trans* fatty acids may contribute to hypercholesterolaemia and because transisomorization will reduce its linoleic and oleic acid content.

Theoretically, a fatty acid which cannot by virtue of its structure be metabolized by the human would be toxic. A model might be Refsum's disease, which occurs in rare individuals who are unable to metabolize phytanic acid which accumulates within their tissues, even though it is present in only small amounts in the diet. It is a fatty acid with a 16 carbon chain like palmitate, but which has additional methyl groups linked to the carbon chain at four sites. The methyl group closest to the carboxyl group blocks the beta position preventing beta-oxidation. A preliminary alpha-oxidation is therefore required before the molecule is susceptible to beta-oxidation. Individuals susceptible to Refsum's disease lack the capacity for this[81] and a syndrome of retinitis pigmentosa, peripheral polyneuropathy and cerebellar ataxia results.

If an unusual fatty acid were to enter the diet in large quantities, there is the possibility that it may have toxic effects even in normal humans by exceeding their capacity to metabolize it. This is thus a subject of concern when oil from unusual sources or which has subsequently been chemically modified is incorporated in cooking oils. The recent production of rapeseed oil in quantity was thus only possible with breeding of a variety which does not contain the substantial quantities of erucic acid (C22 : 1) present in wild brassica (rapeseed) and which is largely replaced by oleic and linoleic acid[82].

## Cholesterol

There has been much more controversy about how much effect dietary cholesterol has on the serum cholesterol concentration. This may seem strange to those unfamiliar with the subject, since a diet termed the 'low cholesterol diet' is frequently what is recommended for the management of hypercholesterolaemia.

The more appropriate term is 'cholesterol-lowering diet' and, as we have previously discussed, a considerable element of such a diet and probably the most important element in the great majority of patients will be a reduction in saturated fat.

The reason for the usually small and rather variable influence of dietary cholesterol on serum cholesterol levels is not entirely known, but germane to the issue must be the efficiency of intestinal absorption of dietary cholesterol. The digestion and absorption of triglycerides and phospholipids is virtually complete; only around 30–60% of cholesterol is absorbed. At high dietary intakes of cholesterol the absorptive capacity of the intestine may be exceeded and this may explain the lack of effect of adding cholesterol to the diet when substantial quantities were already present[83,84]. The type of fat in the diet might be expected to influence the absorption of cholesterol, because the bile composition may be different on a diet which is largely saturated compared with one rich in polyunsaturates, but there is little experimental evidence for this[33,85]. Also, the quantity of fat in the diet might influence the absorption of cholesterol since phospholipid, monoglycerides and fatty acids are required for the formation of mixed micelles in the gut. Certainly diets low in total fat quite often reduce the serum cholesterol to very low levels, perhaps in part due to limited absorption.

Some of the variation in the effect of dietary cholesterol and, indeed diet in general, on serum cholesterol and lipoprotein levels is also genetic. People with apo $E_4$ alleles absorb cholesterol more efficiently than those with apo $E_3$ and those with apo $E_3$ more so than those with the $E_2$ allele[86]. This may be part of the explanation for the effect of apo E phenotype on serum cholesterol levels in people consuming high as opposed to low fat diets[87] (Chapter 2, page 51).

Considering numerous experiments on the effects of dietary cholesterol on serum cholesterol, a figure of around 4–5 mg/dl (0.1–0.13 mmol/l) seems likely for the change in serum cholesterol for each 100 mg alteration in dietary cholesterol up to about 500 mg/day[33]. Keys developed the following formula for predicting the response of serum cholesterol to dietary cholesterol using data from 39 experiments, which is broadly in agreement:

Change in serum cholesterol = $1.5(\sqrt{X_2} - \sqrt{X_1})$

where $X_1$ and $X_2$ are the dietary cholesterol in mg/1000 cal before and after. The formula predicts an increase of 6.2 mg/dl (0.16 mmol/l) for a change from 100 to 200 mg/1000 cal, 4.8 mg/dl (0.12 mmol/l) from 200 to 300 mg/1000 cal, and 4.1 mg/dl (0.01 mmol/l) from 300 to 400 mg/dl. Thus, changes in serum cholesterol due to alterations in dietary cholesterol are on average relatively small and a more potent dietary means of reducing serum cholesterol is by decreasing the intake of saturated fat. In practice, however, cholesterol-rich foods are generally rich in saturated fat and a diet intended to decrease saturated fat will thus decrease the intake of both and their effects in reducing serum cholesterol will summate.

The effect of altering dietary cholesterol intake on serum cholesterol is largely due to changes in the serum LDL concentration. These are brought about by two mechanisms. First, the rate of synthesis of LDL apo B increases with increasing cholesterol ingestion[88]. It has been suggested that this might be due to a concurrent decrease in the clearance of IDL from the circulation, leaving more to be converted to LDL[35]. Secondly, there is a decrease in the rate of LDL catabolism. Experiments with cyclohexanedione-blocked LDL suggest that this is due to a decrease in receptor-mediated catabolism[88]. This seems very plausible, since the hepatic cholesterol content would be expected to rise as the liver receives the increased quantities of cholesterol-laden chylomicron remnants and thus LDL receptor synthesis would be down-regulated. There is evidence that the individual response to dietary cholesterol may be related to the contribution of the LDL receptor to cholesterol homeostasis[89]. A decrease in the receptor-mediated catabolism of LDL even without any increase in serum LDL concentration might be deleterious, since a greater quantity of LDL must then enter non-receptor-mediated pathways, which may be atherogenic (Chapter 2, page 33). Also, continued suppression of hepatic LDL receptor expression by habitually high cholesterol intakes may permanently imprint itself on the individual. This has been suggested to account for the rise in serum cholesterol, which occurs with advancing age in people consuming a high cholesterol diet but not in, for example, rural Africans (Chapter 3, page 85) or perhaps life-long vegetarians[90]. The rise with age appears to be related at least in part to a decrease in LDL receptor activity[91] and thus the rate of LDL catabolism[92].

Cholesterol-feeding experiments have also shown that increments in the serum HDL cholesterol concentration occur with increasing cholesterol intake in some individuals[10]. Furthermore, in the Lipid Research Clinics Study Prevalence Programme a positive correlation was present between dietary cholesterol intake and the serum HDL cholesterol level in school-age boys[93]. Qualitative changes in serum HDL have been reported in one study, even in individuals where serum HDL cholesterol concentration was relatively unaffected by increases in dietary cholesterol[94]. This was due to an increase in the apo E-containing fraction of HDL, designated HDLc

We need to know a great deal more about the reason for the tendency for HDL cholesterol to rise with dietary cholesterol, but clearly it cannot be assumed that an increase in HDL cholesterol is necessarily beneficial and this should be remembered in other contexts, for example, the insulin-treated diabetic (Chapter 11, page 306).

## Carbohydrate

Carbohydrate, when it comprises a substantial proportion of dietary energy, has been shown in many experiments to produce an increase in serum triglycerides. There is variation in individual susceptibility. Often, however, the effect is greatest in patients with pre-existing hypertriglyceridaemia. It is also more marked when carbohydrate is added to the diet, rather than substituted isocalorically for fat, so that there is a concomitant increase in dietary energy. In experiments with isocaloric diets, it is likely that any reduction in saturated fat intake will counteract to a considerable extent the tendency for serum triglycerides to rise and that the effect may be abolished or reversed if unsaturated fat as well as carbohydrate is fed[25,37,95].

The most consistent increase in serum triglycerides occurs when carbohydrate comprises 65% or more of the dietary energy. There is an enormous literature, suggesting that refined carbohydrates, which usually means sucrose, are more potent in raising serum triglycerides than starch. There is, however, a dearth of properly conducted experiments to support this view and metabolic ward studies indicate that sucrose and starch do not differ greatly in this respect[96].

The effect on serum triglycerides of dietary carbohydrate occurs in three phases[97]. The first occurs within a few hours of starting a high carbohydrate diet and is a transitory fall in serum triglycerides[98]. The effect may be mediated via temporary increase in insulin secretion, decreasing fatty acid release for adipose tissue (Chapter 1, page 11) and perhaps hepatic VLDL secretion[99]. This is followed within about 2–3 days by a rise[100,101], which is at its peak in about 1–5 weeks[22,102] and which in one series of experiments with normal people was about two and a half times the basal level[100]. The rise is generally considered to be due to increased hepatic triglyceride synthesis and secretion secondary to *de novo* fatty acid synthesis, but there may also be a decrease in triglyceride catabolism[99,100,103]. Interestingly, carbohydrate delivered intravenously does not produce a rise in serum triglycerides in individuals in whom a similar amount given orally does do so[104]. Presumably this is either because the liver receives less glucose when given intravenously than it does via the portal vein when given orally, or because some signal from the intestine or pancreas is important.

In the majority of individuals there is a third phase of carbohydrate induction, which is a decline in the serum triglyceride concentration back to the initial level. In experiments with prisoners in South Africa, baseline values were resumed after 17 weeks in blacks and 32 weeks in whites[22]. Observations such as this have led some to question whether or not dietary carbohydrate is ever a contributory factor to hypertriglyceridaemia[101,105,106]. It is, however, difficult to relate some of the feeding experiments to real life because generally a sustained high carbohydrate intake was maintained throughout the experiments. Presumably the chosen diet of hypertriglyceridaemic individuals would be more variable and it is not known whether this would make adaptation more or less likely. It can, however, reasonably be concluded that a low carbohydrate diet should no longer be considered to have a place in the management of hypertriglyceridaemia.

There is one circumstance in clinical practice which appears to mimic the middle phase of carbohydrate induction. This occurs in the patient with severe hypertriglyceridaemia with chylomicronaemia (Fredrickson type I or V), who is given a diet which is low in total fat (Chapter 7, page 208, and this chapter, page 245). If a deficit in energy intake is not intended, because the patient is non-obese, a marked increase in carbohydrate intake is required. Thus, although the diet will abolish the chylomicronaemia and, when it is first introduced, may produce a rapid decrease in serum triglycerides towards normal, at a later stage there will be a rise in endogenous triglycerides (VLDL), particularly if, as is generally the case in these patients, the clearance of circulating triglycerides is impaired. The problem may be difficult to overcome and it is important to recognize that it may not need to be, since the patient may remain free of attacks of pancreatitis, because even though the triglyceride level is still markedly elevated, it is nevertheless usually lower than originally.

As has previously been discussed (page 226), substituting carbohydrate for dietary saturated fat decreases the serum LDL cholesterol. Interestingly this effect may be more marked when the carbohydrate is given intravenously rather than orally[104] and this may apply even in homozygotes for familial hypercholesterolaemia[107].

One effect of a high proportion of dietary energy as carbohydrate is to decrease serum HDL cholesterol and, unlike the effect on serum triglycerides, this seems much more commonly to be sustained. It is of the order of 4 mg/dl (0.1 mmol/l) for replacement of about 10% dietary fat energy by carbohydrate[10]. Between populations, the proportion of dietary energy derived from carbohydrate is inversely related to the HDL cholesterol and this is true for boys from different populations (Figure 9.1) in whom the effects of alcohol, cigarettes and obesity which also affect HDL levels are not evident[75]. This effect is also observed within the North American population, since in the Lipid Research Clinics study HDL was negatively related to starch and sucrose intake[108]. It also probably explains the low levels of HDL in vegetarians[109–111].

## Alcohol

The effects of alcohol on lipoprotein metabolism are dealt with in Chapter 11 (pages 322–325).

## Dietary fibre

Major differences exist in the quantities of non-absorbable vegetable matter in the diets of different nations[112]. Thus, for example, in the UK the average per capita consumption of dietary fibre is around 20 g daily[113] and in many people this is from white bread! In Africa, in particular, the intake is substantially greater, between say 50 and 100 g daily in maize-eating populations in for example Swaziland, Malawi and rural South Africa, and as high as 150 g daily in Uganda where plantains are the staple food. When populations are compared there is, as might be anticipated, a relationship between the average intake of dietary fibre and the prevalence of ischaemic heart disease: populations such as those of the UK having little dietary fibre and being at high coronary risk and populations in rural Africa being at the other end of the spectrum. As we have seen in earlier sections of the chapter, however, this is largely explicable on the basis of dietary fat and carbohydrate intake: a high fibre intake is almost inevitably the result of a diet low in fat and rich in carbohydrate, since unrefined carbohydrate-rich foods are also rich in vegetable fibre.

   Much time and energy has been expended in addressing the question of whether dietary fibre has any effect of its own in decreasing coronary risk by, for example, lowering the concentration of plasma lipids. Unfortunately a great part of the literature consists of poorly designed experiments over short time intervals, with little attempt to control the intake of other nutrients. It is, however, possible to gain an overall impression of the influence of fibre *per se* on lipoprotein metabolism[114,115]. There seems to be very little evidence that non-mucilaginous fibre, when added to a diet such as that in the UK or America, has any influence on serum VLDL, LDL or HDL concentration. This generalization applies to lignin, cellulose, bagasse and cereal bran from wheat and corn. Oat bran, which is partly mucilaginous, may be an exception[116]. Mucilaginous fibre, like non-mucilaginous fibre seems to have no influence on serum VLDL and probably HDL concentrations, but it does decrease serum LDL levels[117,118]. The two mucilaginous fibres which have been most studied are pectin, a substantial component of the connective tissue of citrus fruits and apples and pears, and guar gum derived from the seeds of the Indian cluster bean (*Cyamopsis tetragonolabata*). The cholesterol-lowering effect, however, only occurs when quantities of several grammes are ingested and so it is difficult to see how the quantities of mucilaginous vegetable fibre present in any natural diet can be of any major importance in determining the serum cholesterol. In one study for example, we observed an 8% decrease in serum cholesterol when pectin 10 g daily was consumed; a similar dietary intake could only have been achieved if some 2.5 kg of apples had been eaten every day[10]. Both pectin and guar are quite unpalatable in their extracted forms in the quantities necessary to influence cholesterol. There have been a number of attempts to make them more palatable, particularly guar, which may also have a favourable effect on glycaemic control in diabetes[119,120], but its place in patient management should be evaluated alongside pharmacological agents of proven efficacy and should not be considered in a nutritional context.

In addition to the effect of adding extracted vegetable fibre to the pre-existing diet, attempts have also been made to determine the effects of fibre in whole foods on serum cholesterol. Such experiments, which involve the introduction of cereals, fruit or pulses into the diet in place of other nutrients, are clearly very difficult to design, if the effect of the fibre is to be seen in isolation from any alteration in fat, carbohydrate or energy intake. In general, evidence that fibre in fruits and vegetables has some hypocholesterolaemic effect is better than for most of the cereals so far studied, as might be expected from experiments with fibre extracts.

The overall impression must be that effects of dietary fibre on serum lipids are seldom more than marginal. It should not therefore be assumed that one aim of a lipid-lowering diet must be to increase fibre intake. The effects of decreasing saturated fat consumption are much greater and are the first priority. Where dietary energy is to be replaced, an increase in carbohydrate should replace at least part of the energy deficit. This will inevitably increase fibre intake, but evidence that specific advice to increase fibre intake beyond that will produce any additional lipid-lowering is poor. As part of a reducing diet, low energy, fibre-rich foods may prove helpful to some patients and the suggestion that fibre can be an obstacle to energy intake[121] is probably not without foundation. In the energetic lean patient, for example a youngster who is a heterozygote for FH, this may be a positive disadvantage, however. Also many patients do not like eating lots of vegetable fibre and it is important to see that they do not have any misconceptions about the most important aim of their diet: a reduction in saturated fat consumption. Fibre can also be an obstacle to dietary compliance. In the 'cholesterol-lowering diet stakes' it probably also trails behind decreasing dietary cholesterol, and increasing unsaturated fats, which although coming home behind reduction in saturated fat, will not be far out of the finishing frame.

## Dietary antioxidants and pro-oxidants

With the current interest in oxidative modification of LDL as an important process in atherogenesis and plaque rupture attention has focused on nutrients that might influence the susceptibility of LDL to oxidation. At the present time we do not have hard evidence that antioxidants can alter the natural history of human atheroma. We do, however, have excellent evidence that lowering LDL cholesterol whether by diet or drugs does reduce both IHD morbidity and mortality (Chapter 6, page 148). This should therefore remain a primary aim of nutritional therapy. Furthermore, a more effective means of decreasing oxidatively modified LDL is probably to lower the levels of LDL so that it is not there to be oxidized rather than leaving the LDL level unchanged and trying to protect it against oxidation.

There is epidemiological evidence that plasma vitamin E is inversely related to IHD both from intra- and inter-population studies[122,123]. The most biologically active vitamin E, alpha-tocopherol, is the most abundant on LDL, although another lipid-soluble non-vitamin antioxidant, ubiquinol-10 is also present in substantial quantity[124]. When LDL is subjected to oxidizing conditions experimentally, the initial lag phase before conjugated dienes are detectable is thought to relate to its antioxidant components. This phase can be extended by dietary supplementation with vitamin D. However, it does not correlate well with the alpha-tocopherol content of LDL. Other factors such as ubiquinol-10 and also the degree of unsaturation of the fatty acyl groups of its lipids may also be important. So also may other as yet unknown factors and it must not be forgotten that *in vivo* the water-soluble antioxidant systems, such as vitamin C, will also be on hand to replenish the antioxidant capacity of the first-line fat-soluble antioxidants present in LDL. It is also not necessarily the case that delaying conjugated diene formation by a few minutes would have any influence on lipid-peroxide formation over several hours[125]. The possibility that a relatively innocuous substance such as vitamin E might confer protection from IHD is, however, worthy of clinical trials.

The more double bonds in a fatty acyl group theoretically the more susceptible a fat containing it should be to oxidation. This is why fish oils rapidly deteriorate unless they are stored in the presence of antioxidants or air is excluded. Linoleic acid too is more susceptible than oleic acid to oxidation. There is now some experimental evidence to suggest that diets differing only in their relative proportions of oleic and linoleic acid alter the susceptibility of LDL to lipid peroxidation[126,127]. Fish oil might be expected to make LDL even more susceptible, but this would depend on whether it actually was incorporated into LDL lipids in sufficient quantity. Considerations such as that and also the effect of a fat on the LDL concentration and other risk factors mean that we are not yet in a position to recommend the use of a particular fat on the basis of its susceptibility to oxidation. The Mediterranean diet is not simply rich in olive oil, but also in polyunsaturated fats, fruit, vegetables and antioxidants.

## Other nutrients and dietary constituents

Only the constituents of our diet reviewed so far have been shown to have any major influence on lipoprotein metabolism. Experiments with protein are hard to perform, if alterations in the intake of other macronutrients are to be avoided. Such experiments as have been reported suggest only marginal effects[128–130]. Lecithin too, a popular panacea from health food shops for the patient with coronary disease, may have some effect in decreasing cholesterol absorption[131,132], but its effect on serum lipids is trivial[131,133,134]. Garlic[135], walnuts and perhaps almonds[136], vitamin C[137] and trace elements[138] all have their advocates. Unfortunately they are supplied by health food shops at smaller doses than that used in trials suggesting an effect on serum lipid levels. I do not stop patients from taking any of these, but it is important to point out to them that the benefit they will derive from other measures is more certain. Coffee has its critics[139], but its effect is too small to advise limitation of its intake on present evidence.

# Background considerations to dietary recommendations for the general population and for patients with hyperlipidaemia

Most people in the world live on a diet which is much richer in carbohydrate and contains much less fat (and often energy) than the populations of countries of predominantly Northern European descent. Such a diet is associated with lower rates of both ischaemic heart disease and diabetes mellitus. Despite this, the view was promulgated in the post-war years that carbohydrate was in some way harmful. This is, of course, understandable since during the war and in the immediate post-war years the nutritional crisis facing many populations in Northern Europe was a deficiency of dietary energy. It was sensible to transport fatty foods into Europe from countries outside, since a ship-load of fat contains vastly more energy than a ship-load of grain. This is because, as was discussed in Chapter 1 (page 8), fat yields 9 cal/g whereas even refined carbohydrate yields only 4 cal/g, and cereals and potatoes and other natural carbohydrate foods much less than that. In the post-war years the production of fat by farmers was greatly encouraged by premiums on fatty livestock and fatty milk, and the egg industry was organized on an unprecedented scale. At one stage, even soap was rationed in Britain so that the fat that might normally have been used in its manufacture could be diverted into margarine and cooking oil. Later, premium bonds were given as prizes to people found eating eggs for breakfast. In fact, fat has historically occupied a special place in the cuisine of Northern Europe, with a great variety of ways of conserving fat and improving its flavour practised by the good mother and the restaurateur: sausages, pâté, fatty hams (smoked, preserved, rancified, etc.), cheeses of all kinds, etc. This was, of course, eminently sensible when frequent wars, revolutions, crop failures and so on meant that a substantial proportion of the European population was undernourished and vulnerable to infections much of the time. Indeed, the provision of more fatty foods would be advantageous in those countries facing similar problems today where only inadequate supplies of rice or maize are available.

It is no longer sensible in countries with a Northern European culture to persist with a high dietary fat intake, particularly saturated fat, when this is the cause of the greater part of our premature mortality and serious morbidity. Also, with central heating and motor cars, two major sources of energy expenditure, heat conservation and exercise, are not part of our routine existence and our energy needs are even less. We can afford the luxury of a diet which contains foods which are chosen for their flavour and variety, rather than their energy content. It is important to remember that what is frequently described as a traditional diet is neither traditional nor even natural. It has arisen out of necessity and often deliberate nutrition policy by our governments. The various mutations that have been bred into our modern cows, pigs and sheep, and the rich nourishment which they receive throughout the year as a result of modern agricultural methods, mean that the meat they produce can bear little relationship to the 'roast beef of Old England' or their high fat milk to the 'curds and whey' Miss Muffet consumed. The 'traditional' cow was leaner and accustomed to grazing on poorer pasture and covering more ground in so doing. Its milk contained less fat (triglycerides) and its carcass much less depot fat (triglycerides) and proportionately more structural fat (phospholipid). The suggestion that the adipose tissue running through the flesh of modern meat or left untrimmed before cooking improves its flavour is incorrect, since a greater contribution to its flavour comes from the phospholipid present largely in the membranes of the myocytes of the flesh. Meats such as venison, from an animal that has not gone through the same intensive breeding, remain as they always have been, low in triglycerides.

There does not appear to be any case on medical grounds for retaining saturated fat in our diet. None of the saturated fatty acids is essential and we are capable of synthesizing them ourselves. It would be hard to argue that the fall in HDL cholesterol which accompanies their removal is harmful, when one makes comparison with those parts of the world where coronary disease is uncommon. In the UK, the average consumption of fat is about 85 g/day, equivalent to 41% of dietary energy intake[140]. The great bulk of this is in the form of triglycerides. The next most common dietary fat is phospholipid and then cholesterol which is less than 1 g/day and seldom more than 500 mg. Of the fatty acids in these fats, some 40% are saturated. Most dietary unsaturated fatty acid is the mono-unsaturated fatty acid oleic acid. The most common polyunsaturated fatty acid is linoleic, often less than 10% of the total fat. The bulk of the saturated fats and oleic acid come from dairy products, spreads and cooking fats, meats and meat products, cakes and biscuits. Clearly, any attempt to reduce the intake of saturated fat will reduce dietary energy intake and another source must be substituted (except in the obese). It is usually recommended that a substantial part of this energy deficit should be met by carbohydrate.

There is very little evidence that carbohydrate is harmful. It seems to improve glucose tolerance rather than cause it to deteriorate (see Chapter 11, page 295). How frequently the rise in VLDL with carbohydrate is sustained is unknown, but it is likely that it is not very significant in terms of atherosclerosis risk. Refined carbohydrate, in particular sucrose, has received much condemnation[141,142], but it should be remembered that Cuba, which has the highest per capita consumption of sucrose, also has one of the lowest rates of coronary disease, and that the hypothesis linking sucrose with ischaemic heart disease has been refuted in detail[1]. Nevertheless, it does not seem sensible to encourage the use of sucrose, since it may have other disadvantages such as tooth decay. Any realistic increase in dietary carbohydrate, in any case, involves the greater consumption of foods such as potatoes, beans, pasta, rice, flour and other vegetables. Inevitably this will cause some increase in dietary fibre. Dietary fibre may be beneficial in preventing some diseases other than coronary disease, but it should be remembered, particularly in advising the patient with hyperlipidaemia, that an increase in dietary fibre is not a primary aim of the diet. Some patients do not like high fibre diets and their resentment may make them rebel against more important goals such as the reduction of saturated fat intake. There is no good evidence that cereal fibre influences serum lipids, there is some evidence which would support a small cholesterol-lowering effect of fibre in fruit and pulses. The epidemiological evidence linking high fibre intake with low coronary risk is most likely to result from its association with high carbohydrate and low fat intakes.

Substitution of saturated fat energy entirely with carbohydrate is not to the taste of many people and it imposes a limitation on the variety of meals. More importantly, in medical practice it may also not be feasible in, for example, the vigorous lean younger patients who are heterozygotes for familial hypercholesterolaemia. A 20-year-old man with FH actively engaged in sports can expend 2000 cal/day or more and, if he truly follows advice to decrease his saturated fat intake substantially, he will waste away, if only carbohydrate is offered as an energy source (unless, that is, he spends most of his day munching away). Polyunsaturated fat, particularly linoleic acid, present in sunflower oil, safflower oil, corn oil and soya bean oil, is one alternative source of calories. It can be consumed in cooking, dressings, margarine, cakes, biscuits, etc. For some odd reason, patients and sometimes dieticians seem to identify lipid-lowering diet with throwing out the chip pan, whereas in fact chips fried in linoleic acid-rich oils are an excellent source of calories. Oleic acid too may be included in the cholesterol-lowering diet. Olive oil may be a major source of calories in the diet of the Mediterranean countries, which enjoy relatively low levels of ischaemic heart disease, and the case for its wider use in lipid-lowering has recently been argued[37,74]. Most of the oleic acid consumption in populations such as those with a Northern Europe background is from animal fats, so switching to a diet low in saturated fat and increasing carbohydrate and linoleic acid consumption will not bring about any increase in oleic acid consumption: it may even decrease it[143]. One way to increase oleic acid consumption is to do as the Mediterranean population do and consume olive oil, which at the present time is expensive. The cheapest cooking oil is, however, rapeseed oil (called Canola in the USA and Canada). This can be produced in the cooler parts of Europe and North America and is almost as rich as olive oil in oleic acid (Table 9.1). This must be seriously regarded as an alternative to olive oil and answers the criticism that a healthy diet must necessarily be expensive.

There has been much discussion of fish oils (page 228) and, whatever the merits of the ω3 fatty acid in pharmacological doses, fish in the diet may be encouraged in most patients on a low saturated fat diet as the fatty fish are a valuable source of energy and non-fatty fish are helpful food for those trying to lose weight.

Since many populations habitually consume more fish than the UK currently does, side-effects from dietary consumption of fish (as opposed to the pharmacological consumption of fish oil) would seem to be remote. A similar argument may be advanced for the greater consumption of olive oil. In the case of linoleic acid, however, doubts linger about possible adverse effects, if it is consumed in large quantities for a protracted period of time. This is not because of any good evidence for any harmful effect[145,146], but because we know of no natural population in which it is a major source of dietary energy. It seems reasonable, therefore, to encourage its use as a substitute for only part of the saturated fat in our national diet. In the case of the hyperlipidaemic patient, who is at much greater risk than

**Table 9.1 The percentage of fatty acids in various fats[144]**

| | % fatty acids | | |
|---|---|---|---|
| | Saturated | Oleic | Linoleic |
| Spreads | | | |
| Polyunsaturated margarine | 18 | 20 | 50 |
| Butter | 69 | 28 | 3 |
| Cooking fats | | | |
| Sunflower oil | 12 | 25 | 63 |
| Corn oil | 12 | 30 | 54 |
| Beef fat | 51 | 39 | 2 |
| Lard (pork) | 39 | 45 | 10 |
| Rapeseed oil | 7 | 62 | 31 |
| Olive oil | 14 | 76 | 9 |

the general population, the same restraint need not apply, since the benefit of reducing the serum lipids will be greater and can be expected to outweigh any potential disadvantages. This is the major reason why bodies such as COMA (Committee on Medical Aspects of Food Policy)[147,148] and the National Institutes of Health Consensus Conference[149] made a distinction between diets which may reasonably be advocated for the population as a whole and individuals at greater than average risk of coronary disease. One advantage of including linoleic acid in a low saturated fat diet, rather than relying on carbohydrate as an energy source, is that it prevents the rise in serum triglycerides which might occur with carbohydrate alone[37]. This may not be so important in people whose serum triglyceride levels are not raised, because in them the carbohydrate-induced rise in serum triglycerides is probably not sustained. In patients with hypertriglyceridaemia, a decrease in saturated fat intake is a potent means of lowering triglycerides. In this circumstance, however, increased carbohydrate intake would tend to nullify this advantage and substitution of polyunsaturated fat has been shown to be clearly more effective in lowering serum triglycerides (much more so than the low carbohydrate diet[25,95], the use of which should be discontinued in clinical practice). Avoiding refined dietary sugars, certainly those containing fructose (fruit sugar, sucrose), may reduce the tendency to hyperuricaemia which is a feature of hypertriglyceridaemia[150].

## Specific dietary recommendations

### General population

The recommendations of the COMA panel for the diet in the UK would seem very reasonable based on present evidence: they represent a decrease in total fat intake on average from around 40% of dietary energy to 35% and a decrease in saturated fat intake of about one-quarter (Table 9.2). This policy could be pursued by promoting it to the general public, altering the composition of manufactured foods and adjusting the goals of the farming industry. The problem in instituting the diet does not seem to lie with the general public, who seem ready to follow the recommendations when they are properly presented[151,152]. This diet is not intended as a diet for an individual known to have a raised cholesterol. In the USA, the view has formed that dietary recommendations aimed at coronary prevention are likely to prove more successful if much more attention is paid to the individual, and they are therefore linked with an active programme to persuade the public to have their serum cholesterol measured[153].

**Table 9.2 Dietary recommendations of the Committee on Medical Aspects of Food Policy[147]**

| Dietary components | General population | High risk |
|---|---|---|
| Proportion of dietary energy* from: | | |
|   (i)   Fat | 35% | <30% |
|   (ii)  Saturated fat plus *trans* unsaturated fat | 15% | <10% |
|   (iii) P : S | 0.24 | towards 1 |
|   (iv) Unrefined carbohydrate | increase | increase |
| Cholesterol | decrease secondary to (i) and (ii) | <100 mg/1000 cal |
| Dietary fibre | increase secondary to (iv) | >30 g/day |

\* Excluding energy from alcohol.

## Patients with hypercholesterolaemias

There is general agreement about the diet which should be recommended for people found to have hyperlipidaemia. When serum cholesterol exceeds 200 mg/dl (5.2 mmol/l), dietary advice is required[154–156]. All agree that obesity when present should, if possible, be corrected. Dietary recommendations might be in the form of a simple diet sheet initially, and for patients whose cholesterol does not exceed 240 mg/dl in the USA or 6.5 mmol/l in Europe, a diet of the type recommended by COMA might suffice. For people with additional risk factors or more severe hypercholesterolaemia, a more stringent diet of the type described by COMA for the high risk individual would be applicable (Table 9.2). This might be explained by the physician or a nurse. This is broadly similar to the Step 1 diet of the National Cholesterol Education Program[153] developed from the American Heart Association Diet[157–159]. This programme recommends a further reduction of saturated fat intake (down to 7% of total dietary energy), the Step 2 diet, for those whose cholesterol remains elevated. However, my own view, which accords with that of the European Atherosclerosis Society[155] and the British Hyperlipidaemia Association[156], is that for patients whose cholesterol exceeds 260 mg/dl (6.5 mmol/l) despite the institution of the COMA high risk diet, the time has come to refer the patient to a qualified dietitian. This is because a dietary history is necessary to establish the individual's particular likes and dislikes and to design for him or her an enjoyable and acceptable diet. In the case of a male patient, it is important that the wife be present and her own culinary skills, household budget and the needs of the rest of the family be considered. It is also essential to discuss any misconceptions about the aims of the diet.

Mothers are frequently worried about sharing the diet with their children, but as long as it provides sufficient energy for growth there is no need for concern. Obviously in the younger child fat in milk is an essential source of energy, but certainly for children over 5 years old a low saturated fat diet is not harmful[147] and for those with familial hypercholesterolaemia it may with the cooperation of parents be instituted even sooner. Fortunately it is becoming much easier to adopt a low saturated fat diet with improvements in the quality and availability of vegetables and other low saturated fat foods, and as attitudes among cookery writers and teachers change. Against this must be set a growth in the market for instant foods, although this would be less worrying if manufacturers would follow recommendations such as those of COMA. More insidious is the growth of the use of the appellation 'healthy' to describe foods which have little to recommend them. For example, to describe a chip cooked in lard as healthy, because it contains vitamin C, is misleading. To label a margarine as 'low cholesterol' is also to mislead. Most oils and fats, since they come from the adipose tissue of animals or from plants, are low in cholesterol (in a steak, the fat actually contains less cholesterol than the lean meat, because cholesterol is a component of cell membranes which are more plentiful in muscle than in adipose tissue). The real question is whether they are low in saturated fat, and a glance at the label will often reveal the presence of substantial quantities of saturated fat or that the polyunsaturated fat present has been substantially hydrogenated.

Another myth is that whole milk is essential for health. Many people believe that without a pint of it each day, women will develop osteoporosis. In fact, skimmed milk contains more calcium than whole milk!

Recipe books, too, may frequently mislead. Many with the stated aim of cooking for healthy hearts contain recipes loaded with saturated fat. Often there is an undue preoccupation with dietary fibre and the more important advice about fat intake is flouted, many recipes containing large amounts of cheese and fatty meats such as lamb, pork and sausage.

Eating out generally remains a disaster for patients on a lipid-lowering diet. Even Italian, Greek, Turkish, Spanish, Japanese and Chinese restaurants may have Anglicized their menu so that these representatives of cuisines, which should be ideal, cannot invariably be trusted to have used the right oils or not to have smothered everything in cheese. Indeed Greek take-aways (doner kebabs) were among the worst for high fat content in one survey[160]. Set against this, fish and chips cooked in corn oil or sunflower oil will be much better. Indian restaurants provide probably the highest fat cuisine. People originating from the Indian subcontinent and living in Britain have about twice the risk of ischaemic heart disease of the indigenous population; part of the explanation for this may be a high intake of oxides of cholesterol formed in the production of ghee[161], although further evidence for this suggestion is needed. For the patient who is forced to entertain, be entertained or to spend time away from home for his or her living, dietary compliance may be a great problem. For the rest, if they are to remain reasonably sociable and not to be labelled as food freaks, they will have to compromise with their diet on occasions. Clearly the exception must not become the rule and this will not become the case if the home diet is right.

The diet in Table 9.3 is based on information from a variety of sources and references[39,162–165] and is intended to be rather more detailed than might be suitable for giving directly to patients. However, it is hoped that it will prove useful in planning individual diets and answering specific questions.

It should be emphasized that failure of a patient to achieve a low plasma cholesterol level by diet is not, in itself, a reason to introduce drug therapy. That decision will depend on a judgement of that individual's particular risk of ischaemic heart disease. It should also be emphasized that dietary treatment seldom is a failure: a decrease in serum cholesterol of only 1% represents a 2% decrease in ischaemic heart disease risk (Chapter 6, page 157). Thus, for example, in a patient with a serum cholesterol of 280 mg/dl (7 mmol/l) a decrease of only 7% to 260 mg/dl (6.5 mmol/l) represents a 14% reduction in risk. Since the first edition of this book an over-view of dietary trials of cholesterol-lowering diets has been published[166]. This suggests that the effect of the Step 1 diet on serum cholesterol is marginal and that more stringent dietary therapy is required to achieve clinically relevant decreases in cholesterol. To some extent this argument revolves around exactly how one decides whether a particular study used a diet which was more or less strict than the Step 1 diet[167]. The most important point, however, made by Ramsay and his colleagues, is that the effect of diet has been grossly overestimated in some of the guidelines for the management of hypercholesterolaemia. The most recent EAS ones[168] state that the vast majority of people with serum cholesterol levels of 7.8 mmol/l (300 mg/dl) will be able to achieve levels of 6.5 mmol/l (250 mg/dl) or from 6.5 mmol/l (250 mg/dl) to 5.2 mmol/l (200 mg/dl). The danger is that patients who fail to do this (in actual fact the majority) may be prescribed lipid-lowering drugs for this reason alone. This will, of course, not happen if the statement at the beginning of this paragraph, unaltered from the earlier edition of this book, is followed.

## Patients with hypertriglyceridaemia

*Serum triglycerides between 180 and 1000 mg/dl (2 and 11 mmol/l)*

Patients with serum triglycerides in this range should generally be treated by diet in the same way as has been discussed in the foregoing section: weight reduction for the obese by a diet in which fat intake, particularly saturated fat, is decreased, with replacement of energy in the non-obese by unrefined carbohydrate foods and polyunsaturated and mono-unsaturated fats.

*Serum triglyceride exceeding 1000 mg/dl (11 mmol/l)*

Most patients in this group will have chylomicronaemia (usually type V or more rarely type I hyperlipoproteinaemia) (Chapter 7, page 197). If the cholesterol is also high, type III hyperlipoproteinaemia should be excluded (Chapter 8).

Patients with severe hypertriglyceridaemia of this type are at risk of acute pancreatitis, certainly when the levels exceed 2000–3000 mg/dl (20–30 mmol/l). Various secondary causes should always be excluded (Chapter 11). Alcohol may frequently be a major factor in the aetiology of the condition and it is essential to dramatically reduce or abolish its intake. Obesity too is often present and weight reduction, as in the other hyperlipoproteinaemias, is an essential part of management. The diet for patients with chylomicronaemia, however, differs from that for the other hyperlipoproteinaemias in that it must be low in fat of all types. This is because the triglyceride-rich chylomicrons are formed by the gut in response to all long-chain fatty acids in the diet, regardless of whether they are saturated. In some patients, a decrease of fat intake to 30–35 g/day is sufficient, but in others further reductions may be necessary. Diets containing 10 g/day or less of fat are extremely difficult, since they require meticulous compliance and weighing of food items by the patient, but they are only rarely required. Admission to a metabolic ward is very helpful for the patient whose dietary fat intake must be 30 g/day or less, for instruction and to assess its effectiveness. Carbohydrate is the only nutrient which can realistically be substituted for the fat. This may cause an endogenous hypertriglyceridaemia in its own right due to carbohydrate induction (page 235). A careful balance may thus have to be drawn between exogenous and endogenous hypertriglyceridaemia when arriving at a satisfactory diet. Fortunately, normal levels of triglyceride do not have to be achieved to abolish attacks of acute pancreatitis, and many patients will be free of attacks even with levels as high as 2000–3000 mg/dl (20–30 mmol/l).

Medium-chain triglycerides and fish oils are frequently discussed in the context of hyperchylomicronaemia. It should be remembered that both of these, like fat restriction itself, are double-edged swords. In the case of medium-chain triglycerides, in theory they may be used as energy supplements since they do not lead to chylomicron formation (Chapter 1, page 22). In practice, however, the products containing them may also contain fatty acids of chain length greater than 10, which will enter chylomicrons, and the medium-chain triglycerides, themselves, when they arrive at the liver via the portal blood, may be taken up by the liver and, if the patient is not starving, they will be synthesized into long-chain triglycerides and secreted as VLDL, which will contribute to the hypertriglyceridaemia. Fish oils which are rich in highly polyunsaturated fatty acids, such as eicosapentaenoic acid, have also been used in the treatment of type V hyperlipoproteinaemia. They would, however, be expected to contribute to chylomicronaemia, just as much as

**Table 9.3 A lipid-lowering diet which embodies most of the principles discussed in this chapter***

| | Eat/drink regularly | Eat/drink in moderation | Avoid eating/drinking |
|---|---|---|---|
| CEREAL FOOD | Wholemeal flour<br>Oatmeal<br>Wholegrain bread<br>Wholegrain cereals<br>Crispbreads<br>Wholegrain, rice and pasta<br>Popcorn, (without butter or sugar), sweetcorn<br>*Homemade cakes, biscuits, pastries and pizzas, using permitted oils*<br>*Chapatis made without fat* | *White flour*<br>*White bread*<br>*Sugar-coated breakfast cereals*<br>*White rice*<br>*Pasta without added egg*<br>*Muesli without coconut or fat (consult label)*<br>Water biscuits | Fancy breads, e.g. croissants, Danish pastries, sponges, choux pastry, and all bought cakes.<br>Savoury cheese biscuits, cream crackers, biscuits |
| FRUIT, VEGETABLES AND SALAD | All fresh, frozen, dried, *bottled or tinned fruit*, vegetables and salad, especially peas, beans, lentils, pulses and potatoes (baked or boiled)<br>Olives<br>*Ratatouille made with permitted oil* | *Chips and roast potatoes in permitted oil*<br>*Avocado pears* | Potato crisps and savoury snacks.<br>Chips and roast potatoes cooked in unsuitable oil or fat |
| NUTS | *Walnuts*<br>*Almonds*<br>*Pecan nuts*<br>*Chestnuts*<br>*Hazel (filbert) nuts* | *Brazil nuts*<br>*Peanuts*<br>*Pistachio nuts*<br>*Cashew nuts*<br>*Macadamia nuts*<br>(If you are a vegetarian you must eat more regularly) | Coconut |
| FISH | All fresh, frozen, canned, smoked, soused fish<br>Avoid battered fish<br>Watch tinned fish (olive oil, sunflower oil, brine, tomato sauce permitted, but not vegetable oil)<br>*Avoid oily fish and fried fish only if you are on a weight-reducing diet* | Shellfish:<br>(a) Crustaceans (crabs, lobsters, crayfish, langoustines, shrimps, prawns, etc.) in modest amounts<br>(b) Molluscs (oyster, mussels, whelks, winkles, scallops, coquilles, clams, abalone, squid, octopus) a little more generously | Fish roe<br>Taramasalata, caviar<br>Fish paste (unless made with permitted oils only)<br>Potted fish<br>Sweetbreads<br>Fish fried in unsuitable oil or smothered in cheese |

| | | | |
|---|---|---|---|
| MEAT | Chicken and turkey (without skin) Veal Well-trimmed grilled steak Rabbit, hare, grouse, partridge, pheasant Venison Soya protein meat substitute | Lean mince beef, boiled and fat skimmed off before draining *and frying in permitted oil, to use in chilli, spaghetti sauce, etc.* | Ham, beef, pork, lamb, bacon, duck, goose, offal, liver, kidney, tripe, sweetbreads, heart, brain. Crackling and skin Sausage Salami Luncheon meat Paté, corned beef Scotch eggs, meat pies and pasties |
| PREPARED FOODS AND MADE-UP DISHES | Home made is the basic rule Jelly, sorbet | Ice cream | All bought frozen, tinned, dried or packet prepared meals and dishes, soups and sauces |
| SWEETS, PRESERVES, JAMS AND SPREADS | Chutneys and pickles Sugar-free artificial sweetners, *jam, marmalade, honey* | *Added sugar (sucrose), fruit sugar (fructose), boiled sweets, fruit pastilles and jellies, peppermints* | Chocolates, chocolate spreads and sweets Toffees, fudge Butterscotch, lemon curd, mincemeat, meat and fish pastes, spreads, coconut bars, etc. |
| DRINKS | Marmite, Bovril, tea, coffee, mineral water *Avoid fruit juice, fizzy drinks and squashes if on a weight-reducing diet unless they are low in calories or sugar* | Alcohol-containing drinks (there may be no reason for you to be more zealous in this regard than the general population unless you receive specific advice from your doctor) *Avoid beer, sweet sherry, wine and mixers containing sugar if on a weight-reducing diet* | Wholemilk drinks, bought soups, cream-based liqueurs Malted milk or hot chocolate drinks – check fat content even when label says 'low fat' |

**Table 9.3** continued

| | Eat/drink regularly | Eat/drink in moderation | Avoid eating/drinking |
|---|---|---|---|
| EGGS AND DAIRY PRODUCE | Skimmed milk<br>Dried skimmed milk<br>Soya milk<br>Low fat yoghurt<br>Cottage cheese<br>Low fat curd cheese<br>Egg white (meringue) (3 eggs yolks per week only) | | Whole milk, cream, imitation cream, full fat yoghurt<br>Evaporated or condensed milk<br>Excess eggs<br>Hard cheese, cream cheese or processed cheese (most hard cheeses 31–35 g/100 g fat of which two-thirds is saturated fat). Lymeswold is the worst (41% fat); Edam, Gouda, Brie, Camembert, Feta and proprietary low fat hard cheeses have lower than average fat content<br>Quiche, soufflé, Welsh rarebit, Crocque monsiuer, cheese pizza, cooked cheese dishes |
| FATS | All fats should be limited | *Corn oil, sunflower oil, safflower oil, soya oil, olive oil, rapeseed oil, wheatgerm oil, sesame seed oil, poppyseed oil, grapeseed oil*<br>*Margarine labelled 'high in polyunsaturates' or 'high in linoleic acid'*<br>*Ignore 'low in cholesterol'. Saturated fat should be less than 15 g/100 g*<br>Low fat spreads | Butter, dripping, suet, lard, margarine, shortening, ghee, cocobutter, cooking oil, or vegetable oil of unspecific origin.<br>Palm oil, coconut oil, cotton seed oil, peanut oil<br>Peanut butter (especially if hydrogenated) |

SAUCES AND DRESSINGS

| | | |
|---|---|---|
| Herbs, spices, garlic, watercress<br>Lemon and lemon juice<br>Tomato purée and sauce, brown sauce,<br>  Tabasco, soy, anchovy, Worcestershire,<br>  Tandoori sauces (made with yoghurt)<br>Mint sauce and jelly<br>Redcurrant jelly<br>Vinegar, chutneys and pickles,<br>  Cumberland sauce, olive oil<br>Home-made dressings with permitted<br>  oils, e.g. French dressing, vinaigrette<br>  dressing, etc.<br>Low fat yoghurt dressings, sweet and<br>  sour sauce, Portugaise and Provençale<br>  sauce<br>Bechamel (white or veloute) sauce made<br>  with permitted oil or margarine in<br>  place of butter, which may then be<br>  converted to a variety of sauces, e.g.<br>  parsley, caper, mussel, mustard, curry,<br>  wine, mushroom, veronique, anchovy,<br>  etc. | Sprinkling of Parmesan cheese<br>Bought low fat or low calorie salad<br>  dressings | Mayonnaise, ordinary salad cream or<br>  other cream dressings and sauces<br>  including Hollandaise, tartare and<br>  Aioli<br>Gravy<br>Brandy butter<br>Watch stuffings which may contain<br>  unsuitable ingredients |

* The three columns are based on the original idea of the Family Heart Association diet, but their contents is modified. In general, to occupy the 'Eat/drink regularly' column a food must contain less than 5 g/100 g saturated fat and, to be in the 'Avoid eating/drinking' column, more than 15 g/100 g saturated fat or more than 120 mg/100 g cholesterol. Some allowance has, however, been made for the quantities of foods to be eaten, to avoid senseless restrictions or liberalizations. The foods in italics should be avoided if the patient is attempting to lose weight. Conversely, the patient with a high energy expenditure or who becomes underweight may need to eat more of these foods.

any other long-chain fatty acid, and their triglyceride-lowering effect must be due to a decrease in the hepatic production of triglyceride. In a patient in the early phase of treatment, where chylomicronaemia still contributes substantially to the hypertriglyceridaemia, fish oil might therefore exacerbate it further. Later, when the patient has adapted to a very low fat, high carbohydrate diet and any persisting hypertriglyceridaemia is due to hepatic VLDL production, they may have a role in lowering serum triglyceride levels further. Care must therefore be exercised in their use in patients subject to recurring attacks of acute pancreatitis.

## Elevated serum lipoprotein (a)

There have been several publications suggesting that lipoprotein (a) levels can be decreased when they are initially high by various dietary means. Almost certainly the apparent changes were due to biological variation which is more marked when serum Lp(a) levels are high. In a well-conducted trial comparing diets which clearly altered serum cholesterol levels no parallel changes in serum Lp(a) were seen (169).

## References

1. Keys, A. Coronary heart disease – the global picture. *Atherosclerosis*, **22**, 149–192 (1975)
2. Keys, A. (ed.) Coronary heart disease in seven countries. *Circulation*, **41** (Suppl. 1), I1–21 (1970)
3. Report of a WHO Study Group. *Diabetes Mellitus. World Health Organization Technical Report Series* 727. WHO, Geneva (1985)
4. Editorial. New thoughts on the British diet. *Lancet*, **ii**, 143–144 (1984)
5. Hubert, H. B., Feinleib, M., McNamara, P. M. and Castelli, W. P. Obesity as an independent risk factor for cardiovascular disease: a 26 year follow-up of participants in the Framingham Heart Study. *Circulation*, **67**, 968–977 (1983)
6. Rabkin, S. W., Mathewson, F. A. L. and Hsu, P. H. Relation of body weight to development of ischaemic heart disease in a cohort of young North American men after a 26 year observation period: the Manitoba study. *Am. J. Cardiol.*, **39**, 452–455 (1977)
7. Cook, L. and the Pooling Project Research Group. Relationship of blood pressure, serum cholesterol, smoking habit, relative weight and ECG abnormalities to incidence of major coronary events: final report of the Pooling Project. *J. Chron. Dis.*, **31**, 201–311 (1978)
8. Leelarthaepin, B., Woodhill, J. M., Palmer, A. J. and Blackett, R. B. Obesity, diet and type II hyperlipidaemia. *Lancet*, **ii**, 1217–1221 (1974)
9. Wolf, R. N. and Grundy, S. M. Influence of weight reduction on plasma lipoproteins in obese patients. *Arteriosclerosis*, **3**, 160–169 (1983)
10. Katan, M. B. Diet and HDL. In *Clinical and Metabolic Aspects of High-density Lipoproteins* (eds N. E. Miller and G. J. Miller), Elsevier, Amsterdam, pp. 103–131 (1984)
11. Ahrens, E. H., Hirsch, J., Insull, W. and Peterson, M. L. Effects of dietary fats on serum lipid levels in man. *Trans. Assoc. Am. Phys.*, **70**, 224–233 (1957)
12. Hegsted, D. M., McGundy, R. B., Myers, M. L. and Stare, F. J. Quantitative effects of dietary fat on serum cholesterol in man. *Am. J. Clin. Nutr.*, **17**, 281–295 (1965)
13. Keys, A., Anderson, J. T. and Grande, F. Serum cholesterol response to changes in the diet. IV Particular saturated fatty acids in the diet. *Metabolism*, **14**, 776–787 (1965)
14. Grande, F., Anderson, J. T. and Keys, A. Comparison of the effects of palmitic and stearic acids in the diet on serum cholesterol in man. *Am. J. Clin. Nutr.*, **23**, 1184–1193 (1970)
15. Grande, F., Anderson, J. T. and Keys, A. Diets of different fatty acid composition producing identical serum cholesterol levels in man. *Am. J. Clin. Nutr.*, **25**, 53–60 (1972)
16. Bonanome, A. and Grundy, S. M. Effect of dietary stearic acid on plasma cholesterol and lipoprotein levels. *N. Engl. J. Med.*, **318**, 1244–1248 (1988)

17. Lichtenstein, A.H., Ausman, L.M., Carrasco, W., Jenner, J.L., Ordovas, J.M. and Schaefer, E.J. Hypercholesterolaemic effect of dietary cholesterol in diets enriched in polyunsaturated and saturated fat. *Arterioscler. Thromb.*, **14**, 168–175 (1994)

18. Mitropoulos, K.A., Miller, G.J., Martin, J.C. and Cooper, R.J. Dietary fat induces changes in factor VII coagulant activity through effects on plasma free stearic acid concentration. *Arterioscler. Thromb.*, **14**, 214–222 (1994).

19. Hashim, A., Artega, S. A. and van Itallie, T. B. Effects of a saturated medium-chain triglyceride on serum lipids in man. *Lancet*, **i**, 1105–1108 (1960)

20. Ahrens, E. J., Tsaltas, T. T., Hirsch, J. and Insull, W. Effects of dietary fat on the serum lipids of human subjects. *J. Clin. Invest.*, **34**, 918 (1955)

21. Ahrens, E. H., Hirsch, J., Insull, W., Tsaltas, T. T., Blomstrand, R. and Peterson, M. L. The influence of dietary fats on serum-lipid levels in men. *Lancet*, **i**, 943–953 (1957)

22. Antonis, A. and Bersohn, I. Influence of diet on serum triglycerides in South African White and Bantu prisoners. *Lancet*, **i**, 3–9 (1961)

23. Beveridge, J. M. R., Jogannathan, S. N. and Connel, W. F. The effect of the type and amount of dietary fat on the level of plasma triglyceride in human subjects and in the post-absorptive state. *Canad. J. Biochem. Physiol.*, **42**, 999 (1964)

24. Nestel, P. J., Carroll, K. F. and Havenstein, N. Plasma triglyceride response to carbohydrates, fats and caloric intake. *Metabolism*, **19**, 1–18 (1970)

25. Chait, A., Onitiri, A., Nicoll, A., Rabaya, E., Davies, J. and Lewis, B. Reduction of serum triglyceride levels by polyunsaturated fat. Studies on the mode of action and on very low density lipoprotein composition. *Atherosclerosis*, **20**, 347–364 (1974)

26. Durrington, P. N., Bolton, C. H., Hartog, M., Angelinetta, R., Emmett, P. and Furniss, S. The effect of a low-cholesterol, high-polyunsaturate diet on serum lipid levels, apolipoprotein B levels and triglyceride fatty acid composition. *Atherosclerosis*, **27**, 465–475 (1977)

27. Uzama, H., Schlierf, G., Chirman, S., Michals, G., Wood, P. and Kinsell, L. W. Hyperglyceridaemia resulting from intake of medium chain triglycerides. *Am. J. Clin. Nutr.*, **15**, 365–369 (1964)

28. Grande, F., Anderson, J. T. and Keys, A. Diets of different fatty acid composition producing identical serum cholesterol levels in man. *Am. J. Clin. Nutr.*, **25**, 53–60 (1972)

29. Malmros, H. and Wigand, G. The effect on serum cholesterol of diets containing different fats. *Lancet*, **ii**, 1–8 (1957)

30. Keys, A., Anderson, J. T. and Grande, F. Prediction of serum cholesterol responses of man to changes in fats in the diet. *Lancet*, **ii**, 959–966 (1957)

31. Keys, A., Anderson, J. T. and Grande, F. Effect on serum cholesterol in men of mono ene fatty acid (oleic acid) in the diet. *Proc. Soc. Exp. Biol. Med.*, **98**, 387–393 (1958)

32. Thomasson, H. J., de Boer, J. and De Inogh, H. Influence of dietary fats on plasma lipids. *Pathol. Microbiol.*, **30**, 629–647 (1967)

33. McGandy, R. B. and Hegsted, D. M. Quantitative effects of dietary fat and cholesterol on serum cholesterol in man. In *The Role of Fats in Human Nutrition* (ed. A. J. Vergroesen), Academic Press, London, pp. 211–230 (1975)

34. Mattson, F. H. and Grundy, S. M. Comparison of effects of dietary saturated, monounsaturated and polyunsaturated fatty acids on plasma lipids and lipoproteins in man. *J. Lipid Res.*, **26**, 194–202 (1985)

35. Mensink, R.P. and Katan, M.B. Effect of monounsaturated fatty acids versus complex carbohydrates on high-density lipoproteins in healthy men and women. *Lancet*, **i**, 122–125 (1987)

36. Valsta L.M. *et al.* Effects of monounsaturated rapeseed oil and polyunsaturated sunflower oil diet on lipoprotein levels in humans. *Arteriosclerosis*, **12**, 50–57 (1992)

37. Grundy, S. M. Dietary therapy of hyperlipidaemia. *Ballière's Clin. Endocrinol. Metabol.*, **1**, 667–698 (1987)

38. Mensink, R.P. and Katan, M.B. Effect of dietary trans fatty acids on high-density and low-density lipoprotein cholesterol levels in healthy subjects. *N. Engl. J. Med.* **323**, 439–445 (1990)

39. Hilditch, T. P. and Williams, P. N. *The Chemical Constitution of Natural Foods*, 4th edn, Chapman and Hall, London (1964)

40. Bang, H. O. and Dyerberg, J. Lipid metabolism and ischaemic heart disease in Greenland Eskimos. In *Advances in Nutrition Research* (ed. H. H. Draper), Plenum Press, New York, pp. 1–22 (1980)

41. Harris, W. S., Connor, W. E. and McMurry, M. P. The comparative reduction of the plasma lipids and lipoproteins by dietary polyunsaturated fats: salmon oil versus vegetable oils. *Metabolism*, **32**, 179–184 (1983)

42. Phillipson, B. E., Rothrock, D. W., Connor, W. E., Harris, W. S. and Illingworth, D. R. The reduction of plasma lipid, lipoproteins and apolipoproteins in hypertriglyceridaemic patients by dietary fish oils. *N. Engl. J. Med.*, **312**, 1210–1216 (1985)

43. Sandars, T. A. B. Fish and coronary artery disease. *Br. Heart J.*, **57**, 214–219 (1987)

44. Saynor, R., Verel, D. and Gillot, T. The long term effect of dietary supplementation with fish lipid concentrate on serum lipids, bleeding time, platelets and angina. *Atherosclerosis*, **50**, 3–10 (1984)

45. Schmidt, E.B. Kristensen, S.D., Caterina, R.D. and Illingworth, D.R. The effects of n-3 fatty acids on plasma lipids and lipoproteins and other cardiovascular risk factors in patients with hyperlipidaemia. *Atherosclerosis*, **103**, 107–121 (1993)

46. Mackness, M.I., Bhatnagar, D., Durrington, P.N. *et al*. Effects of a new fish oil concentration on plasma lipids and lipoproteins in patients with hypertriglyceridaemia. *Eur. J. Clin. Nutr.* (in press)

47. Sullivan, D. R., Sandars, T. A. B., Trayner, I. M. and Thompson, G. R. Paradoxical elevations of LDL apoprotein B levels in hypertriglyceridaemia patients and normal subjects ingesting fish oil. *Atherosclerosis*, **61**, 129–134 (1986)

48. Illingworth, D. R., Harris, W. S. and Connor, W. E. Inhibition of low density lipoprotein synthesis by dietary omega-3-fatty acids in humans. *Arteriosclerosis*, **4**, 270–275 (1984)

49. Bradlow, B. A., Chetty, N., Van der Westhuyzen, J., Mendelsohn, D. and Gibson, J. E. The effects of mixed fish diet on platelet functions, fatty acids and serum lipids. *Thromb. Res.*, **29**, 561–568 (1983)

50. Goodnight, S. H., Harris, W. S. and Connor, W. E. The effects of dietary ω3 fatty acids on platelet composition and function in man. A prospective, controlled study. *Blood*, **58**, 880–885 (1981)

51. Burr, M.L., Fehily, A.H., Gilbert, J.F. *et al*. Effects of change in fat, fish and fibre intakes on death and myocardial reinfarction: death and reinfarction trial (DART). *Lancet*, **ii**, 757–760 (1989)

52. Nichols, A. V., Dobbin, Y. and Gofman, J. W. Influence of dietary factors upon human serum lipoprotein concentrations. *Geriatrics*, **12**, 7–31 (1957)

53. Spritz, N. and Mishkel, M. A. Effects of dietary fats on plasma lipids and lipoproteins – an hypothesis for the lipid-lowering effect of unsaturated fatty acids. *J. Clin. Invest.*, **48**, 78–86 (1969)

54. Vega, G. L., Groszek, E., Wolf, R. and Grundy, S. M. Influence of polyunsaturated fats on composition of plasma lipoproteins and apolipoproteins. *J. Lipid Res.*, **23**, 811–822 (1982)

55. Glomset, J. A. The plasma lecithin: cholesterol acyltransferase reaction. *J. Lipid Res.*, **9**, 155–167 (1968)

56. Grundy, S. M. and Ahrens, E. H. The effects of unsaturated dietary fats on absorption, excretion, synthesis and distribution of cholesterol in man. *J. Clin. Invest.*, **49**, 1135–1152 (1970)

57. Wood, P. D. S., Lee, Y. L. and Kinsell, L. W. Determination of dietary cholesterol absorption in man. *Fed. Proc.*, **26**, 261 (1967)

58. Moore, R. B., Anderson, J. T., Taylor, H. L., Keys, A. and Frant, I. D. Effect of dietary fat on the fecal excretion of cholesterol and its degradation products in man. *J. Clin. Invest.*, **47**, 1517–1534 (1968)

59. Connor, W. E., Witiak, D. T., Stone, D. B. and Armstrong, M. L. Cholesterol balance and fecal neutral steroid and bile acid excretion in normal man fed dietary fats of different fatty acid composition. *J. Clin. Invest.*, **48**, 1363–1375 (1969)

60. Grundy, S. M. Effects of polyunsaturated fats on lipid metabolism in patients with hypertriglyceridaemia. *J. Clin. Invest.*, **55**, 269–282 (1975)

61. Kinsell, L. W., Wood, P. D. S., Shioda, R., Schlierf, R. and Lee, Y. L. Effect of diet on plasma, bile and fecal steroids. *Prog. Biochem. Pharmacol.*, **4**, 59–73 (1968)

62. Nestel, P. J., Havenstein, N., Whyte, H. M., Scott, T. J. and Cook, J. Lowering of plasma cholesterol and enhanced sterol excretion with the consumption of polyunsaturated ruminant fats. *N. Engl. J. Med.*, **288**, 379–382 (1973)

63. Nestel, P. J. and Barter, P. J. Metabolism of palmitic and linoleic acids in man: differences in turnover and conversion to glycerides. *Clin. Sci.*, **40**, 345–350 (1971)

64. Cortese, C., Levy, Y., Janus, E. D., Turner, P. R., Rao, S. N. *et al.* Modes of action of lipid-lowering diets in man: studies of apolipoprotein B kinetics in relation to fat consumption and dietary fatty acid composition. *Eur. J. Clin. Invest.*, **13**, 79–85 (1983)

65. Harris, W.S., Connor, W.E., Illingworth, D.R., Rothrock, D.W. and Foster, D.M. Effects of fish oil on VLDL triglyceride kinetics in humans. *J. Lipid. Res.*, **31**, 1549–1558 (1990)

66. International Collaborative Study Group. Metabolic epidemiology of plasma cholesterol. Mechanisms of variation of plasma cholesterol within populations and between populations. *Lancet*, **ii**, 991–996 (1986)

67. Nestel, P. J., Connor, W. R., Rearden, M. F., Connor, S., Wong, S. and Boston, R. Suppression by diets rich in fish oil of very low density lipoprotein production in man. *J. Clin. Invest.*, **74**, 82–89 (1984)

68. Spady, D.K. and Wollett, L.A. Interaction of dietary saturated and polyunsaturated triglycerides in regulating the processes that determine plasma low density lipoprotein concentrations in the rat. *J. Lipid Res.*, **31**, 1809–1819 (1990)

69. Thornburg, J.T. and Rudel, L.L. How do polyunsaturated fatty acids lower lipids? *Curr. Opin. Lipidol.*, **3**, 17 21 (1992)

70. Shepherd, J., Packard, C. J., Grundy, S. M. *et al.* Effects of saturated and polyunsaturated fat diets on the chemical composition and metabolism of low density lipoproteins in man. *J. Lipid. Res.*, **21**, 91–99 (1980)

71. Shepherd, J., Packard, C. J., Patsch, J. R., Gotto, A. M. and Taunton, O. D. Effects of dietary polyunsaturated and saturated fat on the properties of high density lipoproteins and the metabolism of apolipoprotein AI. *J. Clin. Invest.*, **61**, 1582–1592 (1978)

72. Pietinen, P. and Huttunen, J. K. Dietary determinants of plasma high-density lipoprotein cholesterol. *Am. Heart J.*, **113**, 620–625 (1987)

73. Grundy, S. M. Comparison of monounsaturated fatty acids and carbohydrates for plasma cholesterol lowering. *N. Engl. J. Med.*, **314**, 745–748 (1986)

74. Mensink, R. P. and Katan, M. B. Effect of monounsaturated fatty acids versus complex carbohydrates on high density lipoproteins in healthy men and women. *Lancet*, **i**, 122–125 (1987)

75. Kruiman, J., Westenbrink, S., Van der Hyeyden, L., West, C. E., Burema, J. *et al.* Determinants of total and high density lipoprotein cholesterol in boys from Finland, The Netherlands, Italy, The Philippines and Ghana with special reference to diet. *Human Nutr. Clin. Nutr.*, **37C**, 237–254 (1973)

76. Carlsen, L. A. and Kolmodin-Hedman, B. Decrease in alpha-lipoprotein cholesterol in men after cessation of exposure to chlorinated hydrocarbon pesticides. *Acta Med. Scand.*, **201**, 375–376 (1977)

77. Durrington, P. N. Effect of phenobarbitone on plasma apolipoprotein B and plasma high-density lipoprotein cholesterol in normal subjects. *Clin. Sci.*, **56**, 501–504 (1979)

78. Luoma, P. V., Sotaniemi, E., Pelkonen, R. O., Arranto, E. and Elnolm, C. Plasma high density lipoproteins and hepatic microsomal enzyme induction. Relation to histological changes in the liver. *Eur. J. Clin. Pharmacol.*, **23**, 275–282 (1982)

79. Fraser, H. S., Bulpitt, C. J., Kahn, C., Mould, G., Mucklow, J. C. and Dollery, C. T. Factors affecting antipyrine metabolism in West African villagers. *Clin. Pharmacol Ther.*, **20**, 369–376 (1976)

80. British Nutrition Foundation Task Force. *Report on Trans Fatty Acids*. The British Nutrition Foundation, London (1987)

81. Steinberg, D. Phytanic acid storage disease (Refsum's disease). In *The Metabolic Basis of Inherited Disease*, 5th edn (eds J. B. Stanbury, J. B. Wyngaarden, D. S. Fredrickson, J. L. Goldstein, and M. S. Brown), McGraw-Hill, New York, pp. 731–747 (1983)

82. Vles, R. O. P. Nutritional aspects of rapeseed oil. In *The Role of Fats in Human Nutrition* (ed. A. J. Vergroesen), Academic Press, London, pp. 433–477 (1975)

83. Beveridge, J. M. R., Connell, W. F., Mayer, A. G. and Haust, H. L. The response of man to dietary cholesterol. *J. Nutr.*, **71**, 61–65 (1960)

84. Connor, W. E., Hodges, R. E. and Bleiler, R. A. The serum lipids in men receiving high cholesterol and cholesterol-free diets. *J. Clin. Inves.*, **40**, 894–901 (1961)

85. Keys, A. Serum cholesterol response to dietary cholesterol. *Am. J. Clin. Nutr.*, **40**, 351–359 (1984)

86. Kesaniemi, A.Y., Ehnholm, C. and Miettinen, T.A. Intestinal cholesterol absorption efficiency in man is related to apoprotein E phenotype. *J. Clin. Invest.*, **80**, 578–581 (1987)

87. Dreon, D.M. and Krauss, R.M. Gene-diet interactions in lipid metabolism. In *Molecular Genetics of Coronary Artery Disease. Candidate Genes and Processes in Atherosclerosis* (eds A. J. Lusis, J. I. Rotter, and R. S. Sparkes), Karger, Basle, 14, pp. 325–349 (1992)

88. Packard, C. J., McKinney, L., Carr, K. and Shepherd, J. Cholesterol feeding increases low density lipoprotein synthesis. *J. Clin. Invest.*, **72**, 45–51 (1983)

89. Mistry, F., Miller, N. E., Laker, M., Hazzard, W. B. and Lewis, B. Individual variation in the effects of dietary cholesterol on plasma lipoproteins and cellular homeostasis in man. *J. Clin. Invest.*, **67**, 493–502 (1981)

90. Thorogood, M., Carter, R., Benfield, L., McPhewn, K. and Mann, J. I. Plasma lipids and lipoprotein cholesterol concentrations in people with different diets in Britain. *Br. Med J.*, **295**, 351–353 (1987)

91. Miller, N. E. Why does plasma low density lipoprotein in adults increase with age? *Lancet*, **i**, 263–266 (1984)

92. Grundy, S. M., Vega, G. L. and Bilheimer, D. W. Kinetic mechanisms determining variability in low density lipoprotein levels and their rise with age. *Arteriosclerosis*, **5**, 623–630 (1985)

93. Glueck, C. J., Waldman, G., McClish, D. K. *et al.* Relationships of nutrient intake of lipids and lipoproteins in 1234 white children. *Arteriosclerosis*, **2**, 523–536 (1982)

94. Mahley, R. W., Innerarity, T. L., Bersot, T. P., Lipson, A. and Margolis, S. Alterations in human high-density lipoproteins with or without increased plasma cholesterol, induced by diets high in cholesterol. *Lancet*, **ii**, 807–809 (1978)

95. Sommariva, D., Scotti, L. and Fasoli, A. Low-fat diet versus low-carbohydrate diet in the treatment of type IV hyperlipoproteinaemia. *Atherosclerosis*, **29**, 43–51 (1978)

96. Mann, J. I. and Truswell, A. S. Effects of isocaloric exchange of dietary sucrose and starch on fasting serum lipids, postprandial secretion and alimentary lipaemia in human subjects. *Br. J. Nutr.*, **27**, 395–405 (1972)

97. Lewis, B. Influence of diet, energy balance and hormones on serum lipids. In *The Hyperlipidaemias. Clinical and Laboratory Practice*, Blackwell, Oxford, pp. 131–180 (1976)

98. Havel, R. J. Early effects of fasting and of carbohydrate ingestion on lipids and lipoproteins of serum in man. *J. Clin. Invest.*, **36**, 855–859 (1957)

99. Durrington, P. N., Newton, R. S., Weinstein, D. B. and Steinberg, D. Effects of insulin and glucose on very low density lipoprotein triglyceride secretion by cultured rat hepatocytes. *J. Clin. Invest.*, **70**, 63–73 (1982)

100. Mancini, M., Mattock, M., Rabaya, E., Chait, A. and Lewis, B. Studies in the mechanism of carbohydrate-induced lipaemia in normal man. *Atherosclerosis*, **17**, 445–454 (1973)

101. Glueck, C. J., Levy, R. I. and Fredrickson, D. S. Immunoreactive insulin, glucose tolerance and carbohydrate inducibility in type II, III, IV and V hyperlipoproteinaemia. *Diabetes*, **18**, 739–747 (1969)

102. Ahrens, E. H., Hirsch, J., Oette, W., Farquhar, J. W. and Stein, Y. Carbohydrate-induced and fat-induced lipemia. *Trans. Assoc. Am. Phys.*, **74**, 134–146 (1961)

103. Fallon, H. J. and Kemp, E. L. Effect of diet of hepatic triglyceride synthesis. *J. Clin. Invest.*, **47**, 712–719 (1968)

104. Den Besten, L., Reyna, R. H., Connor, W. E. and Stegiuk, L. D. The different effects on the serum lipids and fecal steroids of high carbohydrate diets given orally or intravenously. *J. Clin. Invest.*, **52**, 1384–1393 (1973)

105. Schonfeld, G. and Kudzma, D. J. Type IV hyperlipoproteinaemia. *Arch. Intern. Med.*, **132**, 55–62 (1973)

106. Hall, Y., Stamler, J., Cohen, D. B., Majonnier, L., Epstein, M. B. *et al.* Effectiveness of a low saturated fat, low cholesterol, weight-reducing diet for the control of hypertriglyceridaemia. *Atherosclerosis*, **16**, 389–403 (1972)

107. Torsvik, H., Feldman, H. A., Fischer, J. E. and Lees, R. S. Effects of intravenous hyperalimentation on plasma-lipoproteins in severe familial hypercholesterolaemia. *Lancet*, **i**, 601–604 (1975)

108. Ernst, N., Fisher, M., Smith, W., Gordan, T., Rifkind, B. M. *et al.* The association of plasma high-density lipoprotein cholesterol with dietary intake and alcohol consumption. The Lipid Research Clinics Program Prevalence Study. *Circulation*, **62**, (Suppl. IV), 41–52 (1980)

109. Sacks, F. M., Castelli, W. P., Donner, A. and Wass, E. H. Plasma lipids and lipoproteins in vegetarians and controls. *N. Engl. J. Med.*, **292**, 1148–1151 (1975)

110. Kruiman, J. T. and West, C. E. The concentration of cholesterol in serum and in various serum lipoproteins in macrobiotic, vegetarian and non-vegetarian men and boys. *Atherosclerosis*, **43**, 71–82 (1982)

111. Thorogood, M. Vegetarianism, coronary disease risk factors and coronary heart disease. *Curr. Opin. Lipidol.*, **5**, 17–21 (1994)

112. Eastwood, M. A. and Passmore, R. Dietary fibre. *Lancet*, **i**, 202–206 (1983)

113. Wenlock, R. W., Buss, D. H. and Agater, I. B. New estimates of fibre in the diet in Britain. *Br. Med. J.*, **228**, 1873 (1984)

114. Kay, R. M. and Truswell, A. S. Dietary fiber: effects on plasma biliary lipids in man. In *Medical Aspects of Dietary Fiber* (eds G. A. Spiller and R. M. Kay), Plenum, New York, pp. 153–173 (1980)

115. Story, J. A. Dietary fiber and lipid metabolism: an update. In *Medical Aspects of Dietary Fiber* (eds G. A. Spiller and R. M. Kay), Plenum, New York (1980)

116. Anderson, J. W., Story, L., Sieling, B., Chen, W-J. L., Petro, M. S. and Story, J. Hypocholesterolaemic effects of oat-bran or bean intake for hypercholesteraemic men. *Am. J. Clin. Nutr.*, **40**, 1146–1155 (1984)

117. Durrington, P. N., Manning, A. P., Bolton, C. H. and Hartog, M. Effect of pectin on serum lipids and lipoproteins, wholegut-transit-time and stool weight. *Lancet*, **ii**, 394–396 (1976)

118. Jenkins, D. J. A., Leeds, A. R., Slavin, B., Mann, J. and Jepson, E. M. Dietary fibre and blood lipids: reduction of serum cholesterol in type II hyperlipidaemia by guar gum. *Am. J. Clin. Nutr.*, **32**, 16–18 (1979)

119. Anderson, J. W. *The Role of Dietary Carbohydrate and Fibre in the Control of Diabetes*, Year Book, St Louis, pp. 67–96 (1980)

120. Simons, L. A., Gayst, S., Balasubramanian, S. and Ruys, J. Long-term treatment of hypercholesterolaemia with a new palatable formulation of guar gum. *Atherosclerosis*, **45**, 101–108 (1982)

121. Heaton, K. W. Food fibre as an obstacle to energy intake. *Lancet*, **ii**, 1418–1420 (1972)

122. Riemersma, R.A., Wood, D.A., MacIntyre, C.C.A., Elton, R.A., Gey, K.F. and Oliver, M.F. Risk of angina pectoris and plasma concentrations of vitamins A, C and E and carotene. *Lancet*, **337**, 1–5 (1991)

123. Gey, K.F., Puska, P., Jordan., P. and Maser, U.K. Inverse correlation between plasma vitamin E and mortality from ischaemic heart disease in cross-cultured epidemiology. *Am. J. Clin. Nutr.*, **53**, 326S–334S (1991)

124. Stocker, R., Dowry, V.W. and Frei, B. Ubiquinol-10 protects human low density lipoproteins more efficiently against lipid peroxidation than does alpha tocopherol. *Proc. Natl Acad. Sci. USA*, **88**, 1646–1650 (1991)

125. Mackness, M.I., Abbott, C.A., Arrol, S. and Durrington, P.N. The role of high-density lipoprotein and lipid soluble anti-oxidant vitamins in inhibiting low-density lipoprotein oxidation. *Biochem. J.*, **294**, 829–834 (1993)

126. Reaven, P., Parthasarathy, S., Grasse, B.J., Miller, E., Almazan, F. *et al.* Feasibility of using an oleate-rich diet to reduce the susceptibility of low-density lipoprotein to oxidative modification in humans. *Am. J. Clin. Nutr.*, **54**, 701–706 (1991)

127. Bonanome, A. *et al.* Effect of dietary monounsaturated and polyunsaturated fatty acids on the suseptibility of plasma low density lipoproteins to oxidative modification. *Atherosclerosis*, **13**, 529–533 (1992)

128. Van Raaij, J. M. A., Katan, M. B., Hautvest, J. G. A. J. and Hermus, R. J. Effects of casein versus soy protein diets on serum cholesterol and lipoproteins in young healthy volunteers. *Am. J. Clin Nutr.*, **34**, 1261–1271 (1981)

129. Van Raaij, J. M. A., Katan, M. B., West, C. E. and Hautvast, J. G. A. G. Influence of diets containing Qsein, soy isolate and soy concentrate on serum cholesterol and lipoproteins in middle-aged volunteers. *Am. J. Clin. Nutr.*, **35**, 925–934 (1982)

130. Sacks, F. M., Breslow, J. L., Wood, P. G. and Wass, E. H. Lack of an effect of dairy protein (casein) and soy protein on plasma cholesterol of strict vegetarians. *J. Lipid Res.*, **24**, 1012–1020 (1983)

131. Beil, F. V. and Grundy, S. M. Studies on plasma lipoproteins during absorption of exogenous lecithin in man. *J. Lipid Res.*, **21**, 525–536 (1980)

132. Greten, H., Raetzer, H., Stiehl, A. and Schettler, G. The effect of polyunsaturated phosphatidyl-choline on plasma lipids and fecal sterol excretion. *Atherosclerosis*, **36**, 81–88 (1980)

133. Ter Welle, H. F., Van Gert, C. M., Dekker, W. and Willebrands, A. F. The effect of soya lecithin on serum lipid values in type II hyperlipoproteinaemia. *Acta Med. Scand.*, **195**, 267–271 (1974)

134. Childs, M. T., Bowlin, J. A., Ogilvie, J. T., Hazzard, W. R. and Albers, J. J. The contrasting effects of a dietary soya lecithin product and corn oil on lipoprotein lipids in normolipidemic and familial hypercholesterolic subjects. *Atherosclerosis*, **38**, 217–228 (1981)

135. Neil, A. and Silagy, C. Garlic: its cardio-protective properties. *Curr. Opin. Lipidol.*, **5**, 6–10 (1994)

136. Sabate, J. and Fraser, G.E. Nuts: a new protective food against coronary heart disease. *Curr. Opin. Lipidol.*, **5**, 11–16 (1994)

137. Hemila, H. Vitamin C and plasma cholesterol. *Crit. Rev. Food Sci. Nutr.*, **32**, 33–57 (1992)

138. Klevay, L.M. Elements of atherosclerosis. In *Proceedings of the First International Conference on Trace Elements in Health and Disease with Special Emphasis on Atherosclerosis* (ed. M. Reis), Portuguese Atherosclerosis Society, Lisbon (in press)

139. Editorial. Coffee and cholesterol. *Lancet*, **ii**, 1283–1284 (1985)

140. *Household Food Consumption and Expenditure Survey*, HMSO, London (1991)

141. Yudkin, J. Dietary carbohydrates and ischaemic heart disease. *Am. Heart J.*, **66**, 835–836 (1963)

142. Cleave, T. L., Campbell, G. D. and Painter, N. S. *Diabetes, Coronary Thrombosis and the Saccharine Disease*, J. Wright, Bristol (1969)

143. Durrington, P.N. Fats and the British Diet Lancet, 338, 1329–1330 (1991)

144. Durrington, P.N. Dietary fat and coronary heart disease. Chapter 13 in *Cardiovascular Disease Risk Factors and Intervention* (eds N. Poulter, P. Sever and S. Thom), Radcliffe Medical Press, Oxford, 119–127 (1993)

145. Heyden, S. Epidemiological data on dietary fat intake and atherosclerosis with an appendix on possible side effects. In *The Role of Fats in Human Nutrition* (ed. A. J. Vergroesen), Academic Press, London, pp. 43–113 (1975)

146. Mann, J. I. Fats and atheroma: a retrial. *Br. Med. J.*, **i**, 732–734 (1979)

147. Committee on Medical Aspects of Food Policy. Report of the Panel in Relation to Disease. *Report on Health and Social Subjects No. 28*, Department of Health and Social Security, HMSO, London (1984)

148. Committee on Medical Aspects of Food Policy. Report of the Panel on Dietary Reference Values. Dietary values for food energy and nutrients for the United Kingdom. *Report on Health and Social Subjects No. 41*, Department of Health and Social Security, HMSO, London (1991)

149. Consensus Conference. Lowering blood cholesterol to prevent heart disease. *J. Am. Med. Assoc.*, **253**, 2089–2090 (1985)

150. Bastow, M. D., Durrington, P. N. and Ishola, M. Hypertriglyceridaemia and hyperuricaemia: effects of two fibric acid derivatives (Bezafibrate and Fenofibrate) in a double-blind, placebo-controlled trial. *Metabolism*, **37**, 217–220 (1988)

151. Consumers' Association. *Facts and Health. Which?*, June, pp. 263–266 (1985)

152. Consumers' Association. *Healthy Eating. Which?*, Jan., pp. 16–21 (1986)

153. National Cholesterol Education Program. *Report of the Expert Panel on Detection, Evaluation and Treatment of High Blood Cholesterol in Adults*, National Institutes of Health, Bethesda, Maryland (1987)

154. NCEP (National Cholesterol Education Program) *J. Am. Med. Assoc.*, **269**, 3015–3023 (1993)

155. Pyorala, K., De Backer, G., Graham, I., Poole-Wilson, P. and Wood, D. Prevention of coronary heart disease in clinical practice: recommendations of the Task Force of the European Society of Cardiology, European Atherosclerosis Society and European Society of Hypertension. *Atherosclerosis*, **110**, 121–161 (1994)

156. Betteridge, D. J., Dodson, P. M., Durrington, P. N., Hughes, E. A. *et al.* Management of hyperlipidaemia: guidelines of The British Hyperlipidaemia Association. *Postgrad. Med. J.*, **69**, 359–369 (1993)

157. Grundy, S. M., Bilheimer, D., Blackburn, H., Brown, W. V., Kwiterovich, P. O. *et al.* Rationale of the diet – heart statement of the American Heart Association. Report of Nutrition Committee. *Circulation*, **65**, 839A–854A (1982)

158. Gotto, A. M., Bierman, E. L., Connor, W. E., Ford, C. H., Frantz, I. D. *et al.* Recommendations for treatment of hyperlipidaemia in adults. A joint statement of the Nutrition Committee and the Council on Arteriosclerosis. *Circulation*, **69**, 1067A–1090A (1984)

159. Council on Scientific Affairs of the American Heart Association. Dietary and pharmacologic therapy for the lipid risk factors, *J. Am. Med. Assoc.*, **250**, 1873–1879 (1983)

160. Pascoe, J., Dockerty, J. and Ryley, J. The nutrient composition of some takeaway foods in ethnic menu items. *Hum. Nutr. Appl. Nutr.* (Communication)

161. Jacobson, M. S. Cholesterol oxides in Indian ghee: possible cause of unexplained high risk of atherosclerosis in Indian immigrant populations. *Lancet*, **ii**, 656–658 (1987)

162. Paul, A. A. and Southgate, D. A. T. *McCance and Widdowson's 'The Composition of Foods'*, 4th edn, HMSO, London (1978)

163. Paul, A. A., Southgate, D. A. T. and Russell, J. *First supplement to McCance and Widdowson's 'The Composition of Foods'*, HMSO, London (1980)

164. Turner, D. *Handbook of Diet Therapy*, 3rd edn, University of Chicago Press, Chicago (1959)

165. Feeley, R. M., Griver, P. E. and Watt, B. K. Cholesterol content of foods. *J. Am. Diet Assoc.*, **61**, 134–149 (1972)

166. Ramsay, L.E., Yeo, W.W. and Jackson, P.R. Dietary reduction of serum cholesterol: time to think again. *Br. Med. J.*, **303**, 953–957 (1991)

167. Thompson, G.R. Dietary reduction of serum cholesterol concentration. *Br. Med. J.*, **303**, 1332 (1991)

168. Recommendations of the European Atherosclerosis Society. Prevention of coronary heart disease: scientific background and new clinical guidelines. *Nutr. Metabol. Cardiovasc. Dis.*, **2**, 113–156 (1992)

169. Brown, S.A., Morrisett, J., Patsch, J.R., Reeves, R., Giotto, A M and Patsch, W. Influence of short term dietary cholesterol and fat on human plasma Lp(a) and LDL levels. *J. Lipid Res.*, **32**, 1281–1289 (1991).

# Chapter 10

# Drug therapy of hyperlipidaemias

## Introduction

Drug therapy for lowering serum lipids should only be considered in patients who have failed to achieve satisfactory levels after an adequate trial of dietary treatment. Failure of dietary treatment is, however, not in itself an indication to commence drug therapy. In patients in whom the diagnosis of familial hypercholesterolaemia or type III hyperlipoproteinaemia has been made, persisting hyperlipidaemia after institution of diet almost invariably calls for drug intervention. In other patients, however, other factors are important. These include the extent of hyperlipidaemia, whether there is an adverse family history of coronary disease, the age and sex of the patients, whether they have any manifestations of arterial disease or have undergone coronary artery surgery, and the presence of other risk factors such as hypertension, diabetes and a history of smoking (Chapter 6, page 172). It is also important to arrive at as precise a diagnosis as is possible. Thus it is essential to exclude secondary causes and to have several lipoprotein measurements, including fasting triglycerides, cholesterol and HDL cholesterol, before initiating drug therapy.

Prescribing habits vary considerably throughout the world (Figure 10.1). In Japan and France, it seems that despite their low prevalence of coronary disease more lipid-lowering drugs are used than in any other countries. In Germany and Italy too, which are not among the leaders in ischaemic heart disease prevalence in Europe, treatment with hypolipidaemic agents is commonplace, whereas in the UK, parts of which now lead Europe, if not the world, in coronary disease rates and where it would be expected that attempts at coronary prevention would be most active, the prescription of lipid-lowering drugs is an exceptional practice. This is not because doctors in the UK are generally more conservative in their drug prescribing (Figure 10.2), because large quantities of diuretics and beta-blockers are used in the management of hypertension (which has only a limited place in the prevention of ischaemic heart disease). The rate of prescription of lipid-lowering drugs relative to antihypertensives is staggeringly lower in the UK (Table 10.1). It also cannot be said that worries about long-term safety have stayed the prescribers' hand in other areas of treatment, as witness the enormous number of prescriptions for non-steroidal anti-inflammatory agents, which continue to be a major source of iatrogenic morbidity and mortality. It is also the case that mild hypertension continues to be treated with drugs, despite the evidence that the great majority of patients do not benefit and often agents are employed which have never been shown to be as beneficial as older ones used in clinical trials or more severe hypertension.

That drug treatment in other areas of medicine is in such disarray is, of course, no reason for introducing similar confusion into the management of lipid disorders.

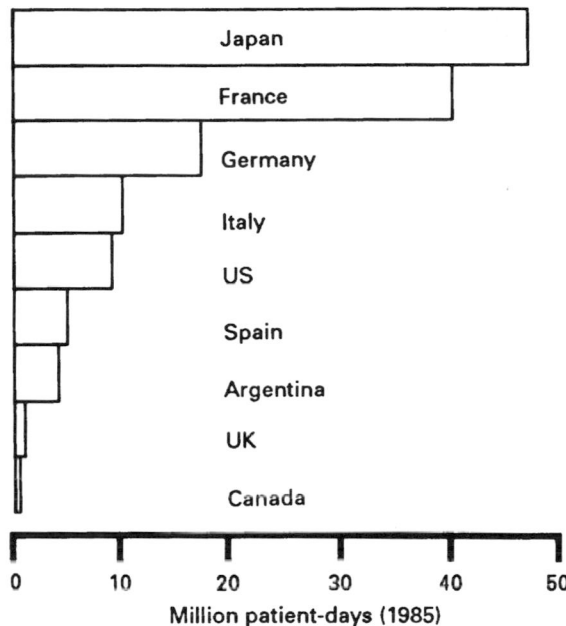

**Figure 10.1**  Number of patients treated for 1 day with lipid-lowering drugs in different countries. It seems that the quantity of prescriptions bears no direct relationship to the prevalence of hyperlipidaemia

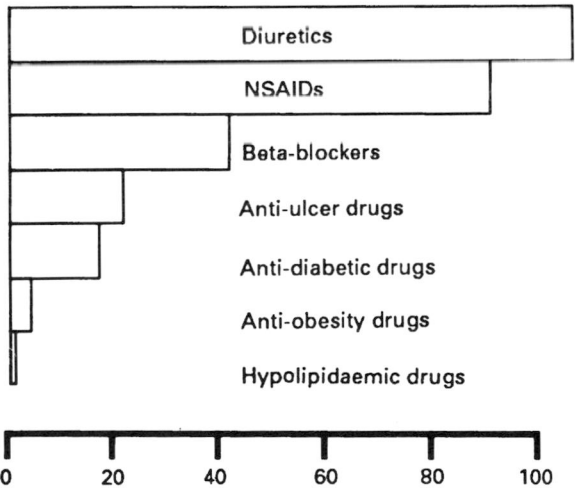

**Figure 10.2**  How prescribing of lipid-lowering drugs compares with the use of other drugs in the UK

**Table 10.1 The ratio of the prescribing (patient days per capita) of antihypertensive to lipid-lowering drugs in different countries**

| Nation | Prescribing of antihypertensive drugs relative to lipid-lowering drugs |
| --- | --- |
| Japan | 2.7 |
| France | 2.8 |
| Canada | 4.3 |
| Spain | 5.0 |
| USA | 5.6 |
| Italy | 6.2 |
| UK | 26.0 |

The precribing rates of antihypertensive agents is relatively constant at around 5 days per capita except in France, which is about double this. The table serves to show the attitude of physicians in different countries to the detection and treatment of hyperlipidaemia as opposed to that of hypertension.

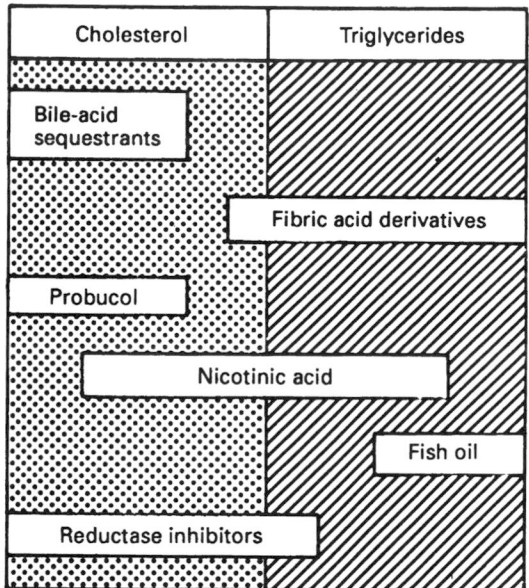

**Figure 10.3** Lipid-modifying drugs grouped according to whether their predominant action is on serum cholesterol or triglycerides

In fact, the conclusive evidence of benefit that has been demanded by the medical profession in many countries before the introduction of antihyperlipidaemic drugs into routine practice may in the long run turn out to be no bad thing. In the UK, however, cholesterol testing rates are low, with only 10% of the middle-aged population ever having had their serum cholesterol measured (as opposed to 40–50% in most countries with a similar level of prosperity). This chapter is intended to review the pharmacology and practical aspects of drug treatment for the hyperlipidaemias. Clearly, as our clinical experience with lipid-lowering agents lengthens and better methods for defining individual risk are developed, the use of these drugs will become more precisely defined and less a matter for clinical judgement.

The predominant effect of the different lipid-lowering drugs on serum cholesterol or triglycerides is shown in Figure 10.3.

## Bile-acid sequestrating agents

The bile-acid sequestrating agents or resins which are currently available are cholestyramine and colestipol. Their mode of action is usually considered to be similar. They are anion exchange resins which bind bile acids in the intestinal lumen. Since neither drug is absorbed, the reabsorption of bile acids, which normally occurs in the terminal ileum, is impeded and those bound are lost to the body with the bile-acid sequestrant in the faeces. The faecal bile-acid output is thus considerably increased[1–3]. Failure of reabsorption of bile acids is compensated by their enhanced hepatic synthesis from cholesterol, which is their precursor, via increased activity of cholesterol-7-hydroxylase, which is rate-limiting for bile-acid synthesis[4]. Therapy with bile-acid sequestrants has been shown to lower LDL cholesterol by increasing catabolism via the receptor-mediated pathway[5]. It is usually assumed that this increased receptor-mediated uptake is into the liver, since it is in this organ that the increased LDL receptor expression would be expected in response to increased demand for cholesterol (for conversion to bile acids).

Bile-acid sequestrating agents are effective in lowering serum LDL cholesterol and even in heterozygotes for FH with only one fully functional LDL receptor gene, they increase receptor-mediated LDL catabolism[5]. Patients who are homozygotes for FH do not respond to bile-acid sequestrants as would be anticipated, since by definition neither of their LDL receptor genes operates effectively. Until patients with heterozygous FH unable to tolerate either cholestyramine or colestipol did not usually achieve satisfactory cholesterol levels despite the use of other lipid-lowering agents. With the advent of the better tolerated HMG-CoA reductase inhibitors this situation has changed. The place of bile-acid sequestrants in current medical practice is currently undergoing considerable revision.

It is wrong to assume that HMG-CoA reductase inhibitors are more efficacious than bile-acid sequestrating agents. In patients with heterozygous FH who tolerate bile-acid sequestrating agents the cholesterol-lowering response is as good as with an HMG-CoA reductase inhibitor[6] (see Figure 5.3).

The principal advantages of bile-acid sequestrants are the knowledge that in FH they correct the basic defect by increasing LDL receptor expression and that they would appear to be free of serious side-effects even in the long term. They were introduced in the 1960s, so there is considerable experience in their use; furthermore, cholestyramine was the drug employed in the Lipid Research Clinics Study, in which the participants were observed for 7 years or more for adverse effects[7]. Indeed, it might be expected that drugs not absorbed into the body would be relatively safe. Finally, of course, there is good evidence that by its action (Chapter 6, page 156) it does reduce the morbidity of coronary artery disease[8].

Weighed against all these points is the disadvantage that bile-acid sequestrants are awkward to take and frequently unpalatable. They are dry powders which attract water and cannot be taken unless they are well soaked in liquid. Probably they should be allowed to soak for at least 15–20 min before they are swallowed and adequate liquid, usually water or fruit juice, must be taken with them to avoid an unpleasant feeling of fullness or bloating. Initially they may also produce other upper gastrointestinal symptoms such as nausea and heartburn. However, these symptoms usually subside, although for patients with hiatus hernia or peptic ulcer they may prove a contraindication. Bile-acid sequestrants should never be prescribed for a trivial reason and always with detailed explanation of how they should be taken. Care must be taken to build up the dose slowly and to discourage the patient from abandoning them at the outset. True resistance to their LDL-lowering effect is rare and the reason for any failure to obtain an initial response, or to maintain it, is non-compliance. It is the case, however, that they do cause an unwanted increase in cholesterol biosynthesis due to stimulation of HMG-CoA reductase in response to increased bile-acid synthesis[3]. In most patients this limits their effectiveness, but does not render them ineffective. It is the reason that their combination with HMG-CoA reductase inhibitor drugs may be a particularly effective therapy[8,9].

It is my own practice to prescribe first a single sachet each day, to be taken before breakfast. If time is at a premium in the morning, the powder can be left in fruit juice in the refrigerator overnight and then shaken and drunk the next morning. The morning seems a particularly good time to begin, since for the drug to be most effective it must mix with bile, and this will have collected in the gall bladder overnight. It is always important to take the bile-acid sequestrant before food to ensure that the gall bladder does contract when the drug is present in the intestine. If patients are not in the habit of having breakfast, they should be advised to at least have some cereal or toast after their morning dose. After 2 weeks or so patients are asked to increase the dose to two sachets, taken together before breakfast. After a further 2 weeks the serum cholesterol is repeated and the dose slowly built up until a satisfactory response is achieved, the patient cannot tolerate any more or a dose of around six sachets per day is achieved. Occasionally there is a further reduction in cholesterol from increasing the dose beyond six sachets. After the two morning sachets, one, then two, sachets before the evening meal are introduced. For patients on more than four sachets, their daily routine will decide whether a lunchtime dose is possible or whether the dose must be split between breakfast and the evening meal. Constipation is a frequent problem with larger doses and attempts to overcome it by increasing dietary fibre or even the prescription of aperients may be appropriate if compliance is to be achieved.

Increasingly, the use of bile-acid sequestrating agents is being confined to lower doses, usually two sachets before breakfast combined with and HMG-CoA reductase taken in the evening in, for example, heterozygous FH. This smaller dose may also be added to fibric acid therapy in patients with combined hyperlipidaemia who, despite a good response in their serum triglyceride and HDL cholesterol levels, are left with an undesirably high LDL cholesterol. It may also be used as monotherapy when it has been decided to lower serum cholesterol by only a relatively modest amount, particularly in a patient who has been alarmed by the misleading publicity surrounding certain erroneous conclusions about the adverse effects of cholesterol-lowering medication. Larger doses are thus needed only in FH heterozygotes who are too young to receive systemically absorbed lipid-lowering agents or are still likely to become pregnant or who have reacted adversely to other lipid-lowering medication.

Two potentially important adverse effects of bile-acid sequestrating agents stand out and these are their effect on the metabolism of other drugs and their effect on triglyceride metabolism. Bile-acid sequestrating agents bind anions non-specifically and thus may interfere with absorption of any substance which is anionic at intestinal pH[10]. This applies most significantly to drugs such as the oral anticoagulants, digoxin, thyroxine and perhaps amiodarone. These drugs should not be administered until at least 4 h have elapsed after the last dose of bile-acid sequestrant. Fortunately they are all given once a day and so their administration at bedtime or lunchtime, if no bile-acid sequestrant is taken then, is the usual solution.

The effect of bile-acid sequestrants on triglyceride metabolism is not favourable. It should be emphasized that their effect is to lower cholesterol in LDL, but that they are not suitable agents for lowering raised cholesterol associated with chylomicrons or VLDL. A slight increase in triglycerides, which is usually clinically unimportant, occurs in hypercholesterolaemic patients even when their triglycerides are initially normal (type IIa)[7]. In patients where both LDL and VLDL levels are raised (type IIb), the cholesterol may be lowered, but there may be an accompanying substantial rise in triglycerides. This difficulty may be overcome by initiating treatment with a fibrate drug, acipimox or nicotinic acid. This generally produces a satisfactory reduction in the triglyceride concentration and any persisting hypercholesterolaemia may then be treated with a bile acid sequestrant. In patients with type III, IV or V hyperlipoproteinaemia, bile-acid sequestrants are contraindicated. This is despite the fact that in both types III and V serum total cholesterol levels may be markedly elevated. A severe hypertriglyceridaemia (and further rise in cholesterol due to increased VLDL) may result and perhaps even precipitate acute pancreatitis.

The reason for the elevation in serum triglycerides is probably an increase in hepatic triglyceride synthesis, perhaps mediated via the phosphatidate phosphohydrolase enzyme[11] (Chapter 1, page 10). Despite the increase in serum triglycerides, there is in type II hyperlipoproteinaemia, at least, a tendency for HDL cholesterol to rise slightly during bile-acid sequestrant therapy[7].

In theory, cholelithiasis might be expected to be an adverse effect of the bile-acid sequestrants, because of depletion of the bile salt pool. In hypercholesterolaemic patients prescribed these drugs, however, this does not appear to be the case[7]. Steatorrhoea and fat-soluble vitamin deficiencies have been reported with their use, but this is really only likely to be encountered in patients with short bowel or terminal ileal disease (which, of course, conversely they can help if cholorrheic enteropathy is causing diarrhoea). Folate supplements should be given to children receiving bile-acid sequestrants[12]. It is also our practice to prescribe folate for patients on cholestyramine contemplating pregnancy. Most patients prefer to stop cholestyramine during pregnancy and some while they are trying to conceive. Cholestyramine is prescribed for pruritus associated with pregnancy, which is reassuring, but it is not a reason to insist that it should be taken during pregnancy despite the spectacular rises in cholesterol that may occur during pregnancy in patients with FH. It can be reintroduced following the pregnancy. Again it should not be forced on a reluctant patient who is breast feeding. A small dose up until weaning might be a satisfactory compromise. The patient who stops her treatment before conception, but then does not conceive, is a more difficult problem, since she may be ineffectively treated for a long while. In those circumstances it seems more appropriate to encourage the patient back on to treatment with a bile-acid sequestrant but not any other lipid-lowering agent.

## Nicotinic acid (niacin) and its derivatives

Nicotinic acid (pyridine-3-carboxylic acid) (Figure 10.4), or niacin as it is known in the USA, lowers both serum cholesterol (LDL) and triglycerides (VLDL) and can also be used in the management of all the hyperlipoproteinaemias except type I. Its hypolipidaemic action has been known since the 1950s[13]. It produces a profound decrease in the release of non-esterified fatty acids from adipose tissue[14] which in turn diminishes hepatic triglyceride synthesis and VLDL secretion[15] (Chapters 1 and 11, pages 11 and 297). A plausible explanation for the reduction in LDL levels would be that they decrease as a consequence of the reduction in secretion of VLDL, its precursor molecule[16]. In addition, there is evidence that nicotinic acid increases faecal neutral sterol excretion (Chapter 1, page 20)[17], an effect which might be due to a separate action rather than secondary to decreased VLDL secretion. HDL cholesterol may increase slightly with nicotinic acid[18].

Nicotinic acid is often described as an ideal lipid-lowering agent were it not for its side-effects. These are so common and so unpleasant as to render it of limited value. To be fair, some authors[19] do find it better than has been our experience and this may be because we tend to introduce it last in patients with severe hypercholesterolaemia which persists despite attempted treatment with other drugs. We may thus have selected a group many of whom are not compliant.

The most troublesome adverse effect of nicotinic acid is flushing of the skin. This is prostaglandin-mediated and can be alleviated, if aspirin is taken at the same time. It is said that the flushing occurs in response to changing serum levels of nicotinic acid, which is probably why it is worse if the drug is taken on an empty stomach, and this has led to numerous slow-release formulations aimed at stabilizing circulating levels. Unfortunately these all too frequently make the flushing occur unpredictably. Many patients prefer to take the ordinary nicotinic acid (niacin) preparation as a single dose with a meal, at home, where they can cope better with the flushing reaction. Generally, 3 g daily is required for any worthwhile therapeutic response and some authorities recommend its use in doses as great as 2.5 g t.d.s.[20]. It is, however, important to build the dose up slowly, starting with as little as 100 mg daily. Other side-effects include headache, postural hypotension, nausea, diarrhoea, exacerbation of peptic ulcer, hepatic dysfunction, hyperuricaemia, gout and an increase in blood glucose. These effects need to be monitored. Also, during its use in the Coronary Drug Project there seemed to be an increase in cardiac dysrhythmias, although there was evidence that it decreased cardiac reinfarction[21]. Pruritus, skin pigmentation, acanthosis nigricans and vascular oedema have also been reported[19,22].

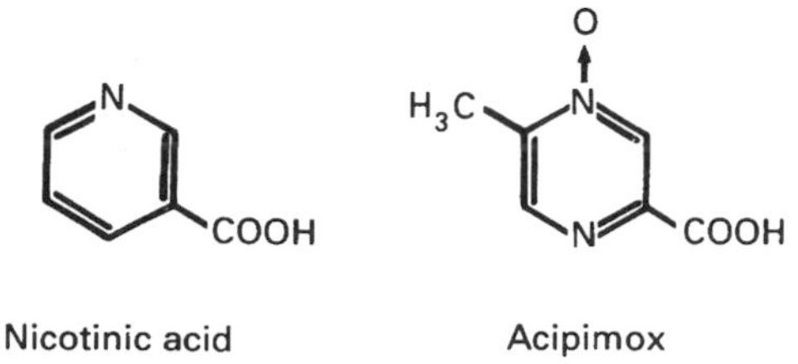

Nicotinic acid                    Acipimox

**Figure 10.4**   Structure of nicotinic acid (niacin) and one of its derivatives, acipimox

Nicotinic acid has frequently been recommended in combination with bile-acid sequestrating agents in the management of FH[19,23]. This combination certainly produces an encouraging decrease in LDL cholesterol and is associated with a decrease in tendon xanthoma size[20]. One fear has been that the combined effects of bile salt depletion and an increased biliary cholesterol might produce rampant cholelithiasis. Unexpectedly, however, it seems that a biliary cholesterol saturation decreases on this combination of drugs[24].

It is surprising how frequently nicotinic acid, usually in combination with a bile-acid sequestrating agent, has been used in the more successful secondary prevention and regression studies (Chapter 6). This probably reflects the fact that for many years and during the period when most of these trials were done, nicotinic acid in combination with a bile acid sequestrating agent was the most effective means of treating type IIa and IIb hyperlipoproteinaemia, the combinations lowering LDL and triglycerides and increasing HDL. It has sometimes, however, been suggested that nicotinic acid may have some special property not shared by other lipid-lowering drugs. Certainly nicotinic acid lowers serum lipoprotein (a)[25,26] and remains the only even vaguely practical drug to have been entirely convincingly shown to do this. The status of Lp(a) as a causative IHD risk factor is not, however, at present, established (Chapter 12, page 364). The suggestion, has also been made that the vasodilator properties of nicotinic acid may be cardioprotective. There is no evidence for this and it should not be forgotten that nicotinic acid has sometimes been considered to potentiate dysrythmias. It is overwhelmingly likely therefore that any benefits due to nicotinic acid are the result of its effects on lipoprotein metabolism.

A recent development has been the introduction into clinical practice of acipimox (5 methylpyrazine carboxylic acid 4-oxide) (Figure 10.4), an analogue of nicotinic acid. It is more potent than nicotinic acid in suppressing NEFA[27] and does so in doses which cause less flushing than does nicotinic acid. Like nicotinic acid it lowers serum triglycerides and raises HDL, but does so at lower doses[28–30]. However, at these doses it has no effect on the serum concentration of LDL cholesterol nor probably of Lp(a). Used alone therefore acipimox may be regarded as having similar clinical indications to fibric acid derivatives[31], particularly those which are less effective in lowering serum LDL cholesterol. Type III hyperlipoproteinaemia has been effectively treated with acipimox[29] as it has been with nicotinic acid and the increased cholesterol, which in this condition is due to β-VLDL, is decreased. In combination with a bile-acid sequestrant, acipimox does appear to augment substantially the reduction in LDL cholesterol[32] and cause the serum triglyceride levels to fall rather than remain unaltered or increase with bile acid sequestrant therapy alone. Acipimox has been shown to increase the affinity of LDL for LDL receptors in patients with hypertriglyceridaemia even when the serum LDL level does not fall[33]. In this respect it may be similar to fibric acid derivatives which appear to divert LDL from non-receptor-mediated to receptor-mediated catabolic pathways by causing a relative decrease in the smaller LDL particles and an increase in the larger LDL particles which are more rapidly cleared by receptor-mediated pathways. This effect may have explained its LDL-lowering action in combination with a bile acid sequestrating agent, because hypertriglyceridaemia was present in some of the hypercholesterolaemic patients studied either before or after treatment with the bile-acid sequestrant, which itself would have increased LDL receptor expression, so that enhanced binding induced by acipimox as a result of a shift in LDL particle size distribution towards larger LDL[34] might under these circumstances have increased its effectiveness in lowering LDL.

Theoretically, lowering serum NEFA would be expected to produce an improvement in glucose tolerance due to a decrease in insulin resistance (Chapter 11). In practice, however, nicotinic acid frequently makes diabetic glycaemic control worse. This is because of its relatively short action in lowering plasma NEFA which is followed by a rebound increase accompanied by a rise in blood glucose. Acipimox, which has a longer duration of action, acutely improves glucose tolerance[35,36]. In the longer term this improvement may have little clinical impact in improving glycaemic control, probably because there is still some rebound of NEFA[37,38], but there is certainly no deterioration in control as occurs with nicotinic acid. A longer acting preparation of acipimox may, however, bring about worthwhile clinical improvement in glycaemic control in the longer term[39,40], although at present this requires further study. So also does the effectiveness of combining acipimox with HMG-CoA reductase inhibitors in type IIa and IIb hyperlipoproteinaemia and with fibric acid derivatives in the management of severe hypertriglyceridaemia whether or not these are associated with frank diabetes.

Etofibrate is the condensation product of clofibric and nicotinic acids. Whether it has any advantage over nicotonic acid or fibrate drugs requires careful clinical evaluation.

## Fibric acid derivatives

The first of these derivatives (Figure 10.5), developed in the 1950s by Thorp and his colleagues, underwent its initial clinical evaluation in 1962[41,42]. Since then, analogues have been developed and attitudes and opinions of the value of this group of drugs have undergone many changes.

Recent developments, such as the Helsinki Heart Study, are a clear indication of their clinical role as lipid-lowering agents and there remains a strong suspicion that we have much yet to learn about their other pharmacological properties, which also may be of immense value.

In terms of their action on lipoprotein metabolism, the predominant effect of all the fibrate drugs is to lower serum triglyceride levels by decreasing VLDL. In addition, for reasons that are still uncertain, they markedly decrease the levels of β-VLDL in type III hyperlipoproteinaemia (Chapter 8, page 215). The mechanism by which VLDL levels are reduced is still somewhat controversial. There seems general agreement that they increase the activity of lipoprotein lipase in adipose tissue and skeletal muscle[43–45] and it is possible, but unproven, that this might result from an increase in apo CII, the activator of this enzyme[46,47]. Consistent with the view that the triglyceride-lowering action of fibrate drugs is due to enhanced VLDL catabolism by lipoprotein lipase, is the slight rise in LDL which occurs in patients with hypertriglyceridaemia whose LDL is initially low[48]. This explanation has not, however, been supported by kinetic studies which suggest that the increase in serum LDL may be due to the fibrate-induced decrease in the accelerated non-receptor-mediated LDL catabolism in hypertriglyceridaemia[49–52].

In patients with an elevation in both LDL and VLDL (type IIb hyperlipoproteinaemia), the usual response to fibrate drugs is a decrease in VLDL, but with a relatively smaller decrease in LDL cholesterol[49,53]. The decrease in total serum

Clofibrate

Ciprofibrate

Gemfibrozil

Fenofibrate

Bezafibrate

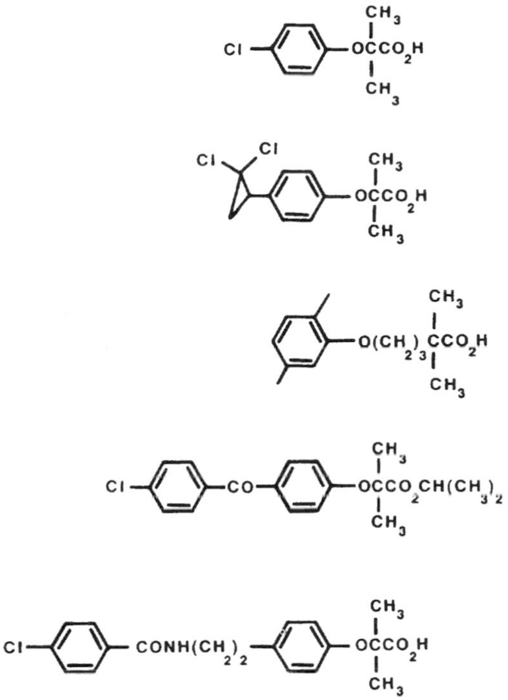

**Figure 10.5** Structure of fibric acid derivatives, which are currently in use on a wide scale

cholesterol generally appears much greater than the LDL cholesterol response because it includes the reduction in VLDL cholesterol. The LDL response cannot be explained simply on the basis of an increase in lipoprotein lipase activity, and it has been suggested that the increase in receptor-mediated catabolism observed in some studies[50,51,54] might be responsible for the decrease in serum LDL cholesterol. However, this may not be a primary effect. A fibrate-induced increase in biliary cholesterol excretion might decrease the intrahepatic cholesterol pool and might thus stimulate hepatic LDL receptor expression. However, it is usually stated that not all fibrate drugs increase biliary cholesterol saturation and that clofibrate, which does, may not do so on prolonged administration[55,56]. Thus a decrease in cholesterol synthesis has also been suggested[50,54,57,58]. Another possibility which has gained favour in recent years has, however, been proposed to explain the LDL-lowering action of fibrate in terms of enhanced LDL catabolism. It is suggested that the relatively triglyceride-rich, but relatively dense cholesterol-dependent LDL present in the circulation in patients with hypertriglyceridaemia is poorly cleared by receptors. Its binding to LDL receptors is enhanced by lowering the serum triglyceride concentration by fibrate therapy[59] or other means[33]. It has been shown in patients that there is a shift in the LDL particle distribution from small LDL towards larger LDL under this circumstance and that LDL receptor-mediated catabolism is enhanced[49–51]. The shift away from non-receptor-mediated catabolic pathways may in its own right be antiatherogenic[60]. The tendency for serum LDL to rise or remain unaltered in type IV hyperlipoproteinaemia may be because of the enhanced VLDL conversion to large LDL by the fibrate-induced increase in lipoprotein lipase. In type IIb hyperlipoproteinaemia, however, in addition to the shift in particle distribution towards large LDL there is usually a decrease in the serum LDL concentration[61] and this is probably because in this type of patient a more profound LDL catabolic defect is contributing to the hypercholesterolaemia.

In patients with type IIa hyperlipoproteinaemia a decrease in serum LDL with fibrate therapy generally occurs whereas the increase encountered in some hypertriglyceridaemic states is not. Generally the decrease is small and it is usual to initiate therapy with a bile-acid sequestrant or a HMG-CoA reductase inhibitor and to use fibrate drugs only if those are poorly tolerated or ineffective. However, it is undoubtedly the case that some patients, usually those with relatively mild increases in serum cholesterol, but occasionally also those with FH clinical syndrome (Chapter 5) do show a worthwhile clinical response[62,63]. This is most likely with fenofibrate, ciprofibrate or bezafibrate.

There is a tendency for serum HDL cholesterol to rise with fibrate drugs, which has been reviewed in detail[64]. The effect is most consistently seen in type III hyperlipoproteinaemia. In other hyperlipoproteinaemias, the effect is more variable and may depend on the particular drug and on the type of hyperlipoproteinaemia. All of the fibrates show the effect to some extent when hypertriglyceridaemia is present and to a lesser extent in type IIa hyperlipoproteinaemia.

It would be valuable to have much more information about the comparative effect of the different fibrate drugs on different lipoprotein disorders obtained by careful cross-over studies of the different fibrate drugs in large numbers of closely defined patients.

An increase in HDL cholesterol would be expected from an increase in lipoprotein lipase activity because of the release of HDL components during the lipolysis of triglyceride-rich lipoproteins (Chapter 2). There may also be a direct effect of some fibrates on HDL production[65]. Perhaps the most interesting reason for an increase in the circulating HDL cholesterol concentration with fibric acid therapy was, however, until recently overlooked. That is the effect of fibrates in decreasing the transfer of cholesteryl ester out of HDL in exchange for triglyceride into VLDL[66,67] (Figure 10.6) whence it may contribute to LDL cholesterol and increase atheroma risk rather than complete its passage back to the liver (Chapter 2, page 58).

Furthermore, a similar movement of cholesteryl out of LDL back to VLDL would account for the small triglyceride-rich, cholesteryl ester-depleted LDL present in hypertriglyceridaemia. A decrease in this latter process would thus account for the effect of fibrates in decreasing the concentration of small LDL by a similar mechanism to that by which HDL cholesterol is raised. Increased transfer of cholesteryl ester out of HDL to VLDL is probably atherogenic because it is increased in IHD[68] and genetic deficiency of CETP is associated with relative freedom from IHD whereas CETP expression in mice increases susceptibility to atheroma[69]. The decrease seen with fibric acid drugs is due to a reduction in the circulating triglyceride pool and to a decrease in free cholesterol in VLDL are increased in hypertriglyceridaemia. Whether fibrates have any more specific effect on cholesteryl ester remains to be investigated.

Many statements have been made about the relative efficacy of the different fibrates, often on inadequate evidence – for example, that clofibrate is more effective than the others in type III hyperlipoproteinaemia, which has no foundation.

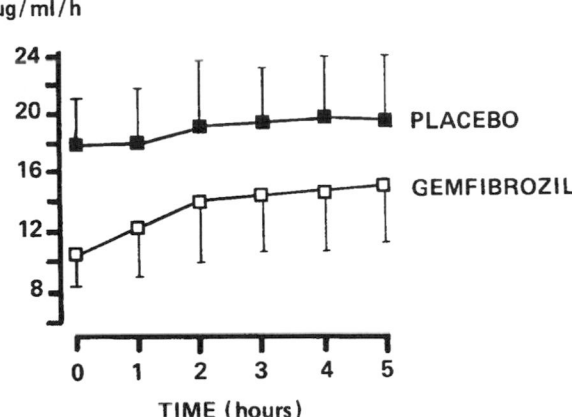

**Figure 10.6** The effect of gemfibrozil was to decrease the transfer of cholesteryl ester from HDL to VLDL and LDL fasting (time zero) and for 5 h after a mixed meal in a placebo controlled, cross-over trial of patients with primary hypertriglyceridaemia[66]

A review of the literature in 1987[53] produced conclusions that have tended to be supported by subsequent publications[61,70–74]. The greatest LDL-lowering effect occurs with bezafibrate, ciprofibrate and fenofibrate, with the latter two probably having most effect. There does not appear to be any consistent evidence that they differ in their effectiveness in lowering serum triglyceride levels, raising HDL cholesterol or in raising LDL cholesterol when it is initially low. The trials do, however, show considerable variation in these effects and this must serve to emphasize that it may occasionally be helpful to try another fibrate drug when a patient shows an inadequate response or is intolerant of one. The fibrates also have a wide range of properties other than their effect on serum lipoproteins and the clinician should be aware of these in choosing a particular agent. Indeed the fibrate drugs may show considerable variation in some of these other effects. Some of the considerations in choosing a fibrate are as follows.

### (a) Efficacy

If one views efficacy as the ability of a lipid-lowering drug to decrease morbidity from coronary disease in middle-aged men with modestly increased serum lipids, then both clofibrate[75] and gemfibrozil[76] would pass this test. A 25% decrease in non-fatal myocardial infarction was produced by clofibrate in 5000 men treated for 5.3 years and a 34% decrease in coronary and end points by gemfibrozil in 2000 men treated for 5.4 years.

### (b) Serious side-effects

### (i) Side-effects in clinical trials

All of the fibrate drugs are well tolerated, which is a considerable relief for patient and physician alike, if one considers some of the other currently available lipid-lowering agents. The WHO clofibrate trial[75] did, however, raise serious doubts about longer term, more serious side-effects of fibrate drugs. In the trial, the administration of clofibrate was associated with 4.9 deaths per 1000 compared with 3.8 deaths per 1000 in a control group with similar initial cholesterol levels who received an olive oil 'placebo'. This was statistically significant, but not when standardized for differences in age. There are also three other considerations in evaluating these findings. The clofibrate-treated group was chosen because they came from the upper third of the cholesterol distribution. What, one wonders, would have been the outcome of a trial of an antihypertensive drug or a hypogly-caemic agent, if it had been evaluated in people whose blood pressure or blood glucose was in the upper tercile of the population? Almost certainly such a study could only have revealed side-effects and no benefits. The WHO clofibrate trial must thus be regarded as of very limited relevance to clinical practice, in which clofibrate would be given to patients with more marked hyperlipidaemia who had failed to respond to diet and in whom, because of the steeper relationship between cholesterol and ischaemic heart disease risk at higher levels, the benefits of treat-ment would be greatest. Furthermore, when one analyses the excess deaths in the clofibrate-treated patients in the WHO trial, these were not related to effective reduction of cholesterol. In clinical practice, where a patient's hyperlipidaemia does not respond to a drug, such as clofibrate, it would be discontinued, so that only patients in whom the therapeutic balance was favourable would be exposed to the drug for long periods.

The third problem in interpreting whether the WHO trial really established that clofibrate was unsafe results from the method that was used in analysing the results. The most worrying statistic to emerge from the trial was that it was reported that 4 years after its completion – 9.6 years after it commenced – there was a statistically significant excess of deaths in those who received clofibrate. It has since emerged, although not with the publicity attending the earlier finding, that this apparent excess of deaths due to clofibrate was a statistical aberration due to the exclusion of men who had withdrawn from the trial of their own volition. Now that the intention-to-treat analysis has finally been published[77], it is clear that there was no increase in mortality in the clofibrate-treated group even after they had been followed for 9.6 years. There were 484 deaths in the clofibrate group and 469 in controls matched for their serum cholesterol at randomization. Deaths due to neoplasms were 131 in the clofibrate group and 142 in the controls.

One specific complication during the trial itself, however, which did clearly emerge was clofibrate-related cholelithiasis. Cholecystectomy was performed at rates of 2.1 per 1 000 in the clofibrate-treated group and 0.9 per 1000 in the placebo group. Clofibrate-induced changes in the composition of bile (see later) would account for this.

The WHO clofibrate study should be viewed alongside the Helsinki Heart Study of gemfibrozil[76]. That study was conducted in men whose non-HDL cholesterol exceeded 200 mg/dl (5.2 mmol/l), and diet advice was given to both the gemfibrozil-and placebo-treated groups. Despite this, the patients treated and their manner of treatment was not very close to clinical practice. Nevertheless, the findings with regard to side-effects over 5 years of treatment are very relevant to the present discussion. Malignancies were identical in the treatment and placebo groups (5.4 per 1000 in both) and cholecystectomies, although numerically greater in the gemfi-brozil group (18 vs 12), were not significantly so. The reason for the absence of a significant decrease in all-cause mortality, despite favourable effects on coronary disease morbidity in the Helsinki Heart Study and other lipid-lowering studies, is discussed in Chapter 6, page 158. It is not the case, however, that there is any evidence that favourable effects on ischaemic heart disease mortality are counter-acted by an increase in mortality from some unrelated disease.

At the present time it must be concluded that treatment with clofibrate should not be initiated without good reason when other drugs of similar class are avail-able because of the undoubted risk of cholelithiasis associated with its use. Of these, only gemfibrozil has been observed under clinical trial conditions for suffi-ciently long for us to be reasonably reassured about its long-term side-effects compared with its benefits.

## (ii) Effects on bile composition

The results of investigations of the effects of different fibrate drugs on the choles-terol saturation index of bile[55–57,78–87] need to be interpreted with caution for three reasons. First, there have been few cross-over studies, making comparison difficult. Secondly, the well-known increase in cholesterol saturation associated with many of the drugs may not be sustained beyond the initial few months of therapy. Thirdly, many studies have been carried out in healthy volunteers and yet the drugs are to be used in patients who, by virtue of their hypertriglyceridaemia and other clinical features, may already have abnormalities of biliary lipid metabolism[82].

The effect of bezafibrate[85,86] and fenofibrate[87] are thus unclear and the issue is further confused by gemfibrozil, which appeared not to have the side-effect supposedly associated with clofibrate[76], but which has been shown to affect the lithogenic index unfavourably[84]. This does not indicate that the effect of fibrates on bile composition is irrelevant, but, perhaps, that the lithogenic index is an outmoded way of examining their true lithogenic potential, which may relate to their effects on other biliary components such as mucus or apolipoproteins.

## (iii) Peroxisomes

Fibrate drugs induce proliferation of liver peroxisomes in rats and so also, it is suggested, does clofibrate in man[88]. Whether differences in the propensity of different fibrate drugs to do this really exist[89,90], and whether they relate to any potential long-term side-effects, such as hepatic neoplasia, is at present uncer-tain[91]. It is the case, however, that clofibrate has been in use for over 35 years and bezafibrate, fenofibrate and gemfibrozil for more than 15 years.

## (iv) Other side-effects

Without doubt, the most potentially serious side-effect of the fibric acid drugs which presents a common problem is their potentiation of oral anticoagulants. Serious haemorrhage can be provoked by their inadvertent prescription to patients on such treatment, and it is essential that the introduction of fibrate drug therapy when a patient is anticoagulated is carried out under the closest laboratory scrutiny. It is my practice to admit patients to hospital to accomplish this. None of the currently available fibrate drugs has any conspicuous advantage in this respect.

The fibrate drugs should not be prescribed for the hyperlipidaemia of obstruc-tive jaundice, for example primary biliary cirrhosis, since they may paradoxically exacerbate it (Chapter 11, page 325). Since all the currently available fibrates are at least partly renally excreted, it is generally inadvisable to use them for the hyperlipidaemias in renal disease. Their administration to patients with renal failure results in high drug levels and a severe myositis with marked elevations of muscle enzymes[92]. The occasional patient with normal renal function will complain of muscle-aching on the highest recommended doses and in asymptomatic patients minor increases in creatinine kinase are occasionally encountered[93]. Bezafibrate has sometimes been linked with a further increase in serum creatinine in patients with mild elevation initially. Gemfibrozil, on the other hand, which is structurally rather different from the other drugs classified as fibric acid derivatives, is eliminated largely by the liver. It has been used in patients with nephrotic syndrome and with chronic renal failure, although experience is limited[94].

## (c) Potential advantages of fibric acid derivatives in addition to lipoprotein changes

### (i) Effects on coagulation

Fibrinogen is a major independent risk factor for myocardial infarction, at least in populations already predisposed to atheroma like that of the UK[95,96]. A potentially beneficial action of some of the fibrate drugs is that they lower serum fibrinogen levels. As usual, entirely satisfactory direct comparisons between the different agents do not exist. However, fibrinogen decreases markedly with clofibrate[97,98]. This property seems to be shared with some other fibric acid derivatives such as bezafibrate[85,99–101] and fenofibrate[100,102]. Ciprofibrate may also lower fibrinogen but additional studies are needed to confirm this[103]. Gemfibrozil, however, appears not to lower fibrinogen[104,105] or may even increase it[100,106]. Fibrinogen is the major determinant of blood viscosity, which thus also decreases with fibrate therapy and which, it has been suggested, may improve blood flow in patients with established arteriosclerosis[98]. Other effects of fibrate drugs on the coagulation system have also been reported, for example on platelet aggregation, factor VII or plasminogen activator inhibitor-1, and tissue plasminogen activator. Much more information is required before drawing any conclusions about any such possible effects.

### (ii) Gout and hyperuricaemia

Many patients with hypertriglyceridaemia experience attacks of gout and an even greater number have hyperuricaemia[107]. Despite the close association, treating hypertriglyceridaemia does not usually affect serum urate or vice versa. An exception to this is the drug fenofibrate, which lowers the levels of both the triglycerides and uric acid[108]. The effect is due wholly or in large part to increased renal urate clearance and is frequently of sufficient magnitude to correct hyperuricaemia. Other fibric analogues may be uricosuric in single dose studies, but only with fenofibrate has the effect been sustained on chronic administration.

### (iii) Glucose tolerance

The fibric acid derivatives tend to produce an improvement in glucose tolerance. This has been most extensively documented for bezafibrate[85,109–113] and is, perhaps, most marked with that drug. The effect may be due to a decrease in insulin resistance, possibly mediated by a decrease in circulating levels of NEFA[114].

# Probucol

Probucol or 4,4'-(isopropylidenedithio)bis(2,6-di-*t*-butylphenol) lowers serum cholesterol, but does not usually affect triglyceride levels. The decrease in cholesterol concentration occurs both in LDL and HDL cholesterol. The decrease in LDL cholesterol usually averages around 8–17%[115] and this applies in both polygenic hypercholesterolaemia and FH[116]. The probucol-induced decrement in LDL cholesterol in heterozygous FH is, however, less than with cholestyramine[117]. Nevertheless, some patients achieve a therapeutic reduction in LDL cholesterol with probucol and these tend to be those whose serum HDL cholesterol is high initially and in whom proportionately greater decreases in that lipoprotein also occur[116]. Such patients tend to be younger women, in whom the drug is not recommended for other reasons, which limits its usefulness as a purely LDL-lowering drug or as primary medication. It lowers the serum LDL cholesterol not only in heterozygous FH, but also in some homozygotes[118,119]. This may be explained, because its principal mode of action in reducing the LDL concentration is by increasing its fractional catabolic rate via the non-receptor-mediated route[120]. The non-receptor-mediated route for LDL catabolism is often regarded as potentially harmful. However, it may not be a single route at all and may involve a variety of pathways. A potentially beneficial effect on one of these pathways is illustrated by an elegant series of experiments[120]. Low density lipoprotein when incubated with copper or cultured endothelial cells undergoes oxidation and is then readily taken up by the macrophages in tissue culture (Chapter 2, page 63). This is not the case, however, with LDL taken from patients receiving treatment with probucol, which resists oxidative modification. Probucol is a powerful lipophilic antioxidant. If arterial wall foam cell formation is a prerequisite for atherogenesis (Chapter 2, page 60), then this is a fascinating observation. In Watanabe rabbits (rabbits with inherited hypercholesterolaemia), probucol causes a striking decrease in aortic atheromatous deposits[121]. Trials of probucol as a means of decreasing IHD risk in man have, however, been disappointing so far[122,123]. The reason for this may be that probucol increases the transfer of cholesteryl ester from HDL into VLDL[124], which is potentially atherogenic (Chapter 2, page 59) and might thus counteract its effect in decreasing the oxidative modification of LDL. None the less probucol does sometimes decrease xanthoma size. As was discussed in Chapter 5, page 111, xanthomata have many histological features in common with atheromatous lesions, and from its earliest use there were anecdotes that probucol shrunk xanthomata more than other lipid-lowering drugs did. This was confirmed quantitatively in an investigation using soft-tissue radiography of Achilles tendon xanthomata[125]. The reduction in xanthoma size correlated best with the decrease in serum HDL cholesterol and, as in our earlier study[116], the remaining HDL contained a higher proportion of smaller HDL particles[125].

The mechanism by which probucol lowers serum HDL concentrations is probably partly by a decrease in apolipoprotein AI synthesis[126]. The effect of a decrease in apo AI synthesis on the circulating HDL cholesterol concentration would also be compounded by the accelerated transfer of cholesteryl ester out of HDL into the triglyceride-rich lipoprotein pool[124]. It has been suggested that a decrease in lipoprotein lipase activity might also contribute[127], but neither the Intralipid tolerance test[116] nor the catabolism of VLDL[128] are affected by probucol.

There is a tendency for the serum HDL cholesterol concentration to rise with bile-acid sequestrant therapy, probably due to increased apolipoprotein AI synthesis[129].

**Table 10.2 Effect of probucol 500 mg b.d. for 3 months in a cross-over, placebo control, double-blind trial in five severe familial hypercholesterolaemia heterozygotes receiving bile-acid sequestrant therapy (BAS), either cholestyramine or colestipol 5–6 sachets daily***

| Mean ± SEM | Placebo and BAS | | Probucol and BAS | |
|---|---|---|---|---|
| Total cholesterol | 11.03 ± 1.64 | (430 ± 64) | 8.95 ± 0.77 | (349 ± 30) |
| LDL cholesterol | 9.10 ± 1.48 | (355 ± 57) | 7.40 ± 0.85 | (289 ± 33) |
| HDL cholesterol | 1.31 ± 0.10 | (51 ± 3.9) | 0.97 ± 0.19 | (39 ± 7.4) |
| $HDL_2$ cholesterol | 0.62 ± 0.09 | (24 ± 3.5) | 0.41 ± 0.15 | (16 ± 5.9) |
| $HDL_3$ cholesterol | 0.58 ± 0.05 | (23 ± 2) | 0.63 ± 0.09 | (25 ± 3.5) |

* Before treatment, the average cholesterol level was 14.8 ± 1.4 mmol/l (577 ± 55 mg/dl).
Based on unpublished observations of P.N. Durrington and J.P. Miller

The use of probucol in patients already receiving treatment with bile-acid seques-trants is therefore appealing because not only might the decrease in serum HDL levels be counteracted, but also because of the increased starting level, if the relation-ship between this and the decrease in LDL holds true, a synergistic effect on LDL might be anticipated. In fact, comparative studies do not really allow us to decide how valid either of these predictions might be. We studied a group of patients who were heterozygotes for FH and who were difficult to treat adequately with bile-acid sequestrants, largely because of high initial cholesterol levels[130]. While maintain-ing bile-acid sequestrant therapy they received placebo and probucol each for 3 months. To ensure that they took the bile-acid sequestrants they were admitted to a metabolic ward for 2 weeks at the end of each 3 months. Probucol was associated with reduction in LDL cholesterol of around 20% (Table 10.2). Other studies with heterozygotes for FH gave similar results[131,132]. There is little information avail-able from clinical trials at present about probucol combined with other drugs.

Probucol currently has little place in the management of hypercholesterolaemic patients. It has no place in the management of hypertriglyceridaemia, but does not adversely affect triglyceride levels in patients with type IIb hyperlipopro-teinaemia[133]. It is generally well tolerated, but some 10% of patients have mild gastrointestinal side-effects, usually diarrhoea (which may not be a disadvantage if the patient is constipated due to bile-acid sequestrant therapy). Probucol is both highly lipophilic and incompletely absorbed from the gut. Its incorporation into mixed micelles might interfere with their absorption (Chapter 1, page 20) and explain the increased faecal bile acid excretion in patients receiving it[126,133]. Probucol, however, takes a long time to become fully effective (at least 3 months). This is to be expected of a highly lipophilic drug, if its major site of action is post-absorptive. Probucol has been shown to reduce biliary cholesterol saturation[134], possibly because it inhibits cholesterol biosynthesis[115], but this is speculative in man.

The lipophilic nature of probucol means that it has a long residence time within the body: when it is discontinued, several months may elapse before its influence abates. Probucol also increases the electrocardiographic Q–T interval. The signifi-cance of this is uncertain, but the drug is not recommended in patients with dysrhyth-mias or the potential for dysrhythmias, e.g. those about to undergo cardiac surgery.

## Neomycin

Neomycin at doses of 2 g/day decreases serum LDL cholesterol[135,136]. At this dose it does not usually produce malabsorption syndrome, although diarrhoea commonly occurs[137]. Its effect is frequently ascribed to a decrease in formation of mixed micelles in the gut lumen inhibiting cholesterol absorption[138,139]. This effect is often attributed to precipitation of bile acids which would be expected to bind to its polycationic structure, but other antibiotics also have some hypercholesterolaemic activity and increases in faecal bile acids have not always been demonstrable[140]. Changes in bile salt conversions (Chapter 1, page 20) by bowel flora may also therefore be important[141]. Neomycin has not really found much favour in clinical practice[136], probably because of fears about ototoxicity, nephrotoxicity and bacterial colitis.

## HMG-CoA reductase inhibitors

A major advance in therapy stems from the discovery by Endo and Kuroda[142] of a class of fungal metabolites that inhibit 3-hydroxy,3-methylglutaryl-CoA reductase (HMG-CoA reductase), the rate-limiting enzyme in cholesterol biosynthesis (Chapter 1, page 18). Compactin (subsequently renamed Mevastatin) was the original compound studied, but because of possible adverse effects in animals it did not undergo full clinical evaluation in man. Mevinolin, later named lovastatin, was the first analogue of compactin to have undergone extensive clinical use, but other related compounds have since entered clinical practice. These include simvastatin, a methylated derivative of mevinolin, and pravastatin, a hydroxylated derivative of compactin (Figure 10.7). Fluvastatin, which is produced entirely by chemical synthesis and which is structurally distinct, is also now available on prescription. More than ten other statins are undergoing development.

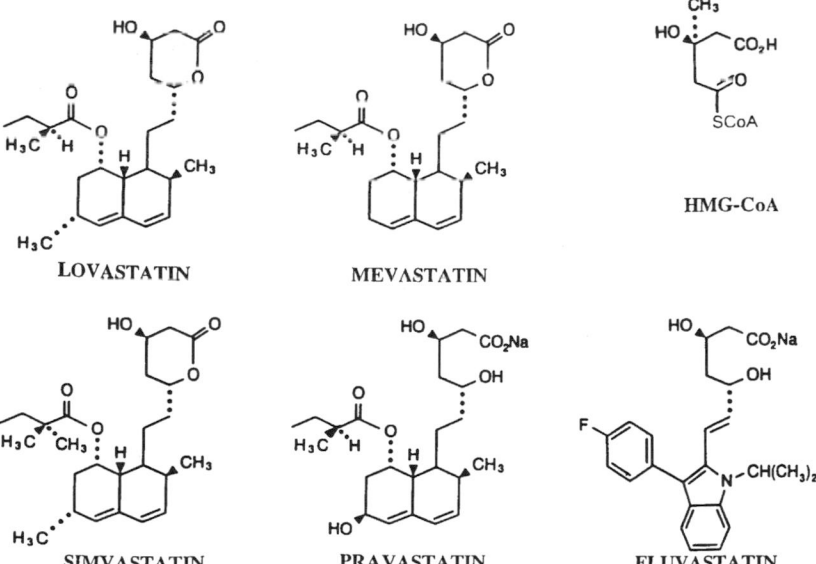

**Figure 10.7**   3-Hydroxy, 3-methylglutaryl-CoA (HMG-CoA) and the drugs which have been developed to block HMG-CoA reductase, the enzyme which converts it to mevalonate (Figures 1.14 and 1.15)

Inhibition of cholesterol biosynthesis with lovastatin leads to an increase in receptor-mediated LDL catabolism[143]. Serum LDL cholesterol and apolipoprotein B levels fall in both heterozygous FH[144] and polygenic hypercholesterolaemia[145]. Decreases in serum LDL cholesterol of 30–40% in both these groups of patients were reported with doses that did not decrease cholesterol biosynthesis to levels which might jeopardize its supply for vital functions[146]. A small decrease in serum triglycerides also occurs with lovastatin and there is a tendency for HDL cholesterol to increase[144,145]. Similar observations were made with simvastatin[147].

The statins can exist in a lactone form or as hydroxy acids. The lactone is insoluble in water and lipophilic, whereas the hydroxy acid is considerably more soluble in water. Lovastatin and simvastatin are administered as lactones, whereas pravastatin and fluvastatin are sodium salts of their hydroxy acids[148]. There is evidence that lovastatin and simvastatin are converted to their hydroxy acids before they become active. They do, however, enter tissues more widely than the drugs administered as the hydrophilic hydroxy acids probably because the lipophilic lactones cross cell membranes more readily. The hydrophilic statins inhibit cholesterol biosynthesis more specifically in the liver, which they enter as the result of an active transport mechanism. This has been hailed both as an advantage and disadvantage. The lactone, simvastatin, is the most potent in decreasing serum LDL cholesterol, whereas pravastatin is less effective (although similar to lovastatin[149]) and fluvastatin least effective. It has, however, been claimed that sleep disturbance may result from lipophilic statins, but not by pravastatin which because of its hydrophilic nature does not cross the blood–brain barrier as readily. This would be analogous to the higher incidence of CNS side-effects with the lipophilic beta-adrenoreceptor blocker, propranolol, contrasted with hydrophilic ones, such as atenolol. It does, however, also have to be considered that potentially antiatherogenic effects of statins other than their serum LDL cholesterol-lowering actions have become a focus of interest now that some studies appear to be showing more rapid changes in coronary events associated with their use than might be explicable on the basis of the decrease of circulating LDL (Chapter 6 page 152). Inhibition of oxidation of LDL by macrophages[150] and inhibition of smooth muscle cell proliferation[151] have, for example, been reported. Obviously a more extensive tissue distribution would be important for such effects to occur *in vivo*.

Since one of the limiting factors in bile-acid sequestrant therapy is considered to be a stimulation of cholesterol biosynthesis, the combination of such therapy with an HMG-CoA reductase inhibitor should prove particularly effective and this appears to be the case in early studies[8,9,19,152]. For similar reasons, HMG-CoA reductase inhibition is a good way of counteracting the tendency for serum LDL to rise after its initial favourable response to partial ileal bypass[152,153].

Although the statins are a relatively new group of lipid-lowering drugs, clinical experience and clinical trial information are building up rapidly with regard to their safety. There were early fears that less opacities might be a side-effect as they had been with triparanol, an early inhibitor of cholesterol biosynthesis[154]. Despite extensive testing, this has not proved to be the case. It should be remembered that unlike triparanol, which blocks at a comparatively late stage of cholesterol synthesis, statins inhibit the physiological rate-limiting enzyme for cholesterol production (Chapter 1, page 18). It is therefore extremely unlikely that we should have evolved with a system for cholesterol synthesis, which permits the accumulation of toxic metabolites proximal to the enzyme at the point of regulation.

Effects of the statin unrelated to their effects on cholesterol biosynthesis are, however, possible. Myositis was encountered with an incidence of around 0.5% with the early use of lovastatin[155,156]. Some episodes were sufficiently severe to cause rhabdomyolysis. The likelihood of myositis was increased by concurrent administration of gemfibrozil or cyclosporin. Reports of myositis with simvastatin or pravastatin have been rare. Perhaps this is because of the avoidance of drug combinations likely to provoke it and because of monitoring of the creatinine kinase (CK) and possible myositic symptoms. The decision to combine a statin with a fibrate drug or to use it in a patient with a cardiac or renal transplant should therefore be made only after balancing the risk of myositis against benefit. It is not known whether gemfibrozil is more likely to provoke myositis than other fibrates. Fluvastatin, the most recently introduced statin, has been claimed to be less likely to provoke myositis with fibric acid therapy.

Drug-related increases in serum CK activity in response to simvastatin are uncommon with simvastatin or pravastatin. It is not uncommon in patients with type IIa and IIb hyperlipoproteinaemias to find that the CK is marginally above the upper limit of normal regardless of whether a statin is being administered. We reported considerable fluctuations up to two to three times the upper limit of normal in heterozygotes for FH on no drug therapy and who are free of cardiac symptoms, have not exercised unduly or had an alcohol binge[157]. It is important therefore that small increases in serum CK activity in patients receiving statins, especially in the absence of symptoms, are not wrongly interpreted and the therapy discontinued. Often repetition of the test reveals that the CK activity will return to normal spontaneously. Also, of course, muscular aches and pains without any increase in CK are common and not likely to be statin-induced. It is important, however, that sensible monitoring to prevent myositis is continued.

I avoid statins in patients who over indulge in alcohol or who have liver dysfunction for other reasons. Statin-induced hepatic dysfunction is, however, uncommon. One benefit of statin therapy is that the biliary lithogenic index is not increased and indeed statins may encourage gallstone dissolution[158,159] They are increasingly employed in the management of dyslipidaemia in renal disease (Chapter 11, page 328) and in diabetes mellitus (Chapter 11, page 313).

The statins are undoubtedly a great advance in the management of severe hypercholesterolaemia. The great majority of patients respond well to them, particularly in combination with bile acid sequestrant treatment. A small number who genuinely take their medication are truly resistant to their cholesterol-lowering effect[160]. The reasons for this are unclear, but the phenomenon could be explained if these patients already have low rates of cholesterol biosynthesis and/or their receptor-mediated hepatic LDL catabolism is already occurring at maximum rates. There is some evidence to suggest that the nature of the mutation of the LDL receptor can influence the response to statin treatment in heterozygous FH[161,162].

## Fish oil

A preparation of marine fish oil (Maxepa) rich in highly polyunsaturated fatty acids, particularly eicosapentaenoic acid (Chapter 1, page 6) is available as liquid or capsules for the treatment of hypertriglyceridaemia. It is less well tolerated than the fibrate drugs. Also, although it is a natural product, it should not be regarded as necessarily free of long-term side-effects when given in pharmacological doses.

Having said that, the 10 g/day, which is the recommended dose, probably provides no more fish oil than is present in some diets habitually consumed. There may be some place for Maxepa in the management of types IV, V and occasionally in combination with cholesterol-lowering medication in type IIb hyperlipoproteinaemia[163,164]. It should, however, not be given to patients with type IIa hyperlipoproteinaemia, particularly FH, since far from decreasing serum LDL cholesterol, it will tend to increase it. The major action of fish oil is to decrease serum triglycerides, which is accompanied by a tendency for HDL cholesterol and LDL levels to rise[165]. The latter effect is seen with other therapy for type IV hyperlipoproteinaemia, particularly in the type of patient who has low levels of LDL initially (Chapter 7, page 196). A more potent preparation of fish oil in which the highly polyunsaturated components are concentrated may prove more acceptable to patients and upset diabetic glycaemic control less than other fish oil preparations[166], but additional clinical trials are needed.

Fish oils may have beneficial effects on the cardiovascular system not mediated through their lipid-lowering effects. However, it should be remembered that evidence for these effects is at present unsubstantiated. The Eskimo data are not entirely reliable (Chapter 9, page 228) and the current epidemiological evidence provides little support for fish oils having an effect in reducing coronary heart disease mortality *per se*[167]. A trial of fish-oil in the prevention of reinfarction in myocardial infarction survivors did, however, have a favourable outcome[168].

## Steroid hormones

Of these, oestrogens in particular have frequently been considered as lipid-lowering agents. High dose oestrogen treatment of men is unsuccessful as a means of coronary prevention[169]. However, lower doses in post-menopausal women reduce levels of LDL cholesterol[170] and also decrease the concentration of β-VLDL in type III hyperlipoproteinaemia[171]. The use of oestrogens is also associated with an increase in HDL, particularly in HDL2 cholesterol[172]. However, there is a tendency for VLDL levels to rise and, certainly in patients with pre-existing hypertriglyceridaemia, oestrogens may precipitate a severe hypertriglyceridaemia, occasionally even leading to acute pancreatitis[173]. None the less, where oestrogen replacement is considered for other reasons then, in the absence of established coronary disease, hyperlipoproteinaemia need not be a contraindication with the exception of severe hypertriglyceridaemia (Chapter 7, page 201). Such indications would almost certainly include premature menopause whether surgical or spontaneous, severe symptoms and risk factors for osteoporosis. Whether a desire to alter serum lipoproteins favourably and to reduce the risk of IHD are satisfactory indications for oestrogen replacement therapy is at present unclear. Overviews of surveys of the health of women receiving oestrogen replacement in comparison with those not receiving it have shown lower overall mortality, largely because of decreased IHD mortality[174–176]. However, all of the studies have been case-control studies and are open to the criticism that control and oestrogen-treated women were not randomly allocated and thus clinical and social considerations related to cardiovascular risk may have influenced the decision to prescribe hormone replacement. For example, women who smoked, had hypertension or hyperlipidaemia or had a bad family history may have been more likely to have been discouraged from taking such treatment and those requesting it may have been from a higher social class.

Thus the women receiving oestrogen replacement may have had a more favourable cardiovascular prognosis even before treatment commenced.

So far as possible, the Lipid Research Clinics Program attempted by statistical adjustment to exclude these possibilities in assessing the risk of oestrogen replacement in over 2000 women aged 48–69 followed for 6.6 years. The effect of the oestrogen *per se* was to decrease cardiovascular risk to about one-third that of women not receiving oestrogen[174]. Nonetheless in the absence of a randomized clinical trial we cannot say that the benefits of oestrogen would outweigh its adverse effects on, for example, coagulation or blood pressure in a typical post-menopausal woman. We certainly cannot conclude that women with established IHD should be advised to have oestrogen therapy for its 'cardioprotective effect'. Clinical trials are required to address these questions.

The other major unanswered question about hormone replacement therapy arises because in women who have not had a hysterectomy unopposed oestrogen cannot be given because it can induce endometrial carcinoma. Endogenous progesterone must therefore be combined with oestrogen replacement in a cyclical fashion to mimic menses by inducing regular shedding of the endometrium. We do not know whether the various progestogens used for this purpose themselves have any adverse effects sufficient to ameliorate the protective benefits from the oestrogen. At least one survey suggested such fears may be groundless[177]. However, that does not amount to a clinical trial. Further research into oestrogen and progestogens and their effects on vascular prognosis is important, particularly as oestrogen has recently been reported to protect LDL against oxidative damage[178] and norethisterone (a progestogen) to decrease serum Lp(a) (see page 280).

## ACAT inhibitors

Both absorbable and non-absorbable inhibitors of acyl-CoA:cholesterol acyltransferase are currently undergoing evaluation. The cholesterol absorbed from the gut into the enterocyte is esterified by ACAT before it is transported out in chylomicrons. Non-absorbable ACAT inhibitors may therefore find a role in preventing absorption[179–182]. Since one of the factors limiting the removal of cholesterol from atheromatous lesions is its esterification, absorbable inhibitors of ACAT are also being investigated as anti-atherogenic drugs[183,184].

## Pantethine

Pantethine is a derivative of pantethenic acid, which in early studies has been shown to modify serum lipoprotein levels favourably[185] and to inhibit LDL oxidation *in vitro*[186].

## Other agents of little clinical significance or without wide application

### D-thyroxine

This effectively lowers serum LDL cholesterol in familial hypercholesterolaemia[187], but at the doses required produces other thyroid hormone effects including angina and arrhythmias. In the Coronary Drug Project it may have increased the incidence of sudden death[188]. Although potentially it could be used in combination with a beta-adrenoreceptor blocking drug, understandably this suggestion has not found favour.

## Plant sterols

Although these are of interest in blocking cholesterol absorption (see Chapter 1, page 20), they do not possess great efficacy[189,190].

## Various formulations of plant fibre

From time to time, such formulations been reported to lower serum cholesterol. In general, a more thorough evaluation has shown their effects to be too small for serious clinical consideration. A more encouraging result with a guar gum preparation was, however, evident in one such study[191]. (See also Chapter 11, page 312.)

## Vitamin C

Vitamin C supplementation probably decreases serum cholesterol[192], but the effect is small and, in a reasonably well-nourished population, without clinical significance.

# Serum lipoprotein (a)

The serum lipoprotein (a) concentration is more difficult to decrease than that of VLDL or LDL. The only drug therapy convincingly shown to decrease its levels has been nicotinic acid[25,26] and perhaps neomycin[26]. It also decreases with plasmapheresis and LDL apheresis[193,194]. Given the markedly skewed frequency distribution of serum Lp(a) levels, changes in its median concentration must be substantial if it is to be more than the coincidence of random fluctuations in the same direction unless huge number of patients are involved. It is probably unaffected by statins[195] and occasional claims that it is either increased or decreased by such therapy remain dubious. Reports that fibrates may decrease Lp(a)[196] require further confirmation. The report that N-acetyl cysteine decreases Lp(a)[197] was not substantiated in a second larger study[198]. The effect is also not shown with carbocisteine[199]. Several studies have hinted that hormone replacement therapy might modestly decrease Lp(a) in postmenopausal women[200]. The results of larger trials are required, but the possibility is plausible because of the effect of larger doses of anabolic steroid hormones[201–203] and norethisterone[204]. The decreases are of course accompanied by increases in serum LDL cholesterol and decreases in HDL cholesterol so they cannot be regarded as beneficial. The combination of small amounts of norethisterone with oestrogen could potentially prevent these disadvantageous effects. Perhaps the lack of response of Lp(a) to therapy is not so bad if one considers that we do not yet know whether it actually is causally involved in IHD or what its true biological role is. The evidence, however, does indicate that a more rigorous approach should be taken to the treatment of other IHD risk factors if serum Lp(a) levels are increased.

# References

1. Moutafis, C.D. and Myant, N.B. The metabolism of cholesterol in two hypercholesterolaemic patients treated with cholestyramine. *Clin. Sci.*, **37**, 443–454 (1969)
2. Moutafis, C.D., Simons, L.A., Myant, N.B., Adams, P.W. and Wynn, V. The effect of cholestyramine on the faecal excretion of bile acids and neutral steroids in familial hypercholesterolaemia. *Atherosclerosis*, **26**, 329–334 (1977)
3. Packard, C.J. and Shepherd, J. Involvement in hepatobiliary axis and regulation of plasma lipoprotein levels. In *Cholesterol-7α-Hydroxylase* (eds R. Fears and L. R. Sabine), CRC Press, Boca Raton, pp. 147–165 (1986)
4. Kwok, C.T., Pillay, S.P. and Hardie, I.R. Molecular control of activity by reversible phosphorylation. In *Cholesterol-7α-Hyroxylase* (eds R. Fears and J. R. Sabine), CRC Press, Boca Raton, pp. 89–102 (1986)
5. Shepherd, J., Packard, C.J., Bicker, S., Lawrie, T. D. V. and Morgan, H. G. Cholestyramine promotes receptor-mediated low-density lipoprotein catabolism. *N. Engl. J. Med.*, **302**, 1219–1222 (1980)
6. Betteridge, D.J., Bhatnagar, D., Bing, D., Durrington, P.N., Evans, G. *et al*. Treatment of familial hypercholesterolaemia. The United Kingdom lipid clinics study of pravastatin and cholestyramine. *Br. Med. J.*, **304**, 1335–1338 (1992)
7. Lipid Research Clinics Program. The Lipid Research Clinics Coronary Primary Prevention Trial Results I. Reduction in incidence of coronary heart disease. *J. Am. Med Assoc.*, **251**, 351–364 (1984)
8. Mabuchi, H., Sakai, T., Sakai, Y., Yoshimura, A., Watanabe, A. *et al*. Reduction in serum cholesterol in heterozygous patients with familial hypercholesterolaemia: additive effects of compactin and cholestyramine. *N. Engl. J. Med.*, **308**, 609–613 (1983)
9. Illingworth, D.R. Mevinolin plus colestipol in therapy for severe heterozygous familial hypercholesterolaemia. *Ann. Intern. Med.*, **101**, 598–604 (1984)
10. Heel, R.C., Brogden, R.N. and Pakes, G.E. Colestipol: a review of its pharmacological properties and therapeutic effficacy in patients with hypercholesterolaemia. *Drugs*, **19**, 161–180 (1980)
11. Angelin, B., Bjorkhem, I. and Einvarsson, W. Cholesterol-7α-hydroxylase and bile acid synthesis in relation to triglyceride and lipoprotein metabolism. In *Cholesterol-7α-Hydroxylase* (eds R. Fears and J. R. Sabine), CRC Press, Boca Raton, pp. 167–177 (1986)
12. West, R.J. and Lloyd, J.K. Effect of cholestyramine on intestinal absorption. *Gut*, **16**, 93–98 (1975)
13. Altschul, R., Hoffer, A. and Stephen, S.D. Influence of nicotinic acid on serum cholesterol in man. *Arch. Biochem. Biophys.*, **54**, 558–599 (1955)
14. Carlson, L.A. Studies on the effect of nicotinic acid on catecholamine stimulated lipolysis in adipose tissue in vitro. *Acta Med. Scand.*, **173**, 719–722 (1963)
15. Carlson, L.A., Oro, L. and Ostman, J. Effect of nicotinic acid on plasma lipids in patients with hyperlipoproteinaemia during the first week of treatment. *J. Atheroscl. Res.*, **8**, 667–677 (1968)
16. Langer, T. and Levy, R.I. The effect of nicotinic acid on the turnover of low density lipoproteins in type II hyperlipoproteinaemia. In *Metabolic Effects of Nicotinic Acid and its Derivatives* (eds K.F. Gay and L.A. Carlson), Huber, Berne, pp. 641–648 (1971)
17. Miettinen, T.A. Effect of nicotinic acid on catabolism and synthesis of cholesterol in man. *Clin. Chim. Acta*, **20**, 43–51 (1968)
18. Shepherd, J., Packard, C.J., Patsch, J.R., Gotto, A.M. and Taunton, O. D. Effects of nicotinic acid therapy on plasma high density lipoprotein subfraction distribution and composition and on apolipoprotein A metabolism. *J. Clin. Invest.*, **63**, 858–867 (1979)
19. Illingworth, D.R. and Gowen, D. Management of lipoprotein abnormalities. In *Recent Advances in Cardiology* (ed. D. J. Rolands), Churchill Livingstone, Edinburgh, pp. 71–100 (1987)
20. Kane, J.P., Malloy, M.J., Tun, P., Phillipis, N.R., Freedman, D.D. *et al*. Normalisation of low-density lipoprotein levels in heterozygous familial hypercholesterolaemia with a combined drug regimen. *N. Engl. J. Med.*, **304**, 251–258 (1981)
21. Coronary Drug Project Research Group. Clofibrate and niacin in coronary heart disease. *J. Am. Med. Assoc.*, **231**, 360–381(1975)
22. Brown, W.V., Goldberg, I.J. and Ginsberg, H.N. Treatment of common lipoprotein disorders. *Progr. Cardiovasc. Dis.*, **27**, 1–20 (1984)

23. Illingworth, G.R., Rapp, J.H., Phillipson, B.E. and Connor, W.E. Colestipol plus nicotinic acid in the treatment of heterozygous familial hypercholesterolaemia. *Lancet*, **i**, 296–298 (1981)

24. Angelin, B., Eriksson, M. and Einarsson, K. Combined treatment with cholestyramine and nicotinic acid in heterozygous familial hypercholesterolaemia: effects on biliary lipid composition. *Eur. J. Clin. Invest.*, **16**, 391–396 (1986)

25. Carlson, L.A., Hamsten, A. and Asplund, A. Pronounced lowering of serum levels of Lp(a) in hyperlipidaemic subjects treated with nicotinic acid. *J. Intern. Med.*, **226**, 271–276 (1989)

26. Gurakar, A., Hoeg, J.H., Kostner, G., Papadopoulos, N.B. and Brewer, H.B. Levels of lipoprotein (a) decline with neomycin and niacin treatment. *Atherosclerosis*, **57**, 293 (1985)

27. Fuccella, L.M., Goldaniga, G., Lovisolo, P., Maggi, E., Musatti, L. *et al.* Inhibition of lipolysis by nicotinic acid and by acipomox. *Clin. Pharmacol. Ther.*, **28**, 790–795 (1980)

28. Sommariva, D., Pogliaghi, I., Bonfiglioli, D., Cabrine, C., Tirrito, M. and Lavezzari, M. Changes in lipoprotein cholesterol and triglycerides induced by acipimox in type IV and type III hyperlipoproteinaemic patients. *Curr. Thera. Res.*, **37**, 363–368 (1985)

29. Stuyt, P.M.J., Stalenhoef, A.F.H., Demacker, P.N.M. and Van't Laar, A. A comparative study of the effects of a acipimox and clofibrate in type III and type IV hyperlipoproteinaemia. *Atherosclerosis*, **55**, 51–62 (1985)

30. Taskinen, M-R. and Nikkila, E.A. Effects of acipimox on serum lipids, lipoproteins and lipolytic enzymes in hypertriglyceridaemia. *Atherosclerosis*, **69**, 249–255 (1988)

31. Anon. Acipimox – a nicotinic acid analogue for hyperlipidaemia. *Drug Thera. Bull.*, **29**, 57–59 (1991)

32. Series, J.J., Gaw, A., Kilday, C., Bedford, D.K., Lorimer, A.R. *et al.* Acipimox in combination with low dose cholestyramine for the treatment of type II hyperlipidaemia. *Br. J. Clin. Pharmacol.*, **30**, 49–54 (1990)

33. Francheschini, G., Bernini, F., Michelagnoli, S., Bellosta, S., Vaccarino, V. *et al.* Increased affinity of LDL for their receptors after acipimox treatment in hypertriglyceridaemia. *Eur. J. Clin. Pharmacol.*, **40**, (Suppl.), S45–S48 (1991)

34. Griffin, B.A., Caslake, M.J., Gaw, A., Yip, B., Packard, C.J. and Shepherd, J. Effects of cholestyramine and acipimox on subfractions of plasma low density lipoprotein studies in normolipidaemic and hypercholesterolaemic subjects. *Eur. J. Clin. Invest.*, **22**, 383–390 (1992)

35. Fulcher, G.R., Farrer, M., Thow, J.C., Johnson, A.B., Davis, S.N. *et al.* The glucose-fatty acid cycle in non-insulin dependent diabetes mellitus: the acute effects of inhibition of lipolysis overnight with acipimox. *Diab. Nutr. Metabol.*, **4**, 285–293 (1990)

36. Fulcher, G.R., Walker, M., Catalano, C., Farrer, M. and Alberti, K.G.M.M. Acute metabolic and hormonal responses to the inhibition of lipolysis in non-obese patients with non-insulin-dependent (type 2) diabetes mellitus: effects of acipimox. *Clin. Sci.*, **82**, 565–571 (1992)

37. Fulcher, G.R., Catalano, C., Walker, M., Farrer, M., Thow, J. *et al.* A double-blind study of the effect of acipimox on serum lipids, blood glucose control and insulin action in non-obese patients with type 2 diabetes mellitus. *Diabetic Med.*, **9**, 908–914 (1992)

38. Dean, J.D., McCarthy, S., Betteridge, D.J., Whataby-Smith, C., Powell, J. and Owens, D.R. The effect of acipimox in patients with type 2 diabetes and persistent hyperlipidaemia. *Diabetic Med.*, **9**, 611–615 (1992)

39. Kumar, S., Durrington, P.N., Laing, I. and Bhatnagar, D. Suppression of non-esterified fatty acids to treat type A insulin resistance syndrome. *Lancet*, **343**, 1073–1074 (1994)

40. Kumar, S., Durrington, P.N., Bhatnagar, D., Mackness, M.I., Gordon, C. *et al.* Improvement in glucose tolerance and insulin sensitivity in Type 2 diabetic patients treated with a long-acting formulation of Acipimox for 8 weeks. *Diabetic Med.*, in press (1995)

41. Thorp, J.M. and Waring, W.S. Modification of metabolism and distribution of lipids by ethyl chlorophenoxyisobutyrate. *Nature*, **194**, 948–949 (1962)

42. Buxton Symposium on Atromid. *J. Atheroscler. Res.*, **3**, 341–753 (1963)

43. Taylor, K.G., Holdsworth, G. and Galton, D.J. Clofibrate increases lipoprotein-lipase activity in adipose tissue of hypertriglyceridaemic patients. *Lancet*, **ii**, 1106–1107 (1977)

44. Nikkila, E.A., Huttunen, J.K. and Ehnholm, C. Effect of clofibrate on post-heparin plasma triglyceride lipase activities in patients with hypertriglyceridaemia. *Metabolism*, **26**, 179–186 (1977)

45. Vessby, B., Lithell, H. and Ledermann, H. Elevated lipoprotein lipase activity in skeletal muscle tissue during treatment of hypertriglyceridaemic patients with bezafibrate. *Atherosclerosis*, **44**, 113–118 (1982)

46. Naruszewicz, M., Szostak, W. B., Cybulska, B., Wozlowska, M. and Chotkowska, E. The influence of clofibrate on lipid and protein components of very low density lipoproteins in type IV hyperlipoproteinaemia. *Atherosclerosis*, **35**, 382–392 (1980)

47. Schwandt, P., Weisweiler, P., Drosner, M. and Janetschek, P. Effects of bezafibrate on the composition of very low density lipoproteins in type IV hyperlipoproteinaemia. *Atherosclerosis*, **42**, 245–249 (1982)

48. Carlson, L. A., Olsson, A. G. and Ballantyne, D. On the rise in low density and high density lipoproteins in response to treatment of hypertriglyceridaemia in type IV and type V hyperlipoproteinaemias. *Atherosclerosis*, **26**, 603–609 (1977)

49. Caslake, M.J., Packard, C.J., Gaw, A., Murray, E., Griffin, B.A. *et al.* Fenofibrate and LDL metabolic heterogeneity in hypercholesterolaemia. *Arteriosclerosis*, **13**, 702–711 (1993)

50. Stewart, J.M., Packard, C.J., Lorimer, A.R., Boag, D.E. and Shepherd, J. Effects of bezafibrate on receptor-mediated and receptor-independent low density lipoprotein catabolism in type II hyperlipoproteinaemic subjects. *Atherosclerosis*, **44**, 355–365 (1982)

51. Shepherd, J., Caslake, M., Gaw, A., Griffin, B., Lindsay, G. and Packard, C. Atherogenicity of triglyceride-rich lipoproteins: clinical aspects. In *Drugs Affecting Lipid Metabolism* (eds A.L. Catapano, A.M. Gotto, L.C. Smith and R. Paoletti), Kluwer Academic Publishers, Dordrecht, pp. 453–466 (1993)

52. Grundy, S.M. and Vega, G.L. Fibric acids: effects on lipids and lipoprotein metabolism. *Am. J. Med.*, **83** (Suppl. 5B), 9–20 (1987)

53. Hunninghake, D.B., Peters, J.R. Effect of fibric acid derivatives on blood lipid and lipoprotein levels. *Am. J. Med.*, **83** (Suppl. 5B), 44–48 (1987)

54. Malmendier, C.L. and Delcroix, C. Effects of fenofibrate on high and low density lipoprotein metabolism in heterozygous familial hypercholesterolaemia. *Atherosclerosis*, **55**, 161–169 (1985)

55. Schlierf, G., Chwat, M., Feverborn, E., Wulfinghof, E., Henck, C.C. *et al.* Biliary and plasma lipids and lipid-lowering chemotherapy. Studies with clofibrate, fenofibrate and etofibrate in healthy volunteers. *Atherosclerosis*, **36**, 323–329 (1980)

56. Hrabak, P., Skorepa, J., Zak, A. and Zeman, M. Effect of long-term bezafibrate treatment on biliary lipid metabolism in patients with endogenous hypertriglyceridaemia: with special reference to the risk of cholelithiasis. In *Pharmacological Control of Hyperlipidaemia*, J. R. Prous Science Publishers, S.A., pp. 343–349 (1986)

57. Grundy, S.M., Ahrens, E.H., Salen, G., Schreibman, Ph.H. and Nestel, P.J. Mechanism of action of clofibrate on cholesterol metabolism in patients with hyperlipidaemia. *J. Lipid Res.*, **13**, 531–551 (1972)

58. Kesaniemi, Y.A. and Grundy, S.M. Influence of gemfibrozil and clofibrate on metabolism of cholesterol and plasma triglycerides in man. *J. Am. Med. Assoc.*, **251**, 2241–2247 (1984)

59. Kleinman, Y., Oschry, Y. and Eisenberg, S. Abnormal regulation of LDL receptor activity and abnormal cellular metabolism of hypertriglyceridaemic low density lipoprotein: normalization with bezafibrate therapy. *Eur. J. Clin. Invest.*, **17**, 538–543 (1987)

60. Austin, M.A., King, M.C., Vranizan, K.M. and Krauss, R.M., Atherogenic lipoprotein phenotype. A proposed genetic marker for coronary heart disease risk. *Circulation*, **82**, 495–506 (1990)

61. Brown, W.V., Dujovne, C.A., Farquhar, J.W., Feldman, E.B., Grundy, S.M. *et al.* Effects of fenofibrate on plasma lipids. Double-blind, multicenter study in patients with type IIA or IIB hyperlipidaemia. *Arteriosclerosis*, **6**, 670–678 (1986)

62. O'Connor, P., Freely, J. and Shepherd, J. Lipid lowering drugs. *Br. Med. J.*, **300**, 667–672 (1990)

63. Illingworth, D.R. Treatment of hyperlipidaemia. *Br. Med. Bull.*, **46**, 1025–1058 (1990)

64. Sirtori, C.R. and Franceschini, G. Drug effects on HDL. In *Clinical and Metabolic Aspects of High-Density Lipoproteins* (eds N. E. Miller and G. J. Miller), Elsevier, Amsterdam, pp. 341–379 (1984)

65. Eisenberg, S. High density lipoprotein metabolism. *J. Lipid Res.*, **25**, 1017–1058 (1984)

66. Bhatnagar, D., Durrington, P.N., Mackness, M.I., Arrol, S., Winocour, P.H. and Prais, H. Effects of treatment of hypertriglyceridaemia with gemfibrozil on serum lipoproteins and the transfer of cholesteryl ester from high density lipoproteins to low density lipoproteins. *Atherosclerosis*, **92**, 49–57 (1992)

67. Mann, C.J., Yen, F.T., Grant, A.M. and Bihain, B.E. Mechanism of plasma cholesteryl ester transfer in hypertriglyceridaemia. *J. Clin. Invest.*, **88**, 2059–2066 (1991)

68. Bhatnagar, D., Durrington, P.N., Channon, K.M., Prais, H. and Mackness, M.I. Increased transfer of cholesteryl esters from high density lipoproteins to low density and very low density lipoproteins in patients with angiographic evidence of coronary artery disesase. *Atherosclerosis*, **98**, 25–32 (1992)

69. Durrington, P.N. How HDL protects against atheroma. *Lancet*, **342**, 1315–1316 (1993)

70. Farrier, M., Truong-Tan, N. and Regy, C. Comparative multicentre trial of the efficacy and tolerability of ciprofibrate and simvastatin in the treatment of mixed type IIb hyperlipoproteinaemia. *J. Drug. Dev.*, **5**, 13–21 (1992)

71. Stohler, R., Keller, U. and Riesen, W.F. Effects of simvastatin and fenofibrate on serum lipoproteins and apolipoproteins in primary hypercholesterolaemia. *Eur. J. Clin. Pharmacol.*, **37**, 199–203 (1989)

72. Monk, J.P. and Todd, P.A. Bezafibrate: a review. *Drugs*, **33**, 539–576 (1987)

73. Todd, P.A. and Ward, A. Gemfibrozil: a review of its pharmacodynamic and pharmacokinetic properties, and therapeutic use in dyslipidaemia. *Drugs*, **36**, 314–339 (1988)

74. Balfour, J.A., McTavish, D. and Heel, R.C. Fenofibrate: a review of its pharmacodynamic and pharmacokinetic properties and therapeutic use in hyslipidaemia. *Drugs*, **40**, 260–290 (1990)

75. Committee of Principal Investigators. A cooperative trial in the primary prevention of ischaemic heart disease using clofibrate. *Br. Heart J.*, **40**, 1069–1118 (1978)

76. Fick, M. H., Elo, O., Haapa, K., Heinonen, O.P., Heinsalmi, P. *et al.* Helsinki Heart Study: primary prevention trial with gemfibrozil in middle-aged men with dyslipidaemia. Safety of treatment, changes in risk factors and incidence of coronary heart disease. *N. Engl. J. Med.*, **317**, 1237–1245 (1987)

77. Heady, J.A., Morris, J.N. and Oliver, M.F. WHO clofibrate/cholesterol trial: clarifications. *Lancet*, **340**, 1405–1406 (1992)

78. Angelin, B., Einarsson, K. and Leijd, B. Effect of ciprofibrate treatment on biliary lipids in patients with hyperlipoproteinaemia. *Eur. J. Clin. Invest.*, **14**, 73–78 (1984)

79. Angelin, B., Einarsson, K. and Leijd, B. Biliary lipid composition during treatment with different hypolipidaemic drugs. *Eur. J. Clin. Invest.*, **9**, 185–190 (1979)

80. von Bergmann, K. and Leiss, O. Effect of short-term treatment with bezafibrate and fenofibrate on biliary lipid metabolism in patients with hyperlipoproteinaemia. *Eur. J. Clin. Invest.*, **14**, 150–154 (1984)

81. Angelin, B., Einarsson, K. and Leijd, B. Clofibrate treatment and bile cholesterol saturation: short-term and long-term effects and influence of combination with chenodeoxycholic acid. *Eur. J. Clin. Invest.*, **ii**, 185–189 (1981)

82. Grundy, S. M. Biliary lipids, gallstones and treatment of hyperlipidaemia. *Eur. J. Clin. Invest.*, **9**, 179–180 (1979)

83. Bateson, M.C., Ross, P.E., Murison, J. and Bouchier, I.A. Reversal of clofibrate-induced cholesterol oversaturation of bile with chenodeoxycholic acid. *Br. Med. J.*, **i**, 1171–1173 (1978)

84. Leiss, O., van Bergmann, K., Gnasso, A. and Angus, J. Effect of gemfibrozil on biliary lipid metabolism in normolipaemic subjects. *Metabolism*, **34**, 74–82 (1985)

85. Monk, J. P. and Todd, P. A. Bezafibrate: a review of its pharmacologic and pharmacokinetic properties and therapeutic use in hyperlipidaemia. *Drugs*, **33**, 539–576 (1987)

86. Eriksson, M. and Angelin, B. Bezafibrate therapy and biliary lipids: effects of short-term and long-term treatment in patients with various forms of hyperlipoproteinaemia. *Eur. J. Clin. Invest.*, **17**, 396–401 (1987)

87. Palmer, R.H. Effects of fibric acid derivatives on biliary lipid composition. *Am. J. Med.*, **83** (Suppl. 5B), 37–43 (1987)

88. Harefield, M., Kemmer, C. and Kadner, E. Relationship between morphological changes and lipid-lowering action of *p*-chlorophenoryisobutyric acid (CPIB) on hepatic mitochondria and peroxisomes in man. *Atherosclerosis*, **46**, 239–246 (1983)

89. Blumcke, S., Schwartzkopff, W., Lobeck, H., Edmondson, M.A., Prentice, D.E. and Blane, G.F. Influence of fenofibrate on cellular and subcellular liver structure in hyperlipidaemic patients. *Atherosclerosis*, **46**, 105–116 (1983)

90. De la Iglesia, F.A., Lewis, J.E., Buchannan, R.A., Marcus, E.L. and McMahon, G. Light and electron microscopy of liver in hyperlipoproteinaemic patients under long-term gemfibrozil treatment. *Atherosclerosis*, **43**, 19–29 (1982)

91. Reddy, J., Azarnoff, D. and Hignite, C.E. Hypolipidaemic hepatic peroxisome proliferators form a novel class of hepatocarcinogens. *Nature*, **283**, 397–398 (1980)

92. Bridgman, J.F., Rosen, S.M. and Thorp, J.M. Complications during clofibrate treatment of nephrotic-syndrome hyperlipoproteinaemia. *Lancet*, **ii**, 506–509 (1972)

93. Langer, T. and Levy, R. I. Acute muscular syndrome associated with administration of clofibrate. *N. Engl. J. Med.*, **279**, 856–858 (1968)

94. Short, C.D. and Durrington, P.N. Hyperlipidaemia and renal disease. *Ballière's Clin. Endocrinol. Metabol.*, **4**, 777–806 (1990)

95. Meade, T. W., Mellows, S., Brozovic, M., Miller, G. J., Chakrabarti, R. R. et al. Haemostatic function and ischaemic heart disease: principal results of the Northwick Park Heart Study. *Lancet*, **ii**, 533–537 (1986)

96. Stone, M.C. and Thorp, J.M. Plasma fibrinogen – a major coronary risk factor. *J. R. Coll. Gen. Pract.*, **35**, 565–569 (1985)

97. O'Brien, J.R., Etherington, M.D., Jamiesson, S. and Susse, J. The effects of ICI 55, 897 and clofibrate on platelet function and other tests abnormal in atherosclerosis. *Thromb. Haemostas.*, **40**, 75–82 (1978)

98. Dormandy, J.A., Gutteridge, J.M.C., Hoare, E. and Dormandy, T.L. Effect of clofibrate on blood viscosity in intermittent claudication. *Br. Med J.*, **ii**, 259–262 (1974)

99. Winocour, P.H., Durrington, P.N., Bhatnagar, D., Ishola, M., Arrol, S. et al. Double-blind placebo controlled study of the effects of bezafibrate on blood lipids, lipoproteins and fibrinogen in hyperlipidaemic type 1 (insulin-dependent) diabetes mellitus. *Diabetic Med.*, **7**, 736–748 (1990)

100. Brianchi, A., Rovellini, A., Gugliandolo, D., Sommariva, D. and Fasoli, A. Comparative evaluation of the effect of 3 fibrates and of 2 HMG-CoA reductase inhibitors on plasma fibrinogen in hypercholesterolaemic patients. (in press)

101. Almer, L.D. and Kjellstrom, T. The fibrinolytic system and coagulation during bezafibrate treatment of hypertriglyceridaemia. *Atherosclerosis*, **61**, 81–85 (1986)

102. Leschke, M., Hoffken, H., Schmidtdroff, A., Blanke, H., Egbring, R. et al. The effect of fenofibrate on fibrinogen concentrations and blood viscosity. *Dtsch. Med. Wochenschr*, **114**, 939–944 (1989)

103. Sirtori, C.R. and Colli, S. Drugs affecting thrombosis and atherosclerosis. In *Drugs Affecting Lipid Metabolism* (eds A.L. Catapano, A. M. Gotto, L.C. Smith and R. Paoletti), Kluwer Academic Publishers, Dordrecht, pp. 215–229 (1993)

104. O'Brien, J.R., Etherington, M.D., Shuttleworth, R.D., Adams, C.M., Middleton, J.E. and Goodland, F.C. Effect of gemfibrozil on some haematological parameters. In *Further Progress with Gemfibrozil* (ed. C. Wood), Royal Society of Medicine, London, pp. 11–14 (1986)

105. Ciuffetti, G., Orecchini, G., Siepi, D., Lupattelli, G. and Vertwa, A. Hemorheological activity of gemfibrozil in primary hyperlipidaemias. In *Drugs Affecting Lipid Metabolism* (eds R. Paoletti et al.), Springer-Verlag, Berlin, pp. 372–375 (1987)

106. Anderson, P., Smith, P., Seljeflot, I., Brataker, S. and Arnesen, H. Effect of gemfibrozil on lipids and haemostasis after myocardial infarction. *Thromb. Haemostas.*, **63**, 174–177 (1990)

107. Wyngaarden, J.B. and Kelly, W.N. Gout. In The *Metabolic Basis of Inherited Disease*, 5th edn (eds J.B. Stanbury, J.B. Wyngaarden, D.S. Fredrickson, J.L. Goldstein and M.S. Brown), McGraw-Hill, New York, pp. 1043–1114 (1983)

108. Bastow, M.D., Durrington, P.N. and Ishola, M. Hypertriglyceridaemia and hyperuricaemia: effects of two fibric acid derivatives (bezafibrate and fenofibrate) in a double-blind placebo-controlled trial. *Metabolism*, **37**, 217–220 (1988)

109. von Volgelberg, K.H., Muller, H.J. and Hubinger, A. Der Somatostatin-infusions test zurberteilung de glukose-utilisation unter bezafibrat-medikation. *Drug Res.*, **34**, 1038–1041 (1984)

110. Wahl, P., Hasslacher, Ch., Lang, P.D. and Vodman, J. Der Lipsenkende effekt von bezafibrat bei patient en mit diabetes mellitus und hyperlipidaemie. *Dtsch. Med Wochenschr.*, **103**, 1233–1237 (1978)

111. Bruneder, H. and Klein, H.J. Behandlung de hyperlipoproteinaemie bei diabetikern. *Dtsch. Med. Wochenschr.*, **106**, 1653–1656 (1981)
112. Volhard, E., Lasch, H.G., Matis, P. and Kruchel, F. Einfluss von bezafibrat auf den kohlenhy-dratstoffwechsel von 17 diabetikern mit hyperlipidaemia. *Med Welt.*, **32**, 268–271 (1981)
113. Ruth, E. and Vollman, J. Verbesserung den diabeteseinstellung unter der therapie mit bezafibrat. *Dtsch. Med Wochenschr.*, **107**, 1470–1473 (1982)
114. Randle, P.J., Garland, P.B., Hales, C.N. and Newsholme, E.A. The glucose fatty-acid cycle. Its role in insulin sensitivity and the metabolic disturbances of diabetes mellitus. *Lancet*, **i**, 785–789 (1963)
115. Glueck, C.J. Colestipol and probucol: treatment of primary and familial hypercholesterolaemia and amelioration of atherosclerosis. *Ann. Intern. Med.*, **96**, 475–482 (1982)
116. Durrington, P.N. and Miller, J.P. Double-blind, placebo-controlled, cross-over trial of probucol in heterozygous familial hypercholesterolaemia. *Atherosclerosis*, **55**, 187–194 (1985)
117. Jones, D.B., Simpson, H.C.R., Slaughter, P., Lounsley, S., Carter, R.D. *et al.* A comparison of cholestyramine and probucol in the treatment of familial hypercholesterolaemia. *Atherosclerosis*, **53**, 1–7 (1984)
118. Baker, S.G., Joffe, B.I., Mendlesohn, D. and Seftel, H.C. Treatment of homozygous familial hypercholesterolaemia with probucol. *S. Afr. Med. J.*, **62**, 7–11 (1982)
119. Yamamoto, A., Matsuzawa, Y., Kishino, B., Kayashi, R., Hayashi, R. *et al.* Effects of probucol on homozygous cases of familial hypercholesterolaemia. *Atherosclerosis*, **48**, 157–166 (1983)
120. Steinberg, D. Studies on the mechanism of action of probucol. *Am. J. Cardiol.*, **57**, 16H–21H (1986)
121. Carew, T.E., Schwenke, D.C. and Steinberg, D. Antiatherogenic effect of probucol unrelated to its hypocholesterolaemia effect: evidence that antioxidants in vivo can selectively inhibit low density lipoprotein degradation in macrophage-rich fatty streaks and slow the progression of atherosclerosis in the Watanabe heritable hyperlipidaemia rabbit. *Proc. Natl Acad. Sci. USA*, **84**, 7725–7729 (1987)
122. Miettinen, T.A., Huttunen, J.K., Naukkaviven, V., Strandberg, T. and Vanhanen, H. Long term use of probucol in the multifactorial primary prevention of vascular disease. *Am. J. Cardiol.*, **57**, 49H–54H (1986)
123. Miettinen, T.A., Huttunen, J.K., Naukkarinen, V., Strandberg, T., Mattila, S. *et al.* Multifactorial primary prevention of cardiovascular disease in middle-aged men. Risk factor changes, incidence and mortality. *J. Am. Med Assoc.*, **254**, 2079–2082 (1985)
124. Franceschini, G., Sirtori, M., Vaccirio, U., Gainfranceschi, G., Rezzonizo, L. *et al.* Mechanisms of HDL reduction after probucol. Changes in HDL subfractions and increased reverse cholesteryl ester transfer. *Arteriosclerosis*, **9**, 462–469 (1989)
125. Yamamoto, A., Matsuzawa, Y., Yokoyama, S., Funahashi, T. and Kishino, B. Effects of probu-col on xanthomata regression in familial hypercholesterolaemia. *Am. J. Cardiol.*, **57**, 29H–35H (1986)
126. Nestel, P.J. and Billington, T. Effects of probucol on low density lipoprotein removal and high density lipoprotein synthesis. *Atherosclerosis*, **38**, 203–209 (1981)
127. Miettinen, T.A., Huttunen, I.W., Kuusi, T., Humlin, T., Makila, S. *et al.* Effect of probucol on the activity of postheparin plasma lipoprotein lipase and hepatic lipase. *Clin. Chim. Acta*, **113**, 59–64 (1981)
128. Lock, D.R., Kuisk, I., Gonen, B., Patsch, W. and Schonfeld, G. Effect of probucol on the compo-sition of lipoproteins and on VLDL apolipoprotein B turnover. *Atherosclerosis*, **47**, 271–278 (1983)
129. Shepherd, J., Packard, C.J., Morgan, H.G., Third, J.L.H.C., Steward, J.H. and Lawrie, T.D.V. The effect of cholestyramine on high density lipoprotein metabolism. *Atherosclerosis*, **33**, 433–444 (1979)
130. Durrington, P.N. and Miller, J.P. Unpublished observation
131. Jackson, J.M. and Lee, H.A. The effect of probucol and cholestyramine combination therapy in severe familial hypercholesterolaemia. *Atherosclerosis*, **51**, 189–197 (1984)
132. Kuo, P.T., Wilson, A.C., Kostis, J.B. and Moreyra, A.E. Effects of combined probucol-colestipol treatment for familial hypercholesterolaemia and coronary artery disease. *Am. J. Cardiol.*, **57**, 43H–48H (1986)

133. Miettinen, T.A. Mode of action of a new hypocholesterolaemic drug (DH-581) in familial hypercholesterolaemia. *Atherosclerosis*, **15**, 163–176 (1971)

134. Bateson, M.C., Fiabane, A.H., Clarke, A. and Bouchier, I.A.D. Probucol and hypercholesterolaemia. *Br. J. Pharmacol.*, **ii**, 531–533 (1981)

135. Miettinen, T.A. Effects of neomycin alone and in combination with cholestyramine on serum cholesterol and faecal steroids in hypercholesterolaemic subjects. *J. Clin. Invest.*, **64**, 1485–1493 (1979)

136. Samuel, P. Treatment of hypercholesterolaemia with neomycin – a time for reappraisal. *N. Engl. J. Med.*, **301**, 595–597 (1979)

137. Faergeman, O. Effects and side-effects of treatment of hypercholesterolaemia with cholestyramine and neomycin. *Acta Med. Scand.*, **194**, 165–167 (1973)

138. Thompson, G.R., Barrowman, J., Gutierrez, L. and Dowling, R.H. Action of neomycin on the intraluminal phase of lipid absorption. *J. Clin. Invest.*, **50**, 319–323 (1971)

139. Kesaniemi Y.A. and Grundy, S.M. Turnover of low density lipoproteins during inhibition of cholesterol absorption by neomycin. *Arteriosclerosis*, **4**, 41–48 (1983)

140. Sedaghat, A., Samuel, P., Grouse, J. R. and Ahrens, E. H. Effects of neomycin on absorption, synthesis and/or flux of cholesterol in man. *J. Clin. Invest.*, **55**, 12–21 (1975)

141. Fears, R. Mode of action of lipid-lowering drugs. *Ballière's Clin. Endocrinol. Metabol.*, **i**, 727–754 (1987)

142. Endo, A. The discovery and development of HMG-CoA reductase inhibitors. *J. Lipid Res.*, **33**, 1569–1582 (1992)

143. Bilheimer, D.W., Grundy, S.M., Brown, M.S. and Goldstein, J.L. Mevinolin and colestipol stimulate receptor-mediated clearance of low density lipoprotein from plasma in familial hypercholesterolaemia heterozygotes. *Proc. Natl Acad. Sci., USA.*, **80**, 4124–4128 (1983)

144. Illingworth, D.R. and Sexton, G.J. Hypocholesterolaemic effects of mevinolin in patients with heterozygous familial hypercholesterolaemia. *J. Clin. Invest.*, **74**, 1982–1988 (1984)

145. The Lovastatin Study Group II. Therapeutic response to lovastatin (Mevinolin) in non-familial hypercholesterolaemia. A multicenter study. *J. Am. Med. Assoc.*, **256**, 2829–2834 (1986)

146. Grundy, S.J. and Bilheimer, D.W. Inhibition of 3-hydroxy-3-methylglutaryl-CoA reductase by mevinolin in familial hypercholesterolaemia heterozygotes: effects on cholesterol balance. *Proc. Natl Acad. Sci., USA.*, **81**, 2538–2542 (1984)

147. Mol, M.J.T.M., Erkelens, D.W., Leuven, J.A.G., Schouten, J.A. and Stalenhoef, A.F.H. Effects of synvinolum (MK-773) on plasma lipids in familial hypercholesterolaemia. *Lancet*, **ii**, 936–939 (1986)

148. Serajuddin, A.T.M., Ranadive, S.A. and Mahoney, E.M. Relative lipophilicites, solubilites, and structive-pharmacological considerations of 3-hydroxy-3-methylglutaryl-coenzyme A (HMG-CoA) reductase inhibitors pravastatin, lovastatin, mevastatin, and simvastatin. *J. Pharmaceut. Sci.*, **80**, 830–834 (1991)

149. Feussner, G. HMG-CoA reductase inhibitors. *Curr. Opin. Lipidol.*, **5**, 59–69 (1994)

150. Girouz, L.M., Davignon, J. and Naruszewics, M. Simvastatin inhibits the oxidation of low-density lipoproteins by activated human monocyte-derived macrophages. *Biochim. Biophys. Acta*, **1165**, 335–338 (1993)

151. Hidaka, Y., Eda, T., Yonemoto, M. and Kanei, T. Inhibition of cultured vascular smooth muscle cell migration by simvastatin (MK-733). *Atherosclerosis*, **95**, 87–96 (1992)

152. Thompson, G.R., Ford, J., Jenkinson, M. and Trayner, I. Efficacy of mevinolin as adjuvant therapy for refractory familial hypercholesterolaemia. *Q. J. Med.*, **60**, 803–811(1986)

153. Illingworth, D.R. and Connor, W.E. Hypercholesterolaemia persisting after distal ilial bypass: response to mevinolin. *Ann. Intern. Med.*, **100**, 850–851 (1984)

154. Laughlin, R.C. and Carey, T.F. Cataracts in patients treated with triparanol. *J. Am. Med. Assoc.*, **181**, 339–340 (1962)

155. McKenney, J.M., Lovastatin. A new cholesterol-lowering agent. *Clin. Pharmacol.*, **7**, 21–36 (1988)

156. Tobart, J.A. Efficacy and long-term adverse effect pattern of lovastatin. *Am. J. Cardiol.*, **62**, 28J–34J (1988)

157. Bhatnagar, D., Durrington, P.N., Neary, R. and Miller, J.P. Elevation of skeletal muscle isoform of creatinine kinase in heterozygous familial hypercholesterolaemia. *J. Intern. Med.*, **228**, 493–495 (1990)

158. Saunders, K.D., Cates, J.A., Abedin, M.Z. and Roslyn, J.J. Lovastatin and gallstone dissolution: a preliminary study. *Surgery*, **113**, 28–35 (1993)
159. Smit, J.W., van Erpecun, K.J., Stolk, M.F., Goerdink, R.A., Chiysenaer, O.J. *et al.* Successful dissolution of cholesterol gallstone during treatment with pravastatin. *Gastroenterology*, **103**, 1068–1070 (1992)
160. Nasumova, R.P., Marais, D., Erkelens, W., Rendell, N.B., Taylor, G.W. and Thompson, G.R. Changes in plasma mevalonate predict responsiveness to HMG CoA reductase inhibitors. *Atherosclerosis*, **103**, 297 (1993)
161. Leitersdorf, E., Eisenberg, S., Eliav, O., Friedlander, Y., Berkman, N. *et al.* Genetic determinants of responsiveness to the HMG-CoA reductase inhibitor heterozygous familial hypercholesterolaemia. *Circulation*, **87** (Suppl. III), 35–44 (1993)
162. September, J.M., van Roggen, F.G., de Villiers, Seftel, H. and Marais, D. Influence of specific mutations at the LDL-receptor gene locus on the response to simvastatin therapy in Afrikaner patients with heterozygous familial hypercholesterolaemia. *Atherosclerosis*, **98**, 51–58 (1993)
163. Simons, L.A., Hickie, J.B. and Balesubramanian, S. On the effects of dietary n-3 fatty acids (Maxepa) on plasma lipids and lipoproteins in patients with hyperlipidaemia. *Atherosclerosis*, **54**, 75–88 (1985)
164. Sanders, T.A.B., Sullivan, D.R., Reeve, J. and Thompson, G.R. Triglyceride-lowering effect of marine polyunsaturates in patients with hypertriglyceridaemia. *Atherosclerosis*, **5**, 459–465 (1985)
165. Sullivan, D.R., Sanders, T.A.B., Traynor, I.M. and Thompson, G.R. Paradoxical elevations of LDL apolipoprotein B levels in hypertriglyceridaemic patients and normal subjects ingesting fish oil. *Atherosclerosis*, **61**, 129–134 (1986)
166. Mackness, M.I., Bhatnagar, D., Durrington, P.N., Prais, H., Haynes, B. *et al.* Effects of a new fish oil concentrate on plasma lipids and lipoproteins in patients with hypertriglyceridaemia. *Eur. J. Clin. Nutr.* (in press)
167. Crombie, I.K., McHoone, P., Smith, W.C.S., Thomson, M. and Tunstall Pedoe, J. International differences in coronary disease mortality and consumption of fish and other food stuffs. *Eur. Heart J.*, **8**, 560–563 (1987)
168. Burr, M.L., Fehily, A.M., Gilbert, J.F., Rogers, S., Holliday, R.M. *et al.* Effects of changes in fat, fish and fibre intake on death and myocardial reinfarction: diet and reinfarction trial (DART). *Lancet*, **ii**, 757–761 (1989)
169. Coronary Drug Project. Findings leading to discontinuation of the 2.5 mg/day oestrogen group. *J. Am. Med Assoc.*, **226**, 652–657 (1973)
170. Tikkanen, M.J., Nikkila, E.A. and Vartiainen, E. Natural oestrogen as an effective treatment for type II hyperlipoproteinaemia in postmenopausal women. *Lancet*, **ii**, 490–501 (1978)
171. Kushwaha, R. S., Hazzard, W. R., Gagne, C., Chait, A. and Albers, J. T. Type III hyperlipoproteinaemia: paradoxical hypolipidaemic response to oestrogen. *Ann. Intern. Med.*, **87**, 517–525 (1977)
172. Tikkanen, M. J., Nikkila, E. A., Kuusi, T. and Sipinen, S. U. High density lipoprotein-2 and hepatic lipase: reciprocal changes produced by estrogen and norgestrel. *J. Clin. Endocrinol. Metabol.*, **54**, 1113–1117 (1982)
173. Glueck, C.J., Scheel, D., Fishback, J. and Steiner, P. Estrogen-induced pancreatitis in patients with previously covert familial type V hyperlipidaemia. *Metabolism*, **21**, 657–666 (1972)
174. Bush, T.L., Rifkind, B.M., Criqui, M.H., Cowan, L.D., Barrett-Connor, E. *et al.* Postmenopausal oestrogen use and cardiovascular mortality in women. In *Myocardial Infarction in Women* (eds. M.F. Oliver, A. Vedin and C. Wilhelmson), Churchill Livingstone, Edinburgh, 130–145 (1980)
175. Grady, D. Rubin, S.M., Petitti, D.B., Fox, C.S., Black, D. *et al.* Hormone therapy to prevent disease and prolong life in postmenopausal women. *Ann. Intern. Med.*, **117**, 1016–1041 (1992)
176. Meade, T.W. and Berra, A. Hormone replacement therapy and cardiovascular disease. *Br. Med. Bull.*, **48**, 276–308 (1992)
177. Falkeborn, M., Persson, I., Adami, H., Bergstrom, R., Eaker, E. *et al.* The risk of acute myocardial infarction after oestrogen-progestogen replacement. *Br. J. Obstet. Gynaecol.*, **99**, 821–828 (1992)
178. Sack, M.N., Rader, D.J. and Cannon III, R.O. Oestrogen and inhibition of oxidation of low-density lipoproteins in postmenopausal women. *Lancet*, **343**, 269–270 (1994)

179. Heider, J.G., Pickens, C.E. and Kelly, L.A. Role of acyl-CoA: cholesterol acyltransferase in cholesterol absorption and its inhibition by 57-118 in the rabbit. *J. Lipid Res.*, **24**, 1127–1134 (1983)

180. Clark, S.B. and Tercyak, A.M. Reduced cholesterol transmucosal transport in rats with inhibited mucosal acyl CoA: cholesterol acyltransferase and normal pancreatic function. *J. Lipid Res.*, **25**, 148–159 (1984)

181. Ross, A.C., Go, K.J., Heider, J.G. and Rothblat, G.H. Selective inhibition of acyl-coenzyme A: cholesterol acyltransferase by compound 58-035. *J. Biol. Chem.*, **259**, 815–819 (1984)

182. Suckling, K.E. and Stange, E.F. Role of acyl-CoA: cholesterol acyltransferase in cellular cholesterol metabolism. *J. Lipid Res.*, **26**, 647–671 (1985)

183. Schmitz, G., Niemann, R., Rennhausen, B., Krause, R. and Assmann, G. Regulation of high density lipoprotein receptors in cultured macrophages: role of acyl-CoA: cholesterol acyltransferase. *EMBO J.*, **4**, 2773–2779 (1985)

184. De Vries, V.G., Schaffer, S.A., Largis, E.E., Dutia, M.D., Wang, C. *et al.* Potential anti-atherosclerotic agents 5. An acyl-coenzyme A: cholesterol O-acyltransferase inhibitor with hypocholesterolaemic activity. *J. Med. Chem.*, **29**, 1131–1133 (1986)

185. Gaddi, A., Descovich, G.C., Noseda, G., Fragiacomo, C., Colombo, L. *et al.* Controlled evaluation of pantethine, a neutral hypolipidaemic compound in patients with different forms of hyper lipoproteinaemia. *Atherosclerosis*, **50**, 73–83 (1984)

186. Bon, G.B., Cazzolato, G., Zago, S. and Avagaro, P. Effects of pantethine on in-vitro peroxidation of low density lipoproteins. *Atherosclerosis*, **57**, 99–106 (1985)

187. Simons, L.A. and Myant, N.B. The effect of D-thyroxine on the metabolism of cholesterol in familial hyperbetalipoproteinaemia. *Atherosclerosis*, **19**, 103–117 (1974)

188. Coronary Drug Project. Findings leading to further modification of its protocol with respect to dextrothyroxine. *J. Am. Med. Assoc.*, **220**, 996–1008 (1972)

189. Heinemann, T., Leisse, O. and von Bergmannk, K. Effect of low-dose sitostanol on serum cholesterol in patients with hypercholesterolaemia. *Atherosclerosis*, **61**, 219–223 (1986)

190. Vahouny, G.V., Conner, W.E., Subramanian, S., Lin, D.S. and Gallo, L.L. Comparative lymphatic absorption of sitosterol, stigmasterol and frucosterol and differential inhibition of cholesterol absorption. *Am. J. Clin. Nutr.*, **37**, 805–809 (1983)

191. Simons, L.A., Gayst, S., Balasubramaniam, S. and Ruys, J. Long-term treatment of hypercholesterolaemia with a new palatable formulation of guar gum. *Atherosclerosis*, **45**, 101–108 (1982)

192. Hemila, H. Vitamin C and plasma cholesterol. *Crit. Rev. Food Sci. Nutr.*, **32**, 33–57 (1992)

193. Schenck, I., Keller, Ch. Hailer, S., Wolfram, G. and Zollner, N. Reduction of Lp(a) by different methods of plasma exchange. *Klin. Wochenschr.*, **66**, 1197–1201 (1988)

194. Armstrong, V.W., Schleef, J., Thiery, J., Much, R., Schuff-Werner, P. *et al.* Effect of HELP-LDL-apheresis on serum concentrations of human lipoprotein (a): kinetic analysis of the post-treatment return to baseline levels. *Eur. J. Clin. Invest.*, **19**, 235–240 (1989)

195. Kostner, G.M., Gavish, D., Leopold, B., Bolzano, K., Weintraub, M.S. *et al.* HMG-CoA reductase inhibitors lower LDL cholesterol without reducing Lp(a) levels. *Circulation*, **80**, 1313–1319 (1989)

196. Bimmerman, A., Boerschmann, C., Schwartzkopff, W., von Baeyer, H. and Schleicher, J. Effective therapeutic measures for reducing lipoprotein (a) in patients with dyslipidaemia. Lipoprotein (a) reduction with sustained-release bezafibrate. *Curr. Ther. Res.*, **49**, 635–643 (1991)

197. Gavish, D. and Breslow, J.J. Lp(a) reduction by N-acetylcysteine. *Lancet*, **337**, 203–204 (1991)

198. Kroon, A.A., Demacker, P.N.M. and Stalenhoef, F.H. N-acetylcysteine and serum concentrations of Lp(a). *J. Intern. Med.*, **230**, 519–526 (1991)

199. MBewu, A.D., Durrington, P.N., Bhatnagar, D., Miller, J.P. and Mackness, M.I. Oral carbocisteine does not lower serum lipoprotein (a) levels. *Atherosclerosis*, **90**, 219–220 (1991)

200. Seed, M. and Crook, D. Post-menopausal hormone replacement therapy, coronary heart disease and plasma lipoproteins. *Curr. Opin. Lipidol.*, **5**, 48–58 (1994)

201. Albers, J.J., Taggart, H.M., Applebaum-Bowden, D., Haffner, S., Chestnut, C.H. and Hazzard, W.R. Reduction of lecithin-cholesterol acyltransferase, apolipoprotein D and the Lp(a) lipoprotein with the anabolic steroid stanozolol. *Biochim. Biophys. Acta*, **795**, 293–296 (1984)

202. Crook, D., Sidhu, M., Seed, M., O'Donnell, M. and Stevenson, J.C. Lp(a) levels in women given danazol, an impeded androgen. *Atherosclerosis*, **92**, 41–47 (1992)
203. Rymer, J., Crook, D., Sidhu, M., Chapman, M. and Stevenson, J.C. Effects of tibolone on serum concentrations of lipoprotein (a) in postmenopausal women. *Acta Endocrinol.*, **128**, 259–262 (1993)
204. Farish, E., Rotton, H.A., Barnes, J.F. and Hart, D.M. Lipoprotein (a) concentrations in postmenopausal women taking norethisterone. *Br. Med. J.*, **303**, 694– (1991).

Chapter 11

# Secondary hyperlipidaemia

Many diseases may be associated with hyperlipidaemia. In some instances they are linked because the hyperlipidaemia is the cause of the disease as, for example, in the case of ischaemic heart disease, cerebral ischaemia, peripheral arterial disease or pancreatitis. Frequently, however, another primary disease affects lipoprotein metabolism in such a way as to increase serum lipid concentrations, and that is the group of disorders which are properly regarded as secondary hyperlipidaemias. They are the subject of this chapter. There are yet other associations between hyperlipidaemia and diseases where no causal link between them has been established and where the treatment of neither affects the other. Perhaps the best example of this is hypertriglyceridaemia and gout. Although not truly a cause of hyperlipidaemia, gout is usually included with the secondary hyperlipidaemias and is thus considered in this chapter.

The secondary hyperlipidaemias are important in clinical practice for three reasons. First, because the primary disease may be an important diagnosis in its own right and it may present as hyperlipidaemia. Certainly the commoner secondary causes must be excluded before a diagnosis of primary hyperlipidaemia can be entertained. Secondly, it is not uncommon for morbidity to arise from a secondary hyperlipidaemia. Thus, for example, in diabetes a main cause of morbidity and the major cause of premature mortality is atherosclerosis, in which the disordered lipoprotein metabolism of diabetes almost certainly has a leading role. In renal disease, too, as survival has been prolonged by techniques for wholly or partially replacing the excretory and homeostatic function of the diseased kidney, atherosclerosis is emerging as a major unresolved complication. Finally, there is also a growing suspicion that lipoproteins have a wider role than simply the transport of lipids (Chapter 2, pages 55–56) and disordered lipoprotein metabolism occurring as a consequence of disease, for example renal or hepatic disease, may have a role in its progression or complications.

Quite apart from clinical considerations, the study of the secondary hyperlipidaemias may lend insight into lipoprotein metabolism of more general importance and improve our understanding of its regulation and the defects involved in the primary hyperlipidaemias.

The impact of the secondary hyperlipidaemias will depend on the milieu in which they occur. Thus diseases causing secondary hyperlipidaemia may be particularly devastating in patients already genetically predisposed to hyperlipidaemia. Diabetes in people who are homozygotes for apolipoprotein E2 or obesity in familial hypercholesterolaemia are obvious examples. The same is almost certainly true, however, of patients with a polygenic tendency to hyperlipidaemia. Thus, populations nutritionally predisposed to hyperlipidaemia may also be more exposed to secondary hyperlipidaemia. Probably the best documented example of this relates to diabetes mellitus in Japan. In the Japanese population, where serum cholesterol is on average low, diabetics have a much lower incidence of atherosclerosis than those in the USA and Northern Europe where the serum cholesterol, probably largely because of the response to diet of genetically predisposed individuals, is in general much greater[1–4].

The secondary hyperlipidaemias are often associated not simply with increases in lipoprotein levels, but also with major alterations in the composition of the different lipoprotein classes. This alters their chemical and physical properties and it must be appreciated that techniques for isolating lipoprotein classes based on these properties developed for use in normal populations or patients with primary disorders may give misleading results. Thus, it is not uncommon in some of the secondary disorders to have lipoproteins in the hydrated density range of VLDL, which are cholesterol rich and behave like LDL on electrophoresis or low density lipoproteins rich in triglycerides. HDL with the electrophoretic properties of LDL

**Table 11.1 Diseases involved in the production of secondary hyperlipidaemia***

| | |
|---|---|
| ENDOCRINE | Diabetes mellitus<br>Thyroid disease<br>Pituitary disease |
| NUTRITIONAL | Obesity<br>Alcohol<br>Anorexia nervosa |
| LIVER DISEASE | Cholestasis<br>Hepatocellular disorders<br>Cholelithiasis<br>Hepatoma<br>Porphyria |
| RENAL DISEASE | Nephrotic syndrome<br>Chronic renal failure |
| DRUGS | |
| IMMUNOGLOBULIN EXCESS | Myeloma<br>Macroglobulinaemia<br>Systemic lupus erythematosus |
| HYPERURICAEMIA | |
| INTESTINAL MALABSORPTION | |
| MISCELLANEOUS | Pregnancy (see Chapter 3)<br>Stress (see Chapter 3)<br>Glycogen storage disease[511]<br>Lipodystrophy[30]<br>Idiopathic hypercalcaemia of infants[512]<br>Hypervitaminosis D[513]<br>Osteogenesis imperfecta[514]<br>Sphingolipodystrophies[515]<br>Progeria[516]<br>Werner's syndrome[517]<br>Cholesterol ester storage disease[518]<br>Carnitine palmityl transferase deficiency[519]<br>Tangier disease (see Chapter 12)<br>Familial LCAT deficiency (see Chapter 12) |

* Those which are not referenced or which are not discussed elsewhere in this book, are included in this chapter.

can also occur and so on. Eventually the study of these lipoproteins may lead to a better understanding of atherogenesis and of the mechanism by which other diseases influence its progression.

The secondary hyperlipidaemias encountered with the greatest frequency in the lipid clinic are shown in Table 4.2. A more comprehensive list, including rare disorders, is found in Table 11.1.

# Endocrine

## Diabetes mellitus

It is frequently overlooked by those responsible for the management of diabetes mellitus that they are dealing with a disorder not only of carbohydrate metabolism, but also (and in many patients more importantly) of lipid and protein metabolism. Two major complications of diabetes, atherosclerosis and ketoacidosis, are disorders of lipid metabolism: the obsession with euglycaemia of recent years may perhaps have led to an underestimation of the involvement of lipids and lipoproteins in other diabetic complications. In the words of E.P. Joslin (1927).

> I believe the chief cause for premature development of arteriosclerosis in diabetes, save for advancing age, is excessive fat; an excess of fat in the body, obesity; an excess of fat in the diet; and an excess of fat in the blood. With an excess of fat diabetes begins and from an excess of fat diabetics die; formerly of coma, recently of arteriosclerosis.

Diabetes mellitus is generally defined in terms of blood glucose concentrations, the arbitrary limits being those below which microvascular complications, particularly retinopathy, are not likely to be encountered[5]. For other complications of diabetes, for example those associated with pregnancy[6] or atherosclerosis, these limits may not pertain. In the case of atherosclerosis, the risk undoubtedly extends to people with blood glucose levels below those currently defined as diabetic[7–9]. It is uncertain whether there is a threshold for glucose intolerance below which the risk ceases to exist.

In both types of diabetes (insulin-dependent and non-insulin-dependent) there is a considerably increased risk of premature arteriosclerosis, particularly coronary artery disease and peripheral arterial disease. Of the clinically identifiable syndromes associated with premature ischaemic heart disease, the risk in diabetes is probably second only to that in FH. Atheroma affecting peripheral arteries in diabetes mellitus not only involves the femoral arteries, as it does, for example, in smokers, but also has a predilection for the smaller popliteal and tibial vessels[10]. Atherosclerosis is thus very much part of the diabetic syndrome. It is a subject of amazement·to the author how frequently diabetics, even when they are known to have severe coronary disease, are described as having mild diabetes or well-controlled diabetes simply because they have blood glucose levels which depart very little from normal. The risk of atherosclerosis within the diabetic population has not been shown to be related to blood glucose or to glycaemic control. There is, however, a much stronger association with serum lipid levels, both in serum cholesterol and in particular the serum triglycerides[11,12]. The risk of IHD is

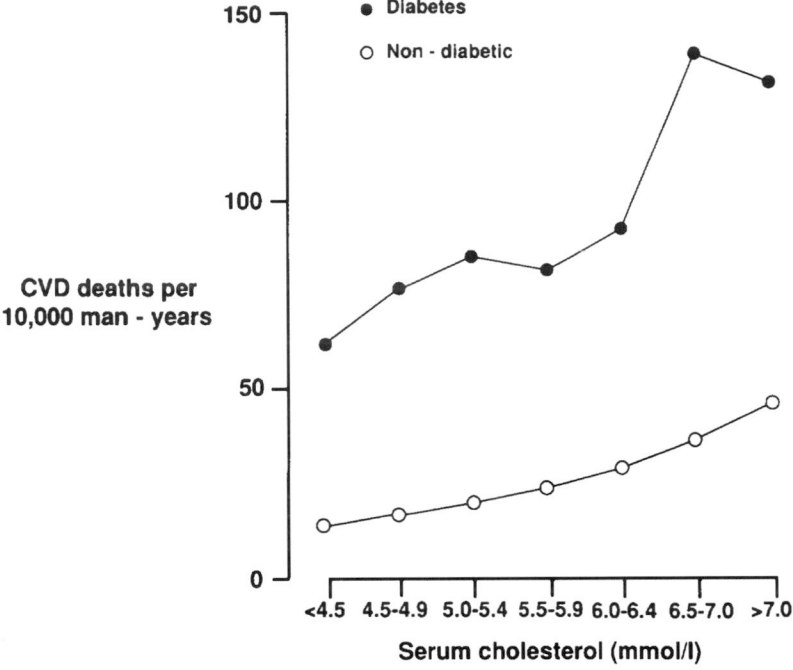

**Figure 11.1**  Age-adjusted cardiovascular death (CVD) rates in men with and without diabetes mellitus according to their serum cholesterol level[13]

greater at any given level of serum cholesterol in diabetes as opposed to the non-diabetic population[13] (Figure 11.1). The stronger association with hypertriglyceridaemia, rather than with hypercholesterolaemia, is different from the general population. This probably relates to the abnormal composition of lipoproteins in diabetes mellitus.

In most other respects, risk factors for vascular disease in diabetes are very similar to those in the general population. Thus, within the diabetic population, hypertension, cigarette smoking and low HDL cholesterol levels all tend to increase the risk[8,9,11–16]. It is noteworthy, too, that the nutritional factors predisposing to a high prevalence of diabetes in a population[17] are very similar to those associated with high rates of ischaemic heart disease, namely a diet which is high in fat and low in carbohydrate (Chapter 9, page 239). Indeed, the use of low carbohydrate diets in the clinical management of diabetes mellitus was a diverticulum from which we are fortunately now emerging. Such diets were until recently widely used despite the widespread recognition that a low carbohydrate diet caused a deterioration in glucose tolerance (starvation diabetes)[18,19]. It was known that the chosen diet of diabetics even before the diagnosis was one which contained on average more fat and less carbohydrate than the general population[17]. The advice to eat less carbohydrate must, therefore, in many cases have not only exacerbated the underlying glucose intolerance[19], but also, if energy intake were not to be decreased, have led to a further increase in fat intake and thus a concomitant increase in the tendency to develop atheroma. The careful and

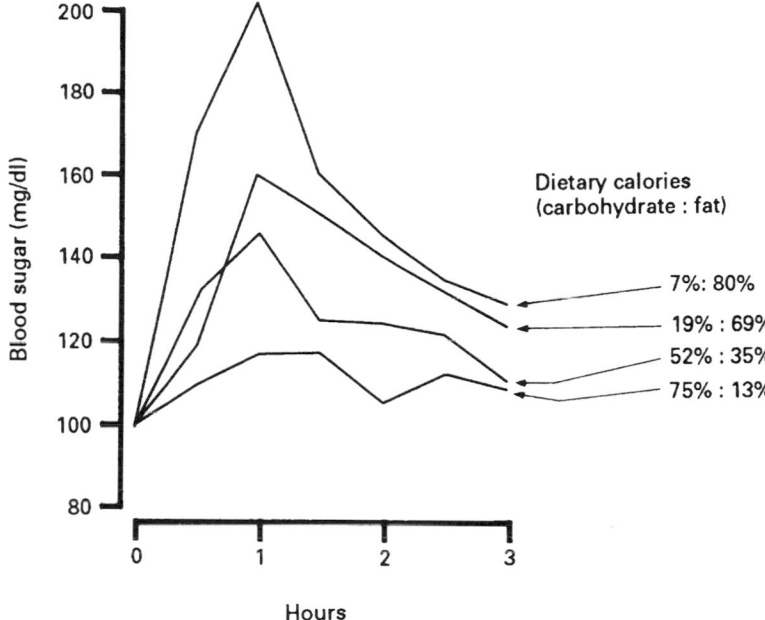

**Figure 11.2**  Blood sugar response to a standard dose of oral glucose after consumption of a diet of equal energy content, but different proportions of fat and carbohydrate. Decreasing glucose tolerance is associated with removal of carbohydrate and addition of fat to the diet (mmol/l = mg/dl × 0.056). (After Himsworth[19])

elegantly designed experiments of Himsworth[19] showing increasing glucose intolerance with increasing fat intake went unheeded (Figure 11.2). It was only through the interest in dietary fibre that the importance of carbohydrate in the diabetic diet was once again discovered[20,21], many of the apparent benefits of fibre-rich foods in improving glucose intolerance being due to the carbohydrate content of the food[22–28].

## Triglyceride metabolism

The dominant hyperlipidaemia in untreated diabetes mellitus is hypertriglyceridaemia[29,30]. In patients attending hospital clinics with reasonably good glycaemic control, the concentration of serum triglycerides in insulin-dependent diabetes mellitus (IDDM) (synonyms: type I diabetes, ketosis-prone diabetes, juvenile onset diabetes) may be similar to or only slightly raised above normal (Table 11.2)[31]. In those with non-insulin-dependent diabetes mellitus (NIDDM) (synonyms: type II diabetes, non-ketosis-prone diabetes, maturity-onset diabetes) there is a great tendency for serum triglycerides to be persistently greater than normal even when good glycaemic control has been achieved[32]. The reason for the greater persistence of hypertriglyceridaemia in NIDDM is probably largely due to the prevalence of factors such as obesity, alcohol intake and concomitant drug therapy, for example with beta-blockers or diuretics which predispose to hypertriglyceridaemia. Occasional patients, perhaps most commonly those with

**Table 11.2 Effect of diabetes on serum lipid and lipoprotein levels compared with healthy control populations\***

|                | NIDDM†   | IDDM     |
|----------------|----------|----------|
| Triglycerides  | ↑        | ↑ or N   |
| Cholesterol    | ↑ or N   | N or ↓   |
| VLDL           | ↑        | ↑ or N   |
| LDL            | ↑ or N   | N or ↓   |
| HDL            | N or ↓   | ↑ or N   |

The author has assumed a degree of glycaemic control reasonable in patients attending a diabetic clinic and has made his own judgement about how closely the reference ranges reported are likely to reflect the levels actually encountered in healthy people. The consensus is gleaned from a number of reports and reviews[31,84,93,138,139,150,520]. The essential point is that the relatively normal serum lipid and lipoprotein lipid concentrations in many diabetics may hide the abnormal composition of the lipoproteins (see text) which may be highly relevant to atherogenesis in diabetes.
Abbreviations: NIDDM, non-insulin dependent diabetes mellitus; IDDM, insulin dependent diabetes mellitus; VLDL, very low density lipoprotein; LDL, low density lipoprotein; HDL, high density lipoprotein; N, within the normal range.

NIDDM, remain markedly hypertriglyceridaemic despite good glycaemic control. In such cases there is often some additional explanation such as hypothyroidism, apo $E_2$ homozygosity or a primary defect in triglyceride clearance.

Diabetes is a disorder which results from inadequate secretion of insulin. In the lean type 1 diabetic, insulin secretion is frequently less than normal, whereas in the type II diabetic, who is often obese, insulin secretion may be increased, but it is nevertheless inadequate to overcome the insulin resistance imposed by the obesity and is less than in a comparably obese non-diabetic[33] (Figure 11.3). It is important to realize that in both IDDM and NIDDM, insulin secretion is inadequate. Patients with NIDDM are frequently described as 'hyperinsulinaemic', creating the impression that all their tissues are exposed to inappropriately high levels of insulin, which is plainly not the case, since, although they may have plasma concentrations of insulin exceeding those in non-diabetic non-obese people, their levels are nevertheless inappropriately low for their degree of insulin resistance[34]. Recently another line of evidence has emerged reinforcing this view. This was as the result of measurement of the serum concentrations of 32–33 split proinsulin and proinsulin[35,36], which suggests that much of the insulin measured in diabetes in earlier studies was not insulin itself, but proinsulin or proinsulin split at its arginine bases at position 32 and 33 in its protein sequence, an intermediate in the conversion of proinsulin to insulin which is a process normally virtually completed within the pancreas. It has been suggested that because proinsulin and partially split proinsulin are less biologically active than

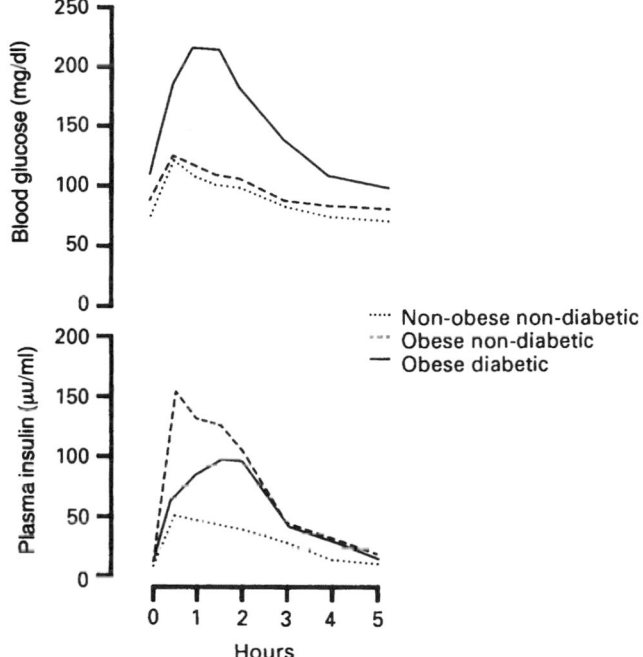

**Figure 11.3**   Blood glucose and plasma insulin responses to a standard dose of oral glucose. Note that although the insulin response of the obese diabetic is greater than the lean non-diabetic, it is nevertheless inadequate when compared with that of the obese non-diabetic (mmol/l = mg/dl × 0.056). (After Perley and Kipnis[33])

insulin that the so called hyperinsulinaemia of NIDDM actually represents a deficiency of true insulin. Against this proinsulin does appear to have at least some biological activity in man[37,38] and it should be remembered that this is not the only case, nor necessarily the strongest case, against hyperinsulinaemia as a concept as the foregoing discussion reveals.

The major actions of insulin on lipoprotein metabolism have previously been reviewed (Chapter 1, page 11). Insulin activates lipoprotein lipase, thus enhancing the clearance from the circulation of the triglyceride component of chylomicrons and VLDL (Figure 11.4). It has the opposite effect on the intracellular lipase of adipose tissue, suppressing the release of non-esterified fatty acids (NEFA) from adipose tissue. This release of NEFA is therefore increased in both types of diabetes[29,30] and may itself contribute to insulin resistance[39].

The physiological basis for the increased release of NEFA from adipose tissue in response to decreased insulin secretion is to provide NEFA as energy substrates during starvation. The delivery of NEFA to the liver increases as their rate of release exceeds the capacity of extrahepatic tissues to oxidize them. In diabetes, as in starvation, the liver partially oxidizes these NEFA to ketone bodies (β-oxidation), which are then released[40]. In starvation, the water-soluble ketone bodies are required because they can enter the Krebs cycle in most tissues, diminishing or abolishing their requirement for glucose. In diabetes, however, the flux of

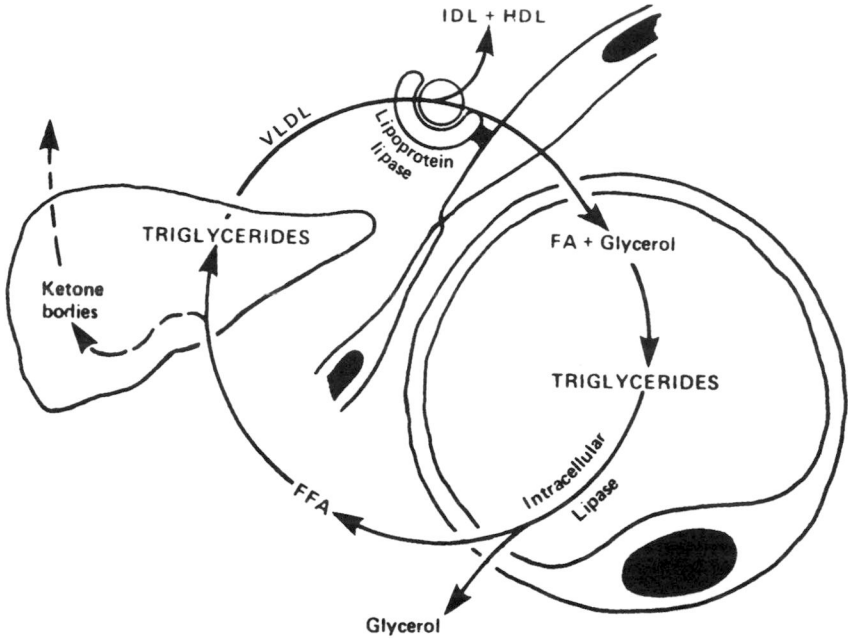

**Figure 11.4**   Triglyceride : fatty acid cycle (see text for explanation)

NEFA to the liver is so great that the hepatic production of ketone bodies far outstrips the ability of extrahepatic tissues to oxidize them completely. This is the process which leads to the ketoacidosis of IDDM[41,42]. In one sense, therefore, diabetic ketoacidosis represents 'starvation gone wrong', which accounts for the appearance of gross undernourishment in many of the patients developing this complication. This concept explains the basis, too, for the starvation therapy discovered by Allen before insulin became available for the treatment of diabetes[43]. He recognized that life might be prolonged if a degree of dietary energy restriction could be imposed on diabetics appropriate to their increased rate of ketone body production, thus permitting their complete oxidation (see reference [44] for graphic accounts of these early days).

There is another response of the liver to the delivery of NEFA, which is to convert them to triglycerides by esterifying them with glycerol (Chapter 1, page 9). Indeed many states, in which the release of NEFA from adipose tissue is increased, lead to hypertriglyceridaemia secondary to increased hepatic production by this mechanism, rather than to ketoacidosis secondary to partial oxidation of fatty acids. Some of the regulatory processes which determine whether fatty acids, synthesized in the liver or transported there, are esterified to form triglycerides (lipogenesis) or converted to ketone bodies (ketogenesis) are understood (Chapter 1, page 13). However, the picture is far from complete. In NIDDM, lipogenesis clearly predominates over ketogenesis and this is the essential difference between the two types of diabetes. To some extent the rate of ketogenesis is related to the severity of the fatty acidaemia, but this is probably not the only factor. In the IDDM patient treated with sufficient insulin to overcome ketogenesis, lipogenesis will, as in NIDDM, predominate.

In untreated diabetes of either type, the decreased activity of lipoprotein lipase will produce a defect in triglyceride catabolism and thus further exacerbate the hypertriglyceridaemic effect of increased hepatic lipogenesis. Indeed the rate of clearance of triglyceride from the circulation is frequently a major determinant of the fasting serum triglyceride concentration in diabetes as well as the postprandial rise in serum triglyceride levels[45]. This accounts for the gross type V hyperlipoproteinaemia not infrequently seen in NIDDM and also sometimes in IDDM receiving inadequate insulin or occasionally even in patients presenting with ketoacidosis[46]. The treatment of diabetes with insulin usually overcomes the triglyceride clearance defects[47]. Indeed, it seems likely that in many patients with relatively good glycaemic control the activity of lipoprotein lipase is increased above normal[48]. It has been suggested that this is due to greater concentrations of free insulin in the systemic circulation of 'well-controlled' insulin-treated diabetics compared with normal people[48]. This is very plausible, because in the insulin-treated diabetic, insulin is administered subcutaneously whence it enters the systemic circulation. Endogenous insulin secretion is, however, into the portal circulation. In the non-diabetic, insulin concentrations in the portal circulation are two to ten times those in the systemic circulation due to the effects of hepatic extraction and dilution[49]. Exogenous insulin administered to diabetics via the systemic circulation, however, arrives at the liver via the hepatic artery. The concentration of insulin in the systemic circulation must therefore be higher, if hepatic metabolism is to be adequately regulated and good glycaemic control achieved[50]. This in turn means that peripheral tissues, such as adipose tissue and skeletal muscle, will be subjected to higher concentrations of insulin than are physiological and that enzymes such as lipoprotein lipase may be more active than normal. Direct evidence for higher levels of free insulin in the peripheral circulation has been hard to obtain because of the presence of high concentrations of insulin bound to antibodies[51]. Furthermore, in many patients retention of some endogenous insulin secretion decreases the necessity for insulin to be delivered to the liver via the systemic circulation in order to regulate its metabolism adequately[52,53]. It is not surprising, therefore, that a wide range of lipoprotein lipase activities, from the subnormal to the supranormal, exist in a diabetic clinic population and that these may not apparently correlate with glycaemic control. Amelioration of the abnormal lipoprotein profile in diabetes with intraperitoneal as opposed to subcutaneous insulin has been reported[54].

Thus far, the effects of diabetes on triglyceride metabolism have been discussed in terms of the peripheral effects of insulin on release of NEFA from adipose tissue or on the clearance of triglycerides from lipoprotein in the peripheral circulation. There remains the question of whether insulin directly influences hepatic triglyceride metabolism and, if so, in what way. It is widely stated that insulin stimulates hepatic triglyceride synthesis and secretion (Figure 11.5). Evidence for this hypothesis has, however, been carefully culled by its proponents and a broader interpretation of the evidence both old and recent might lead to some moderation of this view. Much of the case for a stimulatory effect of insulin on hepatic lipogenesis relies on the observation that hypertriglyceridaemia frequently occurs in conditions where insulin secretion is increased due to insulin resistance and there is so-called 'hyperinsulinaemia'. It has been proposed to account for the hypertriglyceridaemia of carbohydrate induction (Chapter 9, page

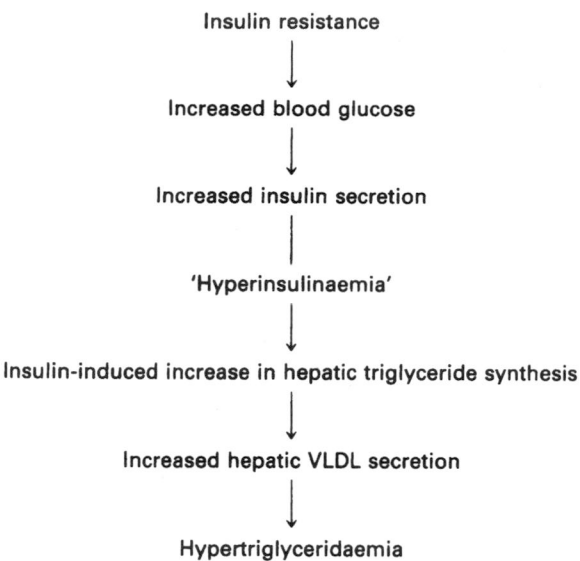

Insulin resistance

↓

Increased blood glucose

↓

Increased insulin secretion

↓

'Hyperinsulinaemia'

↓

Insulin-induced increase in hepatic triglyceride synthesis

↓

Increased hepatic VLDL secretion

↓

Hypertriglyceridaemia

**Figure 11.5**   Postulated events in the hypothesis that insulin is a cause of hypertriglyceridaemia (After Olefsky *et al.*[57])

234), type IV hyperlipoproteinaemia (Chapter 7), NIDDM and obesity[55–58]. One can accept that insulin is a key factor in diverting long-chain fatty acids away from ketogenesis. However, the hypothesis that insulin also directly stimulates triglyceride synthesis and secretion is unsatisfactory on a number of grounds.

First, the experimental evidence in its favour is not confirmed by other similar studies. Thus an inverse relationship between integrated serum insulin and triglycerides in men undergoing carbohydrate induction has been reported, rather than the direct relationship predicted by the hypothesis[59,60]. Furthermore, in type IV hyperlipoproteinaemia, only one-quarter of patients have an increased insulin response to glucose, whereas in more than one-third the insulin response is low[61]. Similarly, in obesity the triglyceride secretory rate was increased not only in patients with high serum insulin responses to glucose, but also in those with lower than normal responses[62].

Secondly, the administration of insulin to both insulin-dependent and non-insulin-dependent diabetics or indeed to non-diabetic subjects, produces a decrease in serum triglyceride levels[63–68]. Insulinoma is associated with low plasma concentrations of serum triglycerides[62]. It could be argued that all these triglyceride-lowering effects of insulin are due to reduction in NEFA levels or to increased triglyceride clearance. However, this would then only allow an insubstantial and unimportant direct role of insulin on hepatic lipogenesis. This would mean the abandonment of the hypothesis that hyperinsulinaemia is a cause of hypertriglyceridaemia.

Thirdly, the hypothesis given in Figure 11.5 is too liberal. It requires that, whereas there is resistance to the effects of insulin on carbohydrate metabolism, this does not apply to hepatic lipid metabolism, which is stimulated. No evidence has ever been obtained that there can be some defect in the post-receptor regulation of

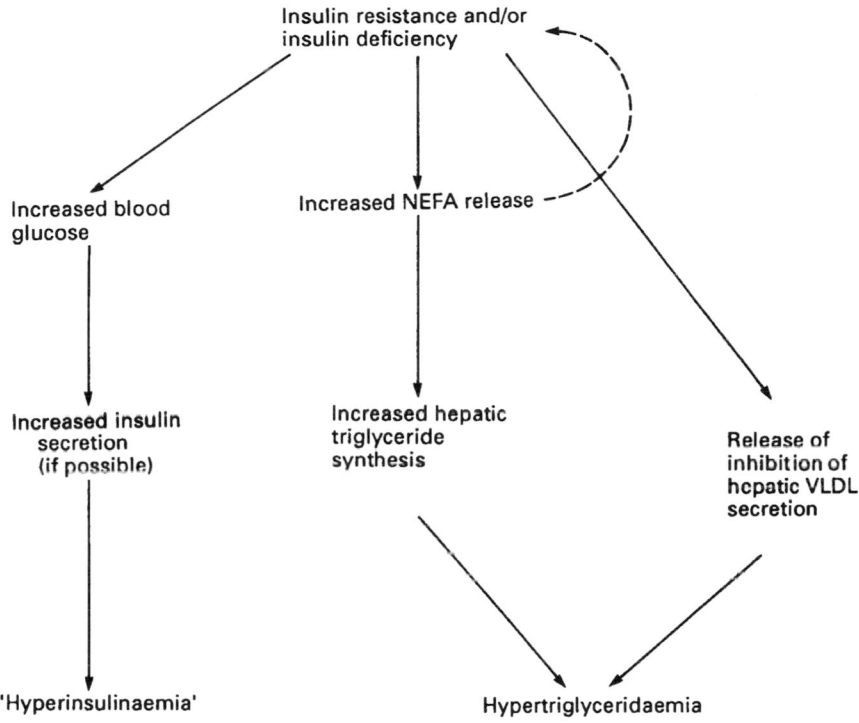

**Figure 11.6** Alternative hypothesis to explain the association between insulin and hypertriglyceridaemia. Insulin resistance causes: (*a*) increased insulin secretion; (*b*) increased flux of non-esterfied fatty acid (NEFA) to the liver, where the stimulate triglyceride synthesis; (*c*) decreased insulin-induced inhibition of hepatic triglyceride secretion (see text for full explanation)

carbohydrate and lipid metabolism whereby there can be inadequate control of carbohydrate metabolism by insulin, but overactivity of insulin with respect to lipid metabolism[34,69]. In certain insulin-resistant states, for example type A insulin resistance, the condition leads to acromegaloid features rather than dwarfism. A possible explanation is that the growth-promoting (mitotic) branch of the postreceptor signalling pathway is functioning in such patients whereas the lipid and carbohydrate metabolic regulatory pathway is resistant[70]. It is, however, possible that this is an effect of the spill-over of the particularly high circulating levels of insulin in this condition on to another functioning receptor such as the IGF1 receptor (insulin-like growth factor 1 receptor). In common-or-garden diabetes and glucose intolerance there is no suggestion of any metabolic diversity of insulin resistance. If, however, one was to abandon the idea that insulin stimulates triglyceride secretion and entertain the possibility that insulin inhibits this process, then a hypothesis is possible which is more conservative and thus more appealing (Figure 11.6).

An inhibitory effect means that in both insulin deficiency and insulin resistance the release of the restraint of insulin on hepatic VLDL secretion would tend to produce hypertriglyceridaemia. The experimental confirmation of this hypothesis requires that insulin inhibits VLDL production by isolated liver preparations.

Experiments with hepatocytes maintained in tissue culture have been remarkably consistent in showing that this is the case. Initially we showed that insulin inhibited VLDL triglyceride secretion from cultured rat hepatocytes when glucose was the synthetic substrate[71] and this was subsequently confirmed using a similar culture system, both when glucose and when fatty acids were the substrate. Not only was triglyceride secretion inhibited, but so also was VLDL apolipoprotein secretion[72,73]. This response to insulin was receptor-mediated[74] and was also present in cultured human hepatoma cells[75]. Recent evidence[76] suggests that insulin inhibits hepatic VLDL secretion by inhibiting the phosphorylation of apolipoprotein $B_{100}$ which must take place before VLDL assembly. Apolipoprotein $B_{100}$ which is not phosphorylated is degraded within the hepatocyte.

Experiments examining the effects of insulin on triglyceride synthesis and/or secretion with rat liver slices, perfused rat liver and with freshly isolated rat hepatocytes in suspension have yielded more conflicting results than tissue culture. In many cases this may be because of the use of radioisotopic methods for assessing triglyceride production as opposed to mass measurements and lack of recovery of tissue from the isolation procedures or from the persistence of other hormonal or substrate effects prevailing in the animal at the time of isolation of the liver. Perhaps the most consistent experiments, in which insulin appeared to stimulate triglyceride production directly, were those reported by one group using the perfused rat liver[77–79]. It must be said, however, that others experimenting with a similar system have found less consistent[80] or opposing results[62]. Certainly it would be untrue to suggest that the consistent results obtained with cultured hepatocytes should be rejected on the grounds that these cells produce VLDL at unphysiological rates[79], since this is manifestly not the case[71].

In experiments with cultured hepatocytes, an increase in the intracellular triglyceride concentration occurred concomitantly with the insulin-induced inhibition of triglyceride secretion. Probably all of this increase in intracellular triglyceride can be accounted for by the decrease in secretion and it is doubtful that the insulin stimulates triglyceride synthesis, which in any case would make little sense because the effect of insulin is to suppress circulating NEFA levels by inhibiting their release from adipose tissue and hence this will decrease hepatic triglyceride synthesis. It would be a remarkably unconcerted regulatory effect if at the same time insulin was stimulating hepatic triglyceride synthesis and simultaneously inhibiting the secretion of VLDL. It has been proposed that insulin might stimulate triglyceride secretion in whole animals because it could oppose a glucagon-mediated inhibition of triglyceride synthesis[71,81]. However, in fact it reinforces the inhibitory action of glucagon in this respect[82,83].

Certainly the insulin-induced inhibition of hepatic VLDL secretion, leading to an accumulation of intracellular triglycerides, is of great interest. It has led us to suggest that insulin might function physiologically to limit the postprandial increase in circulating triglyceride-rich lipoproteins[71]. Postprandially, glucose and other precursors of triglyceride synthesis reach the liver in high concentration and stimulate hepatic triglyceride synthesis at the same time as intestinal fat absorption and chylomicron secretion is at a peak. This latter processs is probably not regulated by insulin. Inhibition of hepatic VLDL secretion and the direction of newly synthesized triglycerides into storage pools by the high concentrations of insulin prevailing at the time would limit the rise in serum triglycerides. Since both VLDL and chylomicron triglycerides are removed by lipoprotein lipase, this temporary decrease in VLDL release facilitates the catabolism of chylomicrons. It would also be expected to relieve the competition between the remnants of chylomicron catabolism and intermediate density lipoproteins (LDL) at the apo E (remnant) receptor. Inadequate suppression of hepatic VLDL secretion postprandially in diabetics might thus be a reason for the accumulation of remnant lipoproteins in the circulation. Later, when insulin levels have fallen and triglycerides are no longer being supplied to peripheral tissues as chylomicrons, the triglycerides stored in the liver will be released as VLDL. Additional evidence in favour of this hypothesis is summarized elsewhere[82,84].

The effects of glucose and insulin on cultured hepatocytes may be relevant to the use of this combination in intravenous feeding regimens. It is possible that such treatment does not satisfy energy requirements as anticipated if the glucose is directed into triglyceride retained within the liver. Indeed, it might cause or contribute to the development of fatty liver (cholesteatosis), and the abnormal liver function which occurs in some seriously ill patients fed in that way[85].

The evidence against the hyperinsulinaemia-induced hypertriglyceridaemia hypothesis makes its extension, the hypothesis that insulin is a cause of atherosclerosis[86], even more tenuous. The relationship between serum insulin and IHD risk observed in a number of studies[87–89] is probably not causal. More likely, both result from another factor. This may well be an increased rate of release of fatty acids from adipose tissue (perhaps secondary to insulin resistance due to obesity or some less clearly defined cause), which would increase hepatic VLDL synthesis and secretion, leading to an increased risk of ischaemic heart disease (see Figure 11.5). At the same time, hyperinsulinaemia would be further exacerbated either by a direct effect of fatty acids on insulin secretion[90] or via a fatty acid-induced insulin resistance or reinforcement of an existing state of insulin resistance by the high NEFA levels[39,70,91,92].

## IDL and LDL metabolism

Serum cholesterol concentrations in diabetes have been the subject of a great number of publications. In summary (see Table 11.2), it appears that in neither NIDDM nor IDDM do they depart greatly from the average levels found in the general population. As with triglycerides, there is a tendency for higher levels in NIDDM patients, who are frequently obese. In IDDM, particularly when good glycaemic control has been achieved, there may however be a decrease in serum cholesterol below that in control populations[93] so that hypercholesterolaemia may be no more prevalent in IDDM than in the general population[31]. This appears to be an effect of insulin[66]. The concentrations of LDL cholesterol measured as the cholesterol in lipoprotein of density 1.006–1.063 g/ml or by the Friedewald formula follow a very similar pattern. Superficially the serum cholesterol levels in diabetes do not therefore seem to offer much in the way of explanation for the greatly increased risk of atheromatous disease in diabetes. As will be seen later in IDDM, the same is true of HDL cholesterol. However, evidence is accumulating that lipid values and lipoproteins isolated in the conventional way may hide the presence of lipoproteins of abnormal composition and physical properties, which may be highly relevant to atherogenesis in diabetes.

Serum apo B levels were reported to be lower than would be anticipated from the LDL cholesterol concentration in IDDM[93]. This resulted in a ratio of LDL cholesterol to apolipoprotein B which was greater than in non-diabetic controls. The explanation for this is that the serum IDL concentration is increased in diabetes[31,94–100]. Because IDL has a high cholesterol content relative to its protein content the effect of an increase in its concentration is to increase the ratio of cholesterol to apolipoprotien B in the LDL fraction as a whole if it is isolated in the ultracentrifuge as the d=1006–1063 g/l lipoprotein or by a precipitation method. The increase in IDL may be even more marked when nephropathy develops[101], but in one report was absent in IDDM in Japan[102], which is intriguing in view of the relatively low rates of atherosclerosis in Japanese diabetics. The increase in IDL in NIDDM, which may be quantitatively as great or greater than in IDDM, is not so clearly reflected in an increased cholesterol to apolipoprotein B ratio in the LDL in the 1006–1063 g/l range, because there is generally a higher concentration of the more dense LDL as well. In fact, in IDDM the small dense LDL may be increased[97] as it is in the primary hypertriglyceridaemias: there is also a relative enrichment of apolipoprotein B with triglycerides compatible with this idea[103]. Possibly this is due to an enhanced transfer of cholesteryl ester from LDL to VLDL (Chapter 2, page 58) consistent with which are reports of an increase in cholesteryl ester transfer activity in diabetes[104–107]. This increased activity may not be present in insulin-treated IDDM, although direct experimental evidence confirming this suggestion is currently lacking.

VLDL in diabetes may also be enriched with cholesterol[66,108] and in a study using radiolabelled VLDL there was increased catabolism of VLDL via lipoproteins less dense than LDL[109]. The increased LDL overlapping with a cholesterol-rich VLDL may be very reminiscent of the β-VLDL or remnant particles of type III hyperlipoproteinaemia (Chapter 8, page 215). In animals, too, the induction of diabetes also appears to lead to the production of a remnant-like lipoprotein[110–113]. The situation in diabetes is thus very different from that in FH (Chapter 5) or hyperapobetalipoproteinaemia (Chapter 6), but parallels more closely that in type III hyperlipoproteinaemia. It is interesting in that context that the anatomical distribution of atheroma in diabetes and type III hyperlipoproteinaemia is so similar. Peripheral arterial disease is, for example, much more frequently found in both of these conditions than in FH. The β-VLDL of type III hyperlipoproteinaemia is readily taken up by cultured macrophages to form foam cells (Chapter 2, page 44), and there are experiments to suggest that avid uptake of the VLDL from diabetics may also occur[114].

In the human, a clearly defined mechanism for the excess production or accumulation of IDL has yet to be demonstrated. Decreased hepatic lipase activity could theoretically be important, particularly in IDDM in which the liver tends to remain relatively deficient in insulin whilst the peripheral tissues are subjected to supranormal insulin levels when treated with exogenous insulin delivered into the systemic circulation. Expression of the apo E2 genotype, usually homozygotic, is required for the development of  primary type III hyperlipoproteinaemia. The apo $E_2$ isoform has less affinity for receptors and this provides a partial explanation for the accumulation of remnant and IDL-like lipoproteins in type III hyperlipoproteinaemia (Chapter 8, page 215). There is an increased prevalence of diabetes in patients with type III hyperlipoproteinaemia: some 4% of them have clinical diabetes[115] which is thus about four times more common than in the general population of the same average age. Glucose intolerance, not amounting to frank diabetes, is also more prevalent in type III than in the general population[116]. This may be relevant to the development of hyperlipoproteinaemia in type III, because the presence of glucose intolerance would be expected to reinforce the effect of the apo $E_2$ genotype. This leaves open the question of whether apo E is relevant to the dyslipoproteinaemia of diabetes. In IDDM, we have found that apo $E_2$ homozygosity, although increased in frequency in diabetic patients, still only affected 7%, so that it could not have been the cause of dyslipoproteinaemia in the majority[117]. The actual gene frequency of apo $E_2$ was also not different from normal. There have been similar findings in non-insulin dependent diabetes[118]. Artefacts due to post-translational glycosylation of apo E, which would increase the acidic apo E isoforms, were avoided in this study by treating the VLDL with hyaluronidase. It was thus a study of the apo E genotype. This is not to say, however, that glycosylation of apo E perhaps affecting its receptor binding might not be important in the generation of remnant-like particles. Several apolipoproteins are known to undergo glycosylation in diabetes[119]. In the case of apo E, increased sialation appears to produce apo E, which is indistinguishable from apo $E_2$ on isoelectric focusing[120,121]. Additional evidence that the apo $E_2$ genotype is not generally involved in hyperlipidaemia in diabetes is our finding that the highest serum cholesterol and apo B levels occur in those with an apo $E_4$ gene[117]. This is similar to the general population. IHD is reported to be more frequent in diabetic patients with an apo $E_4$ genotype[118].

Whatever the relevance of apo E isoforms to diabetic dyslipoproteinaemia, the incidence of apo $E_2$ homozygosity is sufficiently high that the clinician should maintain a high level of suspicion that diabetic patients with obvious hyperlipidaemia may have type III hyperlipoproteinaemia (Chapter 8, page 215). In diabetes, in particular, fasting chylomicronaemia may coexist and mask the usual biochemical features of type III hyperlipoproteinaemia.

It is not essential to speculate that remnant-like particles arise in diabetes by a mechanism involving diminished hepatic lipase activity or abnormal apo E structure. Indeed, the finding that apo E genotypes had an influence on serum cholesterol and LDL cholesterol similar to that in the general population suggests that post-translational glycosylation may not have a major influence on lipoprotein metabolism[117]. Abnormalities of apo CIII metabolism or effects of diabetes on the hepatic remnant receptor[93] might also be important. So, also, might a failure of postprandial inhibition of hepatic VLDL secretion by insulin (page 302), leading to increased pressure on the remnant receptor and, perhaps, accumulation of IDL and chylomicron remnants.

It has been suggested that the catabolism of true LDL ($d$=1.019–1.063 g/ml) might also be abnormal in diabetes, even though this might not be reflected in the LDL cholesterol and serum cholesterol levels in the same way as in FH. There is no direct evidence for this, but two lines of research make it interesting as a hypothesis. First, insulin has been shown to stimulate receptor-mediated entry of LDL into cultured fibroblasts[122–124]. Thus, it is possible that insulin deficiency might decrease the fraction of LDL catabolized by the receptor-mediated pathway. If, however, as has been discussed earlier in this chapter, the peripheral tissues in IDDM are subjected to hyperinsulinaemia, then it would be possible to argue that outside the liver, at least, there might actually be enhanced receptor-mediated LDL degradation. This appears to be the case during euglycaemic insulin clamping[125].

The second line of research involves the demonstration that lipoproteins undergo glycosylation in diabetes. This has been shown for apolipoproteins AI, AII, B, CI and E[119,126,127]. In the non-diabetic about 4% of serum apolipoprotein B is glycosylated and this proportion is about doubled even in reasonably well-controlled diabetes[128]. The absolute concentration of glycosy-lated apolipoprotein B is increased in diabetes because a greater proportion is glycosylated. Interestingly, however, so is it also in familial hypercholestero-laemia, when the LDL concentration is increased, but the proportion glycosylated is normal[128]. Glycosylation of LDL *in vitro* decreases its receptor-mediated catabolism by cultured fibroblasts, but does not affect its cellular uptake by low affinity binding[127,129]. The fractional catabolic rate of glycosylated LDL when it was injected into the circulation of non-diabetic subjects was less than that of unmodified LDL, similar to findings with methylated or cyclohexanedione modified LDL[130,131], which are believed to be catabolized only via the non-receptor pathway (Chapter 2, page 33). This suggests that receptor binding of glycosylated LDL is blocked *in vivo*. Thus, if it is true that non-receptor mediated LDL catabolism is atherogenic, then LDL glycosylation might contribute to premature atheroma in diabetes. There is, however, disagreement about whether the degree of glycosylation which might occur in a diabetic patient is sufficient to affect its rate of catabolism[132,133]. Until that issue, and the one previously discussed (whether the LDL receptor pathway activity is enhanced or decreased in diabetes), have been resolved, the role of the LDL receptor in diabetic atheroma remains largely speculative. Regardless of the outcome, however, glycated LDL may be more susceptible to oxidation[134] or itself represent a modification which is atherogenic. Its uptake by macrophages *in vitro* is enhanced[135]. Free radical damage may be accelerated by diabetes[134].

Another suggestion that might make LDL more atherogenic in diabetes than in non-diabetics involves its binding to collagen. Glycosylated sites on molecules such as collagen can undergo further modification so that cross-linkage occurs (a process known as 'browning' in the food industry). These advanced glycosylation end-products (AGE) have in the case of collagen been shown to bind LDL covalently[136]. Again, this structural modification of collagen has been made *in vitro* and it is not known to what extent it might occur in arterial wall collagen in a diabetic. It is possible, however, that trapping of LDL in such a site would lead to an acceleration of atherogenesis.

### HDL metabolism

Numerous studies have shown that in IDDM, unless glycaemic control is poor, the serum HDL cholesterol concentration is on average either similar to that of comparable non-diabetics or even higher[137–139]. This has not been widely enough appreciated, even by some of those who write reviews. This is probably partly because it is anticipated that HDL cholesterol will be low in diseases associ-ated with premature atheroma and partly because an early paper on the subject appeared to show low levels of HDL in insulin-treated diabetics[140]. That report was, however, unusual in the high proportion of patients who were hypertriglyc-eridaemic, and in the pronounced positive skew of the HDL cholesterol distribu-tion in the control population. In NIDDM, serum HDL cholesterol levels are either normal or decreased[137–139].

Multivariate analysis of the factors determining serum HDL levels in IDDM showed that there was an independent positive effect of that type of diabetes or its treatment[138]. In the case of NIDDM, there was no independent effect of diabetes, the identifiable determinants of serum HDL concentration being similar to those in the non-diabetic population. Thus, in NIDDM the major cause of any decrease in HDL is likely to be obesity, hypertriglyceridaemia, cigarette smoking and abstemiousness from alcohol.

The effect of glycaemic control on serum HDL cholesterol concentration has proved a difficult question to settle. If one looks at the effect of improving glycaemic control in those patients in whom it is worst initially, then increases in serum HDL cholesterol may be the rule. However, widely varying conclusions have been reached when correlations have been sought between the serum HDL cholesterol levels in clinical populations and glycated haemoglobin as an index of glycaemic control. Perhaps there is no linear relationship and, as in the streptozotocin diabetic rat, there is a quadratic relationship, those with the best and worst glycaemic control having lower HDL levels than those in the middle range of control[141].

The distribution of HDL subfractions in diabetes has also given rise to some disagreement. Again glycaemic control may have a bearing, and also the type of diabetes and whether insulin is used in its management. In NIDDM, particularly if not well controlled, the HDL2 subfraction is decreased[96,142] and this accounts for the tendency for low serum levels of total HDL. This is entirely compatible with the conclusion discussed earlier in this section that low HDL in NIDDM is the result of factors such as obesity and hypertriglyceridaemia rather than the diabetes *per se*. Furthermore, it is in just such circumstances that lipoprotein lipase activity is likely to explain the variation in HDL2 concentration[143]. It is very probable too that increases in the activity of this enzyme caused by administration of insulin would lead to a rise in the serum HDL2 concentration[143,144].

In IDDM, three studies employing the ultracentrifuge have found that the $HDL_3$ subfraction is increased, accounting for any rise in total serum HDL, and that the $HDL_2$ subfraction is either decreased or normal[93,145,146]. A fourth investigation[147] showed an insignificant increase in $HDL_3$, but in men in whom total serum HDL cholesterol was raised, the greatest increase was in $HDL_2$. Studies employing precipitation methods for the isolation of HDL subfractions also do not seem to show any increase in $HDL_3$[142]. It is, however, important to realize that a number of observations in diabetes suggest that polyanionic precipitating agents may not bind to the same HDL subspecies as those identified as HDL2 or HDL3 on the basis of their hydrated density[148–150]. Such physical differences between normal HDL and HDL from diabetics suggest that there are changes in the composition of HDL in diabetes. This will certainly be the subject of much future research. Already, however, some discussion of the change in the density of HDL particles in diabetes and of its composition in relation to its role in cholesterol esterification and transfer is possible.

As was mentioned previously, the effect of insulin in enhancing the activity of lipoprotein lipase is to accelerate the removal of triglycerides from VLDL[143]. This generates components of HDL that increase the HDL cholesterol concentration and the average size of HDL particles (Chapter 2, page 56). There is thus a tendency for cholesterol-enriched HDL of lower density to form (i.e. a shift towards $HDL_2$) when insulin is administered and a tendency for $HDL_2$ to be low when insulin deficiency or resistance causes decreased triglyceride clearance. Since in many patients hepatic VLDL production, which is less sensitive to insulin, will still be increased when triglyceride catabolism has been restored to normal, it is possible that the production of HDL components during triglyceride catabolism too may be increased[137]. Lipoprotein lipase activity may contribute even further to this increase in serum $HDL_2$, in patients in whom its activity is greater than normal (page 299). Operating against this tendency for the formation of larger

HDL molecules, however, may be the effect of glycosylation of HDL apolipoproteins AI and AII[119], which appears to accelerate HDL catabolism[151]. Thus there may be more rapid clearance of HDL molecules in diabetics before they have circulated for long enough to acquire sufficient cholesterol to become $HDL_2$. The overall tendency, in insulin-treated IDDM, might therefore be for enhanced generation of HDL due to increased activity in the triglyceride catabolism pathway, but because of concurrent heightened catabolism this will be reflected in increased $HDL_3$ particles because they do not complete their transition to $HDL_2$ molecules[93]. We have recently found that diabetic patients with proteinuria have higher levels of serum $HDL_3$ cholesterol and lower $HDL_2$ than those who have not developed this complication, even before there is any marked deterioration in creatinine clearance[149]. Minor differences in the prevalence of early nephropathy in different diabetic populations might therefore account for some of the opposing findings of different study groups.

Increases in $HDL_3$ and decreases in $HDL_2$ have been reported in primary renal disease with proteinuria[152]. In these patients there was substantial loss of apo AI-containing lipoproteins into the urine and this may have contributed to the increased rate of HDL catabolism observed in other studies[153]. This would apply particularly to the smaller molecular weight $HDL_3$ particles, which might be lost before they had circulated long enough to acquire sufficient cholesterol to become $HDL_2$[152]. A similar mechanism might contribute to the change in the proportion of $HDL_3$ relative to $HDL_2$ in diabetics with proteinuria. Glycosylation of apo AI or of the renal glomerular basement membrane[154] might also increase the ease with which HDL could cross into the urine space. Furthermore, in the early stages of diabetic nephropathy there is an increased renal blood flow and glomerular filtration rate[155]. In the rat there is evidence that the kidney makes a significant contribution to HDL catabolism[156]. If the same is true in man, then an increased renal contribution to apo AI degradation, even at the earliest stage of diabetic nephropathy when proteinuria is minimal, is conceivable. The renal cells responsible for apo AI degradation in the rat are those lining the urine space of the proximal convoluted tubule[156]. To reach them, HDL must cross the glomerular basement membrane and therefore again the greatest catabolic effect would be anticipated to apply to the smaller molecular weight HDL species.

The serum HDL cholesterol concentration continues to act as a factor inversely related to the risk of IHD in IDDM, although set at a higher level than in the non-diabetic and in patients with NIDDM[14,157]. Apart from its effects already discussed, glycosylation of HDL impairs its ability to promote cholesterol efflux from cells *in vitro*[158] (Chapter 2, page 35).

## Cholesterol esterification and transfer

In ketoacidosis, LCAT activity in diabetes is decreased[159]. It probably increases towards normal with improving glycaemic control[160,161] and may even be increased in relatively well-controlled patients[162]. Despite an early contrary report based on a small number of patients[163], there is reasonable agreement that the transfer of cholesteryl ester from HDL to VLDL is increased in NIDDM[104–107]. As has been previously discussed, this in itself is a potentially atherogenic mechanism (Chapter 2, page 58). The increase in cholesteryl ester transfer as in many other situations may not be mediated by a change in the concentration or activity of CETP *per se* but would be expected from the increase in the circulating triglyceride-rich lipoprotein pool which is reflected in the fasting hyper-triglyceridaemia of NIDDM, but is amplified because of the greater rise and presistence throughout much of the day of triglyceride-rich lipoproteins in the circulation postprandially[45]. The effect of IDDM and of insulin therapy on cholesteryl ester transfer requires study.

## Proteinuria in diabetes

Proteinuria in diabetes is well established as a risk factor for premature death[163–166]. In one study, nearly half of the patients with IDDM who developed this complication died within 7 years[164]. Initially the impression was created that these deaths were due to progression to advanced renal failure. However, the great majority of diabetics with proteinuria, who die prematurely, succumb to ischaemic heart disease before their renal failure is advanced. It has been calculated that in IDDM the mortality among patients with proteinuria is 37 times that of the general population, whereas in those who remain free of protein-uria it is only quadrupled[166].

Early in nephropathy, even before progression to overt proteinuria, there may be a rise in blood pressure[167–169]. Hypertension may thus be one factor contributing to premature atherosclerosis. Investigations of lipoproteins after the development of clinically detectable proteinuria, but before the onset of any major impairment of creatinine clearance, have suggested that disturbances of lipoprotein metabolism may also be important[149,170,171]. At this stage, serum levels of triglycerides, and LDL cholesterol, are frequently raised and HDL cholesterol decreased. It is not known whether this lipoprotein pattern was present before the onset of proteinuria or is its consequence. HDL metabolism in proteinuria is discussed in the previous section of this chapter and additional discussion of primary renal effects on triglyceride-rich lipoproteins and LDL are to be found later (page 328).

The premature deaths in diabetics associated with proteinuria are not related to duration of diabetes and this would support the view, expressed earlier, that hyper-glycaemia and hyperinsulinaemia are unlikely to be important[166]. The detection of sustained proteinuria thus calls for intensive management of any associated hypertension or hyperlipidaemia. With the knowledge that the low density lipoproteins in diabetes are of abnormal composition, consensus recommendations (Chapter 6, page 168) have generally set intervention levels for diet and drugs lower than in the general population. The risk from any given level of serum cholesterol in diabetes is greater than that in the general population[13,15] (see Figure 11.1). This may be because cholesterol in diabetes frequently persists in the circulation in lipoproteins of lower density than in the general population. It is well established in diabetes that triglycerides are a risk factor in their own right, which is not the case in the general population, and this too may be because of the accumulation of lower density lipoproteins which tend to have a higher triglyceride content than the low density lipoproteins in which the greater part of the serum cholesterol is contained in health.

## Insulin resistance

The association between IHD and dyslipidaemia termed variously insulin resistance syndrome, syndrome X, chronic cardiovascular risk syndrome, plurimetabolic syndrome, and various epenymous titles most often Reaven syndrome (although he did not claim this title and others are in contention[172]), which almost certainly overlaps (or perhaps embraces) familial combined hyperlipidaemia, and is probably best described as the atherogenic profile[173], has already been discussed in some detail (Chapter 6, page 143 and Chapter 7, page 192). The suggestion that any of the components of the syndrome are due to 'hyperinsulinaemia' as opposed to insulin resistance and a relative deficiency of insulin action is dubious[34,69] (page 296). Increased circulating C peptide levels associated with more severe expression of the syndrome[174] is not necessarily evidence of increased secretion of biologically active insulin[175], but rather evidence that because of the resistance to its action it is 'flogging a dead horse' and that the pancreas cannot meet the demands placed on it[176]. The insulin resistance and the pancreatic endocrine insufficiency may have their roots in antecedents in early childhood, perhaps even *in utero*[177]. Obesity in adulthood should not, however, be overlooked as the major acquired factor leading to the syndrome albeit operating in a susceptible host. The android pattern of obesity is particularly associated with the syndrome (page 317), but it is not clear whether the androgenized pattern of obesity in females seen in its most extreme form in polycystic ovary syndrome is actually the cause or the consequence of insulin resistance leading to diminished sex hormone binding globulin and thence a high circulating free androgen level[178,179]. The issue is important, because it may explain why diabetic women lose much of the protection against IHD enjoyed by other women[180].

Perhaps most fascinating despite the obvious association of the syndrome NIDDM and glucose intolerance diabetes in the sense of a raised blood glucose does not appear essential for the syndrome or the predisposition to IHD. For example, despite an increased incidence of diabetes and obesity Pima Indians are not susceptible to it[34]. Nor are Japanese or West Indian diabetics (despite in the case of West Indians perhaps similar childhood antecedents to those suggested as the cause in the British population). On the other hand, the South Asian Indian migrant population to Britain with their high incidence of diabetes are uniquely susceptible to develop the atherogenic lipoprotein profile and to develop IHD prematurely[181,182].

The author does not find the case for the inclusion of hypertension as a comparent of the syndrome other than through its association with obesity convincing, but a review of this topic is outside the scope of this book.

The full components of the suggested syndrome are shown in Table 11.3. In the author's view the most important question is whether the insulin resistance and

**Table 11.3 The components present in the full syndrome of insulin resistance (chronic cardiovascular risk syndrome; atherogenic profile; syndrome X)**

Insulin resistance
Raised NEFA flux
Hypertriglyceridaemia
Prolonged postprandial lipaemia
Raised IDL
Raised small LDL (without necessarily any increase in LDL cholesterol)
Raised non-receptor-mediated LDL catabolism
Low HDL
Raised cholesteryl ester transfer between lipoproteins

the rest of the syndrome all stem from an increased flux of NEFA, with that being the primary abnormality (all the other features could be secondary to hepatic overproduction of VLDL as a consequence of increased NEFA supply) or whether the insulin resistance/pancreatic endocrine insufficiency is the primary abnormality resulting in the high NEFA and thence increased hepatic VLDL production.

## Lipoprotein (a) in diabetes

There have been many reports concerning the serum concentration of Lp(a) in both NIDDM and IDDM. An overview is probably that evidence for an increase associated with diabetes unless it is complicated by nephropathy has been inconsistent[183–190]. Some reports suggest that even in its early stages nephropathy may be associated with an increased frequency of high serum Lp(a) concentrations. Serum Lp(a) is not associated with IHD in diabetes in case-control[157] or prospective studies[191], but diabetics with nephropathy have not been specifically studied.

## Drugs used in the management of diabetes

### Insulin

As will be evident from the earlier discussion that, whatever view is taken of the case for considering hyperinsulinaemia as a cause of hypertriglyceridaemia or of atheroma rather than an associated epiphenomenon, there is no substantial evidence that insulin therapy is associated with any increased risk of atherosclerosis. In the vast majority of studies with insulin, any effect on lipoproteins has been favourable (decrease in triglycerides and sometimes in LDL cholesterol and a tendency for HDL to rise). The decrease in serum triglyceride and increase in serum HDL in NIDDM following the introduction of insulin therapy with a simple regimen of intermediate-acting insulin twice daily may be equally as good as that with three preprandial injections of soluble insulin against a background of a once daily longer-acting insulin in the evening[192]. Of course, in clinical practice, insulin therapy may lead to excessive weight gain and if this is not controlled it will have unfavourable effects on serum lipoprotein levels. Insufficient attention has been drawn to the weight gain in the patient in the group randomized to maintain lower blood glucose levels with insulin than those on a less demanding insulin regimen in the Diabetes Control and Complications Trial[193]. They weighed 4.6 kg more after 5 years. It remains to be seen whether this will nullify the beneficial effect of higher doses of insulin on the serum lipoprotein profile.

### Sulphonylurea drugs

These are probably too readily prescribed, when more persistent attempts to control diabetes by dietary means or treatment with a biguanide might have been more appropriate. The objection to the use of sulphonylurea drugs is their pronounced tendency to cause weight gain and this may have adverse effects on serum lipoproteins and also counteract any initial favourable glycaemic response. In the diabetic clinic one is faced with a succession of obese diabetics on sulphonylurea treatment. Many will have gained considerable amounts of weight since they presented at the clinic. Many will have poor glycaemic control, high serum triglycerides and LDL cholesterol and low HDL cholesterol. Examination of the hospital records will reveal that some years previously they presented to the clinic with NIDDM and initially showed a brief improvement in their glycaemia and symptoms with diet. Soon, however, it was considered that their blood glucose was perhaps a little too high and so a 'small dose' of a sulphonylurea drug was prescribed. This produced a satisfactory reponse, but on a subsequent return visit the glucose was again raised, the patient by now weighing more than at presentation. The dose of sulphonylurea was increased and the whole cycle was repeated over the years until a hyperglycaemic, dyslipoproteinaemic, grossly obese patient on maximum doses of sulphonylurea drugs had been produced and a decision had to be made about whether to introduce insulin (which is no aid to weight reduction) or, now that the struggle is unequal, whether to add a biguanide. Neither the patient nor the physician has gained from this sequence of events. Indeed one wonders what would have been the outcome had the patient simply been allowed to continue with the marginally 'unacceptable' blood glucose before the sulphonylurea drug was introduced.

This 'sulphonylurea syndrome' helps to explain the paradox that surveys of clinic populations of NIDDM patients show that those on sulphonylureas have low serum HDL cholesterol levels and increased serum triglycerides[194–196], whereas the response to sulphonylurea drugs in controlled trials (either as a consequence of drug action or of control of hyperglycaemia) is often to reduce serum triglycerides and sometimes to increase HDL cholesterol[197,198].

Care should be taken in selecting patients to receive sulphonylurea treatment and escalating dosage should be avoided, particularly without further resort to diet. Otherwise the conclusions of the University Group Diabetes Program (UGDP)[199,200], apparently so thoroughly refuted[201], may be closer to our actual clinical practice than we realize.

### Biguanide drugs

Mefformin, rather than phenformin with its greater risk of lactic acidosis, is the commonly prescribed biguanide. These drugs have the advantage that they do not cause hypoglycaemia and are not associated with weight gain. In the UGDP trial, the blood glucose response was better sustained with phenformin than with the sulphonylurea, tolbutamide. As with tolbutamide, doubts, which have since been refuted[201], were raised about their effects on cardiovascular mortality[199,200]. Their chief limitation in practice is a fairly high incidence of gastrointestinal side-effects. Metformin is thus the first-line agent in patients with persistent hyperglycaemia who remain obese after attempts at dietary therapy.

Metformin therapy is associated with a decrease in both serum triglyceride and cholesterol concentrations, in diabetes[196,202–205]. In non-diabetics with primary hypertriglyceridaemia, a similar response is seen, but metformin has no effect when hypercholesterolaemia is the dominant disorder[206].

### Guar gum

Various experiments suggest that guar, a mucilaginous vegetable fibre made from the powdered seeds of the Indian cluster bean (*Cyamopsis tetragonolabrata*) can decrease postprandial hyperglycaemia and serum cholesterol[205,207]. It might also assist weight reduction. The extent to which any of these benefits are borne out in practice is uncertain[208]. Its effect on serum cholesterol is mediated through a similar mechanism to that of bile-acid sequestrating agents[209] (Chapter 10, page 261).

## Lipid-lowering drugs in the management of diabetes

Dietary treatment must be attempted in the hyperlipidaemic diabetic patient before recourse to lipid-lowering drugs. Weight reduction in the obese is best achieved by a low fat, calorie-restricted diet. For the moderately hypertriglyceri-daemic patient, who is not overweight, substitution of saturated fat with complex carbohydrate and polyunsaturated fat is appropriate (Chapter 9). For those with more severe hypertriglyceridaemia (1000 mg/dl or >11 mmol/l), substantial decreases in total dietary fat may be more effective. If such patients are not obese, increased intake of complex carbohydrate will be required to achieve an adequate energy intake and such patients may be best treated at a centre with specialized facilities. The necessity for drugs likely to exacerbate hyperlipidaemia, particularly beta-blockers, thiazide diuretics and sex steroids[210–212], should also be reappraised before introducing lipid-lowering therapy, and glycaemic control should also be improved as far as reasonably possible.

The great difficulty in recommending the use of lipid-lowering agents in diabetes is the lack of any prospective trial involving clinical events. On the other hand, the strength of the evidence linking dyslipoproteinaemia with premature mortal-ity in diabetics is too great for the clinician to be content to do nothing. On *a priori* grounds, the fibrate drugs, which lower serum triglycerides and often also raise HDL cholesterol, have generally received most attention for the manage-ment of the majority of hyperlipidaemic diabetics[210 215]. These drugs do not upset glycaemic control; they may produce a small improvement (Chapter 10, page 272). They should not be used in patients with reduced creatinine clearance with the possible exception of gemfibrozil in reduced dosage. There is some evidence that bezafibrate can favourably influence the rate of progression of atherosclero-sis in diabetes[216]. The effect of bezafibrate in diabetes is largely in reducing VLDL levels and to some extent IDL. LDL concentration is relatively uneffected[215].

Nicotinic acid, because of its side-effects, particularly flushing, and its unfavourable effect on glycaemic control during the rebound rise in plasma NEFA associated with its fluctuating plasma levels (Chapter 10, page 264), has not found favour in the management of diabetic dyslipidaemia. Longer acting formulations and analogues have been developed. Of these acipimox has a similar effect on serum lipids as the fibrate drugs[217], suppresses NEFA over a longer period thus not unfavourably affecting glycaemic control, and causes less flushing. The devel-opment of even longer acting preparations of this or similar compounds may prove interesting[218].

Fibrate drugs and acipimox do not favourably influence LDL cholesterol levels. It is not known directly whether their action in decreasing non-receptor mediated LDL catabolism and the shift away from circulating smaller LDL particles without their being any overall effect on LDL concentration[219,220] is favourable in decreasing IHD risk. In diabetic patients with elevated LDL levels or in whom it is desired to decrease relatively normal LDL levels, the HMG-CoA reductase inhibitors are valuable. These are effective in lowering both serum LDL and IDL and do not unfavourably affect glycaemic control[221–223]. They may also be used in patients with nephropathy.

Marine fish oils have not proved successful in the management of hyperlipidaemia in diabetes because of deterioration in glycaemic control and exacerbation of hypercholesterolaemia[224–226]. Bile acid sequestrants often provoke an increase in triglycerides in diabetes and the complexity of their administration and frequent gastrointestinal side-effects make them unacceptable to diabetic patients, who are frequently already on multiple drug therapy.

### Antihypertensive drugs and diabetes

Hypertension like hyperlipidaemia is a commonly met problem in diabetes. Again there are no trials of long-term effects of treatment in diabetes on morbidity and mortality to guide us. It does, however, seem sensible to treat it, but to avoid therapy, which is likely to exacerbate hyperlipidaemia. All beta-blockers of any practical value in the treatment of hypertension raise serum triglycerides and lower serum HDL regardless of cardioselectivity (page 333). Indeed, the diabetic with a pre-existing modest increase in serum triglycerides is just the type of patient to develop gross lipaemia, if exposed to beta-blocker therapy. Diuretics too, possibly because of their diabetogenic effects, seem to have a more substantial effect on serum lipids in diabetics than in non-diabetics.

Thus in the management of hypertension in diabetes[227], the use of methyl dopa, calcium antagonists, other vasodilators and angiotensin-converting enzyme inhibitors should be considered before beta-blockers or diuretics. When the latter two drugs are considered essential, the serum lipid response should be monitored and, if necessary, lipid-lowering medication introduced.

# Thyroid disease

## Hypothyroidism

In hypothyroidism there is often an increase in the serum cholesterol concentration[228] due to raised levels of serum LDL and IDL[229]. A high level of suspicion of myxoedema as a cause of hyperlipidaemia particularly in women and diabetics is required in the Lipid Clinic. As many as 20% of women beyond the age of 40 years discovered to have serum cholesterol levels exceeding 320 mg/dl (8.0 mmol/l) had hypothyroidism in one series[230]. Less consistently, there is hypertriglyceridaemia associated with an increase in VLDL and occasionally fasting chylomicronaemia. Decreased receptor-mediated LDL catabolism is the probable cause of the hypercholesterolaemia[231–234]. Decreased triglyceride clearance[235,236], probably mediated via decreased lipoprotein lipase activity, is responsible for the hypertriglyceridaemia[237,238]. The VLDL and IDL in hypothyroidism are rich in cholesterol and apo E[237,239], thus resembling β-VLDL of type III hyperlipoproteinaemia (Chapter 8, page 215). It is not surprising that patients with an underlying tendency to type III hyperlipoproteinaemia may develop the full-blown clinical syndrome if they become hypothyroid[240].

It has been claimed that serum cholesterol may be increased as a result of so-called premyxoedema, by which is meant a phase of autoimmune thyroiditis which precedes the development of hypothyroidism[241]. This was described before the thyroid-stimulating hormone (TSH) assay was available and thus the decision that a patient was euthyroid was perhaps less objective than nowadays. Also, the patients studied were drawn from a population with IHD which must have biased the outcome in favour of finding hyperlipidaemia[241]. Over the years, serum thyroid function tests have been performed on several hundred patients referred to our lipid clinic. A raised TSH in a euthyroid patient has not been a common finding, and when such patients were given thyroxine in a replacement dose there has been little lipoprotein response, suggesting that they actually have a primary hyperlipidaemia and that the raised TSH was a chance finding.

The majority of reports have shown an increased HDL cholesterol level in hypothyroidism, the major component of the increase being in the $HDL_2$ subfraction[242]. The explanation for this may be a decrease in the CETP-mediated transfer of cholesteryl ester out of HDL into VLDL[243].

In contrast to the effect of thyroxine in so-called pre-clinical hypothyroidism, in true hypothyroidism dramatic decreases in serum cholesterol and triglycerides occur. They are accompanied by a marked increase in biliary cholesterol excretion[244], which was previously low. In some studies, serum HDL cholesterol has tended to decrease with thyroid replacement, but this has been a less consistent finding[142,245].

## Hyperthyroidism

There is general agreement that in hyperthyroidism both LDL and HDL cholesterol tend to be decreased[238,246–249]. Serum triglyceride levels are generally normal. An abnormal β-migrating component of HDL has been described[250]. This disappears with treatment of hyperthyroidism and the LDL cholesterol, apolipoprotein B and HDL rise[233,248,249,251].

## Pituitary disease

Clearly, in panhypopituitarism the effect of thyroid hormone deficiency will have a major effect. However, there does appear to be a greater tendency to hypertriglyceridaemia and a lesser tendency to hypercholesterolaemia than in primary hypothyroidism[252]. Serum HDL cholesterol may be reduced[253]. Growth hormone may be important, because in pituitary dwarfism both LDL and VLDL levels are raised[254]. In acromegaly, the LDL levels tend to be low[255]. There is mild hypertriglyceridaemia, but it is presumably related to insulin resistance. The effects of Cushing's syndrome are those of corticosteroid excess (page 335).

# Nutritional

## Obesity

Proneness to obesity may have its origins in an individual's genetic constitution[256] infantile undernourishment – perhaps as early as during fetal development[257] –

and in attitudes to food acquired in the early years when personality is formed. Obesity is a major cause of hyperlipidaemia. Its main effect is to produce hyper-triglyceridaemia[258] and decreased serum HDL cholesterol levels[259]. However, in clinical practice it is frequently also encountered in hypercholesterolaemia and thus in all types of hyperlipoproteinaemia. Regardless of the type of hyper-lipoproteinaemia associated with obesity, the starting point in therapy should always be with the advice to lose weight by dieting[260].

## Recognition of obesity

There has been considerable discussion as to what constitutes obesity[261,262]. By definition, obesity is an excess of body fat of such a degree that is likely to impair health. This definition, it should be noted, is less extensive than would satisfy the cosmetic industry, but the social and psychological implications of obesity need not enter into the definition used in the present context, because we are discussing patients already found to have hyperlipidaemia and there is thus the likelihood that their health will be impaired if their obesity goes untreated.

How is an excess of body fat recognized? Generally this presents more of a problem to the epidemiologist than to the clinician and it is important to realize that fact, if unrealistic therapeutic targets are not to be set for individual patients. The normal 70 kg man contains some 15 kg of adipose tissue triglyc-eride, representing an energy store of 140 000 kcal (compare this with his 6 kg of protein representing 24 000 kcal and 0.225 kg of glycogen equivalent to 900 kcal). The size of the adipose store will vary in health with height and with age, and its anatomical distribution with gender. There are a number of experimen-tal methods for determining body fat in life. These include dilutional methods, which allow the estimation of total body water or intracellular water (which is excluded from triglycerides, see Chapter 1, page 8), using tritiated water or radioactive isotopes of potassium, or the estimation of body fat more directly with fat-soluble substances such as cyclopropane. Other methods involve measurement of body density by weighing in and out of water (triolein has a density of 0.91 g/ml and the remainder of the body about 1.1 g/ml) or by dual-photon absorptiometry[263–265]. Also employed has been skin-fold thickness. The most extensively used method is, however, by the measurement of height and weight. Indices of the adipose mass may be calculated from a knowledge of body weight and height. For a population these indices correlate well with many of the experimental methods for measuring adipose mass (correlation coeffi-cients often in the region of 0.7–0.9), although clearly there will be individuals for whom this will not be so, if they are at the extremes of muscularity, skeletal mass or body habitus.

The indices most frequently studied are weight/height, weight/height$^2$ (Quetelet's index) and weight/height$^3$ (ponderal index). The ponderal index is influenced by height and should no longer be used. In men, Quetelet's index is closest to an estimate of adipose mass, but it may offer no advantage over the use of the weight : height ratio in women[266]. In the Lipid Research Clinics Program Prevalence Study the magnitude of the correlation coefficients with both serum triglyceride and HDL cholesterol concentrations was generally greater with Quetelet's index than with either weight/height or weight/height$^3$[259]. Quetelet's index is thus the most widely used method of comparing the adipose mass of different populations in studies of lipoproteins.

If Quetelet's index is to be a guide in assessing obesity, we must know what should be regarded as the upper range for normality. Ideally, in the context of the management of hyperlipidaemia we should know at what level adipose mass has a significant effect on serum lipid concentrations. Unfortunately this information is not available. It might seem reasonable to turn, therefore, to information about coronary mortality in relation to body mass. Certainly three of the major risk factors for coronary atheroma (hyperlipidaemia, hypertension and diabetes mellitus) are associated with increasing body mass index. As might be anticipated, therefore, in the largest study of men in whom body mass was analysed as a cause of cardiovascular death, there was a positive correlation, the risk increasing progressively steeply after body mass exceeded the average by 10–19%[267]. This, however, has not been the universal experience in numerous smaller studies, which present an inconsistent picture[264]. The reason for this may be because cigarette smoking, itself a major cause of coronary deaths, is associated with lower body weight (on average 5.9 kg less than in non-smokers)[268]. Also, the total adipose mass may not be the most sensitive risk factor for coronary disease. There is an abundance of evidence to suggest that the anatomical distribution of adipose tissue is an important determinant of risk. The male pattern of obesity involves increased adipose tissue principally in the abdominal region, whereas fatness in women is more commonly due to increases in the buttocks and thighs. The upper-body or male pattern of obesity has been termed android and the lower-body or female pattern gynoid[269]. When matched for similar degrees of overall fatness, the android fat distribution, whether it occurs in men or women, is associated with significantly greater blood pressure, serum triglycerides and glucose intolerance[270,271]. It may thus constitute a more discriminating risk factor for ischaemic heart disease (IHD) than an index reflecting total body fat. The ratio of the circumference of the waist to that of the hips may be used to assess whether body fat distribution is of the male or female type. This ratio has been reported to be more closely related to the risk of IHD than the body mass index[272–274]. In men, the risk of IHD was increased when the waist : hip ratio exceeded 1.0 (in women above 0.8).

As opposed to coronary deaths, the relationship between 'all-cause' mortality and obesity has been more consistently reported. There is a U-shaped relationship (Figure 11.7) in both men and women. The increase in mortality at the lower end of the weight distribution is not fully explained by an excess of smokers at this end of the scale. It is on the U-shaped relationship that the tables for desirable weights, which are in such wide use throughout medical practice, are based. The desirable range is thus the range spanning the trough in the U-shaped relationship, and the lower and upper limits of this range should be where the risk of death clearly begins to exceed the minimum risk. There are many limitations on the application of these tables to clinical medicine, and their implicit recommendations should not be slavishly or unthinkingly followed. The widely used tables are based on those constructed by the New York Metropolitan Life Insurance Company. The original Ideal Weight Tables[275] are thought to have been based on the weights of insured 20–29-year-olds. Later tables[276] describing desirable weights were constructed from the initial weight and height of men and women of a higher average age insured between 1935 and 1953 and claims made up until 1954. More recently, the Build Study[277] collated data from 4.2 million policies issued by 25 life insurance companies in the USA and Canada between 1950 and 1971, yielding 106 000 deaths up until 1972. This led to yet more tables[278], which

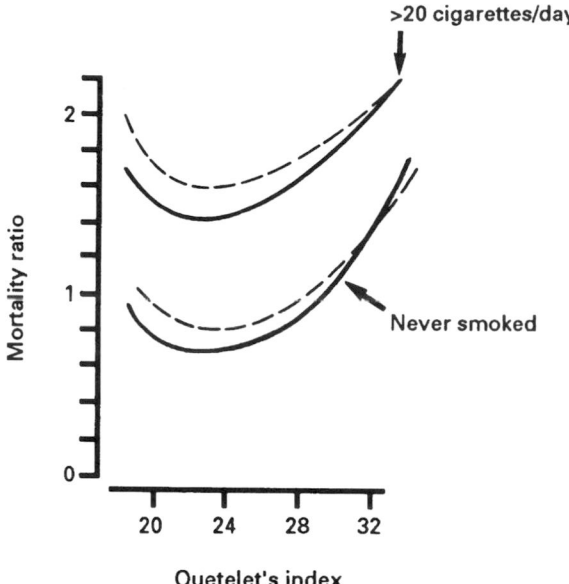

**Figure 11.7**   Effect of obesity on mortality in male (solid line) and female (dashed line) smokers and non-smokers (average mortality = 1) (see reference[261])

have been justifiably criticized because, despite the data available for their construction, they do not improve upon the deficiencies of the earlier ones[279], which are as follows:

1. They retain three separate weight ranges for small, medium and large body frames. It is true that people who are particularly muscular or have large skeletons will, because of the density of muscle and the even greater density of bone, weigh more in relation to their height without necessarily being obese. However, the means of assessing the frame size in the insured population were not designated when the data were recorded and the use of elbow breadth for this purpose does not seem to be widely practised. I have yet to meet an obese patient who did not consider himself or herself to have a large frame and, indeed, in those who have been obese all their lives, this is hardly surprising! They are, however, probably the most 'at risk' group.
2. Age is not taken into account in defining excessive weight. This is particularly unfortunate, since the data show that overweight young people have a much worse prognosis than those in older age ranges[261].
3. Different tables are provided for men and women. This is unnecessary, since once the effect of age has been removed the Quetelet's index with the best prognosis is remarkably similar for men and women[279].

   Various recommendations have been made by different expert committees to remove frame size from height and weight tables. However, these have not generally involved a reanalysis of the data and the other difficulties remain. Andres and co-workers have reanalysed the 1979 data taking all three objections into account,

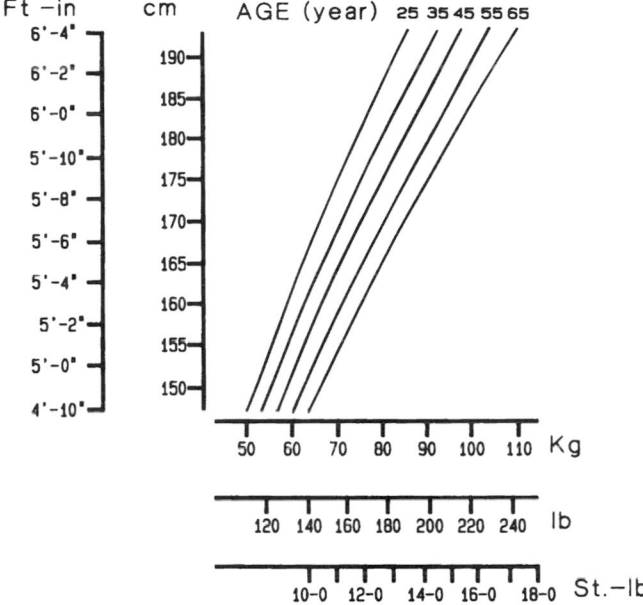

**Figure 11.8**  Ideal body weight in relation to height of different ages (based on tables in Andres *et al.*[279])

and their results agree well with those of 23 other smaller populations collected for non-actuarial purposes[279]. Their tables thus are the same for men and women, leave the clinican free to pass his own judgement on body frame, but are informative as to the effects of age[279]. Figure 11.8 has been constructed from them and may be helpful in the clinic.

In making an assessment of obesity, the importance of the clinical impression of the undressed patient should not be underestimated. Some patients are clearly too fat even though they depart little from the upper limit of the desirable range, whereas others look fit despite their apparent overweight. Hopefully to some extent these anomalies will be less frequent when age-related tables are used, but they cannot be ignored if a sensible assessment is to be made of whether an energy-restricted diet is likely to be helpful in correcting hyperlipidaemia. The clinician is also able to take account of the greater risk conferred by the android (upper body) type of fat distribution when exhorting his or her patient to greater efforts to lose weight.

### Cause of hyperlipidaemia in obesity

The increase in the serum triglyceride concentrations in obesity is related to an increase in the hepatic production of VLDL[258,280–283]. This is due to an increased flux of non-esterified fatty acids out of adipose tissue[284] which is even more pronounced in the android type of obesity[285,286]. The accelerated release of NEFA may be due to the effect of the insulin resistance associated with obesity on the intracellular lipase of adipose tissue[287]. Hepatic VLDL production is frequently greater in obese patients than in non-obese individuals, even when they do not have hypertriglyceridaemia[283]. This is explained by a compensatory increase in the rate of removal of triglycerides from circulating triglyceride-rich lipoproteins due to increased lipoprotein lipase activity[288]. The products of VLDL catabolism will thus be increased even in the absence of hypertriglyceridaemia, and it is perhaps surprising that LDL cholesterol levels are not more strikingly positively associated with obesity in epidemiological surveys. This is particularly so in view of the increase in cholesterol synthesis, which also accompanies obesity[289,290], and the increase in serum cholesterol, which occurs during experimental overfeeding[291].

In clinical practice, however, hypercholesterolaemic patients are frequently found to be obese. The exception is FH (Chapter 5, page 116), in which obesity does not seem to be over-represented. When obesity does occur in FH, particularly when extreme, very high levels of serum LDL cholesterol may occur, which can be extremely resistant to treatment when the patient will not cooperate with advice to lose weight. Figure 11.9 shows the clinical course of a patient with tendon xanthomata and FH whose serum cholesterol was 600 mg/dl (15.4 mmol/l) when she was aged 40 years, weighed 60 kg and was moderately obese. Despite attempts to persuade her to lose weight, she became progressively more obese. Nine years later she was referred to our clinic weighing 82 kg, with a serum cholesterol of 1015 mg/dl (26mmol/l) despite drug therapy. It should be recognized that, occasionally, patients who have definite FH, as shown by the presence of tendon xanthomata, have a type IIb lipoprotein phenotype rather than the more common type IIa hyperlipoproteinaemia. The most common explanation for the hypertriglyceridaemia in these patients is that they have become obese. This is important because

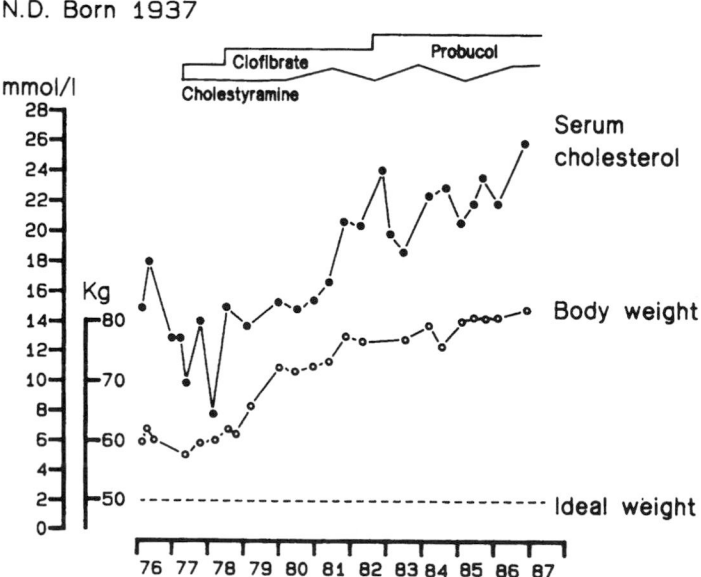

**Figure 11.9**   Disastrous effect of increasing obesity in a patient heterozygous for familial hypercholesterolaemia. Medication was powerless to overcome the rise in serum cholesterol (see text)

they have a worse prognosis (Chapter 5, page 115). Such patients have sometimes been regarded as having familial combined hyperlipidaemia and this must have contributed to the impression that it was a mendelian dominant: the presence of tendon xanthomata identifies such patients as having FH and not familial combined hyperlipidaemia.

Obesity most frequently causes type IV or IIb hyperlipoproteinaemia. It will exacerbate all forms of primary hypertriglyceridaemia, particularly when a clearance defect is present, so that no compensatory increase in catabolism can occur. Obesity may thus provoke gross hyperlipidaemia in patients with type III hyperlipoproteinaemia (Chapter 8, page 215) and patients with pre-existing lipoprotein lipase impairment may develop marked type V hyperlipoproteinaemia (Chapter 7, page 201).

Serum HDL cholesterol concentrations tend to be decreased in obesity and this effect of obesity is independent of other variables known to affect serum HDL cholesterol[292]. It is true to say that serum HDL cholesterol is low in many circumstances in which serum triglyceride levels are increased. The usual explanation for this is that both the high serum triglyceride levels and the low HDL cholesterol concentration are explained by decreased lipoprotein lipase activity[143]. That explanation is, however, unsatisfactory to account for low levels of HDL in obesity, which may occur independently of hypertriglyceridaemia[292] and, as we have already discussed, triglyceride clearance and lipoprotein lipase activity are commonly increased in obesity. The cause of the low HDL cholesterol levels in many obese patients is, therefore, not fully understood.

Furthermore, no increase in serum HDL cholesterol has been shown to occur during weight loss induced by low energy diets[293]. There is some evidence that serum HDL cholesterol will increase if a substantial weight loss is achieved and maintained[294,295]. However, patients who are able to achieve this must be a highly selected group and it would be impossible to dissociate such an effect from other changes in the life-style of the new slim individual.

## Management of obesity in patients with hyperlipidaemia

The management of obesity is by dietary energy restriction. This is discussed in Chapter 10. Increased physical activity may provide some small adjunct to the effect of dietary restriction, but it must be stressed that it is very unlikely to be successful on its own. That is not, of course, to deny that small differences in energy expenditure sustained over a long period may not be the main reason why some individuals are obese and others lean. Adipose cells are almost 90% triglyceride, with a thin rim of cytoplasm. One pound of adipose cells thus contains 3500 kcal (1 kg contains 8000 kcal). Therefore a patient whose daily energy expenditure is 1500 kcal given a 1000 cal diet will lose weight at the rate of 1 lb (0.48 kg) per week. Walking at 4 mph (6.5 km/h) expends 4.7 kcal/min which is only about 3–3.5 kcal/min more than standing or sitting and talking. Thus the diet of 1000 kcal is equivalent to walking for an additional 17 h each week. Fat is an amazingly efficient tissue and patients and doctors frequently have unrealistic expectations of diet and exercise in the treatment of obesity. Claims made for commercial slimming aids are generally downright lies. Most would require that the patient has undergone self-ignition and spontaneous combustion in order to lose weight at the rates quoted.

Drugs for the suppression of appetite have no place in medical practice[296]. Conversely, however, some drugs undoubtedly have the side-effect of increasing body weight and they should be used with caution in the obese. Insulin and sulpho-nylurea drugs have already been discussed in this connection in the section on diabetes. The effects of corticosteroids are, of course, well known. Beta-adrenore-ceptor blocking drugs may also increase body weight[297]. The effects of weight reduction by dieting should always be considered in obese patients with hyper-tension or diabetes mellitus before introducing drug therapy, especially if it may make their obesity more severe.

# Alcohol

Alcohol is a fairly common cause of hyperlipidaemia. Its predominant effect is to produce hypertriglyceridaemia. It should not be forgotten that beer and wine may be major components of dietary energy intake and thus be the cause of obesity. Indeed, these two beverages have probably played an important part in man's social evolution since he forsook the ways of the hunter–gatherer, because they provide a means of storing the nutrients in grain and grape and enhancing their energy content at the same time as ensuring a germ-free water supply! In some regions of Southern Europe the consumption of red wine is high enough for it to be considered as a macronutrient.

## Hypertriglyceridaemia

The increase in serum triglyceride concentration produced by alcohol is largely due to increased hepatic synthesis and secretion. Alcohol decreases the capacity of the liver to oxidize other substrates such as fatty acids, at a time when the supply of precursors of triglyceride synthesis is increased, either because its ingestion coincides with meal times or because of an ethanol-induced enhancement of the release of non-esterified fatty acids from adipose tissue.

Ethanol is oxidized in the liver in preference to all other substrates of oxidative metabolism. Following its ingestion, therefore, there is a decrease in the oxidation of, for example, fatty acids, lactate and glucose[30,298]. The acetate produced by the oxidation of ethanol does not lead directly to increased triglyceride synthesis, since instead it is largely released into the blood stream[298,299].

Carbohydrate is also unlikely to be the substrate for enhanced triglyceride synthesis, because ethanol inhibits gluconeogenesis. Gluconeogenic precursors, such as lactate from the gut, are less readily taken up by the liver in the presence of ethanol[298] and glucose itself may be diverted into glycogen rather than used for de novo fatty acid synthesis. The dominant substrates for the ethanol-induced enhancement of triglyceride synthesis are thus fatty acids either derived from triglycerides stored in adipose tissue or from dietary triglyceride.

Alcohol ingestion often leads to an increase in the rate of lipolysis and release of NEFA from adipose tissue triglycerides. The reason for this effect, which is enhanced by fasting, is not entirely clear[298,300], but it may be so marked as to produce alcoholic ketoacidosis[301].

Ethanol is well known to intensify and prolong the rise in serum triglycerides following a meal[302–305]. Although there is one report of increased intestinal triglyceride production in the rat under these circumstances[306], the predom-inant reason for the increased lipaemia is nevertheless increased hepatic production[307]. Generally, fatty acids are the main oxidative substrate for the liver postprandially[30]. As already discussed, when ethanol is also available it is preferentially oxidized, leaving few alternative directions for the postprandial surge in fatty acid flux to the liver, apart from triglyceride synthesis. The ethanol-induced hepatic conversion of fatty acids to triglyceride occurs at such a pace that it outstrips the ability of the liver to match it with comparable increases in apolipoprotein B production and VLDL secretion[308]. This undoubtedly is the cause of the fatty liver classically associated with heavy drinking.

Clinically one is impressed by the tremendous variation in the serum triglyceride concentrations of different heavy drinkers. This appears to be explained by variation in the capacity of different individuals to clear circulating triglyceride-rich lipoproteins. The chronic effect of alcohol on lipoprotein lipase is to increase its activity[309–313], an effect which reverses on abstinence[310,313]. The result of this increase is to limit the rise in serum triglycerides, which tends to occur due to increased hepatic production and secretion of triglyceride-rich lipoproteins. Those individuals who develop the most severe hypertriglyceridaemia with ethanol have a constitutional limitation in their ability to increase triglyceride clearance and are identifiable by their low catabolic rates for circulating triglycerides both during and after drinking bouts[314].

Alcohol is widely recognized as a cause of pancreatitis. What is less widely recognized is that at least 10% of patients presenting with acute pancreatitis will have severe hypertriglyceridaemia (1800 mg/dl or >20 mmol/l) preceding the onset of abdominal pain. In many patients this is due to the combination of high ethanol ingestion and a partial defect in triglyceride catabolism. The latter defect is identifiable long after the hypertriglyceridaemia has resolved and the patient has recovered and is abstaining from alcohol[315].

## LDL metabolism

The concentration of both serum LDL cholesterol and apolipoprotein B tends to be low in alcoholics[308]. The kinetic explanation for this is not well known. In clinical practice, hypercholesterolaemia is, however, occasionally encountered in association with hypertriglyceridaemia in heavy drinkers, particularly if they are obese or already have a genetic predisposition to hypercholesterolaemia. It must be assumed that in such cases the predominant effect of the alcohol is to increase dietary energy intake.

## HDL metabolism

Alcohol consumption increases serum HDL cholesterol. This is true not only of chronic alcoholics[308], but is also evident in the general population[316,317]. The effect of moderate regular alcohol intake is to increase the serum $HDL_3$ and apo AI and AII concentration[308]. It is possible that this effect is due to increased synthesis and is similar to the increase in serum HDL seen with other hepatic microsomal enzyme-inducing agents[318,319].

Heavy drinking seems to produce a more pronounced increase in serum $HDL_2$, which may be due to accelerated release of surface components from triglyceride-rich lipoproteins[308], because then, as we have previously discussed, VLDL production rates are high and the activity of adipose tissue lipoprotein lipase is frequently increased.

## Clinical considerations

As has already been intimated, ethanol in its own right tends to produce a type IV phenotype. In people whose triglyceride clearance cannot cope with the increased entry of triglyceride-rich lipoproteins, type V hyperlipoproteinaemia will supervene. Never forget that the reason for this may be coexistent diabetes mellitus or the concomitant administration of beta-adrenoreceptor blocking drugs. It should also be realized, however, that patients with an inherent tendency to hypercholesterolaemia may be converted from a type IIa to a type IIb phenotype, if they drink heavily. In any hyperlipidaemia associated with obesity, quite apart from the direct effect of ethanol on lipoprotein metabolism, alcoholic beverages should be considered as a possible cause of excessive dietary energy intake. Although some patients are remarkably revealing, it can be difficult to get a clear history of alcoholism. If alcohol does seem to contribute to a patient's hyperlipidaemia, the usual practice is to ask the patient to abstain completely for a month and then return to the clinic for a further lipid estimation. If this request is met by refusal – or a reaction that most of us would reserve for the imminent ending of the world – it seems reasonable to conclude that alcohol is an important element not only in the genesis of the hyperlipidaemia, but also in the patient's *raison d'être*. Some patients return after 1 month with considerably improved serum lipids and again this is a reasonable indication that alcohol was involved.

Patients who claim to have cooperated, but whose lipid profile is unchanged, pose a problem. Are they lying? To answer this question many might turn to clinical investigations. Certainly the mean cell volume (MCV) can occasionally be helpful[320]. Other tests such as gamma-glutamyl transpeptidase (gamma-GT) or transaminase activities are not always very helpful. Gamma-GT tends to be raised in hypertriglyceridaemia, even when alcohol is not involved[241]. Whether this is because hepatic microsomal enzyme induction is a common feature of hypertriglyceridaemia[318,321] or whether, as in the case of the lactating breast, its release is increased when triglyceride secretory rates are high[322] is unknown. Certainly, however, it would be wrong to attribute the hypertriglyceridaemia in every patient with a raised gamma-GT to alcohol. Severe hypertriglyceridaemia, too, may cause secondary hepatic fatty infiltration (steatosis) and, if there is a severe clearance defect, removal of triglyceride-rich lipoproteins from the circulation by the reticuloendothelial system will lead to hepatosplenomegaly (Chapter 7, page 204). Again the finding of abnormal serum transaminases or even hepatosplenomegaly does not necessarily imply that alcohol is involved. This may pose a problem in treatment, since if liver function is disturbed as the result of some process other than a primary hyperlipidaemia, such as alcohol, then fibrate drugs or nicotinic acid would be inappropriate medication, whereas if the underlying disorder is a primary hyperlipidaemia, then the liver function may improve if it is controlled with such drugs. The judicious use of a small dose of drug gradually building up to a therapeutic dose is sometimes the approach to take.

Thus far, in discussing the clinical aspects of alcohol in hyperlipidaemia, we have considered only the effects of high alcohol consumption. In the case of moderate drinking, epidemiological studies have demonstrated an inverse association with coronary heart disease incidence[323–327]. The evidence that alcohol is protective against IHD falls well short of clinical trial evidence and it should be remembered that people stopping drinking may do so for a reason itself related to IHD[328]. Furthermore not all of the effects of alcohol are beneficial to the cardiovascular system because it is a cause of hypertension and increased risk of death from stroke. Assuming, however, that the balance of evidence is in favour of a beneficial effect in decreasing IHD incidence, it can be calculated that much of the scatter in the relationship between national IHD rates and national fat consumption if adjustment is made for national alcohol consumption[329] – the French paradox – is largely explained. Because of the well-known inverse relationship between serum HDL levels and coronary risk, it is generally supposed that any benefit from ethanol is mediated through its effect on HDL. Were this to be the case, it should be recalled that the effect of moderate amounts of alcohol is to increase the $HDL_3$ subfraction, whereas the subfraction often considered to be protective against ischaemic heart disease is $HDL_2$. This need not detract from the view that the benefit of alcohol is mediated through HDL, since its dynamic effects on HDL metabolism are likely to be more important than its effect on the concentration of any of its individual components. In a clinical context, one might take some comfort from not having to ban reasonable quantities of alcohol from a patient's diet. It would be presumptuous on present evidence, however, to recommend the inclusion of alcohol in a diet from which it was previously absent. The effect of alcohol in moderation is rather small in any case: 10 g of ethanol (equivalent to half a pint (300 ml) of beer or 1½ glasses of wine) seems to raise serum HDL cholesterol only by 1–2 mg/dl (0.03–0.05 mmol/l)[330]. It should also be remembered that heavy drinkers are frequently overwhelmingly coronary prone for other reasons such as cigarette smoking and obesity. They have an increased mortality. The effect of alcoholic liver disease is profoundly to lower serum HDL levels (page 327).

## Anorexia nervosa

Hypercholesterolaemia occurs in one-third or more of women with anorexia nervosa[331–333]. Serum triglyceride levels are in the normal range. The reason for the hypercholesterolaemia is not known with certainty, although decreased catabolism may be the cause, the faecal bile acid excretion being reduced[334].

Patients with anorexia nervosa resemble hypothyroid patients in some respects: low basal metabolic rate, delayed relaxation of tendon jerks, bradycardia, increased serum β-carotene. Serum thyroxine is not usually reduced. It is possible that the ratio of T3 to reverse T3 shifts in favour of reverse T3, however, or that the increased plasma and urinary 11 α-hydroxycorticoids may be relevant to the hypercholesterolaemia[333].

# Liver disorders

The effects of cholestasis and hepatocellular disease are considered separately in order to highlight their different effects on lipoprotein metabolism. In practice, of course, many patients will combine elements of both[335,336].

## Cholestasis

When biliary obstruction occurs with preserved hepatocellular function, for example, in the early stages of primary biliary cirrhosis, the dominant hyperlipidaemia is hypercholesterolaemia. Skin xanthomata such as xanthelasmata frequently develop, but florid planar, tuberoeruptive, striate palmar and even tendon xanthomata may also develop[337]. Indeed, chronic cholestasis due to cholelithiasis was the first cause of xanthomatosis recognized during the last century before surgical treatment was available for gall stones[338]. A xanthomatous peripheral neuropathy may occur when the hyperlipidaemia is marked[339].

The hypercholesterolaemia of cholestasis is characterized by a disproportionate increase in the free cholesterol fraction. In addition to the increase in cholesterol, serum triglycerides may also be elevated. The plasma concentration of lecithin is almost invariably raised, whereas lysolecithin is often low[340,341].

The hyperlipidaemia of cholestasis results from lipoproteins with a hydrated density similar to LDL. Normal LDL, although present, is, however, generally reduced in concentration and the serum apo B is thus lower than would be anticipated from the serum cholesterol concentration. Large quantities of an abnormal lipoprotein designated LpX are present. LpX comprises 25% cholesterol, virtually all of which is free cholesterol. More than 60% of its components are phospholipids. By electron microscopy, it appears as vesicles surrounded by a lipid bilayer, which often stack together in rouleaux so that each assumes a disc-like shape. The protein component is approximately 6%, more than half of which is albumin situated inside the vesicle. There is no apo B or apo E, but apo C and D are present on its surface. One feature of LpX which has occasionally led to the suggestion that it might form the basis of a simple test for cholestasis is that, whereas on agarose gel electrophoresis it migrates, like other lipoproteins, towards the anode, on agar it migrates to the cathode[341,342].

The origin of LpX has been the subject of much speculation. It cannot simply result from the reflux of biliary cholesterol into the circulation, because it is frequently present in larger quantities than such a mechanism would allow. Its presence in patients with familial LCAT deficiency (Chapter 12, page 367) led to the suggestion that a deficiency of that enzyme in liver disorders might be the cause. However, LCAT deficiency is more commonly acquired in hepatocellular disease than in biliary obstruction[340,343], so this cannot be the sole explanation. It seems likely, therefore, that the reflux of biliary phospholipids into the circulation as a result of obstruction may be important[340,344]. In experiments, intravenous infusion of phospholipids attracts cholesterol out of cell membranes and there is a rapid rise in the circulating concentration of free cholesterol[345]. The persistence of such a state might lead to the increase in cholesterol biosynthesis observed in some studies of obstructive jaundice[340].

LpX is degraded by the reticulo-endothelial system. Although hepatocytes do not catabolize LpX, it does appear to interfere with their uptake of chylomicron remnants[346]. LpX, itself, is virtually devoid of triglycerides, but there is often an increase in an LDL-like particle termed lipoprotein-Y[347] or $\beta_2$ lipoprotein[348] which is triglyceride-rich and may represent an accumulation of remnants. Apo E levels may be high[349] and there is frequently an apo E-rich lipoprotein in the more buoyant part of the HDL range which is depleted in apo AI and AII[350]. These particles may be important clinically because they inhibit platelet aggregation and may contribute to a bleeding tendency[351].

Erythrocytes may appear as target cells in cholestasis due to an increase in their membrane cholesterol as the result of the increased circulating free-cholesterol-rich lipoproteins. They may also be seen in states of LCAT deficiency, both primary and secondary, including non-obstructive liver disease[340]. It has been suggested that cell membrane abnormalities may extend to other tissues in liver disease and that these may contribute to some of the morbidity associated with liver disease.

LpX disappears with the relief of biliary obstruction. When this is not possible, in for example primary biliary cirrhosis, the question of therapy to decrease xanthomata may arise in some patients. Diet may be helpful[340]. Cholestyramine, which may in any case be given for pruritus, may be of value. Clofibrate was, however, found to have the paradoxical effect of exacerbating the hypercholesterolaemia, perhaps because of changes in the composition of the bile refluxing into the circulation[340,352]. Recently it has been reported that the hypercholesterolaemia in primary biliary cirrhosis responds to the administration of ursodeoxycholic acid[353]. It also responds to HMG-CoA reductase inhibitor-therapy, but their use has been discouraged because of the risk of their accumulation and of ensuing hepatotoxicity[354]. Occasionally plasmapheresis has been used with success[355] for severe neuropathic symptoms. The hypercholesterolaemia of obstructive jaundice wanes as hepatocellular damage progresses, if the obstruction is chronic. Thus, the xanthomata in many patients with primary biliary cirrhosis will resolve as their liver disease progresses and they may then be found to have rather low levels of serum cholesterol. The question is often asked whether such patients during the hypercholesterolaemic phase of their illness are at increased risk of atherosclerosis[335,336,356]. The question is really unresolved.

# Hepatocellular disease

A moderate hypertriglyceridaemia often accompanies hepatocellular liver disease[342,357]. In some instances an increased flux of fatty acids leading to increased hepatic synthesis of triglycerides may be set against an inability to secrete these adequately into the circulation with resulting fatty liver[30]. The fatty liver of alcoholism and kwashiorkor may be the result of such a mechanism.

The mild hypertriglyceridaemia of primary parenchymal liver disease is not associated with an increase in prebetalipoproteins on lipoprotein electrophoresis, as would be the case in most patients with primary endogenous hypertriglyceridaemia. Instead, the prebeta and beta bands merge to form a single densely staining broad beta band. The alpha band disappears. VLDL levels are decreased and, when isolated in the ultracentrifuge, the VLDL has beta rather than prebeta mobility. LDL is rich in triglycerides[343]. Although total serum cholesterol may not be decreased, the proportion of esterified cholesterol is decreased and this is reflected in the relatively cholesteryl ester-depleted LDL. High density lipoprotein is not absent as might be suggested from lipoprotein electrophoresis, but is present at a stage closer to nascent HDL and may be found as piled-up discs when examined by electron microscopy[341]. It is rich in apo E and possesses beta-mobility, thus explaining the absence of the $\alpha$ band on plasma electrophoresis[358]. Perhaps related to their persistent small size, the fractional catabolic rate of apolipoprotein A-containing lipoproteins is increased[359].

Many of these effects can be explained on the basis of the often profound LCAT deficiency which accompanies hepatocellular failure[343]. Failure to esterify cholesterol by LCAT at its site on HDL prevents the development of the HDL core, and the diminished supply of cholesteryl ester from HDL to VLDL and LDL limits the reciprocal outward flow of triglycerides. In addition a deficiency of the hepatic triglyceride lipase[357,360,361] may influence the removal of remnant-like particles and the abnormal LDL from the circulation. In severe liver disease the whole of the hepatic lipoprotein uptake mechanism may, of course, be put out of action and this too might lead to a build-up of any remnant and IDL-like lipoproteins, still secreted by the gut or liver. As parenchymal disease progresses, serum lipoprotein (a) levels decrease[362].

## Cholelithiasis

There is no agreement about whether cholesterol gall stones are associated with coronary heart disease. The hyperlipidaemia which most predisposes to them is hypertriglyceridaemia rather than hypercholesterolaemia[363], probably because of the relationship which exists between serum triglyceride levels and biliary cholesterol saturation[364]. There is no suggestion that serum triglycerides rise in response to gall stone disease and so where the two conditions coexist some common aetiological factor such as obesity may be the explanation. As might be anticipated from this, HDL cholesterol levels are inversely correlated with bile saturation[365], casting doubt on the suggestion that cholesterol returning to the liver in HDL makes a major contribution to biliary cholesterol[366].

## Hepatoma

Hypercholesterolaemia has been reported in about one-quarter of patients with hepatoma[367,368]. Biliary obstruction may be a partial explanation, but there is also evidence that cholesterol synthesis may not be suppressed in response to dietary cholesterol in hepatomas[369]. Hyperlipidaemia presumably not due to either of these possibilities is also well described in rats with experimental tumours[30].

## Porphyria

Increased serum and LDL cholesterol occurs in about one-third of patients with acute intermittent porphyria[370]. The reason is unknown.

# Renal disease[371,372]

## Nephrotic syndrome

In nephrotic syndrome there is an increase in the serum cholesterol, which often occurs even with only small decreases in the plasma albumin concentration. With more marked decreases in the plasma albumin, hypertriglyceridaemia increasingly frequently accompanies the hypercholesterolaemia. An increase in triglycerides without any accompanying increase in cholesterol is distinctly uncommon in nephrotic syndrome, in contrast to chronic renal failure[373]. The commonest lipoprotein phenotypes are thus IIa, IIb or V. Recently it has become apparent that an increase in the serum Lp(a) concentration is a consistent accompaniment of proteinuria: the levels may increase three- or four-fold in patients with gram range proteinuria[374–376]. They return to normal in patients with minimal-change glomerulonephritis when it remits and the proteinuria subsides[374].

An inhibitory effect of albumin on hepatic VLDL secretion appears to be a basic property of liver evident in hepatocyte tissue culture[377,378]. It has been suggested that the effect of hypoalbuminaemia is mediated via an increase in the unbound NEFA[379]. However, there is no direct evidence for this and in tissue culture studies fatty acids are not required for the effect. The possibility that it is due to osmotic pressure or viscosity is therefore more likely. Although one series of experiments using rat hepatocytes *in vitro* appeared to support the viscosity theory[378], it was not supported by observations in patients in whom osmotic pressure correlated more closely with serum cholesterol, although neither viscosity nor osmotic pressure related to serum triglyceride levels[380].

It is interesting that in man an increase in cholesterol is commoner than hyper-triglyceridaemia and that it is the cholesterol which correlates best with the plasma albumin concentration. This also appears to be the case in analbuminaemia, in which hypercholesterolaemia, but not hypertriglyceridaemia, occurs[381]. In both nephrotic syndrome and analbuminaemia, infusions of albumin or other macro-molecules decrease serum cholesterol[381,382].

The raised serum cholesterol is predominantly due to a raised LDL concentration. Increases in apolipoprotein B accompany the rise in LDL concentration[152,383]. Increased LDL synthesis has been reported[384–386], but, as will be evident from the previous discussion, LDL is unlikely to have arisen as a consequence of conversion from VLDL. Direct hepatic secretion of LDL may be associated with proteinuria, because Lp(a) arises from direct hepatic secretion with no VLDL precursor. Decreased receptor mediated LDL catabolism has also been reported[386] as the explanation. VLDL in nephrotic syndrome also has increased cholesteryl ester content and proportionately less triglycerides[30]. As in so many of the secondary hyperlipidaemias, it is reminiscent of remnant lipoproteins or IDL.

When hypertriglyceridaemia does occur there is frequently an associated decrease in catabolism secondary to a reduction in lipoprotein lipase activity[387,388].

The serum HDL cholesterol and apolipoprotein AI concentrations are usually normal or decreased in nephrotic syndrome. The $HDL_2$ subfraction concentration is, however, commonly decreased and in those patient in whom total HDL remains normal there may be an increase in $HDL_3$[152,383,389]. There appears to be an increase in apo AI production so that enhanced catabolism must explain the normal or low levels present[152,153]. HDL, certainly $HDL_3$, is small enough to leak through the damaged glomerular basement membrane in many patients with nephrotic syndrome and it may be detected in their urine as immunoreactive apo AI[152]. Quantities equivalent to the normal daily production can be detected in the urine of some patients[152]. It is possible, therefore, that although $HDL_3$ is present in the plasma in increased amounts due to increased production, it may be lost into the urine before it has circulated for sufficiently long to acquire enough cholesterol to complete the transition to $HDL_2$. Decreased lipoprotein lipase activity would also be expected to impair the conversion of $HDL_3$ to $HDL_2$[143].

Although it is the everyday experience of renal physicians that their patients with nephrotic syndrome are at increased risk of ischaemic heart disease, this view has been challenged[390]. The probable explanation is that patients with minimal change nephropathy or transient proteinuria were included in that study, diluting the impact of less selective, persistent proteinuria, which carries a high risk for atheroma[372,391].

The management of serum lipids in the nephrotic syndrome has been particularly difficult. The hyperlipidaemia may be compounded by high energy diets, diuretics, beta-adrenoreceptor blocking drugs and steroids used in its therapy. Where possible high energy diets should be rich in polyunsaturated and mono-unsaturated fatty acids rather than saturated ones[392] (Chapter 9, page 239). Cholestyramine has been used to reduce LDL cholesterol, but it will exacerbate any coexisting hypertriglyceridaemia and is unpopular with patients already often on complicated drug regimens. Many fibric acid derivatives, particularly clofibrate, are probably best avoided because of the risk of myositis[393]. However, use of gemfibrozil, which undergoes predominantly hepatic excretion, has been reported[394]. Undoubtedly the most encouraging therapeutic development has been the advent of HMG-CoA reductase inhibitors for the treatment of hyperlipidaemia in patients with proteinuria. Experience with these has generally been good with substantial reductions in serum LDL cholesterol[395–398]. They are probably indicated in the treatment of IIa and IIb hyperlipoproteinaemia associated with nephrotic syndrome except that due to minimal change glomerulonephritis when resolution in the near future is anticipated[372].

## Chronic renal failure without proteinuria

Chronic renal failure *per se* leads to hypertriglyceridaemia. Serum VLDL triglycerides and also LDL triglycerides are increased[371,372,399]. The effect is probably largely due to decreased activity of both hepatic and lipoprotein lipase enzymes. The underlying cause of this is uncertain. Insulin resistance is present in renal failure, but does not appear to lead to an increase in NEFA flux, which normally stimulates hepatic triglyceride synthesis in this circumstance. The significance of raised glucogen and growth hormone levels and of a circulating inhibitor of lipoprotein lipase (possibly parathyroid hormone[400]) are speculative[372].

Serum HDL levels tend to be low in chronic renal failure. This is at least partly due to decreased synthesis of apo AI[401]. Treatment frequently compounds the underlying tendency to hypertriglyceridaemia and this is more readily explicable. Haemodialysis requires the administration of heparin over long periods and this may deplete lipoprotein and hepatic lipase reserves, further exacerbating the defect in the catabolism of triglyceride-rich lipoproteins. Also, a deficiency of apo CII, the activator of lipoprotein lipase, was reported in patients on chronic haemodialysis[402]. Chronic ambulatory peritoneal dialysis (CAPD) leads to absorption from the peritoneum of considerable amounts of glucose, leading to obesity and probably also carbohydrate-induced hypertriglyceridaemia (Chapter 9, page 234). Increases in undoubted remnant particles analogous to type III hyperlipoproteinaemia have been described in patients receiving both types of dialysis[403]. Those receiving CAPD also have more marked increases in their LDL even when LDL cholesterol is not elevated. This is evident from the frequency with which apo B levels are raised, indicating an increase in LDL particles[404].

In patients on dialysis, HDL cholesterol levels tend to be low regardless of the presence of hypertriglyceridaemia[402,405]. This is not necessarily reflected by immunoassay of apo AI because levels of AI unassociated with cholesterol (free apo AI) are often increased[406,407]. An interesting mechanism for this might be that the small molecular weight AI particles accumulate because the normally functioning kidney is a site of their catabolism. There is some evidence for this both in the rat[156] and in man[408]. Decreased LCAT activity in patients on haemodialysis might also be a factor leading to the failure of nascent HDL particles to acquire a cholesterol core[409,410].

Following renal transplantation, many of the abnormalities of lipoprotein metabolism resolve if good renal function is established. Hypertriglyceridaemia tends to improve and HDL to increase[405,411–413]. There is an increase in LCAT activity[385], a decrease in free apo AI[407] and post-heparin lipase activities increase[414]. Hyperlipidaemia does, however, persist in at least one-quarter of patients. The reasons for this are complex and probably involve persisting renal insufficiency[400], weight gain, corticosteroid therapy, antihypertensive therapy and possibly cyclosporin treatment[399,415].

In chronic renal failure serum Lp(a) concentrations are raised[372,416]. Both in patients on haemodialysis and chronic ambulatory peritoneal dialysis[372,417–421] most investigators have reported that the levels of Lp(a) are also increased, probably even more so. After transplantation serum Lp(a) levels may decrease, but generally remain elevated[372,419,422–425]. Important factors in maintaining these high Lp(a) concentration are the degree of post-transplant proteinuria, the function of the graft and the administration of cyclosporin.

The finding of high Lp(a) in renal disease may be particularly important. In patients who have undergone cardiac transplantation serum Lp(a) was highest in those developing transplant atherosclerosis[426].

Cardiovascular disease rather than renal failure is now the leading cause of death in dialysed patients and it continues to be a major problem even following transplantation[427]. Treatment of hyperlipidaemia is in many patients fraught with difficulty. Diet will modify the lipoprotein levels[428] and in some patients, particularly after transplantation, the use of antihypertensive agents, which do not adversely affect lipids, may be advisable. The best immunosuppressive regimen remains controversial. In selected patients, lipid-lowering drugs may be used with caution. It is interesting that there is mounting evidence that lipoprotein abnormalities might contribute to the progression as well as the morbidity of renal disease by decreasing progressive glomerular scarring[429]. Gemfibrozil has been used to control hypertriglyceridaemia both in non-dialysed and dialysed patients with chronic renal failure[430–432] and bezafibrate in those on dialysis[428]. Simvastatin has been employed to regulate hypercholesterolaemia in patients receiving chronic ambulatory peritoneal dialysis[434].

# Drugs

## Overview

Many drugs affect serum cholesterol or triglycerides[435]. In the lipid clinic the most commonly met drugs with adverse effects on serum lipids will be beta-adrenoreceptor blocking drugs and diuretics. Beta-blockers do not affect the cholesterol level, but may markedly increase serum triglycerides, especially in the patient with pre-existing hypertriglyceridaemia. Thiazide diuretics increase both serum triglycerides and cholesterol.

When heart failure is the indication for diuretic therapy it would be absurd to curtail such treatment, because of its lipid effect. Very often the indication for beta-blockers in patients referred to the lipid clinic will be angina. In this circumstance, too, I am reluctant to consider their withdrawal and generally do so only when there is gross hypertriglyceridaemia and then after admission to hospital and after institution of another anti-anginal agent. Also, I would not generally be prepared to withdraw beta-blockers in patients known to have had myocardial infarction, even if they do not have angina, because of the evidence that they may be beneficial in reducing the likelihood of future fatal infarction. Although evidence for rebound acute coronary insuffficiency on cessation of beta-blocker therapy is anecdotal, the author is nevertheless cautious when severe hypertriglyceridaemia does warrant withdrawal of beta-blockade. It is the case, however, that many patients referred to a lipid clinic on beta-blockers or thiazides, because of hypertension, prove not to have hypertension when the medication is withdrawn. The blood pressure should of course be regularly monitored afterwards, because it can take some time to rise again. However, in a great proportion of patients the diagnosis of hypertension may have amounted to no more than one or two casual recordings of diastolic tension of around 100 mmHg. When the blood pressure recording is done properly at rest and off treatment, it is found to be perfectly normal.

Disturbingly, too, many patients with so-called mild hypertension are obese and little consideration has been given to treating them with a reducing diet until their hyperlipidaemia is also discovered. The evidence that treating diastolic blood pressure of less than 110 mmHg has any major influence on subsequent mortality or morbidity is not great. Indeed, evidence for benefit from treatment of polygenic hypercholesterolaemia, certainly in terms of coronary morbidity, is better. Although it is universally agreed that it would be quite wrong to treat every patient with a cholesterol exceeding 260 mg/dl (6.5 mmol/l) with a lipid-lowering drug without considering other factors such as cigarette smoking, blood pressure, obesity, family history and age, it is nevertheless the case that for many years it has been common practice to respond to a mildly abnormal resting diastolic blood pressure by writing a prescription. At long last the concept that cardiovascular risk should determine the need for antihypertensive medication rather than the numerical value of the blood pressure has dawned in the world of hypertension[436]. It should never be forgotten that most hypertensive people will die not from stroke, but from ischaemic heart disease, and that antihypertensive drugs have only limited power to influence this.

Neither hypertension, nor for that matter diabetes, should ever again be treated as a single risk factor without attention to other cardiovascular risk factors. The identification of a patient with hypertension or with diabetes carries with it the necessity to check for other risk factors including the measurement of serum lipids.

The apparently unfavourable effect of thiazides and beta-blockers on serum lipids does not necessarily mean that in our current state of knowledge they should not be used in the management of hypertension. Although there are other antihypertensive drugs, which either do not affect lipoprotein concentrations or perhaps even influence them favourably, there is no evidence from clinical trials that they are effective in decreasing morbidity or mortality. It thus seems reasonable, when the clinical decision to treat mild hypertension is taken, that thiazides, which after all do show some evidence of benefit, should be used[437] and that beta-blockers, for which there is also evidence of benefit in more severe hypertension, should be used when these fail. It is important to treat other risk factors when deciding to institute antihypertensive drugs, to ensure that hypertension actually is present and to consider whether weight reduction should not be the first approach. Alcohol restriction and modification of sodium intake might also be applicable to some patients. If hyperlipidaemia is present, this should be corrected by diet. If it does not respond to diet, then changing the thiazide or thiazide/beta-blocker combination for another antihypertensive agent should be considered, along with the decision as to whether to introduce lipid-lowering medication. It may be premature without clinical trial evidence of benefit to administer antihypertensive agents other than thiazides or beta-blockers as first-line agents, even in patients with hyperlipidaemia[211,438], unless it is severe, although this has been advocated by some authorities[439].

## Beta-adrenoreceptor blocking agents

There is no doubt that beta-blocking drugs are of benefit to many patients. However, as with any drug, when they are prescribed without any clearly established indication, patients will be exposed to their adverse effects without the advantage of their benefits.

There is an enormous literature on the subject of beta-blockers and their effects on serum lipids and lipoproteins. Extensive reviews of the subject have been made[440–445]. There is no convincing evidence that any of the beta-blockers affect LDL levels adversely. Both cardioselective ($\beta_1$ selective) and non-cardioselective beta-blockers do, however, consistently increase VLDL levels. There is also a reduction in serum HDL levels with beta-blocking drugs, an effect most frequently reported with those lacking cardioselectivity (blocking both $\beta_1$ and $\beta_2$ receptors).

Insufficient attention has been paid to several important aspects of the lipid-modifying action of beta-blockers. Some of the inconsistencies in different studies result from heterogeneity among patients with regard to their pretreatment serum triglyceride levels. In Scandinavia, for example, where several studies have been conducted, hypertriglyceridaemia is more common than in the UK or the USA. We have shown that patients with pre-existing hypertriglyceridaemia, when prescribed beta-blockers, may show substantial increases in their serum triglycerides[446], sufficient sometimes to provoke acute pancreatitis[447]. Under these circumstances the rise in triglycerides appears to be due to a beta-blocker-mediated decrease in triglyceride catabolism[447–449]. The rise in serum triglycerides in people with normal initial values is smaller and has not so far been satisfactorily explained. Although the effect on fasting triglycerides may be small, postprandial triglyceride responses may be more obvious[450]. This and the decrease in HDL principally due to $HDL_2$[446,449] could be explained by a decreased rate of lipolysis of triglyceride-rich lipoproteins. Direct evidence for such a mechanism is currently lacking.

Beta-blocking drugs with intrinsic sympathomimetic activity (ISA) have little or no effect on HDL and generally have not been reported to increase triglycerides[441,442]. Often this may, however, have little practical importance since pindolol, which has the most ISA, has found little application as an antihypertensive agent and is unsuitable for the management of angina. Some reports suggest that acebutolol and perhaps oxprenolol, which have about half the ISA of pindolol, have less effect on VLDL and HDL than beta-blockers without ISA[442]. Celiprolol is interesting in that it is a cardioselective $\beta_1$-specific antagonist with $\beta_2$ agonist and vasodilatory properties. It is reported to have an antihypertensive effect without adverse effects on triglycerides and HDL[451,452]. Labetolol, which has both beta- and alpha-blocking activity, may also be without effect[442].

## Thiazide diuretics

Again there have been a large number of studies of thiazide diuretics and serum lipoproteins (see reference [453]). In many respects these investigations are less satisfactory than those with beta-blockers. In general, the thiazides increase VLDL and LDL, but have no effect on HDL. The effect is dose-dependent and it should be remembered that bendrofluazide probably has its maximum antihypertensive effect at 2.5 mg daily, at which dose its effect on lipoproteins is minimal. There is no convincing evidence that loop diuretics, such as frusemide, differ from thiazides in their effects on lipoproteins. The action does not appear to be due to haemoconcentration. Thiazides, of course, produce glucose intolerance, but evidence that this is linked with their effect on plasma lipids is lacking at present. It might be anticipated that their effect on lipids would be most marked when they are administered in diabetes or when they are used in conjunction with beta-blockers.

## Other antihypertensive agents

It seems reasonably established that prazosin[437–439], an alpha blocker, and nifedipine[454–456], a calcium antagonist, are either without effect on lipoproteins or decrease serum triglycerides and total cholesterol and increase HDL. There are fewer studies with other drugs, but the same is probably true of other drugs of their type and also direct-acting vasodilators, such as hydralazine, and angiotensin-converting enzyme inhibitors, such as captopril and enalopril.

## Sex steroids

### Oral contraceptives

Considerable attention has been devoted to the possible harmful effects of oral contraceptive agents. These agents have until recently generally contained a combination of an oestrogen and a progestin. Early reports identified hazards associated with high doses of oestrogen and, more recently, with the decrease in the oestrogen component, the progestin element has come under scrutiny.

In studies of cardiovascular risk in women taking the pill, a significant excess of thromboembolic events was recorded[457–459] attributable to the oestrogen[460,461]. This parallels the effects of oestrogen administration to men[462,463]. In recent years there has been a considerable decrease in the oestrogenic component of oral contraceptive agents. This has undoubtedly reduced the morbidity associated with their use, but precisely by how much is uncertain. There remains, in addition, their effect on blood pressure, glucose tolerance and serum lipoproteins.

Both oestrogens and progestins because of their mineralocorticoid and gluco-corticoid properties tend to raise blood pressure and to impair glucose tolerance. Their effects on serum lipoproteins are different[464,465]. Oestrogens raise VLDL and also increase HDL, usually $HDL_2$. In postmenopausal women they also lower LDL. Even in young women their effect on HDL, considered in isolation, could be interpreted favourably. On the other hand, progestins decrease HDL, especially $HDL_2$, and in addition raise LDL. It is probably wrong to consider progestins as a single class in this context, since there is great diversity among those in current use. Three major classes are: (a) oestranes represented by norethisterone and others, which to be active, must undergo conversion to it (lynoestranol, norethy-nodrel, ethynodiol diacetate); (b) gonanes such as norgestrel and desogestrel; and (c) pregnanes such as cyproterone acetate. As a result of detailed investigation, Wynn[464] has recently recommended the avoidance of progestins stronger than is necessary for contraception or menstrual cycle control. The most favourable combination with regard to glucose tolerance and lipoproteins appear to be progestogen-only formulations or oestrogen in a dose of 30–35 µg combined with desogestrel or low dose (500 µg) norethisterone[466]. The progestogen-only formulations are less certain as a means of contraception and an earlier clinical trial was less favourable to them[467].

## Oestrogen replacement therapy

There have been many studies to investigate the cardiovascular risk associated with oestrogen replacement therapy after the natural menopause. Premature menopause, whether spontaneous or surgical, is known to increase cardiovascular morbidity[468–472]. A major contribution to this increased morbidity may be the rise in serum cholesterol, which occurs immediately following ovarian involution (Chapter 3, page 88). Oestrogens given postmenopausally lower the serum LDL cholesterol[473]. Against this, of course, may be unfavourable effects on blood pressure, glucose tolerance and blood clotting, although there is, in fact, no evidence that the menopause itself has any favourable effect on any of these. Also, evidence for any change in IHD risk due to spontaneous menopause occurring at the normal age is largely lacking, despite the commonly held misconception[474]. Hormone replacement therapy is discussed in Chapter 10, page 278.

## Androgens

The effect of androgens is to reduce serum HDL cholesterol and to raise LDL[475]. The concentration of VLDL tends to fall.

# Corticosteroids

The effect of Cushing's syndrome or exogenous glucocorticoid administration is predominantly to increase serum cholesterol due to increased LDL cholesterol and often VLDL cholesterol. There is often an increase in triglycerides, but this is less marked, unless diabetes is induced[30]. The effect of prednisolone is also to increase serum HDL levels[476].

## Hepatic microsomal enzyme-inducing agents

These include drugs such as phenytoin, phenobarbitone, rifampicin and griseoful-vin and also toxic substances such as chlorinated pesticides, like lindane and DDT. The effect of these is to increase serum HDL concentrations[318,477,478]. There may also be increases in LDL and VLDL cholesterol[479–482], but these have usually been less marked so that the ratio of HDL to total serum cholesterol rises. Exactly how increased cytochrome P450[483] influences HDL metabolism remains a mystery. So also does the answer to whether the lipoprotein changes confer any benefit, although the suggestion has been made that myocardial infarction is uncommon in epilepsy[484,485].

## Retinoic acid derivatives

Increases in the serum triglycerides occur following the administration of vitamin A and its derivatives[486,487]. Etretinate, a synthetic aromatic derivative of retinoic acid, has an important place in the management of psoriasis and ichthyosis. Dietary treatment is recommended for the increase in serum triglyc-erides it provokes. The triglyceride rise should be monitored, because severe lipaemia has been reported with another similar agent, 13-cis-retinoic acid[488], presumably in a patient with some degree of pre-existing hypertriglyceridaemia.

## Amiodarone

Amiodarone treatment causes an increase in the serum cholesterol concentration due to an increase in LDL, which appears to be independent of any changes in thyroid function associated with its use[489,490].

## Cyclosporin

Cyclosporin has an increasing place as immunosuppressive therapy following renal and cardiac transplantation, in the management of skin disorders and autoimmune conditions. Its use is associated with increased serum cholesterol levels due to a rise in LDL[491–493].

# Immunoglobulin excess

Malignancy is generally associated with hypolipidaemia. In myeloma, however, xanthomatosis and sometimes hyperlipidaemia may occur, although hypolipi-daemia is nevertheless more common[30].

Immunoglobulins may influence lipoprotein metabolism in a variety of ways. Disturbances of lipoprotein metabolism may occasionally accompany other immunoglobulinopathies, such as macroglobulinaemia and rarely lymphoma and systemic lupus erythematosis. In most instances complexes between lipoproteins and immunoglobulins lead to the lipoprotein disorder. In one instance this occurred in the intestine even before chylomicron secretion, leading to fat malabsorption[494]. More commonly, however, the disorder is due to immune complexes involving the lipoproteins within the circulation. Planar xanthomata on the neck and thorax are the clinical feature which most frequently indicates that this is occurring[495] (see Plate 10d). Often serum lipid levels are normal or only marginally altered when these occur. Diffuse planar xanthomata in adults should always raise the suspicion of a monoclonal gammopathy[496].

When hyperlipidaemia does occur in myeloma it can mimic type III hyperlipoproteinaemia. There may thus be tuberoeruptive xanthomata and even striate palmar xanthomata. The VLDL is cholesterol-enriched and when isolated by ultracentrifugation the biochemical criteria for the diagnosis of type III hyperlipoproteinaemia may be satisfied. The clinical syndrome seems to result from interference with receptor-mediated clearance of chylomicron remnants, IDL and LDL, by the immunoglobulin attached to those lipoproteins[497].

Clearly a variety of other clinical syndromes will develop depending on the particular part of lipoprotein metabolism most affected, but these are uncommon. Impairment of lipoprotein lipase activity can, for example, occur leading to massive hypertriglyceridaemia[498].

Clearly to a large extent the prognosis in this type of hyperlipidaemia depends on that of the underlying condition. Response to lipid-lowering therapy is often said to be poor. However, it is also the case that vascular disease may not progress rapidly even in the presence of spectacular xanthomatosis[499].

A rare condition associated with paraproteinaemia exists called necrobiotic xanthogranuloma, in which gross periorbital xanthclasmata and subcutaneous hard facial xanthogranulomata so severe as to cause complete closure of the eyes and orbital inflammation, uveitis and corneal ulceration[500]. The lesions consist of foci of collagen necrosis with a heavy infiltration of foamy macrophages resembling histologically most closely lesions such as necrobiosis lipoidica diabeticorum and granuloma annulare. Typically lipoprotein levels are unaffected. Subcutaneous xanthogranulomata may develop elsewhere on the body. The facial ones frequently have telangiectasis overlying and adjacent to them. Its pathogenesis is currently unclear and it may well not respond to measures to lower the paraproteinaemia which is usually an IgG monoclonal gammopathy, either kappa or lamba.

# Hyperuricaemia and gout

Hyperuricaemia commonly accompanies hypertriglyceridaemia[501–506]. It is reasonable to conclude from population surveys that around half of men with hyperuricaemia will also have hypertriglyceridaemia and at least as high a proportion with hypertriglyceridaemia will have hyperuricaemia. Gout is thus frequently met in the lipid clinic, particularly when hyperuricaemia has been further precipitated by thiazide diuretic administration.

The reason for the association is not entirely clear. Obviously hyperuricaemia and hypertriglyceridaemia have aetiological factors in common, such as obesity[503,506] and alcohol consumption[501]. The association, however, appears to be more frequent than might be anticipated from this. Although dealt with in the section of this book on secondary hyperlipoproteinaemias, it is important to remember that there is no evidence that the hyperlipidaemia is dependent on the hyperuricaemia. Thus decreasing the serum urate with allopurinol does not reduce the serum triglyceride level[507,508]. Weight reduction and alcohol restriction may decrease both serum urate and triglycerides, but most lipid-lowering drug therapy does not affect the urate level[509]. Exceptions are nicotinic acid, which raises the serum urate, and fenofibrate, which has a sustained hypouricaemic action[509]. This effect of fenofibrate, which is not possessed by the other fibric acid derivatives, is largely, if not entirely, related to its effect on the kidney where it acts as a uricosuric agent and is not due to its hypolipidaemic effect[509].

Since carbohydrate may induce hypertriglyceridaemia and because some carbohydrates such as fructose also raise serum urate levels, it is possible that this is the common link. Although attractive, this hypothesis requires further evidence. In our experiments, the increment in urate with a single dose of orally administered fructose, although set against a higher basal level in hypertriglyceridaemia, was not different from controls[509]. Furthermore, controversy persists about how commonly dietary carbohydrate contributes to sustained hypertriglyceridaemia (Chapter 9, page 234).

# Intestinal malabsorption

Low concentrations of serum cholesterol, LDL cholesterol and apo B characterize patients with intestinal malabsorption and steatorrhoea. This is likely to be due to malabsorption of cholesterol and bile salts. The serum triglyceride levels are, however, frequently normal and in some patients may be increased[510].

## References

1. Keen, H. Glucose intolerance, diabetes mellitus and atherosclerosis; prospects for prevention. *Postgrad. Med. J.*, **52**, 445–451 (1976)
2. Jarrett, J. Diabetes and the heart: coronary heart disease. *Clin. Endocrinol. Metabol.*, **6**, 389–402 (1978)
3. Kawate, R., Miyanishi, M., Yamikido, M. and Nishimoto, Y. Preliminary studies of the prevalence and mortality of diabetes mellitus in Japanese in Japan and on the island of Hawaii. *Adv. Metabol. Dis.*, **9**, 201–224 (1978)
4. Jarrett R.J., Keen, H. and Chakrabarti, R. Diabetes, hyperglycaemia and arterial disease. In *Complications of Diabetes*, 2nd edn (eds H. Keen and R.J. Jarrett), Edward Arnold, London, pp. 179–204 (1982)
5. WHO Expert Committee on Diabetes Mellitus. Second Report. *WHO Techn. Rep. Ser.*, **656** (1980)
6. Zimmet, P. and King, H. Classification and diagnosis of diabetes mellitus. In *The Diabetes Annual*, vol. 3 (eds K.G.M.M. Alberti and L.P. Krall), Elsevier, Amsterdam, pp. 1–14 (1987)
7. Stout, R.W. Diabetes mellitus and atherosclerosis. In *Hormones and Atherosclerosis*, MTP Press, Lancaster, pp. 19–34 (1982)
8. Fuller, J.H., Shipley, M.J., Rose, G., Jarrett, R.J. and Keen, H. Mortality from coronary heart disease and stroke in relation to degree of glycaemia. The Whitehall Study. *Br. Med. J.*, **287**, 867–870 (1983)
9. Butler, W.J., Ostrander, L.D., Carman, W.J. and Lamphiear, D.E. Mortality from coronary heart disease in the Tecumseh study: long-term effect of diabetes mellitus, glucose tolerance and other risk factors. *Am. J. Epidemiol.*, **121**, 541–547 (1985)
10. Schettler, F.G. and Wollenweber, J. Clinical aspects. In *Atherosclerosis* (eds F.G. Schettler and G.S. Boyd), Elsevier, Amsterdam, pp. 633–672 (1969)

11. West, K.M., Ahuja, M.M., Bennett, P.H., Czyzyk, A., Acosta, O.M. *et al*. The role of circulating glucose and triglyceride concentrations and their interactions with other 'risk factors' as determinants of arterial disease in nine diabetic population samples from the WHO Multinational Study. *Diabetes Care*, **6**, 361–369 (1983)

12. Janka, H.U. Five-year incidence of major macrovascular complications in diabetes mellitus. In *Macrovascular Disease in Diabeta Mellitus: Pathogenesis and Prevention* (eds H.U. Janka, H. Mehnert and E. Standl), Georg Thieme, Stuttgart, pp. 15–19 (1985)

13. Stamler, J., Vaccaro, O., Neaton, J.D. and Wentworth, D. Diabetes, other risk factors, and 12-year cardiovascular mortality for men screened in the Multiple Risk Factor Intervention Trial. *Diabetes Care*, **16**, 434–444 (1993)

14. Reckless, J.P.D., Bettcridge, D.J., Wu, P., Payne, B. and Galton, D.J. High-density and low-density lipoproteins and prevalence of vascular disease in diabetes mellitus. *Br. Med. J.*, **i**, 883–886 (1978)

15. Kannel, W.B. and McGee, D.L. Diabetes and cardiovascular risk factors: the Framingham Study. *Circulation*, **59**, 8–13 (1979)

16. Garcia, M.J., McNamara, P.M., Gordon, T. and Kannel, W.B. Morbidity and mortality in diabetics in the Framingham population. Sixteen year follow-up study. *Diabetes*, **3**, 105–111 (1974)

17. Himsworth, H.P. and Marshall, E.M. The diet of diabetics prior to the onset of the disease. *Clin. Sci.*, **2**, 95–115 (1935)

18. Sweeney, J.S. Dietary factors that influence the detrose tolerance test; preliminary study. *Arch. Intern. Med.*, **40**, 818–830 (1927)

19. Himsworth, H.P. The dietetic factor determining the glucose tolerance and sensitivity to insulin of healthy man. *Clin. Sci.*, **2**, 67–94 (1935)

20. Mann, J.I. Diabetes mellitus: some aspects of aetiology and management. In *Refined Carbohydrate Foods, Dietary Fibre and Disease*, 2nd edn (eds H.C. Trowell, D. Burkitt and K. Heaton), Academic Press, London, pp. 263–295 (1985)

21. Mann, J.I. Diet and diabetes: some agreement, but controversies continue. In *The Diabetes Annual*, vol. 3 (eds K.G.M.M. Alberti and L.P. Krall), Elsevier, Amsterdam, pp. 55–71 (1987)

22. Brunzell, J.D., Lerner, R.L., Hazzard, W.R., Porte, D. Jr and Bierman, E.L. Improved glucose tolerance with high carbohydrate feeding in mild diabetes. *N. Engl. J. Med.*, **284**, 521–524 (1971)

23. Simpson, R.W., Mann, J.I., Eaton, J., Moore, R.A., Carter, R. and Hockaday, T.D. Improved glucose control in maturity-onset diabetes treated with high carbohydrate-modified fat diet. *Br. Med. J.*, **i**, 1753–1756 (1979)

24. Jellish, W.S., Emanuele, M.A. and Abraira, C. Graded sucrose carbohydrate in overtly hypertriglyceridaemic diabetic patients. *Am. J. Med.*, **77**, 1015–1022 (1984)

25. Coulston, A.M., Liu, G.C. and Reaven, G.M. Plasma glucose, insulin and lipid responses to high-carbohydrate low-fat diets in normal humans. *Metabolism*, **32**, 52–56 (1983)

26. Coulston, A.M. and Shishocki, A.L.M. Metabolic effects of high carbohydrate, moderate sucrose diets in patients with non-insulin dependent diabetes mellitus (NIDDM). *Diabetes*, **34**, 34A (1985)

27. Chantelau, E.A., Gosseringger, G., Sonnenberg, G.E. and Berger, M. Moderate intake of sucrose does not impair metabolic control in pump treated diabetic outpatients. *Diabetologia*, **28**, 204–207 (1985)

28. Peterson, D.B., Lambert, J., Gerring, S., Darling, P., Carter, R.D. *et al*. Sucrose in the diet of diabetic patients – just another carbohydrate? *Diabetologia*, **29**, 216–220 (1986)

29. Nikkila, E.A. Triglyceride metabolism in diabetes mellitus. *Progr. Biochem. Pharmacol.*, **8**, 271–299 (1973)

30. Havel, R.J., Goldstein, J.L. and Brown, M.S. Lipoproteins and lipid transport. In *Metabolic Control and Disease*, 8th edn (eds P.K. Bondy and L.E. Rosenberg), W.B. Saunders, Philadelphia, pp. 393–494 (1980)

31. Winocour, P.H., Durrington, P.N., Ishola, M., Hillier, V.F. and Anderson, D.C. The prevalence of hyperlipidaemia and related clinical features in insulin-dependent diabetes mellitus. *Q. J. Med.*, **70**, 265–276 (1989)

32. Durrington, P.N. Secondary hyperlipidaemia. *Br. Med. Bull.*, **46**, 1005–1024 (1990)

33. Perley, M. and Kipnis, D.M. Plasma insulin responses to glucose and tolbutamide of normal weight and obese diabetic and nondiabetic subjects. *Diabetes*, **15**, 867–874 (1966)

34. Durrington, P.N. Is insulin atherogenic? *Diabetic Med.*, **9**, 597–600 (1992)
35. Davies, M.J., Metcalfe, J., Gray, I.P., Day, J.L. and Hales, C.N. Insulin deficiency rather than hyperinsulinaemia in newly diagnosed type 2 diabetes mellitus. *Diabetic Med.*, **10**, 305–312 (1993)
36. Temple, R.C., Carrington, C.A., Luzio, S.D., Owens, D.R., Schneider, A.E. *et al.* Insulin deficiency in non-insulin-dependent diabetes. *Lancet*, **i**, 293–295 (1989)
37. Winocour, P.H., Mallick, T.H., Ishola, M., Baker, R.D., Bhatnagar, D. *et al.* A randomised cross-over study of the effects of proinsulin on lipid metabolism in type II diabetes. *Diabetic Med.*, **8**, 22–27 (1991)
38. Drexel, H., Hopferwieser, Th., Braunsteiner, H. and Patsch, J.R. Effects of biosynthetic human pro-insulin on plasma lipids in type 2 diabetes mellitus. *Klin. Wochenschr.*, **66**, 1171–1174 (1988)
39. Randle, P.J., Garland, P.B., Hales, C.N. and Newsholme, E.A. The glucose fatty-acid cycle. Its role in insulin sensitivity and the metabolic disturbances of diabetes mellitus. *Lancet*, **i**, 785–789 (1963)
40. Cahill, G.F. Starvation in man. *N. Engl. J. Med.*, **282**, 668–675 (1970)
41. Johnston, D.G. and Alberti, K.G. Hormone control of ketone body metabolism in the normal and diabetic state. *Clin. Endocrinol. Metabol.*, **11**, 329–361 (1982)
42. Marshall, S.M. and Alberti, K.G.M.M. Diabetic ketoacidosis. In *The Diabetes Annual*, vol. 3 (eds K.G.M.M. Alberti and L.P. Krall), Elsevier, Amsterdam, pp. 498–526 (1987)
43. Allen, F.M., Stillman, E. and Fitz, R. *Total Dietary Regulation in the Treatment of Diabetes.* Monographs of the Rockefeller Institute for Medical Research, II, New York (1919)
44. Bliss, M. A long prelude. In *The Discovery of Insulin*, Paul Harris, Edinburgh, pp. 20–44 (1982)
45. Winocour, P.H., Mallick, T., Bhatnagar, D., Ishola, M., Arrol, S. *et al.* A comparison of the lipaemic response to a mixed meal and the intravenous fat tolerance test in normolipidaemic and hyperlipidaemic non-insulin-dependent diabetes mellitus. *Diabetes Nutr. Metabol.*, **4**, 213–219 (1991)
46. Nikkila, E.A. and Kekki, M. Plasma triglyceride transport kinetics in diabetes mellitus. *Metabolism*, **22**, 1–22 (1973)
47. Taskinen, M-R. and Nikkila, E.A. Lipoprotein lipase activity of adipose tissue and skeletal muscle in insulin-deficient human diabetes. Relation to high-density and very-low-density lipoproteins and response to treatment. *Diabetologia*, **17**, 351–356 (1979)
48. Nikkila, E.A. and Hormila, P. Serum lipids and lipoproteins in insulin-treated diabetics. Demonstration of increased high density lipoprotein concentrations. *Diabetes*, **27**, 1078–1085 (1978)
49. Field, J.B. Extraction of insulin by liver. *Ann. Rev. Med.*, **24**, 309–314 (1973)
50. Myers, S.R., McGuiness, O.P., Neal, D.W. and Cherrington, A.D. Intraportal glucose delivery alters the relationship between net hepatic glucose uptake and the insulin concentration. J. Clin. Invest., **87**, 930–939 (1991)
51. Munkgaard Rasmussen, S., Heding, L.G., Parbst, E. and Volund, A. Serum IRI in insulin-treated diabetics during a 24 hour period. *Diabetologia*, **11**, 151–158 (1975)
52. Asplin, C.M., Hartog, M., Goldie, D.J., Alberti, K.G.M.M., Binder, C. and Faber, O.K. Diurnal profiles of serum insulin, C-peptide and blood intermediary metabolites in insulin treated diabetics, their relationship to the control of diabetes and the role of endogenous insulin secretion. *Q. J. Med.*, **48**, 343–360 (1979)
53. Winocour, P.H., Durrington, P.N., Kalsi, P., Bhatnagar, D., Ishola, M. *et al.* A one year prospective study of the effects of endogenous insulin reserve (assessed by C-peptide) during a programme of intensified management on metabolic control in insulin dependent (type 1) diabetes mellitus. *Diabetes Nutr. Metabol.*, **3**, 215–224 (1990)
54. Ruotolo, G., Micossi, P., Galimberti, G., Librenti, M.C., Petrella, G. *et al.* Effects of intraperitoneal versus subcutaneous insulin administration on lipoprotein metabolism in Type 1 diabetes. *Metabolism*, **29**, 598–604 (1990)
55. Farquhar, J.W., Frank, A., Gross, R.C. and Reaven, G.M. Glucose, insulin and triglyceride responses to high and low carbohydrate diets in man. J. Clin. Invest., **45**, 1648–1656 (1966)
56. Reaven, G.M., Lerner, R.L., Stern, M.P. and Farquhar, J.W. Role of insulin in endogenous hypertriglyceridaemia. *J. Clin. Invest.*, **46**, 1756–1767 (1967)
57. Olefsky, J.M., Farquhar, J.W. and Reaven, G.M. Reappraisal of the role of insulin in hypertriglyceridaemia. *Ann. J. Med.*, **57**, 551–560 (1974)

58. Reaven, G.M. and Greenfield, M.S. Diabetic hypertriglyceridemia. Evidence for three clinical syndromes. *Diabetes*, **30**, 66–75 (1981)
59. Barter, P.J., Carroll, K.F. and Nestel, P.J. Diurnal fluctuations in triglyceride, free fatty acids and insulin during sucrose consumption and insulin infusions in man. *J. Clin. Invest.*, **50**, 583–591 (1971)
60. Hayford, J.T., Danney, M.M. and Thompson, R.G. Triglyceride integrated concentration: relationship to insulin-integrated concentration. *Metabolism*, **28**, 1078–1085 (1979)
61. Glueck, C.J., Levy, R.J. and Fredrickson, D.S. Immunoreactive insulin, glucose tolerance and carbohydrate inducibility in types II, III, IV and V hyperlipoproteinaemia. *Diabetes*, **18**, 739–747 (1969)
62. Nikkila, E.A. Regulation of hepatic production of plasma triglycerides by glucose and insulin. In *Regulation of Hepatic Metabolism* (eds F. Lundquist. and N. Tygstrup), Munksgaard, Copenhagen, pp. 360–378 (1974)
63. Haahti, E. Effect of insulin in a case of essential hyperlipemia. *Scand. J. Clin. Lab Invest.*, **11**, 305–306 (1959)
63a. Schierf, G. and Kinsell, L.W. Effects of insulin in hypertriglyceridaemia. *Proc. Soc. Exp. Biol. Med.*, **120**, 272–274 (1965)
64. Jones, D.P. and Arky, R.H. Effects of insulin on triglyceride and free fatty acid metabolism in man. *Metabolism*, **14**, 1287–1293 (1965)
65. Dannenburg, W. N. and Burt, R. L. The effect of insulin and glucose on plasma lipids during pregnancy and puerperium. *Am. J. Obstet. Gynecol.*, **92**, 195–201 (1965)
66. Pietri, A.O., Dunn, F.L., Grundy, S.M. and Raskin, P. The effect of continuous subcutaneous insulin infusion on very-low-density lipoprotein triglyceride metabolism in type I diabetes mellitus. *Diabetes*, **32**, 75–81 (1983)
67. Sadur, C.N. and Eckel, R.H. Insulin stimulations of adipose tissue lipoprotein lipase. Use of euglycaemic damp technique. *J. Clin. Invest.*, **69**, 1119–1125 (1982)
68. Lewis, B., Mancini, M., Mattock, M., Chait, A. and Russell Fraser, T. Plasma triglyceride and fatty acid metabolism in diabetes mellitus. *Eur. J. Clin. Invest.*, **2**, 445–453 (1972)
69. Jarrett, R.J. In defence of insulin: a critique of syndrome X. *Lancet*, **340**, 469–471 (1992)
70. Kumar, S., Durrington, P.N., Laing, I. and Bhatnagar, D. Suppression of non-esterified acids to treat type A insulin resistance syndrome. *Lancet*, **343**, 1073–1074 (1994)
71. Durrington, P.N., Newton, R.S., Weinstein, D.B. and Steinberg, D. Effects of insulin and glucose on very-low-density lipoprotein triglyceride secretion by cultured rat hepatocytes. *J. Clin. Invest.*, **70**, 63–73 (1982)
72. Patsch W., Franz, S. and Schonfeld, G. Role of insulin in lipoprotein secretion by cultured rat hepatocytes. *J. Clin. Invest.*, **71**, 1161–1174 (1983)
73. Mangiapane, E.H. and Brindney, D.N. Effects of dexamethasone and insulin on the synthesis of triacylglycerols and phosphatidyl choline and the secretion of very-low-density lipoproteins and lysophosphatidyl choline by monolayer cultures of rat hepatocytes. *Biochem. J.*, **233**, 151–160 (1986)
74. Patsch, W., Gotto, A.M. and Patsch, J. Effects of insulin on lipoprotein secretion in rat hepatocyte cultures. The role of the insulin receptor. *J. Biol. Chem.*, **261**, 9603–9606 (1986)
75. Dashti, N. and Wolfbauer, G. Secretion of lipids, apolipoproteins and lipoproteins by human hepatoma cell line, Hep G2: effects of oleic acid and insulin. *J. Lipid Res.*, **28**, 423–436 (1987)
76. Jackson, T.K., Salhanick, A.I., Elovson, J., Deschman, M.L. and Amatruda, J.M. Insulin regulates apolipoprotein B turnover and phospharylation in rat hepatocytes. *J. Clin. Invest.*, **86**, 1746–1751 (1990)
77. Topping, D.L. and Mayes, P.A. The immediate effects of insulin and fructose on the metabolism of the perfused liver. *Biochem. J.*, **126**, 295–311 (1972)
78. Topping, D.L. and Mayes, P.A. Insulin and non-esterified fatty acids. Active regulators of lipogenesis in perfused rat liver. *Biochem. J.*, **204**, 433–439 (1982)
79. Laker, M.E. and Mayes, P.A. Investigation into the direct effect of insulin on hepatic ketogenesis, lipoprotein secretion and pyruvate dehydrogenase activity. *Biochem. Biophys. Acta*, **795**, 427–430 (1984)
80. Heimberg, M., Wilcox, H.G., Dunn, G.D., Woodside, W.F., Breen, K.J. and Soler-Argilaga, C. Studies on the regulation of secretion of the very low density lipoprotein and on ketogenesis by the liver. In *Regulation of Hepatic Metabolism* (eds F. Lundquist and N. Tygstrup), Munksgaard, Copenhagen, pp. 119–143 (1974)

81. Boyd, M.E., Albright, E.R., Foster, D.W. and McGarry, J.D. In vitro reversal of the fasting state of liver metabolism in the rat. Re-evaluation of the roles of insulin and glucose. *J. Clin. Invest.*, **68**, 142–152 (1981)

82. Arrol, S., Mackness, M.I. and Durrington, P.N. Effects of insulin and glucagon on the secretion of apolipoprotein B-containing lipoproteins and triacylglycerol synthesis by human hepatoma (Hep G2) cells. *Diabetes, Nutr., Metabol.*, **7**, 263–271 (1994)

83. Sparks, C.E. and Gibbons, C.F. The role of pancreatic hormones in the regulation of lipid storage, oxidation and secretion in primary cultures of rat hepatocytes. Short- and long-term effects. *Biochem J.*, **281**, 381–386 (1992)

84. Gibbons, G.F. Hyperlipidaemia of diabetes. *Clin. Sci.*, **71**, 477–486 (1986)

85. Kaminski, D.L., Adams, A. and Jellinek, M. The effect of hyperalimentation on hepatic lipid content and lipogenic enzyme activity in rats and man. *Surgery*, **88**, 93–100 (1980)

86. Stout, R.W. Insulin and atheroma – an update. *Lancet*, **i**, 1077–1079 (1987)

87. Pyorala, K. Relationship of glucose tolerance and plasma insulin to the incidence of coronary heart disease: results from two population studies in Finland. *Diabetes Care*, **2**, 131–141 (1979)

88. Ducimetiere, P., Eschwege, E., Papoz, L., Richard, J.L., Claude, J.R. and Roselin, G. Relationship of plasma insulin levels to the incidence of myocardial infarctions and coronary heart disease mortality in a middle-aged population. *Diabetologia*, **19**, 205–210 (1980)

89. Welborn, T.A. and Wearne, K. Coronary heart disease incidence and cardiovascular mortality in Busselton with reference to glucose and insulin concentrations. *Diabetes Care*, **2**, 154–160 (1979)

90. Crespin, S.R., Greenough, W.B. and Steinberg, D. Stimulation of insulin by infusion of free fatty acids. *J. Clin. Invest.*, **48**, 1934–1943 (1969)

91. Johnson, A.B., Argyraki, M., Thow, J.C., Cooper, B.G., Fulcher, G. and Taylor, R. Effect of increased free fatty acid supply on glucose metabolism and skeletal muscle glycogen synthase activity in normal man. *Clin. Sci.*, **82**, 219–226 (1992)

92. Groop, L.C., Saloranta, C., Shank, M., Bonadonna, R.C., Ferranini, D. and DeFronza, R.A. The role of free fatty acid metabolism in the pathogenesis of insulin resistance in obesity and non-insulin-dependent diabetes mellitus. *J. Clin. Endocrinol. Metabol.*, **72**, 96–107 (1991)

93. Winocour, P.H., Durrington, P.N., Ishola, M. and Anderson, D.C. Lipoprotein abnormalities in insulin-dependent diabetes mellitus. *Lancet*, **i**, 1176–1178 (1986)

94. Schernthaner, G., Kostner, G.M., Dieplinger, H., Prager, R. and Muhlhauser, I. Apolipoproteins (A-I, A-II, B), Lp(a) lipoprotein and lecithin: cholesterol acyltransferase activity in diabetes mellitus. *Atherosclerosis*, **49**, 2M–293 (1983)

95. Gonen, B., White, N., Schonfeld, G., Skor, D., Miller, P. and Santiago, J. Plasma levels of apoprotein B in patients with diabetes mellitus. The effect of glycaemic control. *Metabolism*, **34**, 675–679 (1985)

96. Laakso, M., Voutilainen, E., Sarland, H., Aro, A., Pyorala, K. and Pentilla, I. Serum lipids and lipoproteins in middle-aged non-insulin dependent diabetics. *Atherosclerosis*, **56**, 271–281 (1985)

97. Barakat, H.A., Carpenter, J.W., McLendon, V.D., Khazanie, P., Leggett, N. *et al.* Influence of obesity, impaired glucose tolerance, and NIDDM on LDL structure and composition. Possible link with hyperinsulinaemia and atherosclerosis. *Diabetes*, **39**, 1527–1533 (1990)

98. James, R.W. and Pometta, D. Differences in lipoprotein subfraction composition and distribution between type 1 diabetic men and control subjects. *Diabetes*, **39**, 1158–1164 (1990)

99. Kasama, T., Yoshino, G., Iwatani, I., Iwai, M., Katanaka, H. *et al.* Increased cholesterol concentration in intermediate density lipoprotein fraction of normolipidaemic non-insulin-dependent diabetes. *Atherosclerosis*, **63**, 263–266 (1987)

100. Winocour, P.H., Bhatnagar, D., Durrington, P.N., Ishola, M., Arrol, S. and Mackness, M.I. Abnormalities of VLDL, IDL and LDL characterise insulin-dependent diabetes mellitus. *Artheriosclerosis*, **12**, 920–928 (1992)

101. Winocour, P.H., Durrington, P.N., Bhatnagar, D., Ishola, M., Mackness, M.I., Arrol, S. Influence of early diabetic nephropathy on very low density lipoprotein (VLDL), intermediate density lipoprotein (IDL), and low density lipoprotein (LDL) composition. *Atherosclerosis*, **89**, 49–57 (1991)

102. Yoshino, G., Iwai, M., Kazumi, T., Matsuba, K., Iwatani, I. *et al.* Cholesterol-enrichment of low density lipoprotein fraction is absent in Japanese normolipidemic diabetes. *Hormone Metabol. Res.*, **21**, 152–153 (1987)

103. Schonfeld, G., Birge, C., Miller, J.P., Kessler, G. and Santiago, J. Apolipoprotein B levels and altered lipoprotein composition in diabetes. *Diabetes*, **23**, 927–934 (1974)

104. Dullaart, R.P.F., Groener, J.E.M., Dikkeschi, L.D., Erkelens, D.W. and Doorenboos, H. Increased cholesteryl ester transfer activity in complicated type I (insulin-dependent) diabetes mellitus – its relationship with serum lipids. *Diabetologia*, **32**, 14–19 (1989)

105. Bagdade, J.D., Ritter, M.C. and Subbaiah, P.V. Accelerated cholesteryl ester transfer in patients with insulin-dependent diabetes mellitus. *Eur. J. Clin. Invest.*, **21**, 161–167 (1991)

106. Bagdade, J.D., Lane, J.T., Subbaiah, P.V., Otto, M.E. and Ritter, M.C. Accelerated cholesteryl ester transfer in non-insulin dependent diabetes mellitus. *Atherosclerosis*, **104**, 69–78 (1993)

107. Bhatnagar, D., Durrington, P.N., Kumar, S., Young, C., Winocour, P.H. *et al.* Increased transfer of cholesteryl ester from high density lipoproteins to low density and very low density lipoproteins in patients with type 2 diabetes mellitus not receiving insulin. *Diabetic Med.*, **9** (Suppl. 2), S16 (1992)

108. Weisweiler, P. and Schwandt, P. Type I (insulin-dependent) versus type 2 (non-insulin-dependent) diabetes mellitus: characterisation of serum lipoprotein alterations. *Eur. J. Clin. Invest.*, **17**, 87–91 (1987)

109. Kissebah, A.M., Alfarsi, S., Evans, D.J. and Adams, P.W. Integrated regulation of very low density lipoprotein triglyceride and apolipoprotein B kinetics in non-insulin-dependent diabetes mellitus. *Diabetes*, **31**, 217–225 (1982)

110. Steiner, G. Hypertriglyceridaemia and carbohydrate intolerance: interrelations and therapeutic implications. *Am. J. Cardiol.*, **57**, 27G–30G (1986)

111. O'Looney, P., Irvin, D., Briscoe, P. and Vahouny, G.V. Lipoprotein composition as a component in the lipoprotein clearance defect in experimental diabetes. *J. Biol. Chem.*, **260**, 428–432 (1985)

112. Bar-On, H., Chen, Y.I. and Reaven, G.M. Evidence for a new cause of defective plasma removal of very low density lipoprotein in insulin-deficient rats. *Diabetes*, **30**, 496–499 (1981)

113. Wilson, D.E., Chan, I-F., Elstad, N.L., Peric-Golia, L., Hejazi, J. *et al.* Apolipoprotein E containing lipoproteins and lipoprotein remnants in experimental canine diabetes. *Diabetes*, **35**, 933–942 (1986)

114. Kraemer, F.B., Chan, Y-D., Lopez, R.D. and Reaven, G.M. Effects of non-insulin dependent diabetes mellitus on the uptake of very low density lipoproteins by thioglycolate-elicited mouse peritoneal macrophages. *J. Clin. Endocrinol. Metabol.*, **61**, 335–342 (1985)

115. Brown, M.S., Goldstein, J.L. and Fredrickson, D.S. Familial type 3 hyperlipoprotcinacmia (dysbetalipoproteinaemia). In *The Metabolic Basis of Inherited Disease*, 5th edn (eds J.B. Stanbury, F.B. Wyngaarden, D.S. Fredrickson, J.L. Goldstein and M.S. Brown), McGraw-Hill, New York, pp. 655–671 (1983)

116. Morganroth, J., Levy, R.I. and Fredrickson, D.S. The biochemical, clinical and genetic features of type III hyperlipoproteinaemia. *Ann. Intern. Med.*, **82**, 158–174 (1975)

117. Winocour, P.H., Tetlow, L., Durrington, P.N., Hillier, V. and Anderson, D.C. Apolipoprotein E polymorphism and lipoproteins in insulin treated diabetes mellitus. *Atherosclerosis*, **75**, 167–173 (1989)

118. Laakso, M., Kesaniemi, A., Kervinen, K., Jauhiainen, M. and Pyorala, K. Relation of coronary heart disease and apolipoprotein E phenotype in patients with non-insulin-dependent diabetes. *Br. Med. J.*, **303**, 1159–1162 (1991)

119. Curtiss, L.K. and Witztum, J.L. Plasma apolipoproteins AI, AII, B, CI and E are glucosylated in hyperglycaemic diabetic subjects. *Diabetes*, **34**, 452–461 (1985)

120. Sano, R., Abe, R., Oikawa, S., Fujii, Y. and Toyota, T. Apo E-2/E-3 ratio of very low density lipoprotein in diabetes mellitus. *Tohoku J. Exp. Med.*, **146**, 131–136 (1985)

121. Eto, M., Watanabe, K., Iwashima, Y., Morikawa, A., Oshima, E. *et al.* Apolipoprotein E polymorphism and hyperlipemia in type II diabetics. *Diabetes*, 35, 1374–1382 (1986)

122. Chait, A., Bierman, E.L. and Albers, J.J. Regulatory role of insulin in the degradation of low density lipoprotein by cultured human skin fibroblasts. *Biochim. Biophys. Acta*, **529**, 292–299 (1978)

123. Chait, A., Bierman, E.L. and Albers, J.J. Low-density lipoprotein receptor activity in cultured human skin fibroblasts. Mechanisms of insulin-induced stimulation. *J. Clin. Invest.*, **64**, 1309–1319 (1979)

124. Chait, A., Bierman, E.L. and Albers, J.J. Low density lipoprotein receptor activity in fibroblasts cultured from diabetic donors. *Diabetes*, **28**, 914–918 (1979)
125. Mazzone, T., Foster, D. and Chait, A. In vivo stimulation of low-density lipoprotein degradation by insulin. *Diabetes*, **33**, 333–338 (1984)
126. Schleicher, E., Deufel, T. and Wieland, O.H. Non-enzymatic glycosylation of human serum lipoproteins. *FEBS Letts*, **129**, 1–4 (1981)
127. Witztum, J.L., Mahoney, E.M., Branks, M.J., Fisher, M., Elam, R. and Steinberg, D. Non-enzymatic glucosylation of human low density lipoprotein alters its biologic activity. *Diabetes*, **31**, 283–291 (1982)
128. Tames, F.J., Mackness, M.I., Arrol, S., Laing, I. and Durrington, P.N. Non-enzymatic glycation of apolipoprotein B in the sera of diabetic and non-diabetic subjects. *Atherosclerosis*, **93**, 227–244 (1992)
129. Gonen, B., Baenziger, J., Schonfeld, G., Jacobsen, D. and Farrar, P. Nonenzymatic glycosylation of low density lipoprotein in vivo. *Diabetes*, **30**, 875–878 (1981)
130. Kesaniemi, Y.A., Witztum, J.L. and Steinbrecher, U.P. Receptor-mediated catabolism of low density lipoprotein in man. *J. Clin. Invest.*, **71**, 950–959 (1983)
131. Steinbrecher, U.P., Witztum, J.L., Kesaniemi, Y.A. and Elam, R.L. Comparison of glucosylated LDL with methylated or cyclohexanedione-treated LDL in the measurement of receptor-independent LDL catabolism. *J. Clin. Invest.*, **71**, 960–964 (1983)
132. Schleicher, E., Olgemoller, B., Schon, J., Durst, T. and Wieland, O.H. Limited non-enzymatic glucosylation of low-density lipoprotein does not alter its catabolism in tissue culture. *Biochem. Biophys. Acta*, **846**, 226–233 (1985)
133. Steinbrecher, U.P. and Witztum, J.L. Glucosylation of low density lipoproteins to an extent comparable to that seen in diabetes slows their metabolism. *Diabetes*, **33**, 130–134 (1984)
134. Hunt, J.V. and Wolff, S.P. Oxidative glycation and free radical production: a causal mechanism of diabetic complications. *Free Rad. Res. Commun.*, **12/13**, 115–123 (1991)
135. Creiche, A.G., Dumont, S., Siffert, J.C. and Stahl, A.J.C. *In vitro* glycated low-density lipoprotein interaction with human monocyte-derived macrophages. *Res. Immunol.*, **143**, 17–23 (1992)
136. Brownlee, M., Vlassara, H. and Cerami, A. Non-enzymatic glucosylation products on collagen covalently trap low-density lipoprotein. *Diabetes*, **34**, 938–941 (1985)
137. Nikkila, E.A. High density lipoproteins in diabetes. *Diabetes*, **30**, 82–87 (1981)
138. Durrington, P.N. Serum high density lipoprotein cholesterol in diabetes mellitus: an analysis of factors which influence its concentration. *Clin. Chim. Acta*, **104**, 11–23 (1980)
139. Brunzell, J.D., Chait, A. and Bierman, E. Plasma lipoproteins in human diabetes mellitus. In The *Diabetes Annual*, vol. 1 (eds K.G.M.M. Alberti and L.D. Krall), Elsevier, Amsterdam, pp. 463–479 (1985)
140. Lopes-Virella, M.F.L., Stone, P.G. and Colwell, J.H. Serum high density lipoprotein in diabetic patients. *Diabetologia*, **13**, 285–291 (1977)
141. Durrington, P.N. and Stephens, W.P. The effects of treatment with insulin on serum high-density-lipoprotein cholesterol in rats with streptozocin-induced diabetes. *Clin. Sci.*, **59**, 71–74 (1980)
142. Bergman, M., Gidez, L.I. and Eder, H.A. High-density lipoprotein subclasses in diabetes. *Ann. J. Med.*, **81**, 488–492 (1986)
143. Nikkila, E.A., Taskinen, M-R. and Sane, T. Plasma high-density lipoprotein concentration and subfraction distribution in relation to triglyceride metabolism. *Am. Heart, J.*, **113**, 543–548 (1987)
144. Taskinen, M.-R. and Nikkila, E.A. High density lipoprotein subfractions in relation to lipoprotein lipase activity of tissues in man-evidence for reciprocal regulation of HDL$_2$ and HDL$_3$ levels by lipoprotein lipase. *Clin. Chim. Acta*, **112**, 325–332 (1981)
145. Durrington, P.N. Serum high density lipoprotein cholesterol subfractions in type I (insulin-dependent) diabetes mellitus. *Clin. Chim. Acta*, **120**, 21–28 (1982)
146. Cruickshank, K.J., Orchard, T.J. and Becker, D.J. The cardiovascular risk profile of adolescents with insulin dependent diabetes mellitus. *Diabetes Care*, **8**, 118–124 (1985)
147. Mattock, M.B., Salter, A.M., Fuller, J.H., Omer, T., El-Gohari, R. *et al.* High density lipoprotein subfractions in insulin-dependent diabetic and normal subjects. *Atherosclerosis*, **45**, 67–69 (1982)
148. Durrington, P.N. A comparison of three methods of measuring serum high density lipoprotein cholesterol in diabetics and non-diabetics. *Ann. Clin. Biochem.*, **17**, 199–204 (1980)

149. Winocour, P.H., Durrington, P.N., Ishola, M., Anderson, D.C. and Cohen, H. Influence of protein-uria on vascular disease, blood pressure, and lipoproteins in insulin dependent diabetes mellitus. *Br. Med. J.*, **294**, 1648–1651(1987)
150. Durrington, P.N. High-density lipoprotein cholesterol: methods and clinical significance. *CRC Crit. Rev. Clin. Lab. Sci.*, **18**, 31–78 (1982)
151. Witztum, J.L., Fisher, M., Metro, T., Steinbrecher, V. and Glam, R.I. Non-enzymatic glycosyla-tion of high density lipoprotein accelerates it catabolism in guinea pigs. *Diabetes*, **31**, 1029–1034 (1982)
152. Short, C.D., Durrington, P.N., Mallick, N.P., Hunt, L.P., Tetlow, L. and Ishola, M. Serum and urinary high density lipoproteins in glomerular disease with proteinuria. *Kidney Int.*, **29**, 1224–1228 (1986)
153. Gitlin, D., Comwell, D.G., Natasato, D., Ondey, J.L., Hughes, W.L. and Janeway, C.A. Studies on the metabolism of plasma proteins in the nephrotic syndrome II. The lipoproteins. *J. Clin. Invest.*, **37**, 172–184 (1958)
154. Kverneland, A., Feldt-Rasmussen, B., Vidal, P., Welinder, B., Bent-Hansel, L., Soegaard, U. and Deckert, T. Evidence of changes in renal charge selectivity in patients with type I (insulin-depen-dent) diabetes mellitus. *Diabetologia*, **29**, 634–639 (1986)
155. Mogensen, C.E. Early diabetic renal involvement and nephropathy. In *The Diabetes Annual*, vol. 3 (eds K.G.M.M. Alberti and L.P. Krall), Elsevier, Amsterdam, pp. 306–324 (1987)
156. Glass, C.K., Pittman, R.C., Keller, G.A. and Steinberg, D. Tissue sites of degradation of apopro-tein A-I in the rat. *J. Biol.*, **258**, 7161–7167 (1983)
157. Winocour, P.H., Durrington, P.N., Bhatnagar, D., MBewu, A.D., Ishola, M., Mackness, M.I. and Arrol, S. A cross-sectional evaluation of cardiovascular risk factors in coronary heart diseae associated with Type 1 (insulin-dependent) diabetes mellitus. *Diab. Res. Clin. Pract.*, **18**, 173–184 (1992)
158. Duell, P.B., Oram, J.F. and Beirman, E.L. Nonenzymatic glycosylation of HDL and impaired HDL-receptor-mediated cholesterol efflux. *Diabetes*, **40**, 377–384 (1991)
159. Misra, D.P., Staddon, G., Powell, N., Misra, J. and Crook, D. Lecithin cholesterol acyltransferase activity in diabetes mellitus and the effect of insulin in these cases. *Clin. Chim. Acta.*, **56**, 83–89 (1974)
160. Fielding, C.J., Reaven, G.M. and Fielding, P.E. Human non-insulin-dependent diabetes: identifi-cation of a defect in plasma cholesterol transport normalised *in vivo* by insulin and *in vitro* by selective immunoadsorption of apolipoprotein E. *Proc. Natl Acad Sci. USA*, **79**, 6365–6369 (1982)
161. Fielding, C.J., Reaven, G.M., Liu, G. and Fielding, P.E. Increased free cholesterol in plasma low and very low density lipoproteins in non-insulin-dependent diabetes mellitus: its role in the inhibi-tion of cholesteryl ester transfer. *Proc. Natl Acad Sci. USA.*, **81**, 2512–2516 (1984)
162. Mattock, M.B., Fuller, J.H., Maude, P.S. and Keen, H. Lipoproteins and plasma cholesterol ester-ification in normal and diabetic subjects. *Atherosclerosis*, **34**, 437–449 (1979)
163. Viberti, G.C., Hill, R.D., Jarrett, R.J., Argyroploulos, A., Mahmud, U. and Keen, H. Microalbu-minuria as a predictor of clinical nephropathy in insulin-dependent diabetes mellitus. *Lancet*, **i**, 1430–1432 (1982)
164. Andersen, A.R., Christiansen, J.S., Andersen, J.K., Kreiner, S. and Deckert, T. Diabetic nephropathy in type 1 (insulin dependent) diabetes mellitus: an epidemiological study. *Diabetolo-gia*, **25**, 496–501 (1983)
165. Borch-Johnsen, K., Andersen, P.K. and Deckert, T. The effect of proteinuria on relative mortal-ity in type I (insulin-dependent) diabetes mellitus. *Diabetologia*, **28**, 590–596 (1985)
166. Borch-Johnsen, K. and Kreiner, S. Proteinuria: value as predictor of cardiovascular mortality in insulin dependent diabetes mellitus. *Br. Med. J.*, **294**, 1651–1654 (1987)
167. Wiseman, M., Viberti, G., Macintosh, D., Jarrett, R.J. and Keen, H. Glycaemia, arterial pressure and microaluminuria in type I (insulin-dependent) diabetes mellitus. *Diabetologia*, **26**, 401–405 (1984)
168. Mathieson, E.R., Oxenboll, B., Johansen, K., Svendsen, P.A. and Deckert, T. Incipient nephro-pathy in type 1 (insulin-dependent) diabetics. *Diabetologia*, **26**, 406–410 (1984)
169. Hasslacher, Ch., Stech, W., Wahl, P. and Ritz, E. Blood pressure and metabolic control as risk factors for nephropathy in type 1 (insulin-dependent) diabetes. *Diabetologia*, **26**, 6–11 (1985)

170. Vannini, P., Ciavarella, A., Flammini, M., Bargossi, A.M., Forlani, G. *et al.* Lipid abnormalities in insulin-dependent diabetic patients with albuminuria. *Diabeta Care*, **7**, 151–154 (1984)

171. Eckel, R.H., McLean, E., Albers, J.J., Cheung, M.C. and Bierman, E.L. Plasma lipids and microangiopathy in insulin-dependent diabetes mellitus. *Diabetes Care*, **4**, 447–453 (1981)

172. Crepaldi, G., Manzato, E. and Nosadini, R. Plurimetabolic syndrome or syndrome X. Is it a real syndrome? In *Drugs Affecting Lipid Metabolism* (eds A.L. Catopano, A.M. Gotto, L.C. Smith and R. Paoletti) Kluwer Academic Publishers, Dordrecht, pp. 23–27 (1993)

173. Castelli, W.P. The triglyceride issue: a view from Framingham. *Am. Heart J.*, **112**, 432–437 (1986)

174. Laakso, M., Voutilainen, E., Sarlund, H., Aro, A., Pyorala, K. *et al.* Inverse relationship of serum HDL and HDL$_2$ cholesterol to C-peptide level in middle-aged insulin-treated diabetics. *Metabolism*, **34**, 715–720 (1985)

175. Nagi, D.K., Hendra, T.J., Ryle, A.J., Cooper, T.M., Temple, R.C. *et al.* The relationship of concentrations of insulin, intact proinsulin and 32-33 split proinsulin with cardiovascular risk factors in Type 2 (non-insulin-dependent) diabetic subjects. *Diabetologia*, **33**, 532–537 (1990)

176. Winocour, P.H., Durrington, P.N., Ishola, M., Gordon, C., Jeacock, J. and Anderson, D.C. Does residual insulin secretion (assessed by C-peptide concentration) affect lipid and lipoprotein levels in insulin-dependent diabetes mellitus? *Clin. Sci.*, **77**, 369–374 (1989)

177. Hales, C.N., Barker, D.J.P., Clark, P.M.S., Cox, L.J., Fall, C., Osmond, C. and Winter, P.D. Fetal and infant growth and impaired glucose tolerance at age 64. *Br. Med. J.*, **303**, 1019–1022 (1991)

178. Poretsky, L. On the paradox of insulin-induced hyperandrogenism in insulin-resistant states. *Endocrine. Rev.*, **12**, 3–13 (1991)

179. Nestler, J.E. Sex hormone-binding globulin: a marker for hyperinsulinaemia and/or insulin resistance? *J. Clin. Endocrinol. Metabol.*, **76**, 273–274 (1993)

180. Barrett-Connor, E.L., Cohn, B.A., Wingard, D.L. and Edelstein, S.L. Why is diabetes mellitus a stronger risk factor for fatal ischaemic heart disease in women than in men? The Rancho Bernardo Study. *J. Am. Med. Assoc.*, **265**, 627–631 (1991)

181. McKeigue, P.M. and Keen, H. Diabetes, insulin, ethnicity, and coronary heart disease In *Coronary Heart Disease From Aetiology to Public Health Epidemiology* (eds M. Marmot and P. Elliot), Oxford University Press, Oxford, pp. 217–232 (1992)

182. Mckeige, P.M., Shah, B. and Marmot, M.G. Relation of central obesity and insulin resistance with high diabetes prevalence and cardiovascular risk in South Asians. *Lancet*, **337**, 82–86 (1991)

183. Winocour, P.H., Bhatnagar, D., Ishola, M., Arrol, S. and Durrington, P.N. Lipoprotein (a) and microvascular disease in type 1 (insulin dependent) diabetes mellitus. *Diabetic Med.*, **8**, 922–927 (1991)

184. Kapelrud, H., Bangstad, H.J., Dahl-Jorgensen, K. and Hanssen, K.F. Serum Lp(a) lipoprotein concentrations in insulin-dependent diabetic patients with microalbuminuria. *Br. Med. J.*, **303**, 675–678 (1991)

185. Haffner, S.M., Tuttle, K.R. and Rainwater, D.L. Decrease of lipoprotein (a) with improved glycaemic control in IDDM subjects. *Diabetes Care*, **14**, 302–307 (1991)

186. Levutsky, L.L., Scami, A.M. and Gould, S.H. Lipoprotein (a) levels in black and white children and adolescents with IDDM. *Diabetes Care*, **14**, 283–287 (1991)

187. Davies, M., Rayman, G. and Day, J. Increased incidence of coronary disease in people with impaired glucose tolerance: link with increased lipoprotein (a) concentrations? *Br. Med. J.*, **304**, 1610–1611 (1992)

188. Raminez, L.C., Aranz-Pacheco, O., Lackner, C., Albright, G., Adams, B.V. and Raskin, P. Lipoprotein (a) levels in diabetes mellitus: relationship to metabolic control. *Ann. Intern. Med.*, **117**, 42–47 (1992)

189. Nakata, H., Horita, K. and Eto, M. Alteration of lipoprotein (a) concentration with glycaemic control in non-insulin-dependent diabetic subjects without diabetic complications. *Metabolism*, **42**, 1323–1326 (1993)

190. Ritter, M.M., Loscar, M., Richter, W.O. and Schwandt, P. Lipoprotein (a) in diabetes mellitus. *Clin. Chim. Acta*, **214**, 45–54 (1993)

191. Haffner, S.M., Moss, S.E., Klein, B.E. and Kleen, R. Lack of association between lipoprotein (a) concentrations and coronary heart disease mortality in diabetes: the Wisconsin Epidemiologic Study of Diabetic Retinopathy. *Metabolism*, **41**, 194–197 (1992)

192. Lindstrom, T., Arnqvist, H.J. and Olsson, A. Effect of different insulin regimens on plasma lipoprotein and apolipoprotein concentrations in patients with non-insulin-dependent diabetes mellitus. *Atherosclerosis*, **81**, 137–144 (1990)

193. The Diabetes Control and Complications Trial Research Group. The effect of intensive treatment of diabetes on the development and progression of long-term complications in insulin-dependent diabetes mellitus. *N. Engl. J. Med.*, **329**, 977–986 (1993)

194. Calvert, G.D., Graham, J.J., Mannik, T., Wise, P.H. and Yeates, R.A. Effects of therapy on plasma high density lipoprotein cholesterol concentration in diabetes mellitus. *Lancet*, **ii**, 66–68 (1978)

195. Lisch, H.T. and Sailer, S. Lipoprotein patterns in diet, sulphonylurea and insulin treated diabetics. *Diabetologia*, **20**, 118–122 (1981)

196. Rains, S.G.H., Wilson, G.A., Richmond, W. and Elkeles, R.S. The effect of glibendamide and metformin on serum lipoproteins in type 2 diabetes. *Diabetic Med.*, **5**, 653–658 (1988)

197. Paisey, R., Elkeles, R.S., Hambley, J. and Magill, P. The effects of chlorpropamide and insulin on serum lipids, lipoproteins and fractional triglyceride removal. *Diabetologia*, **15**, 81–85 (1978)

198. Howard, B.V., Xiaoren, P., Harper, I., Foley, J.E., Cheung, M.C. and Taskinen, M.-R. Effects of sulfonylurea therapy on plasma lipids and high-density lipoprotein composition in non-insulin-dependent diabetes mellitus. *Am. J. Med.*, **79** (Suppl. 3B), 79–85 (1985)

199. University Group Diabetes Program. A study of the effects of hypoglycaemia agents on vascular complications in patients with adult-onset diabetes. Sections I and II. *Diabetes*, **19** (Suppl. 2), 747–840 (1970)

200. University Group Diabetes Program. A study of the effects of hypoglycaemic agents on vascular complications in patients with adult-onset diabetes. Section V. Evaluation of phenformin therapy. *Diabetes*, **24** (Suppl. 1), 68–184 (1974)

201. Kilo, Ch. and Williamson, J.R. The controversial American University Group Diabetes Study – a look at sulfonylurea and biguanide therapy. In *Macrovascular Disease in Diabetes Mellitus. Pathogenesis and Prevention* (eds. H.V. Janka, H. Mehnert and E. Standl), Georg Thieme, Stuttgart, pp. 102–104 (1985)

202. Cairns, S.A., Shalet, S., Marshall, A.J. and Hartog, M. A comparison of phenformin and metformin in the treatment of maturity onset diabetes. *Diabete Metabol. (Paris)*, **3**, 183–188 (1977)

203. Taylor, K.G., John, W.G., Matthews, K.A. and Wright, A.D. A prospective study of the effect of 12 months treatment on serum lipids and apolipoproteins A-I and B in type 2 (non-insulin-dependent) diabetes. *Diabetologia*, **23**, 507–510 (1982)

204. Rains, S.G.H., Wilson, G.A., Richmond, W., Elkeles, R.S. The reduction of low density lipoprotein cholesterol by metformin is maintained with long term therapy. *J. R. Soc. Med.*, **82**, 93–94 (1989)

205. Lalor, B.C., Bhatnagar, D., Winocour, P.H., Ishola, M., Arrol, S. *et al.* Placebo-controlled trial of the effects of guar gum and metformin on fasting blood glucose and serum lipids in obese, type 2 diabetic patients. *Diabetic Med.*, **7**, 242–245 (1990)

206. Gustafson, A., Bjorntorp, P. and Fahlen, M. Metformin administration in hyperlipidaemic states. *Acta Med. Scand.*, **190**, 491–494 (1971)

207. Fuessel, H.S., Williams, G., Adrian, T.E. and Bloom, S.R. Guar sprinkled on food. Effect on glycaemic control, plasma lipids and gut hormones in non-insulin dependent diabetic patients. *Diabetic Med.*, **4**, 463–468 (1986)

208. Anon. Guar gum: of help to diabetics. *Drug Ther. Bull.*, **25**, 65–67 (1987)

209. Turner, P.R., Tuomilehto, J., Happonen, P., LaVille, A.E., Shaikh, M. and Lewis, B. Metabolic studies on the hypolipidaemic effect of guar gum. *Atherosclerosis*, **81**, 145–150 (1990)

210. Durrington, P.N. Specific lipid-lowering therapy in the management of diabetes. *Postgrad. Med. J.*, **67**, 947–952 (1991)

211. Durrington, P.N. Diabetes, hypertension and hyperlipidaemia. *Postgrad. Med. J.*, **69** (Suppl. 1), S18–29 (1993)

212. Durrington, P.N. and Winocour, P.H. Therapeutic aspects of hyperlipidaemia in diabetes. *Postgrad. Med. J.*, **65** (Suppl. 1), 33–41 (1989)

213. Prager, R., Schemthaner, G., Kostner, G.M., Muhlhauser, I., Zechner, R. and Dorda, W. Effect of bezafibrate on plasma lipids, lipoproteins, apolipoproteins AI, AII and B and LCAT activity in hyperlipidaemic non-insulin dependent diabetics. *Atherosclerosis*, **43**, 321–327 (1982)

214. Jones, I.R., Swai, A., Taylor, R., Miller, M., Laker, M.F. and Alberti, K.G.M.M. Lowering of plasma glucose concentrations with bezafibrate in patients with moderately controlled NIDDM. *Diabetes Care*, **13**, 855–863 (1990)

215. Winocour, P.H., Durrington, P.N., Bhatnagar, D., Ishola, M., Mackness, M.I. *et al.* The effect of bezafibrate on very low density lipoprotein (VLDL), intermediate density lipoprotein (IDL), and low density lipoprotein (LDL) composition in Type 1 diabetes associated with hypercholestero-laemia or combined hyperlipidaemia. *Atherosclerosis*, **93**, 83–94 (1992)

216. Cesarone, M.R., Laurara, G., de Sanctis, M.T., Pomante, P. and Belcaro, G. Progression of arter-ial wall lesions evaluated by ultrasound biopsy in asymptomatic subjects and in diabetics and hyperlipidaemics with bezafibrate 4 years follow-up. *Minerva Cardioangiol.*, **40**, 15–21 (1992)

217. Dean, J.D., McCarthy, S., Betteridge, D.J., Whately-Smith, C., Powell, J. and Owens, D.R. The effect of acipimox in patients with type 2 diabetes and persistent hyperlipidaemia. *Diabetes Med.*, **9**, 611–615 (1992)

218. Kumar, S., Durrington, P.N., Bhatnagar, D., Mackness, M.I., Gordon, C. *et al.* Improvement in glucose tolerance and insulin sensitivity in Type 2 diabetic patients treated with a long-acting formulation of acipimox for 8 weeks. *Diabetic Med.* (in press) (1994)

219. Shepherd, J., Caslake, M., Gaw, A., Griffin, B., Lindsay, G. and Packard, C. Atherogenicity of triglyceride-rich lipoproteins: clinical aspects. In *Drugs Affecting Lipid Metabolism* (eds A.L. Cataparo, A.M. Gotto L.C. Smith and R. Paoletti), Kluwer Academic Publishers, Dordrecht, pp. 453–466 (1993)

220. Caslake, M.J., Packard, C.J., Series, J.J., Yip, B., Dagen, M.M. and Shepherd, J. Plasma triglyc-eride and low density lipoprotein metabolism. *Eur. J. Clin. Invest.*, **22**, 96–104 (1992)

221. Garg, A. and Grundy, S.M. Treatment of dyslipidaemia in non-insulin-dependent diabetes melli-tus with lovastatin. *Am. J. Cardiol.*, **62**, 44J–49J (1988)

222. Garg, A. and Grundy, S.M. Lovastatin for lowering cholesterol levels in non-insulin-dependent diabetes mellitus. *N. Engl. J. Med.*, **318**, 81–86 (1988)

223. Dean, J.D., Bhatnagar, D., Kumar, S., Mackness, M.I., Young, C. *et al.* The effect of HMG-CoA reducatase inhibition on the transfer of cholesteryl ester from high density lipoproteins to low density and very low density lipoproteins in non-insulin-dependent diabetic patients. *Diabetic Med.*, **10** (Suppl. 3), S18 (1993)

224. Kasim, S.E., Stem, B., Khilnani, S., McLin, P., Baciorowski, S. and Jen, K-L.C. Effects of omega-3 fish oils on lipid metabolism, glycaemic control, and blood pressure in type II diabetic patients. *J. Clin. Endocrinol. Metabol.*, **67**, 1–5 (1988)

225. Glauber, H., Wallace, P., Griver, K. and Brechtel, G. Adverse metabolic effect of omega-3 fatty acids in non-insulin-dependent diabetes mellitus. *Ann. Intern. Med.*, **108**, 663–668 (1988)

226. Borkman, M., Chisholm, D.J. and Furler, S.M. Effects of fish oil supplementation on glucose and lipid metabolism in NIDDM. *Diabetes*, **38**, 1314–1319 (1989)

227. Weidmann, P. and Trost, B.N. Pathogenesis and treatment of hypertension associated with diabetes. In *Macrovascular Disease in Diabetes Mellitus. Pathogenesis and Prevention* (eds H.U. Janka, M. Mehnert and E. Standl), Georg Thieme, Stuttgart, pp. 51–58 (1985)

228. Gardner, J.A. and Gainsborough, H. The relationship of serum cholesterol and basal metabolism. *Br. Med. J.*, **2**, 935–937 (1928)

229. Gofman, J.W., Rubin, I., McGinley, J.P. and Jones, H.B. Hyperlipoproteinaemia. *Am. J. Med.*, **17**, 514–520 (1984)

230. Series, J.J., Biggart, E.M., O'Reilly, D.St.J., Packard, C.J. and Shepherd, J. Thyroid dysfunction and hypercholesterolaemia in the general population of Glasgow, Scotland. *Clin. Chim. Acta*, **172**, 217–222 (1988)

231. Walton, K.W., Scott, P.J., Dykes, P.W. and Davies, J.W.L. The significance of alterations in serum lipids in thyroid dysfunction. II Alterations of the metabolism and turnover of [131]I-low density lipoproteins in hypothyroidism and thyrotoxicosis. *Clin. Sci.*, **29**, 984–994 (1965)

232. Thompson, G.R., Soutar, A.K., Spengel, F.A., Jadhav, A., Gavigan, S. and Myant, N.B. Defects of the receptor-mediated low density lipoprotein metabolism in homozygous familial hypercho-lesterolaemia and hypothyroidism in vivo. *Proc. Natl Acad. Sci. USA.*, **78**, 2591–2595 (1981)

233. Abrams, J.J. and Grundy, S.M. Cholesterol metabolism in hypothyroidism and hyperthyroidism in man. *J. Lipid Res.*, **22**, 323–338 (1981)

234. Chait, A., Kanter, R., Green, W. and Kenny, M. Defective thyroid hormone action in fibroblasts cultured from subjects with the syndrome of resistance to thyroid hormones. *J. Clin. Endocrinol. Metabol.*, **54**, 767–772 (1982)

235. Rossner, S. and Rosenqvist, V. Serum lipoproteins and the intravenous fat tolerance test in hypothyroid patients before and during substitution therapy. *Atherosclerosis*, **20**, 365–381 (1974)

236. Abrams, J.J., Grundy, S.M. and Gisberg, H. Metabolism of plasma triglyceride in hypothyroidism and hyperthyroidism in man. *J. Lipid Res.*, **22**, 307–322 (1981)

237. Porte, D., O'Hara, D.O. and Williams, R.H. The relation between postheparin lipolytic activity and plasma triglyceride in myxedema. *Metabolism*, **15**, 107–113 (1966)

238. Nikkilia, E.A. and Kekki, M. Plasma triglyceride metabolism in thyroid disease. *J. Clin. Invest.*, **51**, 2103–2114 (1972)

239. Clifford, C., Salel, A.F., Shore, B., Shore, V. and Mason, D.T. Mechanisms of lipoprotein alterations in patients with idiopathic hypothyroidism. *Circulation*, (Suppl. II), **18**, 51–52 (1975)

240. Hazzard, W.R. and Biemman, E.L. Aggravation of broad-beta disease (Type III hyperlipoproteinaemia) by hypothyroidism. *Arch. Intern. Med.*, **130**, 822–828 (1972)

241. Fowler, P.B.S., Swale, J. and Andrews, H. Hypercholesterolaemia in borderline hypothyroidism. Stage of premyxoedema. *Lancet*, **ii**, 488–491 (1970)

242. Heimberg, M., Olubadewo, J.O. and Wilcox, H.G. Plasma lipoproteins and regulation of hepatic metabolism of fatty acids in altered thyroid states. *Endocrine Rev.*, **6**, 590–607 (1985)

243. Dullaart, R.P.F., Hoogenberg, K., Groener, J.E.M., Dikkeschei, L.D., Erkelens, D.W. and Doorenbus, H. The activity of cholesteryl ester transfer protein is decreased in hypothroidism: a possible contribution to alterations in high-density lipoproteins. *Eur. J. Clin. Invest.*, **20**, 581–587 (1990)

244. Miettinen, T. Mechanism of serum cholesterol reduction by thyroid hormones in hypothyroidism. *J. Lab. Clin. Med.*, **71**, 537–547 (1968)

245. Verdugo, C., Perrot, L., Ponsin, G., Valentin, C. and Berthezene, F. Time-course of alterations of high density lipoproteins (HDL) during thyroxine administration to hypothyroid women. *Eur. J. Clin. Invest.*, **17**, 313–316 (1987)

246. Agdeppa, D., MaQron, C., Mallik, T. and Schmida, N.D. Plasma high density lipoprotein cholesterol in thyroid disease. *J. Clin. Endocrinol. Metabol.*, **45**, 726–729 (1979)

247. Scottolini, A.G., Bhagavan, N.V., Oshiro, T.H. and Abe, S.Y. Serum high-density lipoprotein cholesterol concentrations in hypo- and hyperthyroidism. *Clin. Chem.*, **26**, 584–587 (1980)

248. Muls, E., Blaton, M., Rosseneu, M., Lesaffre, E., Lamberigts, G. and de Moor, P. Serum lipids and apolipoproteins A-I, A-II and B in hyperthyroidism before and after treatment. *J. Clin. Endocrinol. Metabol.*, **55**, 459–464 (1982)

249. Aviram, M., Luboshitzky, R. and Brook, J.G. Lipid and lipoprotein pattern in thyroid dysfunction and the effect of therapy. *Clin. Biochem.*, **15**, 62–66 (1982)

250. Wieland, H. and Seidel, D. Plasma lipoprotein bei Palienten mit Hyperthyreose. Isolierung und Characterisierung lines abnormen. High-density-lipoproteins. *Z. Klin. Chem. Klin. Biochem.*, **10**, 311–321 (1972)

251. Boberg, J., Dahlberg, P-A., Vessby, B. and Lilhell, H. Serum lipoprotein and apolipoprotein concentrations in patients with hyperthyroidism and the effect of treatment with Carbimazole. *Acta Med. Scand.*, **215**, 453–459 (1984)

252. Summers, V.K., Hipkin, L.J. and Davis, J.C. Serum lipids in diseases of the pituitary. *Metabolism*, **12**, 1106–1113 (1967)

253. Sagel, J., Lopes-Virella, M.F., Levin, J.H. and Colwell, J.A. Decreased high density lipoprotein cholesterol in hypopituitarism. *J. Clin. Endocrinol. Metabol.*, **49**, 753–756 (1979)

254. Merimee, T.J., Hollander, W. and Fineberg, S.E. Studies of hyperlipidaemia in the human growth hormone-deficient state. *Metabolism*, **21**, 1053–1061 (1972)

255. Nikkila, E.A. and Pelkonen, R. Serum lipids in acromegaly. *Metabolism*, **24**, 829–838 (1975)

256. Editorial Born to be fat? *Lancet*, **340**, 881–882 (1992)

257. Law, C.M., Barker, D.J.P., Osmond, C., Fall, C.H.D. and Simmonds, S.J. Early growth and abdominal fatness in adult life. *J. Epidemiol. Commun. Health*, **46**, 184–186 (1992)

258. Albrink, M.J., Meigs, J.W. and Granoff, M.A. Weight gain and serum triglycerides in normal men. *N. Engl. J. Med.*, **226**, 484–489 (1962)

259. Glueck, C.J., Taylor, H.L., Jacobs, D., Morrison, J.A., Beaglehole, R. and Williams, O.D. Plasma high-density lipoprotein cholesterol: association with measurements of body mass. The Lipid Research Clinics Program Prevalence Study. *Circulation*, **62** (Suppl. IV), 62–69 (1980)

260. Leelarthaepin, B., Woodhill, J.M., Palmer, A.J. and Blacket, R.B. Obesity, diet and type II hyperlipidaemia. *Lancet*, **ii**, 1217–1221 (1974)

261. Royal College of Physicians Working Party. Obesity: a report of the Royal College of Physicians. *J. R. Coll. Phys. Lond.*, **17**, 5–65 (1983)

262. National Institutes of Health Consensus Development Conference. Health implications of obesity. *Ann. Intern. Med.*, **103**, 977–1077 (1985)

263. Bray, G.B., Davidson, M.B. and Drenick, E.J. Obesity: a serious symptom. *Ann. Intern. Med.*, **77**, 707–805 (1972)

264. Barrett-Connor, E.L. Obesity, atherosclerosis, and coronary artery disease. *Ann. Intern. Med.*, **103**, 1010–1019 (1985)

265. Mazess, R.B., Poppler, W.W. and Gibbons, M. Total body composition by dual-photon (153 Ga) absorptiometry. *Ann. J. Clin. Nutr.*, **40**, 834–839 (1984)

266. Keys, A., Fidanza, F., Karvonen, M.J., Kimura, N. and Taylor, H.L. Indices of relative weight and obesity. *J. Chron. Dis.*, **25**, 329–343 (1972)

267. Lew, E.A. and Garfinkel, L. Variations in mortality by weight among 750,000 men and women. *J. Chron. Dis.*, **32**, 563–576 (1979)

268. Khosla, T. and Lowe, C.R. Obesity and smoking habits. *Br. Med. J.*, **4**, 10–13 (1971)

269. Vague, J., La Differenciation sexuelle: facteur des formes de l'obesite. *Presse Med.*, **30**, 339–340 (1947)

270. Kissebah, A.H., Vydelingum, N., Murray, R., Evans, D.J., Hartz, A.J., Kallchoff, R.K. and Adams, P.W. Relation of body fat distribution to metabolic complications of obesity. *J. Clin. Endocrinol. Metabol.*, **54**, 254–261 (1982)

271. Krotkiewski, M., Bjorntorp, P., Sjostrom, L. and Smith, U. Impact of obesity on metabolism in men and women. Importance of regional adipose tissue distribution. *J. Clin. Invest.*, **72**, 1150–1162 (1983)

272. Ducimetiere, P., Avons, P., Cambien, F. and Richard, J.L. Corpulence history and fat distribution in CHD etiology: the Paris Prospective Study. *Eur. Heart J.*, **4**, 8 (1983)

273. Lapidus, L., Bengtsson, C., Larsson, B., Pennert, K., Rybo, E. and Sjostrom, L. Distribution of adipose tissue and risk of cardiovascular disease and death: a 12 year follow-up of participants in the population study of women in Gothenburg, Sweden, *Br. Med. J.*, **289**, 1257–1261 (1984)

274. Larsson, B., Svardsudd, K., Welin, L., Wilhelmsen, L., Bjorntorp, P. and Tibblin, G. Abdominal adipose tissue distribution, obesity, and risk of cardiovascular disease and death: 13 year follow-up of participants in the study of men born in 1913. *Br. Med. J.*, **288**, 1401–1404 (1984)

275. Metropolitan Life Insurance Company, New York. Ideal weights for men. *Stat. Bull.*, **24** (June), 6–8 (1943)

276. Metropolitan Life Insurance Company, New York. New weight standards for men and women. *Stat. Bull.*, **40** (Nov–Dec.), 1–3 (1959)

277. Society of Actuaries. *Build. Study.* Associates of Life Insurance Medical Directors of America, Chicago, Illinois (1979)

278. Metropolitan Life Insurance Company, New York. Metropolitan height and weight tables. *Stat. Bull.*, **64** (Jan–June), 2 (1983)

279. Andres, R., Tobin, J.D., Muller, D.C. and Brant, L. Impact of age on weight goals. *Ann. Intern. Med.*, **103**, 1030–1033 (1985)

280. Nestel P. and Goldrick, B. Obesity: changes in lipid metabolism and the role of insulin. *J. Clin. Endocrinol. Metabol.*, **5**, 313–335 (1976)

281. Egusa, G., Belt, W.F., Grundy, S.M. and Howard, B.V. Influence of obesity on the metabolism of apolipoprotein B in humans. *J. Clin. Invest.*, **76**, 596–602 (1985)

282. Howard, B.V., Williams, G. H., Egusa, G. and Taskinen, M.-R. Co-ordination of very low density lipoprotein triglyceride and apolipoprotein B metabolism in humans: effects of obesity and non-insulin dependent diabetes mellitus. *Am. Heart J.*, **113**, 522–526 (1987)

283. Kesaniemi, Y.A. and Grundy, S.M. Increased low density lipoprotein production associated with obesity. *Arteriosclerosis*, **3**, 170–177 (1983)

284. Barter, P.J. and Nestel, P.J. Precursors of plasma triglyceride fatty acids in obesity. *Metabolism*, **22**, 779–785 (1973)
285. Stern, M.P., Olefsky, J., Farquhar, J.W. and Reaven, G.M. Relationship between fasting plasma lipid levels and adipose tissue morphology. *Metabolism*, **22**, 1311–1317 (1973)
286. Bjorntorp, P., Gustafson, A. and Persson, B. Adipose tissue fat cell size and number in relation to metabolism in endogenous hypertriglyceridaemia. *Acta Med Scand.*, **190**, 363–367 (1971)
287. Olefsky, J.M. The insulin receptor. Its role in insulin resistance of obesity and diabetes. *Diabetes*, **25**, 1154–1162 (1976)
288. Pykalisto, O.J., Smith, P.H. and Brunzell, J.D. Determinants of human adipose tissue lipase: effects of diabetes and obesity on basal and diet-induced activity. *J. Clin. Invest.*, **56**, 1108–1117 (1975)
289. Miettinen, T.A. Cholesterol production of obesity. *Circulation*, **44**, 842–850 (1971)
290. Nestel, P.J., Schreibman, P.H. and Ahrens, E.H. Cholesterol metabolism in human obesity. *J Clin. Invest.*, **52**, 2389–2397 (1973)
291. Olefsky, J., Crapo, P.A., Ginsberg, H. and Reaven, G.M. Metabolic effects of increased caloric intake in man. *Metabolism*, **24**, 495–503 (1975)
292. Heiss, G., Johnson, N.J., Reiland, S., Davis, C.E. and Tyroler, H.A. The epidemiology of plasma high-density lipoprotein cholesterol levels: The Lipid Research Clinics Program Prevalence Study Summary. *Circulation*, **62** (Suppl. IV), 116–135 (1980)
293. Katan, M.B . Diet and HDL. In *Clinical and Metabolic Aspects of High-Density Lipoproteins* (eds N.E. Miller and G.J. Miller), Elsevier, Amsterdam, pp. 103–131 (1984)
294. Contaldo, F., Strazzullo, P., Postiglione, A., Riccardi, G., Patti, L. *et al.* Plasma high density lipoprotein in severe obesity after stable weight loss. *Atherosclerosis*, **37**, 163–167 (1980)
295. Streja, D.A., Boyko, E. and Rabkin, S.W. Changes in plasma high-density lipoprotein cholesterol concentration after weight reduction in grossly obese subjects. *Br. Med. J.*, **28**, 770–772 (1980)
296. Garrow, J.S. Treatment of obesity. *Lancet*, **340**, 409–413 (1992)
297. Bai, T.R., Webb, D. and Hamilton, M. Treatment of hypertension with beta-adrenoceptor blocking drugs. *J. R. Coll. Phys. Lond.*, **16**, 239–241 (1982)
298. Wolfe, B.M., Havel, R.J., Marliss, E.B., Kane, J.P., Seymour, J. and Ajhuja, S.P. Effects of a three-day fast and of ethanol on splanchnic metabolism of free fatty acids, amino acids and carbohydrates in healthy young men. *J. Clin. Invest.*, **57**, 329–340 (1976)
299. Hawkins, R.D. and Kalant, H. The metabolism of ethanol and its metabolic effects. *Pharmacol. Rev.*, **24**, 67–157 (1972)
300. Hawkins, J.D. and Foster, D.W. Hormonal control of ketogenesis: biochemical considerations. *Arch. Intern. Med.*, **137**, 495–501 (1977)
301. Cooperman, M.T., Davidoff, F., Spark, R.S. and Pallota, J. Clinical studies of alcoholic keto-acidosis. *Diabetes*, **23**, 433–439 (1974)
302. Talbott, G.D. and Keating, B.M. Effect of preprandial whiskey on post-alimentary lipemia. *Geriatrics*, **17**, 802–808 (1962)
303. Barboriak, J.J. and Meade, R.C. Enhancement of alimentary lipaemia by preprandial alcohol. *Am. J. Med. Sci.*, **225**, 245–251 (1968)
304. Wilson, D.E., Schriebman, P.H., Brewster, A.C. and Arky, R.A. The enhancement of alimentary lipemia by ethanol in man. *J. Lab. Clin. Med.*, **75**, 264–274 (1970)
305. Barboriak, J.J. and Hogan, W.J. Preprandial drinking and plasma lipids in man. *Atherosclerosis*, **24**, 323–325 (1976)
306. Mistilis, S.P. and Ockner, R.K. Effect of ethanol on endogenous lipid and lipoprotein metabolism in small intestine. *J. Lab. Clin. Med.*, **80**, 34–46 (1972)
307. Barona, E., Pirola, R.C. and Leiber, C.S. Pathogenesis of post-prandial hyperlipemia in rats fed ethanol-containing diets. *J. Clin. Invest.*, **52**, 296–303 (1973)
308. Taskinen, M.-R., Nikkila, E.A., Valimaki, M., Sane, T., Kuusi, T., Kesaniemi, A. and Ulikahri, R. Alcohol-induced changes in serum lipoproteins and in their metabolism. *Am. Heart J.*, **113**, 458–464 (1987)
309. Belfrage, P., Berg, B., Hagerstrand, I., Nilsson-Ehle, P., Tornqvist, H. and Wiebe, T. Alterations of lipid metabolism in healthy volunteers during long-term ethanol intake. *Eur. J. Clin. Invest.*, **7**, 127–131 (1977)

310. Eckman, R., Fex, G., Johansson, B.G., Nilsson-Ehle, P. and Wadstein, J. Changes in plasma high density lipoproteins and lipolytic enzymes after long-term, heavy ethanol consumption. *Scand. J. Clin. Lab. Invest.*, **41**, 709–715 (1981)

311. Taskinen, M.-R., Valimaki, M., Nikkila, E.A., Kuusi, T., Ehnholm, C. and Ylikahri, R. High density lipoprotein subfractions and postheparin plasma lipases in alcoholic men before and after ethanol withdrawal. *Metabolism*, **31**, 1168–1174 (1982)

312. Schnieder, J., Liesenfeld, A., Mordasini, R., Schubatz, R., Zofel, P. *et al*. Lipoprotein fractions, lipoprotein lipase and hepatic triglyceride lipase during short-term and long-term uptake of ethanol in healthy subjects. *Atherosclerosis*, **57**, 281–291 (1985)

313. Valamiki, M., Nikkila, E.A., Taskinen, M.-R. and Ylikahri, R. Rapid decrease in high density lipoprotein subfractions and postheparin lipase activities after cessation of chronic alcohol intake. *Atherosclerosis*, **59**, 147–153 (1986)

314. Chait, A., Mancini, M., February, A.W. and Lewis, B. Clinical and metabolic study of alcoholic hyperlipidaemia. *Lancet*, **ii**, 62–63 (1972)

315. Durrington, P.N., Twentyman, O.P., Braganza, J.M. and Miller, J.P. Hypertriglyceridaemia and abnormalities of triglyceride metabolism persisting after pancreatitis. *Int. J. Pancreatol.*, **1**, 195–203 (1986)

316. Ernst, N., Fisher, M., Smith, W., Gordon, T., Rifkind, B.M. *et al*. The association of plasma high-density lipoprotein cholesterol with dietary intake and alcohol consumption. The Lipid Research Clinics Program Prevalence Study. *Circulation*, **62** (Suppl. IV), 41–52 (1980)

317. Razay, G., Heaton, K.W., Bolton, C.H. and Hughes, A.O. Alcohol consumption and its relation to cardiovascular risk factors in British women. *Br. Med. J.*, **304**, 80–83 (1992)

318. Durrington, P.N. Effect of phenobarbitone on plasma apolipoprotein B and plasma high-density-lipoprotein cholesterol in normal subjects. *Clin. Sci.*, **56**, 501–504 (1979)

319. Luoma, P.V., Sotaniemi, E.A., Pelkonen, R.O. and Ehnholm, C. High density lipoproteins and hepatic microsomal enzyme induction in alcohol consumers. *Res. Commun. Chem. Pathol. Pharmacol.*, **37**, 91–96 (1982)

320. Whitehead, R.T., Clarke, C.A. and Whitfield, A.G.W. Biochemical and haematological markers of alcohol intake. *Lancet*, **i**, 978–979 (1978)

321. Martin, P.J., Martin, J.V. and Goldberg, D.M. Gamma-glutamyl transpeptidase, triglycerides and enzyme induction. *Br. Med. J.*, **i**, 17–18 (1975)

322. Binkley, F., Wieseman, M.L., Groth, D.P. and Powell, R.W. Gamma-glutamyl transferase. A secretory enzyme. *FEBS Letts*, **51**, 168–170 (1975)

323. Klatsky, A.L., Friedman, G.D. and Siegelamb, A.G. Alcohol consumption before myocardial infarction. Results from the Kaiser-Permanente epidemiological study of myocardial infarction. *Ann. Intern. Med.*, **81**, 294–301 (1974)

324. Stason, W.B., Neff, R.K., Miettinen, O.S. and Jick, H. Alcohol consumption and non-fatal myocardial infarction. *Am. J. Epidemiol.*, **104**, 603–608 (1976)

325. Marmot, M.G., Rose, G., Shipley, M.J. and Thomas, B.J. Alcohol and mortality: a U-shaped curve. *Lancet*, **i**, 580–583 (1981)

326. Stampfer, M.J., Colditz, G.A., Willet, W.C., Speizer, F.E. and Hennekens, C.H. A prospective study of moderate alcohol consumption and the risk of coronary disease and stroke in women. *N. Engl. J. Med.*, **319**, 267–273 (1988)

327. Boffelta, P. and Garfinkel, L. Alcohol drinking and mortality amongst men enrolled in an American Cancer Society prospective study. *Epidemiol.*, **1**, 342–348 (1990)

328. Lazarus, N.B., Kaplan, G.A., Cohen, R.D., Len, D-J. Change in alcohol consumption and risk of death from all causes and from ischaemic heart disease. *Br. Med. J.*, **303**, 553–556 (1991)

329. Hegsted, D.M. and Ausman, L.M. Diet, alcohol and coronary heart disease in men. *J. Nutr.*, **188**, 1184–1189 (1988)

330. Katan, M.B. Diet and HDL. In Clinical and Metabolic Aspects of High-Density Lipoproteins (eds N.E. Miller and G.J. Miller), Elsevier, Amsterdam, pp. 103–131 (1984)

331. Klinefelter, H.F. Hypercholesterolaemia in anorexia nervosa. *J. Clin. Endocrinol. Metabol.*, **25**, 1520–1521 (1965)

332. Crisp, A.H., Blendis, L.M. and Pawan, G.L.S. Aspects of fat metabolism in anorexia nervosa. *Metabolism*, **17**, 1109–1118 (1968)

333. Mattingly, D. and Bhanji, S. The diagnosis of anorexia nervosa. *J. R. Coll. Phys. Lond.*, **16**, 191–194 (1982)
334. Nestel, P.J. Cholesterol metabolism in anorexia nervosa and hypercholesterolaemia. *J. Clin. Endocrinol. Metabol.*, **38**, 325–328 (1974)
335. Miller, J.P. Dyslipoproteinaemia of liver disease. *Balliere's Clin. Endocrinol. Metabol.*, **4**, 807–832 (1990)
336. Miller J.P., Liver disease. In *Lipoproteins in Health and Disease* (eds D.J. Betteridge, D.R. Illingworth and J. Shepherd), Edward Arnonld, London (in press)
337. Ahrens, E.H. and Kunkel, H.G. The relationship between serum lipids and skin xanthomata in eighteen patients with primary biliary cirrhosis. *J. Clin. Invest.*, **28**, 1565–1574 (1949)
338. Jensen, J. The story of xanthomatosis in England prior to the First World War. *Clio. Medica*, **2**, 289–305 (1967)
339. Thomas, P.K. and Walker, J.G. Xanthomatous neuropathy in primary biliary cirrhosis. *Brain*, **88**, 1079–1088 (1965)
340. MacIntyre, N., Harry, D.S. and Pearson, A.J.G. The hypercholesterolaemia of obstructive jaundice. *Gut*, **16**, 379–391 (1975)
341. Seidel, D. Dyslipoproteinaemia in liver disease. In *Diabetes, Obesity and Hyperlipidaemias*, vol. 11 (eds G. Crepaldi, P.J. LeFebre and D.J. Galton), Academic Press, London, pp. 63–71 (1983)
342. Sabesin, S.M., Bertram, P.D. and Freeman, M.R. Lipoprotein metabolism in liver disease. *Adv. Intern. Med.*, **25**, 117–149 (1980)
343. McIntyre, N. Plasma lipids and lipoproteins in liver disease. *Gut*, **19**, 526–530 (1978)
344. Manzato, E., Fellin, G., Baggio, G., Walch, S., Neubeck, W. and Seidel, D. Formation of lipoprotein-X. Its relationship to bile compounds. *J. Clin. Invest.*, 1248–1260 (1976)
345. Byers, S.O. and Friedman, M. Probable sources of plasma cholesterol during phosphatide induced hypercholesterolaemia. *Lipids*, **4**, 123–128 (1969)
346. Walli, A.K. and Seidel, D. Role of lipoprotein-X in the pathogenesis of cholestatic hypercholesterolaemia. Uptake of lipoprotein-X and its effect on 3-hydroxy-3-methylglutaryl coenzyme A reductase and chylomicron remnant removal in human fibroblasts, lymphocytes, and in the rat. *J. Clin. Invest.*, **74**, 867–879 (1984)
347. Kostner, G.M., Laggner, P., Prexl, H.J., Holasek, A., Ingolic, E. and Geymayer, W. Investigations of the abnormal low-density lipoproteins occurring in patients with obstructive jaundice. *Biochem. J.*, **157**, 401–407 (1976)
348. Muller, P., Fellin, R. and Lambrecht, J. Hypertriglyceridaemia secondary to liver disease. *Eur. J. Clin. Invest.*, **4**, 419–428 (1974)
349. Seidel, D. Lipoproteins in liver disease. In *European Lipoprotein Club: The First Ten Years*, Department of Biochemistry, Glasgow Royal Infirmary, pp. 121–126 (1987)
350. Danilesson, B., Eckman, R., Johansson, B.G., Nilsson-Ehle, P. and Petersson, B.G. Lipoproteins in plasma from patients with low LCAT activity due to biliary obstruction. *Scand. J. Clin. Lab. Invest.*, **38** (Suppl. 150), 214–217 (1978)
351. Desai, K., Mistry, P., Bagget, C. *et al.* Inhibition of platelet aggregation by abnormal high density lipoprotein particles in plasma from patients with hepatic cirrhosis. *Lancet*, **i**, 693–695 (1989)
352. Schaffner, S. Paradoxical elevation of serum cholesterol by clofibrate in patients with primary biliary cirrhosis. *Gastroenterology*, **57**, 253–255 (1969)
353. Poupan, R.E., Ouguerram, K., Chretien, Y. *et al.* Cholesterol-lowering effect of ursodeoxycholic acid in patients with primary biliary cirrhosis. *Hepatology*, **17**, 577–582 (1993)
354. van Buuren, H.R., Baggen, M.G.A., Wilson, J.H.P. and Grundy, S.M. Letters to *N. Engl. J. Med.*, **319**, 1223 (1988)
355. Turnberg, L.A., Mahoney, M.P., Gleeson, M.H., Freeman, C.B. and Gowenlock, A.H. Plasmapheresis and plasma exchange in the treatment of hyperlipaemia and xanthomatous neuropathy in patients with primary biliary cirrhosis. *Gut*, **13**, 976–981 (1972)
356. Crippen, J.S., Linder, K.D., Jorgensen, R. *et al.* Hypercholesterolaemia and atherosclerosis in primary biliary cirrhosis: what is the risk? *Hepatology*, **15**, 858–862 (1992)
357. Muller, P., Fellin, R., Lambrecht, J. Agostini, B., Wieland, H. *et al.* Hypertriglyceridaemia secondary to liver disease. *Eur. J. Clin. Invest.*, **4**, 419–428 (1974)

358. Sabesin, S.M., Hawkins, H.L., Kuiken, L. and Radand, J.B. Abnormal plasma lipoproteins and lecithin-cholesterol acyltransferase deficiency in alcoholic liver disease. *Gastroenterology*, **72**, 510–518 (1977)

359. Nestel, P.J., Tada, N. and Fidge, N.H. Increased catabolism of high density lipoprotein in alcoholic hepatitis. *Metabolism*, **29**, 101–104 (1980)

360. Freeman, M., Kuiken, L., Radand, J.B. *et al.* Hepatic triglyceride lipase deficiency in liver disease. *Lipids*, **12**, 443 (1974)

361. Sauar, J., Bolmhoff, J.P. and Gjone, E. Triglyceride lipase in acute hepatitis. *Clin. Chim. Acta*, **71**, 403–411 (1976)

362. Freely, J., Barry, M., Kccling, P.W.N., Weir, D.G. and Cooke, T. Lipoprotein (a) in cirrhosis. *Br. Med. J.*, **304**, 545–546 (1992)

363. Einarsson, K., Hellstrom, K. and Kallner, M. Gallbladder disease in hyperlipoproteinaemia. *Lancet*, **i**, 484–487 (1975)

364. Ahlberg, J., Angelin, B., Einarsson, K., Hellstrom, K. and Leijd, B. Biliary lipid composition in normo- and hyperlipoproteinaemia. *Gastroenterology*, **79**, 90–94 (1980)

365. Thornton, J.R., Heaton, K.W. and MacFarland, D.G.A Relation between high-density lipoprotein cholesterol and bile saturation. *Br. Med. J.*, **283**, 1352–1354 (1981)

366. Schwartz, C.E., Halloran, L.G., Vlahcevic, Z.R., Gregory, D.H. and Swell, L. Preferential utilization of free cholesterol from high-density lipoprotein for biliary cholesterol secretion in men. *Science*, **200**, 62–64 (1978)

367. Alpert, M.E., Hutt, M.S.R. and Davidson, C.S. Primary hepatoma in Uganda. A prospective clinical and epidemiological study of forty-six patients. *Am. J. Med.*, **46**, 794–802 (1969)

368. Kirayama, C. and Irisa, T. Serum cholesterol and bile acids in primary hepatoma. *Clin. Chim. Acta*, **71**, 21–25 (1976)

369. Siperstein, M.D., Fagan, M.S.R. and Morris, H.P. Further studies on the deletion of the cholesterol feedback system in hepatomas. *Cancer Res.*, **26**, 7–11 (1966)

370. Lees, R.S., Song, C.L., Lever, R.D. and Kappas, A. Hyperbetalipoproteinaemia in acute intermittent porphyria. *N. Engl. J. Med.*, **282**, 432–433 (1970)

371. Short, C.D. and Durrington, P.N. Hyperlipidaemia and renal disease. *Balliere's Clin. Endocrinol. Metabol.*, **4**, 777–806 (1990)

372. Short, C.D. and Durrington, P.N. Lipids and lipoproteins in renal disorders. In *Lipoproteins in Health and Disease* (eds D.J. Betteridge, D.R. Illingworth and J. Shepherd), Edward Arnold, London (in press)

373. Newmark, S.R., Anderson, C.F., Donadio, J.V. and Ellefson, R.D. Lipoprotein profiles in adult nephrotics. *Mayo Clin. Proc.*, **50**, 359–364 (1975)

374. Short, C., Durrington, P.N., Mallick, N., Bhatnagar, D., Hunt, L.P. and MBewu, A.D. Serum lipoprotein (a) in men with proteinuria due to idiopathic membranous nephropathy. *Nephrol., Dial. Transplant.*, (Suppl. 1), 109–113 (1992)

375. Karadi, I., Romics, L., Palos, G., Doman, J., Kaszas, I. *et al.* Lipoprotein (a) lipoprotein concentrations in serum of patients with heavy proteinuria of different origin. *Clin. Chem.*, **35**, 2121–2123 (1989)

376. Thomas, M.E., Freestone, A., Varghese, Z., Parsand, J.W. and Moorhead, J.F. Lipoprotein (a) in patients with proteinuria. *Nephrol. Dial. Transplant.*, **7**, 597–601 (1992)

377. Davis, R.A., Engelhorn, S.C., Weinstein, D.B. and Steinberg, D. Very low density lipoprotein secretion of cultured rat hepatocytes. Inhibition by albumin and other macromolecules. *J. Biol. Chem.*, **255**, 2039–2045 (1980)

378. Yedgar, S., Weinstein, D.B., Patsch W., Schonfeld, G., Casanada, F.E. and Steinberg, D. Viscosity of culture medium as a regulator of synthesis and secretion of very low density lipoproteins by cultured hepatocytes. *J. Biol. Chem.*, **257**, 2188–2192 (1982)

379. Kekki, M. and Nikkila, E.A. Plasma triglyceride metabolism in the adult nephrotic syndrome. *Eur. J. Clin. Invest.*, **1**, 345–351 (1971)

380. Appel, G.B., Blum, C.B., Chien, S., Kunis, C L. and Appel, A.S. The hyperlipidaemia of nephrotic syndrome. Relation to plasma albumin concentration, oncotic pressure, and viscosity. *N. Engl. J. Med.*, **312**, 1544–1548 (1985)

381. Waldmann, T.A., Gordon, R.S. and Rosse, W. Studies on the metabolism of serum proteins and lipids in a patient with analbuminaemia. *Am. J. Med.*, **37**, 960–968 (1964)

382. Baxter, J.H., Goodman, H.C. and Allen, J.C. Effects of infusions of serum albumin on serum lipids and lipoproteins in nephrosis. *J. Clin. Invest.*, **40**, 490–498 (1961)

383. Muls, E., Rosseneu, M., Daneels, R., Schurgers, M. and Boelaert, J. Lipoprotein distribution and composition in the human nephrotic syndrome. *Atherosclerosis*, **54**, 225–237 (1985)

384. Vega, G.L. and Grundy, S.M. Lovastatin therapy in nephrotic hyperlipidaemia: effects on lipoprotein metabolism. *Kidney Intern.*, **33**, 1060–1068 (1988)

385. Joven, J., Villabona, C., Vilella, E., Masana, L., Alberti, R. and Valles, M. Abnormalities of lipoprotein metabolism in patients with nephrotic syndrome. *N. Engl. J. Med.*, **323**, 579–584 (1990)

386. Warwick, G.L., Caslake, M.J., Boulton-Jones, J.M., Dagen, M., Packard, C.J. and Shepherd, J. Low density lipoprotein metabolism in the nephrotic syndrome. *Metabolism*, **39**, 187–192 (1990)

387. Yamada, M. and Matsuda, I. Lipoprotein lipase in clinical and experimental nephrosis. *Clin. Chim. Acta*, **30**, 787–794 (1970)

388. Kashyap, M.L., Srivastava, L.S., Hynd, B.A., Brady, D., Perisutti, G. *et al.* Apolipoprotein C11 and lipoprotein lipase in human nephrotic syndrome. *Atherosclerosis*, **35**, 29–40 (1980)

389. Gherardi, E., Rota, E., Calandra, S., Genova, R. and Tamborino, A. Relationship among the concentrations of serum lipoproteins and changes in their chemical composition in patients with untreated nephrotic syndrome. *Eur. J. Clin. Invest.*, **7**, 563–570 (1977)

390. Wass, V.J., Jarrett, R.J., Chilvers, C. and Cameron, J.S. Does the nephrotic syndrome increase the risk of cardiovascular disease? *Lancet*, **ii**, 664–667 (1979)

391. Mallick, N.P. and Short, C.D. The nephrotic syndrome and ischaemic heart disease. *Nephron*, **27**, 54–57 (1981)

392. d'Amico, G., Gentile, M.G., Manna, G., Fellin, G., Ciceri, R. *et al.* Effect of vegetarian soy diet on hyperlipidaemia in nephrotic syndrome. *Lancet*, **339**, 1131–1134 (1992)

393. Bridgman, J.F., Rosen, S.M. and Thorp, J.M. Complications during clofibrate treatment of nephrotic syndrome. *Lancet*, **ii**, 506–509 (1972)

394. Groggel, G.C., Cheung, A.K., Ellis-Benigni, K. and Wilson, D.E. Treatment of nephrotic syndrome with gemfibrozil. *Kidney Intern.*, **36**, 266–271 (1989)

394a. Bridgman, J. F., Rosen, S. M. and Thorp, J. M. Complications during clofibrate treatment of nephrotic syndrome. *Lancet*, **ii**, 506–509 (1972)

395. Rabelink, A.J., Hene, R.J., Erkelens, D.W., Joles, J.A. and Koomans, K.A. Effects of simvastatin and cholestyramine on lipoprotein profile in hyperlipidaemia of nephrotic syndrome. *Lancet*, **ii**, 1335–1338 (1988)

396. Golper, T.A., Illingworth, D.R., Morris, C.D. and Bennett, W.M. Lovastatin in the treatment of multifactorial hyperlipidaemia associated with proteinuria. *Am. J. Kidney Dis.*, **13**, 312–320 (1989)

397. Chan, P.C.K., Robinson, J.D., Yeung, W.C., Cheng, I.K.P., Yeung, H.W.D. and Tsang, M.T.S. Lovastatin in glomerulonephritis patients with hyperlipidaemia and heavy proteinuria. *Nephrol. Dial. Transplant.*, **7**, 93–99 (1992)

398. Warwick, G.L., Packard, C.J., Murray, L., Grierson, D., Stewart, J.P. *et al.* Effect of simvastatin on plasma lipid and lipoprotein concentrations and low-density lipoprotein metabolism in the nephrotic syndrome. *Clin. Sci.*, **82**, 701–708 (1992)

399. Chan, M.K., Varghese, Z. and Moorhead, J.F. Lipid abnormalities in uremia, dialysis, and transplantation. *Kidney Int.*, **19**, 625–637 (1981)

400. Akmal, M., Kasim, S.E. and Soliman, A.R., Massry Excess parathyroid hormone adversely affects lipid metabolism in chronic renal failure. *Kidney Int.*, **37**, 854–858 (1990)

401. Fuh, M.M.T., Lee, C-M., Jeng, C-Y., Shen D-C., Sheieh, S-M. *et al.* Effect of chronic renal failure on high-density lipoprotein kinetics. *Kidney Int.*, **37**, 1295–1300 (1990)

402. Rapoport, J., Aviram, M., Chaimovitz, C. and Brook, J.G. Defective high-density lipoprotein composition in patients on chronic haemodialysis. A possible mechanism for accelerated atherosclerosis. *N. Engl. J. Med.*, **299**, 1326–1329 (1978)

403. Nestel, P. J., Fidge, N. H. and Tan, M. H. Increased lipoprotein remnant formation in chronic renal failure. *N. Engl. J. Med.*, **307**, 329–333 (1982)

404. Sniderman, A., Cianflone, K., Kwiterovich, P.O., Hutchinson, T., Barre, P. and Prichard, S. Hyperapobetalipoproteinaemia. The major dyslipoproteinaemia in patients with chronic renal failure treated with chronic ambulatory peritoneal dialysis. *Atherosclerosis*, **65**, 257–264 (1987)

405. Nicholls, A.J., Cumming, A.M., Catto, G.R.D., Edward, N. and Engest, J. Lipid relationships in dialysis and renal transplant patients. *Q. J. Med.*, new ser., **L**, 149–160 (1981)
406. Gebhardt, D.O.E., Schicht, I.M. and Paul, L.C. The immunochemical determination of apolipoprotein A, total apolipoprotein A-l and 'free' apolipoprotein A-1 in serum of patients on chronic haemodialysis. *Ann. Clin. Biochem.*, **21**, 301–305 (1984)
407. Neary, R.H. and Gowland, E. The effect of renal failure and haemodialysis on the concentrations of free apolipoprotein A-1 in serum and the implications for the catabolism of high-density lipoproteins. *Clin. Chim. Acta*, **171**, 239–246 (1988)
408. Segal, P., Gidez, L.I., Vega, G., Edelstein, D., Eder, H.A. and Roheim, P.S. Apoprotein of high density lipoproteins in the urine of normal subjects. *J. Lipid Res.*, **20**, 784–788 (1979)
409. McLeod, R., Reeve, C. E. and Frohlick, J. Plasma lipoproteins and lecithin: cholesterol acyltransferase distribution in patients on dialysis. *Kidney Int.*, **25**, 683–688 (1984)
410. Chan, M.K., Ramidial, L., Varghese, Z., Persand, J.W., Fernando, O.N. and Moorhead, J.F. Plasma LCAT activities in renal allograft recipients. *Clin. Chim. Acta*, **124**, 187–193 (1982)
411. Beaumont, J.E., Galla, J.H., Luke, R.G., Rees, E.D. and Siegel, R.R. Normal serum lipids in renal-transplant patients. *Lancet*, **i**, 599–601 (1975)
412. Gokal, R., Mann, J.I., Moore, R.A. and Horns, P.J. Hyperlipidaemia following renal transplantation. *Q. J. Med.*, **192**, 507–517 (1979)
413. Kasiske, B.L. and Umen, A.J. Persistent hyperlipidaemia in renal transplant patients. *Medicine*, **66**, 309–316 (1987)
414. Crawford, G.A., Sardie, E. and Stewart, J.H. Heparin-released plasma lipases in chronic renal failure and after renal transplantation. *Clin. Sci.*, **57**, 155–165 (1979)
415. Editorial. Hyperlipidaemia after renal transplantation. *Lancet*, **i**, 919–920 (1988)
416. Kandoussi, A., Cachera, C., Pagniez, D., Dracon, M., Fruchart, J.C. and Tacquat, A. Plasma level of lipoprotein (a) is high in pre-dialysis or haemodialyis but not in CAPD. *Kidney Int.*, **42**, 424–425 (1992)
417. Anwar, N., Bhatnagar, D., Short, C.D., Mackness, M.I., Durrington, P.N., Prais, H. and Gokal, R. Serum lipoprotein (a) in patients undergoing continuous ambulatory peritoneal dialysis. *Nephrol. Dial. Transplant.*, **8**, 71–74 (1993)
418. Barbagallo, C.M., Avena, M.R., Scafidi, V., Galione, A. and Notarbartolo, A. Increased lipoprotein (a) levels in subjects with chronic renal failure on haemodialysis. *Nephron*, **62**, 471–472 (1992)
419. Murphy, B.G. and McNamee, P.T. Apolipoprotein (a) concentrations decrease following renal transplantation. *Nephrol. Dial. Transplant.*, **7**, 174–175 (1992)
420. Shoji, T., Nishizawa, Y., Nishitani, H., Yamakawa, M. and Morii, H. High serum lipoprotein (a) concentrations in uraemic patients treated with CAPD. *Clin. Nephrol.*, **38**, 271–276 (1992)
421. Haffner, S.M., Gruber, K.K., Aldrete, G., Morales, P.A., Stern, M.P. and Tuttle, K.R. Increased lipoprotein (a) concentrations in chronic renal failure. *J. Am. Soc. Nephrol.*, **3**, 1156–1162 (1992)
422. Brown, J.H., Anwar, N., Short, C.D., Bhatnagar, D., Mackness, M.I., Hunt, L.P. and Durrington, P.N. Lipoprotein (a) level in renal transplant recipients receiving cyclosporin monotherapy. *Nephrol. Dial. Transplant.*, **8**, 863–876 (1993)
423. Black, I.W. and Wilcken, D.E.L. Decreases in apolipoprotein (a) after renal transplantation: implications for lipoprotein (a) metabolism. *Clin. Chem.*, **38**, 353–357 (1992)
424. Webb, A.T., Plant, M., Reaveley, D.A., O'Donnell, M., Luck, V.A. *et al.* Lipid and lipoprotein (a) concentrations in renal transplant patients. *Nephrol. Transplant. Dial.*, **7**, 636–641 (1992)
425. Heimann, P., Josephson, M.A., Fellner, S.K., Thistlewante, R.J., Stuart, F.P. and Dasgupta, A. Elevated lipoprotein (a) levels in renal transplantation and hemodialysis patients. *Am. J. Nephrol.*, **11**, 470–474 (1991)
426. Barbir, M., Khushwaha, S., Hunt, B., Macken, A., Thompson, G.R. *et al.* Lipoprotein (a) and accelerated coronary arterial disease in cardiac transplant recipients. *Lancet*, **340**, 1500–1501 (1992)
427. Wing, A.J., Brunner, F.P., Brynger, H., Jacobs, C., Kramer, P., Selwood, N.H., Gretz, N. Cardiovascular-related causes of death and the fate of patients with cardiovascular disease. *Contr. Nephrol.*, **41**, 306–311 (1984)
428. Gokal, R., Mann, J.I., Oliver, D.O. and Ledingham, J.G.G. Dietary treatment of hyperlipidaemia in chronic haemodialysis patients. *Am. J. Clin. Nutr.*, **31**, 1915–1918 (1978)

429. Moorhead, J.F., Chan, M.K., El-Nahas, M. and Varghese, Z. Lipid nephrotoxicity in chronic progressive glomerular and tubulo-interstitial disease. *Lancet*, **ii**, 1309–1311 (1982)

430. Manninen, V., Malkonen, M. and Eisalo, A. Gemfibrozil treatment of dyslipidaemia in renal failure with uraemia or in the nephrotic syndrome. *Res. Clin. Forum*, **4**, 113–117 (1982)

431. Pasternack, A., Vanttinen, T., Solakiri, T., Kuusi, T. and Korte, T. Normalisation of lipoprotein lipase and hepatic lipase by gemfibrozil results in correction of lipoprotein abnormalities in chronic renal failure. *Clin. Nephrol.*, **27**, 163–168 (1987)

432. Chan, M.K. 1989 Gemfibrozil improves abnormalities of lipid metabolism in patients on CAPD. *Metabolism*, **38**, 939–945 (1989)

433. Pelegri, A., Romero, R., Serti, M., Nogues, X., Pedro-Botet, J. and Rubies-Prat, J. Effect of bezafibrate on lipoprotein (a) and triglyceride-rich lipoproteins, including intermediate-density lipoproteins, in patients with chronic renal failure receiving haemodialysis. *Nephrol. Dial. Transplant.*, **7**, 623–626 (1992)

434. Wanner, C., Lubrich-Birkner, I., Summ, O., Widard, H. and Schollmeyer, P. Effect of simvastatin on qualitative and quantitative changes of lipoprotein metabolism in CAPD patients. *Nephron*, **62**, 40–46 (1992)

435. Henkin, Y., Como, J.A. and Oberman, A. Secondary dyslipidaemia: inadvertent effects of drugs in clinical practice. *J. Am. Med. Assoc.*, **267**, 961–968 (1992)

436. Jackson, R. Which hypertensive patients should be treated? *Lancet*, **343**, 496–497 (1994)

437. Medical Research Council Working Party. MRC trial of treatment of mild hypertension. Principal results. *Br. Med. J.*, **291**, 97–104 (1985)

438. Swales, J.D. First line treatment in hypertension. Still β-blockers and diuretics. *Br. Med. J.*, **301**, 1172–1173 (1990)

439. Grimm, R.H. and Hunninghake, D.B. Lipids and hypertension. Implications of new guidelines for cholesterol management in the treatment of hypertension. *Am. J. Med.*, **80** (Suppl. 2A), 56–63 (1986)

440. Leren, P., Eide, I., Foss, P.O., Helgeland, A., Hjermann, I. *et al.* Antihypertensive drugs and blood lipids. The Oslo Study. *J. Cardiovasc. Pharmacol.*, **3** (Suppl. 3), 5187–5192 (1981)

441. Van Brummelen, P. The relevance of intrinsic sympathomimetic activity for β-blocker induced changes in plasma lipids. *J. Cardiovasc. Pharmacol.*, **5** (Suppl. 1), 551–555 (1983)

442. Ames, R.P. The effect of antihypertensive drugs on serum lipids and lipoproteins: II Non-diuretic drugs. *Drugs*, **32**, 335–357 (1986)

443. Lithell, H. Hypertension and hyperlipidaemia. A review. *Am. J. Hypertension*, **6**, (Suppl.) 303S 308S (1993)

444. Krone, W. and Nagele, H. Effect of antihypertensives on plasma lipids and lipoprotein metabolism. *Am. Heart J.*, **116**, 1729–1734 (1988)

445. Johnson, B.F. and Danylchuk, M.A. The relevance of plasma lipid changes with cardiovascular drug therapy. *Med. Clin. North Am.*, **73**, 449–473 (1989)

446. Durrington, P.N., Brownlee, W.C. and Large, D.M. Short-term effects of β-adrenoceptor blocking drugs with and without cardioselectivity and intrinsic sympathomimetic activity on lipoprotein metabolism in hypertriglyceridaemic patients and in normal men. *Clin. Sci.*, **69**, 713–719 (1985)

447. Durrington P.N. and Cairns, S.A. Acute pancreatitis. A complication of beta-blockade. *Br. Med. J.*, **284**, 1016 (1982)

448. Day, J.L., Metcalfe, J. and Simpson, C.N. Adrenergic mechanisms in control of plasma lipid concentrations. *Br. Med. J.*, **284**, 1145–1148 (1982)

449. Murphy, M.B., Sugrue, D., Trayner, I., Kaufman, S., Yasuhara, H. *et al.* Effect of short term beta adrenoceptor blockade on serum lipids and lipoproteins in patients with hypertension or coronary heart disease. *Br. Med. J.*, **51**, 589–594 (1984)

450. Peden, N.R., Dow, R.H., Isles, T.E. and Martin, B.T. Adrenoreceptor blockade and response of serum lipids to a meal and to exercise. *Br. Med. J.*, **288**, 1788–1790 (1984)

451. Fogari, R., Zoppi, A., Pasotti, Poletti, L., Tettamanti, F., Malamani, G. and Corradi, L. Plasma lipids during chronic antihypertensive therapy with different β-blockers. *J. Cardiovasc. Pharmacol.*, **14** (Suppl. 7) S28–S32 (1989)

452. Dujovne, C.A., Eff, J., Ferraro, L., Goldstein, R.J., Gotto, A.M. *et al.* Comparative effects of atenolol versus caliprolol on serum lipids and blood pressure in hyperlipidaemic and hypertensive subjects. *Am. J. Cardiol.*, **72**, 1131–1136 (1993)

453. Ames, R.P. The effects of antihypertensive drugs on serum lipids and lipoproteins. 1. *Diuretics Drugs*, **32**, 260–278 (1986)
454. Landmark, K. Antihypertensive and metabolic effects of long-term therapy with nifedipine slow-release tablets. *J. Cardiovasc. Pharmacol.*, **7**, 12–17 (1985)
455. Zusman, R., Christensen, D., Federman, E., Kochar, M. S., McCarron, D. *et al*. Comparison of nifedipine and propranolol used in combination with diuretics for the treatment of hypertension. *Am. J. Med.*, **82** (Suppl. 3B), 37–41 (1987)
456. Sasaki, J. and Araka va, K. Effect of nifedipine on serum lipids, lipoproteins, and apolipoproteins in patients with essential hypertension. *Curr. Ther. Res.*, **41**, 845–851 (1987)
457. Vessey, M.P. and Doll, R. Investigation of the relation between use of oral contraceptives and thromboembolic disease. *Br. Med. J.*, **2**, 199–205 (1968)
458. Sartwell, P.E., Masi, A.T., Arthes, F.G., Greene, G.R. and Smith, H.E. Thromboembolism and oral contraceptives. An epidemiologic case-control study. *Am. J. Epidemiol.*, **90**, 365–380 (1969)
459. Inman, W.H.W., Vessey, M.P., Westerholm, B. and Engelind, A. Thromboembolic disease and the steroidal content of oral contraceptives. A report to the Committee on Safety of Drugs. *Br. Med. J.*, **2**, 203–209 (1970)
460. Coope, J., Thompson, J.M. and Poller, L. Effects of 'natural oestrogen' replacement therapy on menopausal symptoms and blood clotting. *Br. Med. J.*, **iv**, 139–143 (1975)
461. Bonnar, J., Hadden, M., Hunter, D.H., Richards, D.H. and Thornton, C. Coagulation system changes in postmenopausal women receiving oestrogen preparations. *Postgrad. Med. J.*, **52**, (Suppl. 6), 30–44 (1976)
462. Blackard, C.E., Doe, R.P., Mellinger, G.T. and Byar, D.P. Incidence of cardiovascular disease and death in patients receiving diethylstilbestrol for carcinoma of the prostrate. *Cancer*, **26**, 249–256 (1970)
463. Coronary Drug Project Research Group. The Coronary Drug Project. Findings leading to discontinuation of the 2.5 mg/day estrogen group. *J. Am. Med. Assoc.*, **226**, 652–657 (1973)
464. Wynn, V. Adverse metabolic effects of oral contraceptives. In *Myocardial Infarction in Women* (eds M.F. Oliver, A. Vedin and C. Wilhelmsson), Churchill Livingstone, Edinburgh, pp. 103–116 (1986)
465. Nikkila, E.A., Tikkanen, M.-J. and Kuusi, T. Gonadal hormones, lipoprotein metabolism and coronary heart disease. In *Myocardial Infarction in Women* (eds M.F. Oliver, A. Vedin and C. Wilhelmsson), Churchill Livingstone, Edinburgh, pp. 341–43 (1986)
466. Godsland, I.F., Crook, D., Simpson, R., Proudler, T., Felton, C. *et al*. The effects of different formulations of oral contraceptive agents on lipid and carbohydrate metabolism. *N. Engl. J. Med.*, **323**, 1375–1381 (1990)
467. Burkman, R.T., Robinson, J.C., KruszMoran, D., Kimball, A.W., Kwiterovich, P. and Burford, R.G. Lipid and lipoprotein changes associated with oral contraceptive use. A randomised clinical trial. *Obstet. Gynecol.*, **71**, 33–38 (1988)
468. Sznajderman, M. and Oliver, M.F. Spontaneous premature menopause, ischaemic heart disease and serum lipids. *Lancet*, **i**, 962–965 (1963)
469. Robinson, R. W., Higano, N. and Cohen, W.D. Increased incidence of coronary heart disease in women castrated prior to the menopause. *Arch. Intern. Med.*, **104**, 908–913 (1959)
470. Parrish, H.M., Carr, C.A., Hall, D.G. and King, T.M. Time interval from castration in premenopausal women to development of excessive coronary atherosclerosis. *Am. J. Obstet. Gynecol.*, **99**, 155–162 (1967)
471. Bengtsson, C. Ischaemic heart disease in women. A study based on a randomised population sample of women and women with myocardial infarction in Goteberg, Sweden. *Acta Med. Scand.*, **549** (Suppl.), 1–128 (1973)
472. Gordon, T., Kannel, W.B., Hjortland, M.C. and McNamara, P.M. Menopause and coronary heart disease. The Framingham Study. *Ann. Intern. Med.*, **89**, 157–161 (1978)
473. Tikkanen, M.J., Nikkila, E.A. and Vartiainen, E. Natural oestrogen as an effective treatment for type II hyperlipoproteinaemia in postmenopausal women. *Lancet*, **ii**, 490–501 (1978)
474. Godsland, I.F., Wynn, V., Crook, D. and Miller, N.E. Sex, plasma lipoproteins and atherosclerosis. Prevailing assumptions and outstanding questions. *Am. Heart J.*, **114**, 1467–1503 (1987)
475. Furman, R.H., Alaupovic, P. and Howard, R.P. Hormones and lipoproteins. *Progr. Biochem. Pharmacol.*, **2**, 215–258 (1967)

476. Zimmerman, J., Fainaru, M. and Eisenberg, S. The effects of prednisone therapy on plasma lipoproteins and apolipoproteins. A prospective study. *Metabolism*, **33**, 521–526 (1984)

477. Nikkila, E.A., Kaste, M., Ehnholm, C. and Viikari, J. Increase of serum high-density-lipoprotein in phenytoin users. *Br. Med. J.*, **ii**, 99 (1978)

478. Carlson, L.A. and Kolmodin-Hedman, B. Hyperalpha-lipoproteinaemia in men exposed to chlorinated hydrocarbon pesticides. *Acta Med. Scand.*, **192**, 29–32 (1972)

479. Miller, N.E. and Nestel, P.J. Altered bile acid metabolism during treatment with phenobarbitone. *Clin. Sci.*, **45**, 257–262 (1973)

480. Pelkonen, R., Fogelholm, R. and Nikkila, E.A. Increase in serum cholesterol during phenytoin treatment. *Br. Med. J.*, **iv**, 85 (1978)

481. Durrington, P.N., Roberts, C.J.C., Jackson, L., Branch, R.A. and Hartog, M. Effects of phenobarbitone on plasma lipids in normal subjects. *Clin. Sci. Mol. Med.*, **50**, 349–353 (1976)

482. Luoma, P.V., Myllyla, V.V., Sotaniemi, E.A., Lehtonen, A. and Hokkanen, E.J. Plasma high density lipoprotein cholesterol in epileptics treated with various anticonvulsants. *Eur. Neurol.*, **19**, 69–72 (1980)

483. Luoma, P.V., Sotanieni, E.A., Pelkonen, R.O., Arranto, A. and Ehnholm, C. Plasma high density lipoproteins and hepatic microsomal enzyme induction. Relation to histological changes in the liver. *Eur. J. Clin. Pharmacol.*, **23**, 275–282 (1982)

484. Linden, V. Myocardial infarction in epileptics. *Br. Med. J.*, **ii**, 87 (1975)

485. Livingston, S. Phenytoin and serum cholesterol. *Br. Med. J.*, **i**, 586 (1976)

486. Michaelsson, G., Bergqvist, A., Vahlquist, A. and Vessby, B. The influence of 'Tigason' (ro 10-9359) on the serum lipoproteins in man. *Br. J. Dermatol.*, **105**, 201–205 (1981)

487. Gerber, L.E. and Erdman, J.W. Changes in lipid metabolism during retinoid administration. *J. Am. Acad. Dermatol.*, **6**, 664–672 (1982)

488. Dicken, C.H. and Connolly, S.M. Eruptive xanthomas associated with isotretinoin (13-cis-retinoic acid). *Arch. Dermatol.*, **116**, 951–952 (1980)

489. Kasim, S.E., Bagchi, N., Brown, T.R., Khilnani, S., Jackson, K. *et al.* Amiodarone-induced changes in lipid metabolism. *Horm. Metabol. Res.*, **22**, 385–388 (1990)

490. Wiersinga, W.M., Trip, M.D., van Beeren, M.H., Plomp, T.A. and Oosting, H. An increase in plasma cholesterol independent of thyroid function during long-term amiodarone therapy. *Ann. Intern. Med.*, **114**, 128–132 (1991)

491. Kasiske, B.L., Tortorice, K.L., Heim-Duthoy, K.L., Awni, W.M. and Rao, K.V. The adverse impact of cyclosporin on serum lipids in renal transplant recipients. *Am. J. Kidney Dis.*, **17**, 700–707 (1991)

492. Raine, A.E.G., Carter, R., Mann, J.I. and Morris, P.J. Adverse impact of cyclosporin on plasma cholesterol in renal transplant recipients. *Nephrol. Dial. Transplant*, **3**, 458–463 (1988)

493. Ballantyne, C.M., Podet, E.J., Patsch, W.P. *et al.* Effects of cyclosporin therapy on plasma lipoprotein levels. *J. Am. Med. Assoc.*, **262**, 53–56 (1989)

494. Linscott, W.D. and Kane, J.P. The complement system in cryoglobulinaemia: interaction with immunoglobulins and lipoproteins. *Clin. Exp. Immunol.*, **21**, 510–519 (1975)

495. Slack, J. and Borrie, P. Xanthomatosis. In *Modern Trends in Dermatology* (ed. P. Borrie), Butterworths, London, pp. 194–213 (1971)

496. Lynch, P.J. and Winkelmann, R.K. Generalised plane xanthoma and systemic disease. *Arch. Dermatol.*, **93**, 639–646 (1960)

497. Cortese, C., Lewis, B., Miller, N.E., Peyman, M.A., Rao, S.N. *et al.* Myelomatosis with type III hyperlipoproteinaemia. Clinical and metabolic studies. *N. Engl. J. Med.*, **307**, 79–83 (1982)

498. Glueck, C.J., Kaplan, A.P., Levy, R.I., Greten K., Gralnick, H. and Fredrickson, D.S. A new mechanism of exogenous hyperglyceridaemia. *Ann. Intern. Med.*, **71**, 1051–1062 (1969)

499. Lewis, L.A., de Wolfe, V.G., Butkus, A. and Page, I.H. Autoimmune hyperlipidaemia in a patient. Atherosclerotic course and changing immunoglobulin pattern during 21 years of study. *Am. J. Med.*, **59**, 208–218 (1975)

500. Cornblath, W.T., Dotan, S.A., Trobe, J.D. and Headington, J.T. Varied clinical spectrum of necrobiotic xanthogranuloma. *Ophthalmology*, **99**, 103–107 (1992)

501. Gibson, T. and Grahame, R. Gout and hyperlipidaemia. *Am. Rheum. Dis.*, **33**, 298–303 (1974)

502. Wyngaarden, J.B. and Kelly, W.N. *Gout and Hyperuricaemia*, Grune and Stratton, New York, pp. 21–27 (1976)

503. Yano, K., Rhoads, G.G. and Kagan, A. Epidemiology of serum uric acid among 8,000 Japanese-American men in Hawaii. *J. Chron. Dis.*, **30**, 171–184 (1977)
504. Myers, A., Epstein, F.H., Dodge, H.J. and Mikkelsen, W.M. The relationship of serum uric acid to risk factors in coronary heart disease. *Am. J. Med.*, **45**, 529–536 (1968)
505. Bayliss, R., Clarke, C., Whitehead, T.P. and Whitfield, A.G.W. The management of hyperuricaemia. *J. R. Coll. Phys.*, **18**, 144–146 (1984)
506. Scott, J.T. Obesity and hyperuricaemia. *Clin. Rheum. Dis.*, **3**, 25–35 (1977)
507. Gibson, T., Kibbourn, K., Horner, I. and Simmonds, J.H. Mechanism and treatment of hypertriglyceridaemia in gout. *Ann. Rheum. Dis.*, **38**, 31–35 (1979)
508. Fox, I.H., John, D., DeBruyne, S., Dwosh, I. and Marliss, E.B. Hyperuricacmia and hypertriglyceridaemia: metabolic basis for the association. *Metabolism*, **34**, 741–746 (1985)
509. Bastow, M.D., Durrington, P.N. and Ishola, M. Hypertriglyceridaemia and hyperuricaemia. Effects of two fibric acid derivatives (bezafibrate and fenofibrate) in a double-blind, placebo-controlled trial. *Metabolism*, **37**, 217–220
510. Thompson, G.R. and Miller, J.P. Plasma lipid and lipoprotein abnormalities in patients with malabsorption. *Clin. Sci. Mol. Med.*, **45**, 583–592 (1973)
511. Howell, R.R. and Williams, J.C. The glycogen storage disease. In *The Metabolic Basis of Inherited Disease*, 5th edn (eds J.B. Stanbury, J.B. Wyngaarden, D.S. Fredrickson, J.L. Goldsein and M.S. Brown), McGraw-Hill, New York, pp. 141–166 (1983)
512. Forfar, J.O., Tompsett, S.L. and Forshall, W. Biochemical studies in idiopathic hypercalcaemia of infancy. *Arch. Dis. Child.*, **34**, 525–537 (1959)
513. Fleischman, A.I., Bierenbaum, M.L., Reichelson, R., Hayton, T. and Watson, P. Vitamin D and hypercholesterolaemia in adult humans. In *Atherosclerosis*, vol. II (ed. R.L. Jones), Springer-Verlag, Berlin (1970)
514. Eustace, P. Hypercholesterolaemia in osteogenesis imperfecta. *Br. J. Clin. Pract.*, **27**, 225–227 (1973)
515. Knight, J.A. and Meyers, G.G. Type IV hyperlipidaemia in the GM1, gangliosidoses. *Am. J. Clin. Pathol.*, **59**, 124 (1973)
516. Vilee, D.B., Nichols, G. and Talbot, N.B. Metabolic studies in two boys with classical progeria. *Pediatrics*, **42**, 207–216 (1969)
517. Epstein, C.J., Martin, G.M., Schultz, A.L. and Motulsky, A.G. Werner's syndrome. A review of its symptomatology, natural history, pathological features, genetics and relationship to the natural aging process. *Medicine*, **45**, 177–221 (1966)
518. Beaudet, A.L., Ferry, G.D., Nichols, B.L. and Rosenberg, H.S. Cholesterol ester storage disease. Clinical, biochemical and pathological studies. *J. Paediat.*, **90**, 910–914 (1977)
519. Bank, W.J., DiMauro, S., Bonilla, E., Capuzzi, D.M. and Rowland, L.P. A disorder of muscle lipid metabolism and myoglobulinuria. Absence of carnitine palmityl transferase. *N. Engl. J. Med.*, **192**, 443–449 (1975)
520. Saudek, C.D. and Eder, H.A. Lipid metabolism in diabetes mellitus. *Am. J. Med.*, **66**, 843–852 (1979)

# Chapter 12

# Genetics of lipoprotein disorders and coronary atheroma

## Introduction

In recent years, considerable resources have been devoted to research into the genetics of coronary heart disease. The outstanding discovery in this area has been the elucidation of the role of the LDL receptor in familial hypercholesterolaemia (FH). However, even the most liberal estimate would attribute fewer than 1 in 20 heart attacks under the age of 60 to FH[1]. That premature ischaemic heart disease (IHD) runs in families far more commonly than this is the everyday experience of physicians and cardiologists. Prospective epidemiological studies employing multivariate analysis suggest that this familial clustering of IHD can be largely explained on the basis of the established risk factors: serum cholesterol, blood pressure, cigarette smoking and glucose intolerance[2]. Clearly much of the association of coronary atheroma with family history is therefore likely to be the result of a shared family environment and dietary and social habits. It might also be concluded that any genetic influence not operating through these risk factors must make only a small contribution to premature coronary disease. This, however, need not be the case if it is considered that the genetic component of IHD frequently involves the combined effect of more than a single gene (polygenic).

This hypothesis would predict that only when the harmful combination of genes was present in one or both parents would a parental history of premature coronary disease be forthcoming. Perhaps more commonly, potentially atherogenic genes in harmful combinations might be inherited by some offspring from both parents neither of whom individually have sufficient to develop IHD at any early age (Figure 12.1). This would not be apparent from epidemiological studies. Using a model of polygenic inheritance, genetic factors have been estimated to contribute as much as 60% to the risk of coronary death in men under 55 years of age and almost 70% in women under 65[3]. In twin studies, about 40% of monozygotic twins are concordant for IHD and about half this number of dizygotic twins, supporting the hypothesis that genes as well as non-genetic familial factors are important[3,4].

The influence of genes on serum lipid and lipoprotein levels has been the subject of several studies[5]. It has been estimated from twin studies[6] that the heritability of serum cholesterol is about 40%. A similar figure was also found in family studies[7] of first-degree relatives. The lack of any substantial correlation between serum cholesterol levels in spouses is evidence that the correlation between parents and children and siblings is not entirely due to non-genetic familial factors. On the other hand, the assumption that factors more closely correlated in monozygotic as opposed to dizygotic twins necessarily have a genetic basis has been challenged[8] and the importance of intrauterine and early nutritional influences on future development of coronary risk factors, such as hyperlipidaemia, which would previously have been regarded as genetic, are receiving great attention at present[9].

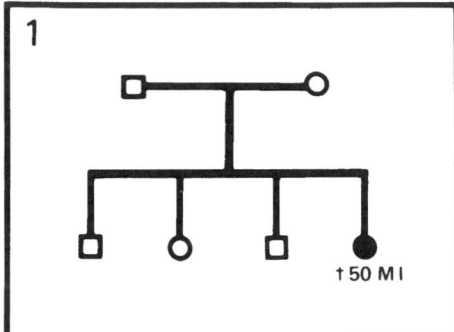 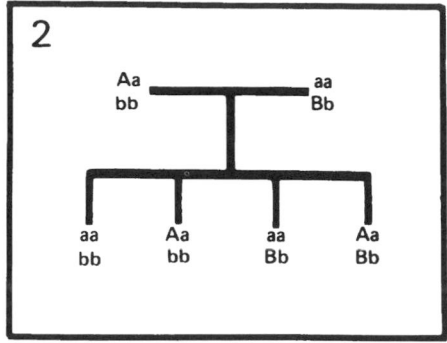

**Figure 12.1**   Involvement of genes in early-onset ischaemic heart disease (IHD) may be underestimated if two or more must combine to produce the disease, i.e. polygenic inheritance. In the sample family shown, neither parent nor any of the siblings of the man dying at the age of 50 of a myocardial infarction (MI) gave a history of IHD (panel 1). However, if susceptibility to premature MI requires the expression of two dominant genes (A and B), for example, neither parent is at risk (one is a heterozygote for A and the other for B), but one in four of their children will be heterozygotes for both A and B and thus be at risk (panel 2)

It is important not to misunderstand the meaning of the statistics relating to the genetic component of hypercholesterolaemia. Heritability is an estimate of the contribution of inherited factors to the variation in serum cholesterol not the mean cholesterol. The impression is frequently created that genes might explain 40% or so of the cholesterol concentration. This is not so. Thus, Slack[3] calculated that the children of a man of 30 with a serum cholesterol of 300 mg/dl (7.7 mmol/l) would be expected to have on average cholesterol levels only about 16 mg/dl (0.4 mmol/l) above the population mean, assuming heritability of 38% and a standard deviation for cholesterol of 42 mg/dl (1.1 mmol/l).

There is also a danger in over-emphasizing the likely impact of genetic research in disease prevention. At present, substantial resources are being devoted to attempts to find genetic factors, more often polymorphisms rather than the mutations actually likely to be directly involved in the disease process. It is true that a genetic polymorphism linked with atherosclerosis might improve our assessment of an individual's risk of coronary disease. This might be enormously helpful in deciding how actively to treat risk factors such as hyper-cholesterolaemia. However, as coronary disease is multifactorial it is unlikely that any single polymorphism will emerge as sufficiently important and a battery of several will be required, reducing the value of this type of approach. It is unlikely in the extreme that any of these polymorphisms will have any place in primary screening for coronary risk, nor is it likely that their discovery will lead to any new preventive measures. It is important, therefore, that the impression is not created that genetic research will in some way remove the necessity for public health programmes aimed at coronary risk factors such as smoking and possibly exercise or for the promotion of individual screening for hypercholes-terolaemia and hypertension supported by an adequate clinical service. Any practical outcome from genetic research presupposes the existence of clinics such as lipid clinics. A recent study of people undergoing coronary angiography failed

**Table 12.1 Inborn errors of lipoprotein metabolism**

*Definitely linked with accelerated atherogenesis*
    Familial hypercholesterolaemia
    Familial defective apolipoprotein B (apolipoprotein $B_{100}$3500 variant)
    Type II hyperlipoproteinaemia
    Apolipoprotein AI-CIII deficiency
    Raised serum lipoprotein (a) concentration
    Familial lecithin: cholesterol acyltransferase deficiency
    Phytosterolaemia (β sitosterolaemia)
    Cerebrotendinous xanthomatosis

*No definite link with atherosclerosis established*
    Tangier disease (analphalipoproteinaemia)
    Fish-eye disease
    Familial lipoprotein lipase deficiency
    Familial apolipoprotein CII deficiency
    Familial hepatic lipase deficiency

*Possibly protective against atherosclerosis*
    Abetalipoproteinaemia
    Familial hypobetalipoproteinaemia
    Hyperalphalipoproteinaemia
    Familial cholesteryl ester transfer protein deficiency

*Contenders for inborn errors of metabolism definitely linked with atherosclerosis*
    Familial combined hyperlipidaemia
    Hyperapobetalipoproteinaemia
    Familial dyslipidaemic hypertension

to find an association between IHD and any of twelve apolipoprotein gene polymorphisms previously proposed, on the basis of smaller case-studies, to be risk markers[10].

The inborn errors of lipoprotein metabolism are important, not only because some of the commoner ones frequently require medical attention, but also because they provide an insight into which areas of lipoprotein metabolism are likely to be involved in atherogenesis. In addition some of the genetic polymorphisms of the apolipoproteins are acquiring interest beyond that of markers for coronary disease, since some of them are beginning to emerge as mutations, or closely linked to mutations, which directly affect lipoprotein metabolism. Inborn errors of lipoprotein metabolism (Table 12.1) and the apolipoprotein variants will therefore be briefly surveyed.

# Inborn errors of lipoprotein metabolism

## Definitely linked with accelerated atherogenesis

### Familial hypercholesterolaemia

Autosomal dominant inheritance (Chapter 5).

### Familial defective apolipoprotein B (apolipoprotein $B_{100}$3500 variant)

Autosomal dominant inheritance with variable penetrance (Chapter 5)

## Type III hyperlipoproteinaemia

Commonly autosomal recessive inheritance with reduced penetrance. Rarely autosomal dominant (Chapter 8). Apolipoprotein E polymorphisms and mutations are discussed on pages 51–53 and pages 375–376.

## Apolipoprotein AI-CIII deficiency and other apolipoprotein A1 deficiencies

Two sisters in their early thirties and, from another unrelated family, a 45-year-old woman have been described with markedly decreased serum HDL levels due to an absence of apo A1 and apo CIII[11–13]. Severe atherosclerosis and mild corneal opacities characterized all three women. Heterozygotes from both families had approximately half the normal levels of serum apo A1 and CIII. The genes of apo A1 and CIII are part of the same cluster on chromosome 11 (page 375) and it thus appears that there is no transcription of either gene. In the first family a rearrangement of the DNA in the apo A1/apo CIII gene cluster has been demonstrated[14] and in the other, deletion of the gene cluster[15].

A few cases of severe apo A1 deficiency due to mutations of the apo A1 gene due to deletion, insertion or introduction of stop codes have been described which produce a profound A1 deficiency and should be distinguished from apo A1 variants (page 375) and are different from Tangier disease because they do not result from increased HDL catabolism. Some have been associated with corneal opacities, xanthamotosis and premature IHD[16].

## Raised serum lipoprotein (a) concentration

An association between the serum concentration of Lp(a) and IHD has long been known[17–21]. Recent evidence reveals that apo(a), the unique apolipoprotein of this lipoprotein (Chapter 2, page 53) is a genetic mutant of plasminogen[22]. The serum concentration of Lp(a) distribution is markedly positively skewed in Caucasian populations[19–21] and the work of Berg and later workers strongly suggests that the higher levels arise as the result of autosomal dominant inheritance[23–27]. This was reinforced by the finding that the serum concentration of Lp(a) is determined by its molecular weight which varies from 300 000–700 000 daltons[28,29]. This in turn is determined by a series of alleles of the apolipoprotein (a) gene. Initially there were thought to be six of these[28,30], giving rise to the possibility of six homozygotes and 15 heterozygotes. Later, however, it became clear that there were more than 20 alleles[31], giving rise to the possibility of more than 20 different homozygotes and 200 or so different heterozygotes. The variation in the alleles was largely due to the length of the sequences coding for the chain of kringle 4 repeats[32]. People with the highest levels of Lp(a) tend to have the lowest molecular weight isoforms, probably because these are synthesized and secreted more rapidly than higher molecular weight isoforms. Secretory rather than catabolic rate is the main determinant of the serum Lp(a) concentration. Also in favour of a substantial genetic component in the determination of the serum Lp(a) concentration is the association between this and a parental history of premature myocardial infarction in several studies[21,24–26,33,34].

Estimates of the extent to which the serum concentration of Lp(a) is determined by the apo (a) gene locus are high in the general population, probably 40–90%. However, other genetic and acquired factors can undoubtedly influence the Lp(a) concentration and may do so to an even greater extent. These include familial hypercholesterolaemia, apolipoprotein E polymorphism, renal disease, hepatic disease, drugs such as anabolic steroids and alcohol, race and coronary heart disease itself.

In Europid populations the frequency distribution of serum Lp(a) concentrations is markedly skewed, with concentrations ranging from <1 mg/dl to 100 mg/dl or more, but with a median value of around 10 mg/dl[35]. In Africans and their descendants[33,36,37], people from the Indian subcontinent[38] and some from China[39], the levels have a more Gaussian distribution, with median levels 1.5–2 times those of Europids. We do not know the true biological function of Lp(a) although a reasonable guess is that it may have some part to play in wound healing or in coagulation, but despite intense effort no convincing confirmation of this has been found *in vivo*. This leads to speculation that we have maybe, by looking in Europids, been studying a population in whom it is a protein contributing little if anything to survival potential. The enormous range of mutations, with the relative lack of conservation of those giving rise to high levels and the generally low serum levels of Lp(a) in Europids would do much to support the view that it is a biological vestige. With the exception of the hedgehog[40], Lp(a) is expressed in the serum only in primates. It may well have important intracellular functions in other non-primate species and indeed it is part of a family of proteins some of which are secreted and some of which appear to perform their function within, for example, hepatocytes. The gene for Lp(a) is located close to that for plasminogen, with which it has the closest homology, giving rise to speculation that it might interfere with fibrinolysis[37]. The serum level of Lp(a) does not, however, appear to influence thrombolytic therapy for acute myocardial infarction[41,42] nor to be related to venous thrombosis[43].

The suggestion that Lp(a) in Europids is a biochemical vestige is not an argument against it being an important cause of pathology any more than regarding the vermiform appendix or the plantaris muscle as vestigial means that they may not cause disease. Case-control studies of patients with and without premature IHD have been reasonably consistent in showing higher serum levels of Lp(a) in myocardial infarction survivors[36,37]. Indeed a substantial component of the influence of family history in differentiating between middle-aged men with and without IHD is explained by variation in serum Lp(a) concentration and by apo (a) isoforms[21]. It was therefore something of a surprise when prospective studies did not inconsistently find that Lp(a) was a risk factor for myocardial infarction; some did[44,45], but others did not[46–48]. A possible explanation of this is that Lp(a) increases in men sustaining acute myocardial infarction closer to the time of the event than it was measured in at least some of the prospective studies[49]. This would not necessarily make Lp(a) of no clinical or scientific interest in the context of atherosclerosis. Whereas, for example, cholesterol retains its association with coronary events for 30 years or more[50], fibrinogen, another dependent risk factor, is linked more strongly to IHD the nearer to the event it is measured[51]. It is easy to see how fibrinogen, which may increase as the burden of atheroma increases in a patient, might herald an acute event and because of its involvement in thrombosis might increase the likelihood of this occurring should an atheromatous plaque rupture. On the other hand, we also know that early in the development substantial amounts of fibrinogen are present in the evolving atheromatous lesion, despite which the circulating level of fibrinogen may not at that stage be raised in an individual destined to sustain an acute myocardial infarction in the distant future. Lp(a) too is present in atheromatous lesions both in native vessels and venous bypass grafts: indeed it may be the predominant apolipoprotein B-containing lipoprotein found in them[52–54]. Because of its adhesiveness to connective tissue matrices and blood clots and its recognition by the macrophage plasminogen receptor its retention in the arterial wall for longer periods than LDL is likely and thus its greater exposure to oxidant damage. Lp(a) which has been oxidatively modified experimentally is rapidly taken up by macrophage receptors[37]. Because so many other factors may be important at this stage of atherogenesis, however, Lp(a) may not figure as a risk factor in prospective studies, but nearer the acute event, perhaps because of its participation in some other process perhaps related to thrombosis, it may.

It is known that Lp(a) levels are high in patients with acute myocardial infarction from the earliest time it can be measured after the onset of symptoms[41,42,55]. It is also known that it does not increase significantly after a myocardial infarction, except perhaps in a subpopulation of patients, and that this rise is not immediate (unlike acute phase reactant such as C-reactive protein), but takes place in the second week after myocardial infarction and is unsustained[55]. Any rise associated with an impending heart attack is therefore likely to have occurred before the event.

That Lp(a) can rise precipitously with certain acquired diseases is well illustrated by renal disease. In renal disorders associated with proteinuria or with chronic renal failure the serum Lp(a) level is raised two to four times that in the general population. This increase persists during an ambulatory peritoneal dialysis, haemodialysis and after renal transplantation (Chapter 11, page 328). This is highly relevant to the debate about the relationship of Lp(a) to atheroma because of the increased risk of IHD events in renal patients. Furthermore the concept that Lp(a) may rise in response to vascular dysfunction is supported by minimal change nephrosis in which the Lp(a) levels are high in patients with active disease, but normal in those in whom it has remitted[56]. In diabetes too evidence for an increase in serum Lp(a) has been most consistent in patients with evidence of nephropathy (Chapter 11, page 311). Interestingly, in patients who have undergone cardiac transplantation, Lp(a) is raised and the extent to which it is raised is related to the development of accelerated coronary artery disease in the transplanted heart[57]

Serum Lp(a) levels can be influenced by other diseases. They are, for example, decreased in cirrhosis[58]. Alcohol and perhaps diet can also influence its concentration. So also can steroid hormones and cyclosporin (Chapter 10, page 280). Genes other than the apolipoprotein (a) gene also influence its concentration, most notably the LDL receptor gene (and the apolipoprotein E gene (Chapter 5, page 122)). It is uncertain whether variation in serum Lp(a) levels in familial hypercholesterolaemia, a condition in which they are generally raised, especially in patients with an apo $E_4$ gene[59], explains the variation in the IHD risk in the condition. Case-control studies are about 2 to 1 in favour of an increased risk in FH associated with high serum Lp(a) levels[60–62], but given the uncertainties already discussed and the difficulty of differentiating between patients with and without coronary atheroma when patients at such high risk as those with FH are matched for age a prospective study is needed to settle this important clinical question.

The higher serum Lp(a) levels in ethnic groups such as Black Africans, already mentioned, despite their low incidence of IHD, also has to be explained. It is usually said that the low LDL cholesterol in the Africans is the explanation. Fibrinogen too is higher in rural African populations than anywhere else in the world, but it has not been dismissed as a IHD risk factor for this reason. Again, a high LDL cholesterol may be a permissive factor if fibrinogen is to operate as an IHD risk factor. Even in Black people in the USA, who retain their high Lp(a), LDL levels are lower than in Europids in the USA. In case-control studies in Europids Lp(a) is most closely associated with the presence of IHD when the serum LDL levels are also high[20,21]. Indians in the UK have LDL levels as high as the Europid population, but higher Lp(a) and their IHD rates are higher than the Europids.

Lp(a), which has for so long appeared to be the paradigm of a genetic IHD risk factor, should not be relegated to the status of a loser, but must be seen as still under starter's orders[63].

## Familial lecithin: cholesterol acyltransferase deficiency

The clinical syndrome caused by LCAT deficiency (Chapter 2, page 57) was first identified by Glomset and co-workers in Norway in 1966[64] and the largest number of patients with the condition have been Scandinavian[64–66]. It is autosomal recessive and probably results, in different parts of the world, from at least eight different mutations[16], perhaps explaining some of the heterogeneity of reported cases.

The absence of LCAT results in a marked decrease in the concentration of cholesteryl ester in the plasma. As expected there is a relative increase in free cholesterol and lecithin. The total cholesterol level is generally somewhat increased. Serum triglyceride levels are variable, but the fasting plasma is often turbid. Serum HDL concentration is greatly reduced. The lipoproteins are all grossly abnormal. Those in the VLDL range possess beta rather than prebeta electrophoretic mobility due to a decrease in their negative charge resulting from a deficiency in apo CII and CIII. The rest of their composition, including the presence of apo $B_{48}$ and apo E, suggests they are remnants of chylomicron metabolism, but the reason for their persistence is unexplained. The LDL contains LpX-like particles, similar to those in obstructive liver disease (Chapter 11, page 325). Cholesterol-poor disc-like particles resembling nascent HDL and small globular particles resembling AI-only particles[67] are found within the HDL range.

Corneal opacities are evident by adolescence and it is interesting how frequently these occur in conditions characterized by abnormality and deficiency of HDL (apo A1/CIII deficiency, Tangier disease, fish-eye disease, familial LCAT deficiency).

Moderate normochromic anaemia with target cells is commonly found. Both this appearance and the anaemia, which is due to an inadequate haemopoietic response to a decreased red cell life span, are associated with an increase in the free cholesterol and lecithin in erythrocyte membranes. In the marrow are found sea-blue histiocytes, containing lamellar structures within their cytoplasm, probably indicating that they are overwhelmed in their attempts to remove excess free cholesterol and lecithin.

Proteinuria is commonly present from childhood. Deterioration of renal function may occur in middle age. The renal content of free cholesterol and phospholipid is increased and biopsy shows a variety of appearances, but almost invariably the presence of foam cells in the glomerular tufts.

Accelerated atherosclerosis is a feature of LCAT deficiency. However, although the appearances of the arterial lesions is consistent with atheroma, their cholesterol content is only about 35% esterified as compared with 75% in atheroma from other causes[64–66]. This makes it doubtful that variations in LCAT activity has a major role in atherogenesis, except when profound, as in the familial deficiency.

### Phytosterolaemia (β sitosterolaemia)

Phytosterolaemia is a rare autosomal recessive disorder[68,69]. For reasons which are not clear, it has predominantly been reported in women. It results from absorption of plant sterols from the intestine (normally these are not absorbed, see Chapter 1, page 20). This may in some way be linked to a defect in cholesterol biosynthesis[70,71], if it were present in intestinal cells and affected their ability to exclude other sterols. As a result, there is an increase in circulating plant sterols, predominantly β-sitosterol, but also campesterol and a host of others including stigmasterol and cholestanol. The total serum cholesterol and LDL cholesterol are raised at least by enzymatic assays, which give values 15–30% higher than gas chromatographic methods.

Xanthomata in the Achilles tendons and tuberose xanthomata develop in childhood. There is impaired growth and arthralgia. Anaemia and thrombocytopenia may occur. Atherosclerosis also develops prematurely. Central nervous system manifestations have not been reported. The disorder can be treated with a diet low in phytosterol and with bile-acid sequestrating agents.

### Cerebrotendinous xanthomatosis

Cerebrotendinous xanthomatosis is a rare autosomal recessive condition, which results from a defect in sterol 27-hydroxylase[72,73], a mitochondrial enzyme of the cytochrome P450 family which hydroxylates sterols, for example, in the pathway leading from cholesterol to bile acids. As a result cholestanol is produced in large quantities and accumulates in the Achilles tendons as xanthomata and in the brain and lungs. Juvenile cataract and osteoporosis are other features. There is a progressive neurological disorder involving behaviour disturbance, dementia, epilepsy and generalized neural involvement producing pyramidal, cerebellar, brain stem, spinal and peripheral nerve dysfunction. Plasma cholesterol levels are low or normal. There are reports of premature atherosclerosis[74]. Amelioration of the neurological disorder may result from suppression of cholesterol biosynthesis with statins and suppression of the early stages of bile salt synthesis with chenodeoxycholate[75,76].

### No definite link with atherosclerosis established

### Tangier disease (analphalipoproteinaemia)

So named because the first patient and his similarly affected sister were from Tangier Island, Chesapeake Bay, Virginia, this disorder is characterized by a complete, or virtually complete, absence of HDL and deposition of cholesterol ester in foam cells in the reticuloendothelial system[77]. The most frequent clinical finding has been enlarged orange–yellow tonsils and adenoids. Deposition of cholesteryl ester also leads to lymph node enlargement, studding of the rectal mucosa with orange–brown spots, hepatosplenomegaly, corneal cloudiness, intermittent peripheral neuropathy and bone marrow infiltration. Thrombocytopenia frequently occurs. Total serum cholesterol is reduced to less than

125 mg/dl (3.2 mmol/l) (often much lower), not only because of the absence of HDL cholesterol, but also because LDL levels are low. Low density lipoprotein is deficient in cholesteryl ester, presumably because there is no HDL from which it might be transferred to VLDL. The triglyceride levels are often increased, due to increases in triglyceride-rich lipoproteins, and LDL itself is enriched in triglyceride.

Serum apo AI levels are reduced to about 1% of normal and AII to 5% of normal. The apo AI which is present is a molecular variant known as apo AI$_{Tangier}$. Rapid catabolism of this apo AI is responsible for the disorder[78].

There is no convincing evidence for accelerated atherogenesis in Tangier disease[79], but this is not to deny HDL a role in atheroma in the wider context, since it must be remembered that the influence of LDL and platelets in promoting arterial disease will also be much reduced in Tangier disease.

Heterozygotes have been identified in the families of patients with Tangier disease because their serum apo AI levels are about half normal. They do not appear to develop any harmful complications. The inheritance of Tangier disease is thus autosomal recessive.

A family has been described with as marked a deficiency of HDL and apolipoprotein AI and AII as in Tangier disease, but with normal tonsils and LDL and apo CIII levels and diffuse yellow planar xanthomata[80].

### Fish-eye disease

Another familial, but less profound deficiency of HDL and apo AI and AII (all approximately 10% of normal) with increased plasma triglycerides has been identified, in which severe corneal opacities resemble fish-eyes[81]. The condition is associated with LCAT deficiency, but differs from familial LCAT deficiency (page 367) because it is absent only from HDL (αLCAT), but is active on VLDL and LDL (βLCAT)[16].

### Familial lipoprotein lipase deficiency

Autosomal recessive (Chapter 7).

### Familial apolipoprotein CII deficiency

Autosomal recessive (Chapter 7).

### Familial hepatic lipase deficiency

Hepatic lipase is located on chromosome 15 and lipoprotein lipase on chromosome 8. Members of two families have been described with extremely low hepatic lipase activity but normal lipoprotein lipase activity. In one marked hypertriglyceridaemia, β-VLDL and triglyceride-enrichment of VLDL and HDL were present and there was associated atherosclerosis[82]. In the other lipoprotein abnormalities were less severe and premature IHD was not present[83]. In the more severely affected family, affected members were compound heterozygotes for two massive mutations of the hepatic lipase gene[84,85].

A third family with a combined defect in hepatic lipase and lipoprotein lipase has also been described[86].

## Possibly protective against atherosclerosis

### Abetalipoproteinaemia

It is perhaps misleading to include abetalipoproteinaemia as being protective against atheroma, since the evidence for such a view would be difficult to obtain because most of those affected have, at least until recently, died prematurely as a result of a progressive neurological disorder resembling Friedreich's ataxia before they could benefit from any such protection. However, it is the most severe manifestation of apolipoprotein B deficiency and it is therefore logical to review it briefly, before mentioning less profound genetic deficiencies of LDL, which may reduce the likelihood of atheroma developing.

Abetalipoproteinaemia was first described as a syndrome comprising retinitis pigmentosa, unusually shaped erythrocytes, a syndrome resembling Friedreich's ataxia and steatorrhoea[87]. It was later shown to be due to a profound deficiency of LDL and has since been extensively reviewed[66,77,88].

Serum triglyceride levels are profoundly reduced, chylomicrons are not produced in response to meals and VLDL and LDL are virtually absent. Plasma cholesterol is present in HDL. Its concentration is usually less than 50 mg/dl (1.3 mmol/l). HDL2 cholesterol levels are usually normal, but HDL3 is decreased. The HDL is richer in apo E and this resembles $HDL_C$ (Chapter 2, page 53). It is deficient in apo CIII and CIII-1.

Fat from the diet accumulates both in the small intestinal mucosal cells, whence it cannot be transported in the absence of apo $B_{48}$, and in the liver as a result of apo $B_{100}$ deficiency. There is an unusually high ratio of sphingomyelin to lecithin in HDL and in cell membranes. Associated with this is the unusual appearance of the red blood cells, more than 50% of which have multiple thorn-like projections and are described as acanthocytes (Gk *akantha* = thorn).

The most devastating effect of the disease is spinocerebellar degeneration, which may be evident in childhood, with combined sensory and cerebellar ataxia too severe to permit standing invariably present by the fourth decade. Diabetes mellitus, frequently associated with Friedreich's ataxia, is rare in abetalipoproteinaemia. Retinitis pigmentosa, which would be unusual in Friedreich's ataxia, is common. As a consequence, night blindness and decreased visual acuity may begin in childhood and nystagmus is often due to this rather than cerebellar ataxia. The spinocerebellar neuropathic features are probably due to fat soluble vitamin transport deficiency and respond to the administration of vitamin A and E.

Neither parent is identifiable from their lipoproteins and the condition is thus an autosomal recessive. Hepatic levels of mRNA for apo B are increased in abetalipoproteinaemia[89] and apo B haptotypes in affected members of the same family may differ[90]. The defect does not therefore appear to be in the apo B gene itself. Recent evidence suggests that it is due to a defect in a microsomal lipid transfer protein involved in the assembly of triglyceride-rich lipoproteins[91,92].

### Hypobetalipoproteinaemia

Occasional patients occur with a syndrome similar to abetalipoproteinaemia, but whose parents both have decreased LDL levels. The parents are regarded as heterozygotes for a dominantly inherited condition, hypoapobetalipoproteinaemia, and the patient as having homozygous hypobetalipoproteinaemia.

Heterozygotes for hypobetalipoproteinaemia are encountered on population screening with a frequency of about 1 in 10 000[93]. Secondary causes including intestinal malabsorption, hyperthyroidism, severe liver disease and anaemia, myeloma and other malignancies should be considered as possible causes. The primary genetic disorder is rarely symptomatic in the heterozygote and has been reported to increase longevity[94], as might be expected from a disorder which decreases one of the major risk factors for atheroma[95].

Primary hypobetalipoproteinaemia usually results from decreased production of both apo $B_{48}$ and apo $B_{100}$[77]. Variants of the more common type of hypobetalipoproteinaemia have been described[96–99] which may be due to diminished production of apo $B_{100}$ but not apo $B_{48}$. The genetic defect in hypobetalipoproteinaemia is in the apo B gene itself and results from a premature stop codon arising in the gene due to mutation[100]. A truncated apo B protein is thus produced. Adopting similar terminology to that used for apo $B_{100}$ and apo $B_{48}$ (48% of the molecular mass of apo $B_{100}$), some 17 truncated apo B variants have been described thus far, ranging from apo $B_9$ to apo $B_{89}$[101]. The shorter truncated apo B molecules lack the lipid-binding domain resulting in the inability of the shortest to form lipoproteins. The formation of apo B-containing LDL is presented with the somewhat larger ones, but with the largest the abnormal apo B appears in VLDL and in LDL. Interestingly, in heterozygous hypobetalipoproteinaemia in addition to decreased formation of VLDL containing the truncated apo B, the secretory rate of apo $B_{100}$-containing VLDL is also diminished, suggesting the truncated apo B somehow interferes with the assembly of the apo $B_{100}$ VLDL. In addition to the decrease in synthetic rate, there may be increased catabolism of the larger truncated apo B variants such as $B_{75}$, $B_{87}$ and $B_{89}$. This is despite the absence of the LDL receptor-binding domain, suggesting either another receptor is involved such as the LRP or that LDL has a LDL receptor-binding site elsewhere in its structure which is somehow exposed in the truncated molecule.

The homozygotes described are now revealed to be true homozygotes in some cases (both parents have the same mutation) or compound heterozygotes (each parent has a different mutation). The most severe expression of the condition (indistinguishable from abetalipoproteinaemia) is in patients who are homozygotes for mutation shorter than apo $B_{48}$ or compound heterozygotes in whom both of these different mutations are shorter than apo $B_{48}$. Steatorrhoea is then a feature of the disorder. Acanthocytosis may be the only clinical manifestation apart from decreased LDL cholesterol levels, even in homozygotes when the truncated apo B mutations are long. It is also the case that in heterozygotes the shorter mutations have a more profound effect on the serum LDL concentration which is more than halved when a shorter mutation is expressed and reaches about half the normal level with a larger mutation.

## Hyperalphalipoproteinaemia

A familial increase in HDL has been described[102,103]. Primary hyperalphalipoproteinaemia is said to occur when the serum HDL cholesterol or apo AI levels are in the highest decile for a population of men or women after exclusion of causes such as alcohol abuse, medication which increases HDL, such as anticonvulsants or oestrogen, pesticide exposure, or extreme physical activity. Clustering of such people occurs in some families and this may have a genetic basis, although available evidence is insufficient to suggest monogenic inheritance. Longevity has been reported[94]. It does, however, not appear to be an especially common cause of longevity[104].

*Familial cholesteryl ester transfer protein deficiency*

A genetic deficiency of cholesteryl ester transfer protein (CETP) has been discovered in humans[105]. The mutation responsible interferes with RNA processing and is a true nul allele resulting in neither CETP activity nor protein production[106–108]. In homozygotes total serum cholesterol is moderately increased due to an increase in the HDL concentration. There are low levels of LDL cholesterol. The increase in HDL is entirely in the $HDL_2$ fraction and the serum apolipoprotein AI concentration is approximately doubled[109]. The ratio of $HDL_2$ and $HDL_3$ is six to ten times normal. The HDL particles are larger than normal and some have the buoyancy of LDL. They are rich in apolipoprotein E. Apolipoprotein CII and CIII levels are also increased. Because of the apo E enrichment, the HDL from CETP deficient individuals will compete with LDL for fibroblast LDL receptors[110]. Theoretically, it might also be taken up by the hepatic remnant receptor. In fact, however, HDL catabolism is decreased in CETP deficiency. Stimulation of reverse cholesterol transport by enhanced removal of HDL from the circulation does not therefore appear to explain the probable reduced risk of IHD and resulting increase in life-span in people with CETP deficiency. This may result from the decreased transfer of cholesteryl ester from HDL back into the VLDL pool whence it may contribute to the atherogenic LDL pool and form a greater tendency for HDL to give up its cholesteryl ester directly to the liver with the whole HDL particle being catabolized. This would partly explain the low LDL cholesterol[111]. In addition, CETP may also be responsible for the transfer of cholesteryl ester from LDL back to VLDL in exchange for triglyceride, a process, which in hypertriglyceridaemia (Chapter 7, page 192) and hyperapobetalipoproteinaemia (Chapter 6, page 179), results in the production of small, dense, cholesterol-depleted, triglyceride-rich, readily oxidizable LDL which is rapidly cleared from the circulation, but not via the LDL receptor. This process would be expected to be decreased in CETP deficiency. Enhanced transfer of cholesteryl ester has been reported in IHD[112] and so the finding that in CETP deficiency there is a decreased incidence of IHD would be logical.

Heterozygotes for CETP deficiency have raised or normal total serum and HDL cholesterol concentrations with an increase in apolipoprotein AI.

## Contenders for inborn errors of metabolism definitely linked with atherosclerosis

These are described as contenders only because their genetic component is ill-defined.

*Familial combined hyperlipidaemia*

Chapter 6, page 142.

*Hyperapobetalipoproteinaemia*

Chapter 6, page 179.

*Familial dyslipidaemia hypertension*

It has been proposed that there is an inherited syndrome in which hypertension developing before the age of 60 years is associated with dyslipidaemia (serum triglycerides >90th percentile, LDL cholesterol >90th percentile, and HDL cholesterol <10th percentile)[113]. It is undoubtedly the case that dyslipidaemia is prevalent in hypertensive patients and that frequently more than one family member is involved. This does not mean that the association is largely genetic in origin because the most common reason for the link is that dyslipidaemia and hypertension are both caused by obesity. Obesity clearly runs in families, but is likely to do so because of attitudes to food and life style learnt in a shared home environment. The dyslipidaemia in hypertensive people frequently predates the development of hypertension[114,115]. Because obesity causes an increase in insulin resistance and thus – in order to maintain euglycaemia – an increase in serum insulin, the association between serum insulin and dyslipidaemic hypertension is not surprising. Whilst there are plausible theories for insulin resistance causing hypertriglyceridaemia and low HDL (Chapter 11, page 293), the evidence that either insulin resistance or hyperinsulinaemia causes hypertension is not yet convincing. It has been suggested that insulin can affect renal tubular sodium reabsorption[116] or the sympathetic nervous system[117] to produce hypertension, but it is not clear that this is the case when insulin is produced endogenously in response to insulin resistance. Twin studies are not reassuring about a genetic basis for hypertensive dyslipidaemia[118,119]. The relationship between serum insulin and hypertension may only apply in obesity[120]. If the association between hypertension and dyslipidaemia could be consistently found in lean families, the case for familial dyslipidaemic hypertension would be considerably strengthened.

# Genetic variants of apolipoproteins

Polymorphisms of apolipoproteins have been extensively investigated by electrophoretic and isoelectric focusing techniques, immunological methods and by restriction enzyme analysis using apolipoprotein complementary deoxyribonucleic acid (cDNA) probes. This latter approach has undergone radical expansion since the first edition of this book due to the introduction of the polymerase chain reaction method[121]. Although some of the polymorphisms are related to IHD in case-control studies, their associations are weak and inconsistent in different populations. It is generally concluded that they provide some support for the hypothesis that genes are involved in coronary heart disease, but that the apolipoprotein and DNA polymorphisms thus far discovered are not sufficiently closely linked to the disease to fulfil the promise implicit in such research that they will have any clinical value in assessing an individual's coronary risk. Probably of greater immediate interest is a more fundamental approach, which attempts to link some of the polymorphisms to variations in different aspects of lipoprotein metabolism. This might ultimately free us from the present constraints of being able only to measure serum concentrations of lipoproteins in the majority of our patients, because polymorphisms may act as markers indicating activity in different metabolic pathways.

## Chromosome 1

There is a restriction-fragment length polymorphism (RFLP) of the apo AII gene with the enzyme MspI. Despite an early report that it had a small influence on the serum concentration of apo AII[122], its effect was not significant in a later study[123]. The relationship of apo AII with atherosclerosis is currently confused because, whilst a case-control study in man showed a possible protective effect[124], the expression of the human apo AII gene in mice increased their susceptibility to atheroma[125]. Two sisters aged 59 and 62 years with no detectable apo AII, who were homozygotes for a mutation preventing functional mRNA transcription, had normal serum concentrations of lipoproteins including HDL, and IHD was absent[126].

## Chromosome 2

Apo B is the most likely apolipoprotein to be involved in atherosclerosis (Chapter 6, page 179). Factors which influence its serum concentration and metabolism, whether they be genetic or acquired, are therefore likely to be of major importance. The elucidation of its structure has been more recent[127,128, Chapter 2, page 48] than that of the more soluble apolipoproteins. Familial defective apo $B_{100}$, in which the substitution glycine for arginine at position 3400 occurs due to a point mutation in the codon CGG to CAG, is undoubtedly the most important apo B mutation thus far described[129]. It is the only apo B mutation, which has been found, which decreases binding of LDL to its receptor without truncation of the protein. It was not found using the candidate gene approach widely advocated, but by the discovery of an unusual phenotype for familial hypercholesterolaemia in which autologous LDL was catabolized more slowly than heterologous LDL[130]. It is discussed in detail in Chapter 5 (page 132).

Even before molecular biological techniques were available, however, polymorphisms of apo B were detectable. The earliest description of any apolipoprotein polymorphisms were in the apo B of multiply transfused patients[131]. Later this antigenic variation in apo B was named the Ag system and five pairs of antigens, each pair of which acted as alleles at a single locus, were identified (a1 and d; c and g; t and z; h and i; x and y)[132]. The molecular basis of all of these polymorphisms has been elucidated[100]. There is an association between the t allele and IHD, but the mechanism is unclear[100], otherwise no association of any of these with atherosclerosis has been firmly established.

Using cDNA probes, RFLPs of apo B have been detected with restriction enzymes. The EcoRI polymorphism shows a weak association with atherosclerosis[133] and its presence is coincident with the Ag(t) allotype and its absence with Ag(z). Another, which can only be detected as a restriction-fragment length polymorphism, is detectable with XbAI. It has been reasonably consistently reported in association with variation in the serum cholesterol concentration[100]. It only explains 3–8% of the variance in the serum cholesterol level (<0.1 mmol/l, <4 mg/dl). Individuals homozygous for the 3.5 kilobase XbaI restriction fragment (called X+X+) have been shown to have slight decreases in the fractional catabolic rate of their LDL[134–136]. The base change which creates the XbaI cutting site does not alter the amino acid for which it codes and thus cannot be the cause of the presumably decreased binding of apo B to the LDL receptor. Another sequence variation, which is responsible, must be linked with it.

## Chromosome 11

Twenty-two variants of apo AI have currently been identified[16]. It has been estimated that at least one person in 400–500 will be a heterozygote for one or other of these polymorphisms[137,138] and multiple bands for apo AI on isoelectric focusing are commonly encountered on isoelectric focusing (Plate 1). Homozygotes for an apo AI polymorphism have only been detected for $AI_{Norway}$. Originally the variants were classified according to the part of the world from which the affected families emanated. Now they are classified according to the amino acid changes. Heterozygotes for only three of the variants have clearly been shown to have diminished serum HDL cholesterol levels. These are AI ($Arg_{173} \rightarrow Cys$) (formerly $AI_{Milano}$), AI ($Pro_{165} \rightarrow Arg$) and AI ($Gly_{26} \rightarrow Arg$) (formerly $AI_{Iowa}$). No association with IHD has been described for any of the AI polymorphisms thus far reported[78]. The AI ($Gly_{26} \rightarrow Arg$) variant is found in familial amyloid with polyneuropathy[139].

The apo AI–CIII–AIV gene cluster is highly polymorphic. cDNA probes for apo AI have been available for a long while and associations between coronary heart disease and RFLPs have been demonstrated in this gene cluster in various populations using the enzymes Sstl, Pstl, Xmnl and Pvul[133,140,141]. The findings are, however, inconsistent between different populations and/or research groups. The effect of multiple statistical tests and small sample sizes is a major consideration in the interpretation of some of the results, but there remains the possibility that there is a potentially atherogenic gene or genes in this cluster, which is variably linked with some of the RFLPs reported in different populations or which requires the presence of some other gene or environmental factor for its expression. An Xmnl RFLP has recently been described by two groups linked to familial combined hyperlipidaemia. This is discussed in more detail elsewhere in this book (Chapter 6, page 142).

## Chromosome 19

The genes for apo CII and apo E are located on chromosome 19. Mutations of apolipoprotein CII when both genes are affected lipoprotein lipase activity. Heterozygotes for apo CII mutations have so far shown normal lipid levels. Apo CII mutations are discussed in Chapter 17, page 198).

Apo E polymorphisms detected by isoelectric focusing (Plate 1) have been the most rewarding apolipoprotein variants studied. The association of apo $E_2$ homozygosity with type III hyperlipoproteinaemia was discussed previously (Chapter 8, page 215). In a wider context, the apo $E_4$ phenotype has been found to relate to increases in the concentration of serum LDL cholesterol and apo B in a wide variety of healthy populations[142,143] and in diabetes[144,145]. Its prevalence in Finland may help to explain the relative hypercholesterolaemia of Finns and its relative infrequency in Italians, their lower serum cholesterol levels[146]. Its effect may be due to down-regulation of the hepatic LDL receptor in response to higher rates of entry of cholesterol contained in chylomicron remnants as a consequence of the higher affinity of apo E4 for the remnant receptor[143] or it may be due to enhanced intestinal cholesterol absorption[147,148]. Opinions are divided as to whether the presence of the $E_4$ phenotype alone is sufficient in the general population to predispose to IHD[143,149–152], but it does appear to hasten the development of coronary disease in patients heterozygous for

FH[153]. The synthesis of apo E in the nervous system as judged by mRNA levels is second only to that in the liver. Apo E is found in the Golgi complexes of brain astrocytes and of non-myelinating glial cells in the peripheral nerves. Apo B-containing lipoproteins are absent from the cerebrospinal fluid. Instead lipid transport is mediated by HDL-like lipoproteins containing apo E as well as apo AI and capable of binding to LDL receptors. Injury to, for example, the peripheral nerves, the optic nerve or the spinal cord results in a considerable increase in apo E synthesis and it is believed that local secretion of apo E-rich lipoproteins by macrophages is responsible for macrophage uptake of cholesterol from damaged Schwan cells and redelivery to regenerating Schwan cells[154,155]. However, peripheral nerve regeneration is reported to be unimpaired in apo E-deficient mice[156].

Thus the physiological role of apo E in the nervous system is unsettled. Considerable interest has, however, recently been generated by the discovery of an association between the apo $E_4$ genotype and both the familial and sporadic late-onset (after the age of 60 years) types of Alzheimer's disease[157–160]. The association is strong enough to suggest direct involvement of the apo E variant in the pathological process. The strongest association is with $E_4$ homozygosity, but the risk is also clearly increased in $E_{4/3}$ heterozygotes[158].

Two cardinal histological features of the brain in Alzheimer's disease are extracellular amyloid deposits and intracellular neurofibrillary tangles. Apo E is localized in both the amyloid plaques and cells possessing neurofibrillary tangles. Similar histological pictures are seen in Down's syndrome and in Creutzfeldt–Jacob disease, but there is no association between these and the apo E genotype[157] nor is there with early-onset Alzheimer's disease. The amyloid deposits are principally amyloid β peptide, a peptide of 39–42 residues which is derived by an unknown process from a large membrane-sparing protein of 695–770 amino acid residues the function of which is unknown. It is termed amyloid precursor protein and its gene is on chromosome 21. This may explain the presence of amyloid deposits in the brain in Down's syndrome (trisomy 21) and also the linkage with markers on chromosome 21 of some cases of the early-onset form of Alzheimer's disease (which accounts for less than 5% of the total number of patients with this disease). Apo $E_4$ appears to associate more avidly with amyloid β protein than other apo E isoforms[161], but it is unclear why this would encourage the development of such plaques in the elderly.

The intracellular neurofibrillary tangles comprise filaments derived from the Tau protein which is normally associated with microtubules, and may be important for their assembly and stability. The Tau protein in the neurofibrillary tangles is extensively phosphorylated. Whereas apo $E_3$ binds to Tau protein with high affinity, apo $E_4$ does not. This has given rise to speculation that apo $E_4$ may fail to protect Tau against phosphorylation *in vivo* and thus lead to cellular microtubular damage in the brain[162].

## References

1. Burn, J., Durrington, P.N. and Harris, R. Genetics and cardiovascular disease. In *Recent Advances in Cardiology* (ed.D.J. Rowlands), Churchill Livingstone, Edinburgh, pp. 27–47 (1987)
2. Epstein, F.H. Genetics of ischaemic heart disease. *Postgrad. Med. J.*, **52**, 477–480 (1976)
3. Slack, J. The genetic contribution to coronary heart disease through lipoprotein concentrations. *Postgrad. Med J.*, **51** (Suppl. 8), 27–32 (1975)

4. Harvald, B. and Hauge, M. Coronary occlusion in twins. *Acta Genet. Gemellog.*, **19**, 248–250 (1970)
5. Segal, P., Rifkind, B.M. and Schull, W.J. Genetic factors in lipoprotein variation. *Epidemiol. Rev.*, **4**, 137–160 (1982)
6. Pikkarainen, J., Takkunen, J. and Kulonen, E. Serum cholesterol in Flemish twins. *Am. J. Hum Genet.*, **18**, 115–126 (1966)
7. Adlersberg, D., Schaefer, L.E. and Steinberg, A.G. Studies on genetic and environmental control of serum cholesterol levels. *Circulation*, **16**, 487–488 (1957)
8. Phillips, D. Twin studies in medical research: can they tell us whether diseases are genetically determined? *Lancet*, **341**, 1008–1009 (1993)
9. Barker, D.J.P. The fetal origins of cardiovascular disease. Chapter 3 in *Cardiovascular Disease. Risk Factors and Intervention* (eds N. Poulter, P. Severn and S. Thom), Radcliffe Medical Press, Oxford, pp. 25–36 (1993)
10. Marshall, H.W., Morrison, L.C., Wu, L.L., Anderson, J.L., Corneli, P.S. *et al*. Apolipoprotein polymorphisms fail to define risk of coronary artery disease. Results of a prospective angiographically controlled study. *Circulation*, **89**, 567–577 (1994)
11. Norum, R.A., Lakier, J.B., Goldstein, S., Anfi, A., Goldberg, R.B. *et al*. Familial deficiency of apolipoproteins AI and C-III and precocious coronary artery disease. *N. Engl. J. Med.*, **306**, 1513–1519 (1982)
12. Schaefer, E.J., Heaton, W.H., Wetzel, M.G. and Brewer, H.B. Plasma apolipoprotein A-I absence associated with marked reduction in high density lipoproteins and premature coronary artery disease. *Arteriosclerosis*, **2**, 16–26 (1982)
13. Schaefer, E.J., Ordovas, J.M., Law, S.W., Ghiselli, G., Kashyap, M.I. *et al*. Familial apolipoprotein A-I and C-III deficiency. Variant II. *J. Lipid Res.*, **26**, 1089–1101(1985)
14. Karathanasis, S.W., Ferris, E., Haddad, I.A. DNA inversion within the apolipoproteins AI/CIII/AIV encoding gene cluster of certain patients with premature atherosclerosis. *Proc. Natl Acad. Sci. USA.*, **84**, 7198–7202 (1987)
15. Ordovas, J.M., Cassidy, D.K., Civeira, F., Bisgaier, C.L. and Schaefer, E.J. Familial apolipoprotein AI, CIII, and AIV deficiency and premature atherosclerosis due to deletion of a gene complex on chromosome 11. *J. Biol. Chem.*, **264**, 16339–16342 (1989).
16. Assmann, G., von Eckardstein, A. and Funke, H. High density lipoproteins, reverse transport of cholesterol, and coronary artery disease. Insights from mutations. *Circulation*, **87** (Suppl. III), III-28–III-34 (1993)
17. Berg, K., Dahlen, G. and Frick, H. Lp(a) lipoprotein and pre-lipoprotein in patients with coronary heart disease. *Clin. Genet.*, **6**, 230–235 (1974)
18. Kostner, G.M., Avogaro, P., Cazzolato, G., Marth, G., Bittolo-Bon, G. and Quinci, G.B. Lipoprotein Lp(a) and the risk for myocardial infarction. *Atherosclerosis*, **38**, 51–61(1981)
19. Dahlen, G.H., Guyton, J.R., Attar, M., Farmer, J.A., Kautz, J.A. and Goko, A.M. Association of levels of lipoprotein Lp(a), plasma lipids, and other lipoproteins with coronary artery disease documented by angiography. *Circulation*, **74**, 758–765 (1986)
20. Armstrong, V.W., Cremer, P., Eberle, E., Manke, A., Schulze, F. *et al*. The association between serum Lp(a) concentration and angiographically assessed coronary atherosclerosis. Dependence on serum LDL levels. *Atherosclerosis*, **62**, 249–257 (1986)
21. Durrington, P.N., Ishola, M., Hunt, L., Arrol, S. and Bhatnagar, D. Apolipoproteins (a), AI and B and parental history in men with early onset ischaemic heart disease. *Lancet*, **i**, 1070–1073 (1988)
22. McLean, J.W., Tomlinson, J.E., Kuang, W.-J., Eaton, D.L., Chen, E.Y. *et al*. cDNA sequence of human apolipoprotein (a) is homologous to plasminogen. *Nature*, **330**, 132–137 (1987)
23. Berg, K. A new serum type system in man. The LP-system. *Acta Pathol. Microbiol. Scand.*, **59**, 369–382 (1963)
24. Berg, K., Dahlen, G. and Borresen, A.L. Lp(a) phenotypes, other lipoprotein parameters, and a family history of coronary heart disease in middle-aged males. *Clin. Genet.*, **16**, 347–352 (1979)
25. Sing, C.F., Schultz, J.S. and Shremer, D.C. The genetics of the LP antigen II A family study and proposed models of genetic control. *Ann. Hum. Genet.*, **38**, 47–56 (1974)
26. Hassted, S.J., Wilson, D.E., Edwards, C.Q., Connon, W.N., Carmelli, D. and Williams, R.R. The genetics of quantitative plasma Lp(a). Analysis of a large pedigree. *Ann. J. Med. Genet.*, **16**, 179–188 (1983)

27. Wilcken, D.E.L., Wang, X.L. and Dudman, N.P.B. The relationship between infant and parent Lp(a) levels. *Chem. Phys. Lipids*, **67/68**, 299–304 (1994)
28. Utermann, G., Kraft, H.G., Menzel, H.J., Hopferwieser, T. and Seitz, C. Genetics of the quantitative Lp(a) lipoprotein trait 1. Relations of Lp(a) glycoprotein phenotypes to Lp(a) lipoprotein concentrations in plasma. *Hum. Genet.*, **78**, 41–46 (1988)
29. Fless, G.M., Rolith, C.A. and Scanu, A.M. Heterogenicity of human plasma lipoprotein (a). *J. Biol. Chem.*, **259**, 11470–11478 (1984)
30. Utermann, G., Menzel, H.J., Kraft, H.G., Duba, H.C., Kemmler, H.G. and Seitz, C. Lp(a) glycoprotein phenotypes. Inheritance and relation to Lp(a)-lipoprotein concentrations in plasma. *J. Clin. Invest.*, **80**, 458–465 (1987)
31. Lackner, C., Boerwinkle, E., Leffert, C.C., Rahmig, T. and Hobbs, H.H. Molecular basis of apolipoprotein (a) isoform size heterogeneity as revealed by pulsed-field gel electrophoresis. *J. Clin. Invest.*, **87**, 2077–2086 (1991)
32. Gavish, D. Azrolan, N. and Breslow, J. Plasma Lp(a) concentration is inversely correlated with the ratio of Kringle IV/Kringle V encoding domains in the apo (a) gene. *J. Clin. Invest.*, **84**, 2021–2027 (1989)
33. Srimivasan, S.R., Dahlen, G.H., Jarpa, R.A., Webber, L.S. and Berenson, G.S. Racial (black–white) differences in serum lipoprotein (a) distribution and its relation to parental myocardial infarction in children. Bogalusa Heart Study. *Circulation*, **84**, 160–167 (1991)
34. Vella, J.C. and Jover, E. Relation of lipoprotein (a) in 11- to 19-year-old adolescents to parental cardiovascular heart disease. *Clin. Chem.*, **39**, 477–480 (1993)
35. Editorial. Lipoprotein (a). *Lancet*, **337**, 397–398 (1991)
36. Uterman G. The mysteries of lipoprotein (a). *Science*, **246**, 904–910 (1989)
37. MBewu, A.D. and Durrington, P.N. Lipoprotein (a): structure, properties and possible involvement in thrombogenesis and atherogenesis. *Atherosclerosis*, **85**, 1–14 (1990)
38. Bhatnagar, D., Mackness, M.I., Britt, R., Anand, I.S. and Durrington, P.N. Serum lipids and apolipoproteins in South Asians living in the UK and their siblings in India. *Atherosclerosis*, **103**, 296 (1993)
39. Bhatnagar, D., Mackness, M.I., Arrol, S. and Durrington, P.N. Preliminary result of a survey of lipid-related coronary risk factors in the Chinese community in Greater Manchester. *Cardiovasc. Risk Factors*, **2**, 302–306 (1992)
40. Laplaud, P.M., Beaubalie, L., Rall, S.J., Lue, G. and Saboweau, M. Lipoprotein (a) is the major apo B-containing lipoprotein in the plasma of a hibernator, the hedgehog (*Erinaceus europalus*). *J. Lipid Res.*, **29**, 1157–1170 (1988)
41. Hodenberg, E., Kreuzer, J., Hautman, M., Nordt, T., Kubler W. and Bode, C. Effects of Lp(a) on success rate of thrombolytic therapy in acute myocardial infarction. *Am. J. Cardiol.*, **67**, 1349–1353 (1991)
42. MBewu, A.D., Durrington, P.N., Mackness, M.I., Hunt, L., Turkie, W. and Creamer, J.E. Serum lipoprotein (a) concentration and the outcome of throbolytic therapy for myocardial infarction. *Br. Heart J.*, **71**, 316–321 (1994)
43. Marz, W., Trommlitz, M., Scharrer, I. and Gross, W. Apolipoprotein (a) concentrations are not related to the risk of venous thrombosis. *Fibrinolysis*, **2**, 595–599 (1991)
44. Rosengren, A., Wilhelmson, L., Eriksson, E., Risberg, B. and Wedel, H. Lipoprotein (a) and coronary heart disease: a prospective case-control study in a general population sample of middle-aged men. *Br. Med. J.*, **301**, 1248–1251 (1990)
45. Sigurdsson, G., Baldursdottir, A., Sigvaldson, H., Agnarsson, U., Thorgeirsson, G. and Sigfusson, N. Predictive value of apolipoproteins in a prospective survey of coronary artery disease in men. *Am. J. Cardiol.*, **69**, 1251–1254 (1992)
46. Jauhiainen, M., Kastinen, P., Ehnholm, C., Frick, M.H., Martari, M., Mannienn, V. and Huttenen, J.K. Lipoprotein (a) and coronary heart disease risk: a selected case-control study of the Helsinki Heart Study Participants. *Atherosclerosis*, **89**, 59–67 (1991)
47. Haffner, S.M., Moss, S.E., Klein, B.E. and Kleen, R. Lack of association between lipoprotein (a) concentrations and coronary heart disease mortality in diabetes: the Wisconsin Epidemiologic Study of Diabetic Retinopathy. *Metabolism*, **41**, 194–197 (1992)
48. Ridker, P.M., Hennekens, C.H. and Stampfer, M.J. A prospective study of lipoprotein (a) and the risk of myocardial infarction. *J. Am. Med. Assoc.*, **270**, 2195–2199 (1993)

49. Bhatnagar, D. and Durrington, P.N. Does measurement of apolipoproteins add to the clinical diagnosis and management of dyslipidaemias? *Curr. Opin. Lipidol.*, **4**, 299–304 (1993)

50. Anderson, K.M., Castelli, W.P., Levy, D. *et al.* 30 years of follow-up from the Framingham study *J. Am. Med. Assoc.*, **257**, 2176–2180 (1987)

51. Meade, T.W. Fibrinogen and other clotting factors in cardiovascular disease with particular reference to smoking. Chapter 20 in *Cardiovascular Disease. Risk Factors and Intervention* (eds N. Poulter, P. Sever and S. Thom), Radcliffe Medical Press, Oxford, pp. 185–199 (1993)

52. Smith, E.B. and Cochran, S. Factors influencing the accumulation in fibrous plaques of lipid derived from low density lipoprotein II: preferential immobilisations of lipoprotein (a) (Lp(a)). *Atherosclerosis*, **84**, 173–181 (1990)

53. Cushing, G.L., Gaubatz, J.W., Nava, M.L., Burdick, B.J., Bocan, T.M.A. *et al.* Quantitation and localisation of apolipoproteins (a) and B in coronary artery bypass vein grafts resected at reoperation. *Arteriosclerosis*, **9**, 593–603 (1989)

54. Rath, M., Niendorf, A., Reblin, T., Dietel, M., Krebber, H.J. and Beisiegel, U. Detection and quantitation of lipoprotein (a) in the arterial wall of 107 coronary bypass patients. *Arteriosclerosis*, **9**, 579–592 (1989)

55. MBewu, A.D., Durrington, P.N., Bulleid, S. and Mackness, M.I. The immediate effect of streptokinase on serum lipoprotein (a) concentration and the effect of myocardial infarction on serum lipoprotein (a), apolipoproteins A1 and B, lipids and C-reactive protein. *Atherosclerosis*, **103**, 65–71 (1993)

56. Short, C., Durrington, P.N., Mallick, N., Bhatnagar D., Hunt, L.P. and MBewu, A.D. Serum lipoprotein (a) in men with proteinuria due to idiopathic membranous nephropathy. *Nephrol. Dial. Transplant.*, Suppl. 1, 109–113 (1992)

57. Barbir, M., Khushwaha, S., Hunt, B., Macken, A., Thompson, G.R. *et al.* Lipoprotein (a) and accelerated coronary arterial disease in cardiac transplant recipients. *Lancet*, **340**, 1500–1501 (1992)

58. Feely, J., Barry, M., Keeling, P.W.N., Weir, D.G. and Cooke, T. Lipoprotein (a) in cirrhosis *Br. Med. J.*, **304**, 545–546 (1992)

59. Bhatnagar, D., Durrington, P.N., MBewu, A.D., Mackness, M.I. and Miller, J.P. Unpublished observation

60. Wiklund, O., Angelin, B., Oloffson, S., Eriksson, M., Fager, G. *et al.* Apolipoprotein (a) and ischaemic heart disease in familial hypercholesterolaemia. *Lancet*, **ii**, 1360–1363 (1990)

61. Seed, M., Hopplicher, F., Reaveley, D., McCarthy, S., Thompson, G. *et al.* Relation of serum lipoprotein (a) concentration and apolipoprotein (a) phenotype to coronary heart disease in patients with familial hypercholesterolaemia. *N. Engl. J. Med.*, **322**, 1494–1499 (1990)

62. MBewu, A.D., Bhatnagar, D., Durrington, P.N., Hunt, L., Ishola, M. *et al.* Serum lipoprotein (a) in patients heterozygous for familial hypercholesterolaemia, their relatives, and unrelated control populations. *Arteriosclerosis*, **11**, 940–946 (1991)

63. Barnathan, E.S. Has lipoprotein 'little' (a) shrunk? *J. Am. Med. Assoc.*, **270**, 2224–2225 (1993)

64. Glomset, J.A., Norum, K.A. and Gjone, E. Familial lecithin: cholesterol acyltransferase deficiency. In *The Metabolic Basis of Inherited Disease*, 5th edn (eds J.B. Stanbury, J.B. Wyngaarden, D.S. Fredrickson, J.L. Goldstein and M.S. Brown), McGraw-Hill, New York, pp. 643–654 (1983)

65. Norum, K.R. Familial lecithin: cholesterol acyltransferase deficiency. In *Clinical and Metabolic Aspects of High Density Lipoproteins* (eds N.E. Miller and G.J. Miller), Elsevier, Amsterdam, pp. 297–432 (1984)

66. Myant, N.B. Disorders of cholesterol metabolism. The hypolipoproteinaemia. In *The Biology of Cholesterol and Related Steroids*, Heinemann Medical, London, pp. 773–815 (1981)

67. Fielding, C.J. and Felding, P.E. Evidence for a lipoprotein carrier in human plasma catalysing sterol efflux from cultured fibroblasts and its relationship to lecithin : cholesterol acyltransferase. *Proc. Natl Acad. Sci. USA.*, **78**, 3911–3914 (1981)

68. Bjorkhem, I. and Skrede, S. Familial diseases with storage of sterols other than cholesterol : cerebrotendinous xanthomatosis and phytosterolaemia. In *The Metabolic Basis of Inherited Disease* (eds C.R. Scriver, A.L. Baeudet, W.S. Sly and D. Valle), McGraw-Hill, New York, pp. 1283–1302 (1989)

69. Berger, G.M.B., Deppe, W.M., Marais, A.D. and Biggs, M. Phytosterolaemia in three unrelated South African families. *Postgrad. Med. J.* (in press)

70. Salen, G., Shefer, S., Nguyen, L., Ness, G.C., Tint, G.S. and Shore, V. Sitosterolemia. *J. Lipid Res.*, **33**, 945–955 (1992)
71. Nguyen, L.B., Shefer, S., Salen, G., Ness, G.S., Tint, G.S. and Zaki, I. Molecular defect in cholesterol synthesis in sitosterolaemia with xanthomatosis. *J. Clin. Invest.*, **86**, 926–931 (1990)
72. Leitersdorf, E. and Meiner, V. Cerebrotendinous xanthomatosis. *Curr. Opin. Lipidol.*, **5**, 138–142 (1994)
73. Cali, J.J., Hsieh, C.L., Francke, U. and Russell, D.W. Mutations in the bile acid biosynthetic enzyme sterol 27-hydroxylase underlie cerebrotendinous xanthomatosis. *J. Biol. Chem.*, **266**, 7779–7783 (1991)
74. Fujiyama, J., Kuriyama, M., Arima, S., Shibata, Y., Nagara, K. *et al.* Atherogenic risk factors in cerebrotendinous xanthomatosis. *Clin. Chim. Acta*, **200**, 1–11 (1991)
75. Nakamura, T., Matsuzawa, Y., Takemura, K., Kubo, M., Miki, H. and Tarui, S. Combined treatment with chenodeoxycholic and pravastatin improves plasma cholesterol levels associated with marked regression of tendon xanthomas in cerebrotendinous xanthomatosis. *Metabolism*, **40**, 741–746 (1991)
76. Peynet, J., Laurent, A., De Liege, P., Lecoz, P., Gambert, P. *et al.* Cerebrotendinous xanthomatosis: treatment with simvastatin, lovastatin, and chenodeoxycholic acid in 3 siblings. *Neurology*, **41**, 434–436 (1991)
77. Herbert, P.N., Assman, G., Gotto, A.M. and Fredrickson, D.S. Familial lipoprotein deficiency. Abetalipoproteinaemia, hypobetalipoproteinaemia and Tangier disease. In *The Metabolic Basis of Inherited Disease*, 5th edn (eds J.B. Stanbury, J.B. Wyngaarden, D.S. Fredrickson, J.L. Goldstein and M.S. Brown), McGraw-Hill, New York, pp. 589–621 (1983)
78. Brewer, H.B., Gregg, R.E., Bojanovski, D., Law, S.A. and Zech, L.A. Genetic disorders of HDL apolipoprotein metabolism. In *Clinical and Metabolic Aspects of High-Density Lipoproteins* (eds N.E. Miller and G.J. Miller), Elsevier, Amsterdam, pp. 273–287 (1984)
79. Schaefer, E.J., Zech, L.A., Schwartz, D.E. and Brewer, H.B. Coronary heart disease prevalence and clinical features in familial high density lipoprotein deficiency (Tangier disease). *Ann. Intern. Med.*, **93**, 261–266 (1980)
80. Gustafson, A., McConathy, W., Alaupovic, P., Curq, M. D. and Persson, B. Identification of apoprotein families in a variant of human plasma apolipoprotein A deficiency. *Scand. J. Clin. Lab. Invest.*, **39**, 377–388 (1979)
81. Carlson, L.A. Fish-eye disease. A new familial condition with massive corneal opacities and dyslipoproteinaemia. *Eur. J. Clin. Invest.*, **12**, 41–53 (1981)
82. Breckenridge, W.C., Little, J.A., Alaupovic, P., Wang, C.S., Kuksis, A. *et al.* Lipoprotein abnormalities associated with a familial deficiency of hepatic lipase. *Atherosclerosis*, **45**, 161–179 (1982)
83. Carlson, L.A., Holmquist, L. and Nilsson-Ehle, P. Deficiency of hepatic lipase activity in post-heparin plasma in familial hyper-alpha-triglyceridaemia. *Acta Med. Scand.*, **219**, 435–447 (1986)
84. Hegele, R.A., Vezna, C., Moorjani, S., Lupien, P.J., Gagne, C. *et al.* A hepatic lipase gene mutation associated with heritable lipolytic deficiency. *J. Clin. Endocrinol. Metabol.*, **72**, 730–732 (1991)
85. Hegele, R.A., Little, J.A. and Connelly, P.W. Compound heterozygosity for mutant hepatic lipase in familial hepatic lipase deficiency. *Biochem. Biophys. Res. Commun.*, **179**, 78–84 (1991)
86. Auwerz, J.H., Babirak, S.P., Hokanson, J.E., Stahnke, G., Will, H. *et al.* Co-existence of abnormalities of hepatic lipase and lipoprotein lipase in a large family. *Am. J. Hum. Genet.*, **46**, 470–477 (1990)
87. Bassen, F.A. and Kornzweig, A.L. Malformation of the erythrocytes in a case of atypical retinitis pigmentosa. *Blood*, **5**, 381–387 (1950)
88. Lloyd, J.K. Lipoprotein deficiency disorders. *Clin. Lnd. Metab.*, **2**, 127–147 (1973)
89. Ross, R.S., Gregg, R.E., Law, S.W., Monge, J.C., Grant, S.M. *et al.* Homozygous hypobetalipoproteinaemia: a disease district from abetalipoproteinaemia at the molecular level. *J. Clin. Invest.*, **81**, 590 (1999)
90. Talmud, P.J., Lloyd, J.K., Muller, D.P.R., Collins, D.R., Scott, J. and Humphries, S. Genetic evidence from two families that the apolipoprotein B gene is not involved in abetalipoproteinaemia. *J. Clin. Invest.*, **82**, 1803– (1988)
91. Rader, D.J. and Brewer, H.B. Abetalipoproteinaemia. New insights into lipoprotein assembly and vitamin E metabolism from a rare genetic disease. *J. Am. Med. Assoc.*, **270**, 865–869 (1993)

92. Wetterau, J.R., Aggerbeck, L.P., Bouma, M-E, Eisenberg, C., Munck, A. *et al.* Absence of microsomal triglyceride transfer protein in individuals with abetalipoproteinaemia. *Science*, **258**, 999–1001 (1992)

93. Wagner, R.D., Krul, E.S., Tang, J., Parhofer, K.G., Garlock, K. *et al.* Apo B 54.7, a truncated apolipoprotein found primarily in VLDL is associated with a nonsense mutation in the apo B gene and hypobetalipoproteinaemia. *J. Lipid Res.*, **32**, 1001 (1991)

94. Glueck, C.J., Gartside, P., Fallat, R.W., Sielski, J. and Steiner, P.M. Longevity syndromes. Familial hypobeta- and familial hyperalphalipoproteinaemia *J. Lab. Clin. Med.*, **88**, 941–957 (1976)

95. Kahn, J. A. and Glueck, C. J. Familial hypobetalipoproteinaemia. Absence of atherosclerosis in a post-mortem study. *J. Am. Med. Assoc.*, **240**, 47–48 (1978)

96. Steinberg, D., Grundy, S.M., Mok, H.Y.I., Turner, J.D., Weinstein, J.B. *et al.* Metabolic studies in an unusual case of asymptomatic familial hypobetalipoproteinaemia with hypoalphalipoproteinaemia and fasting chylomicronaemia. *J. Clin. Invest.*, **64**, 292–301 (1979)

97. Malloy, M.J., Kane, J.P., Hardman, D.A., Hamilton, R.L. and Dalal, K.B. Normotriglyceridaemic abetalipoproteinaemia. Absence of the $B_{100}$ apolipoprotein. *J. Clin. Invest.*, **67**, 1441–1450 (1981)

98. Takashima, Y., Kodama, T., Iida, H., Kawamura, M., Aburatani, H. *et al.* Normotriglyceridemic abetalipoproteinaemia in infancy. An isolated apolipoprotein B-100 deficiency. *Paediatrics*, **75**, 541–546 (1985)

99. Herbert, P.N., Hyams, J.S., Bernier, D.N., Berman, M.M., Saritelli, A.L. *et al.* Apolipoprotein B-100 deficiency. Intestinal steatosis despite apolipoprotein B-48 synthesis. *J. Clin. Invest.*, **76**, 403–412 (1985)

100. Talmud, P. Detection and physiological relevance of mutations in the apoprotein E, C-II and B genes. Chapter 5 in *Structure and Function of Apolipoproteins* (ed M. Rosseneu), CRC Press Inc., Boca Raton, pp. 123–158 (1992)

101. Gabelli, C. The lipoprotein metabolism of apolipoprotein B mutants. *Curr. Opin. Lipidol.*, **3**, 208–214 (1992)

102. Avogaro, P. Familial hyperalphalipoproteinaemia. In *Clinical and Metabolic Aspects of High-Density Lipoproteins* (eds N.E. Miller and G.J. Miller), Elsevier, Amsterdam, pp. 289–295 (1984)

103. Glueck, C.J., Fallat, R.W., Millett, F., Gartside, P., Elston, R.C. and Go, R.C.P. Familial hyperalphalipoproteinaemia. Studies on 18 kindreds. *Metabolism*, **24**, 1243–1265 (1975)

104. Heckers, H., Burkard, W., Schmahl, F.W., Fuhrmann, W. and Platt, D. Hyperalphalipoproteinaemia and hypobetalipoproteinaemia are not markers for a high life expectancy. Serum lipid and lipoprotein findings in 103 randomly selected nonagenarians. *Gerontology*, **28**, 176–202 (1982)

105. Koizumi, J., Mabuchi, H., Yoshimura, A., Michishita, I., Takeda, M. *et al.* Deficiency of serum cholesteryl-ester transfer activity in patients with familial hyperalphalipoproteinaemia. *Atherosclerosis*, **58**, 175–186 (1985)

106. Brown, M.I., Inazu, A., Hesler, C.B., Agellon, L.B., Mann, C. *et al.* Molecular basis of lipid transfer protein deficiency in a family with increased high-density lipoproteins. *Nature*, **342**, 448–451 (1989)

107. Yamashita, S., Hui, D.Y., Sprecher, D.L., Matsuzawa, Y. *et al.* Total deficiency of plasma cholesteryl ester transfer protein in subjects homozygous and heterozygous for the intron 14 splicing defect. *Biochem. Biophys. Res. Commun.*, **170**, 1346–1351 (1990)

108. Inazu, A., Brown, M.L., Hesler, C.B., Agellon, L.B., Koizumi, J. *et al.* Increased high-density lipoprotein levels caused by a common cholesteryl-ester transfer protein gene mutation. *N. Engl. J. Med.*, **323**, 1234–1238 (1990)

109. Yamashita, S., Hui, D.Y., Wetterau, J.R., Sprecher, D.L., Harmony, J.A.K. *et al.* Characterisation of plasma lipoproteins in patients heterozygous for human plasma cholesteryl ester transfer protein (CETP) deficiency: plasma CETP regulates high density lipoprotein concentration and composition. *Metabolism*, **40**, 756–763 (1991)

110. Yamashita, S., Sprecher, D.L., Sakai, N., Matsuzawa, Y., Tarui, S. and Hui, D.Y. Accumulation of apolipoprotein E-rich high density lipoproteins in hyperalphalipoproteinaemic human subjects with plasma cholesteryl ester transfer protein deficiency. *J. Clin. Invest.*, **86**, 688–695 (1990)

111. Bisgaier, C.L., Siebenkas, M.V., Brown, M.L., Inazu, A., Koizumi, J. *et al.* Familial cholesteryl ester transfer protein deficiency is associated with triglyceride-rich low density lipoprotein containing cholesteryl esters of probable intracellular origin. *J. Lipid Res.*, **32**, 21–33 (1991)

112. Bhatnagar, D., Durrington, P.N., Channon, K.M., Prais, H. and Mackness, M.I. Increased transfer of cholesteryl esters from high density lipoproteins to low density and very low density lipoproteins in patients with angiographic evidence of coronary artery disease. *Atherosclerosis*, **98**, 25–32 (1992)

113. Williams, R.R., Hunt, S.C., Hopkins, P.N., Stutts, B.M., Wu, L.L. *et al.* Familial dyslipidaemic hypertension. *J. Am. Med. Assoc.*, **259**, 3579–3586 (1988)

114. Haffner, S.M., Ferrannini, E., Hazuda, H.P. and Stern, M.P. Clustering of cardiovascular risk factors in confirmed prehypertensive individuals. *Hypertension*, **20**, 38–45 (1991)

115. Haffner, S.M., Valdez, R.A., Hazuda, H.P., Mitchell, B.D., Morales, P.A. and Stern, M.P. A prospective analysis of the insulin resistance syndrome (syndrome X). *Diabetes*, **41**, 715–722 (1992)

116. Skott, P., Vaog, A., Bruun, N.E., Hottier-Nielsen, O., Gall, M-A. *et al.* Effect of insulin on renal sodium handling in hyperinsulinaemia Type 2 (non-insulin-dependent) diabetic patients with peripheral insulin resistance. *Diabetologia*, **34**, 275–281 (1991)

117. Rowe, J.W., Young, J.B., Ninaker, K.L., Stevens, A.L., Pallota, J. and Landsberg, L. Effect of insulin and glucose infusions on sympathetic nervous system activity in normal man. *Diabetes*, **30**, 219–225 (1981)

118. Selby, J.V., Newman, B., Quiroga, J., Christian, J.C., Austin, M.A. and Fabsitz, R.R. Concordance for dyslipidemic hypertension in male twins. *J. Am. Med. Assoc.*, **265**, 2079–1084 (1991)

119. Newman, B., Selby, J.V., Quesenberry, C.P., King, M.C., Friedman, G.D. and Fabsitz, R.R. Non genetic influences of obesity on other cardiovascular disease risk factors: an analysis of identical twins. *Am. J. Publ. Health*, **80**, 675–678 (1990)

120. Baba, T., Kodama, T., Tomiyama, T., Sohn, D-R. and Ishizaki, T. Serum insulin level versus blood pressure: a cross-sectional, case-controlled study in non-obese, middle-aged Japanese subjects with normal glucose tolerance. *Diabetic Med.*, **11**, 42–49 (1994)

121. Talmud, P., Tybjaerg-Hansen, A., Bhatnagar, D., MBewu, A., Miller, J.P. *et al.* Rapid screening for specific mutations in patients with a clinical diagnosis of familial hypercholesterolaemia. *Atherosclerosis*, **89**, 137–141 (1991)

122. Scott, J.M., Knott, T.J., Priestly, L.M., Robertson, M.E., Mann, D.V. *et al.* High-density lipoprotein composition is altered by a common DNA polymorphism adjacent to apoprotein AII gene in man. *Lancet*, **i**, 771–773 (1985)

123. Kessling, A.M., Rajput, J., Bainton, D., Scott, J., Miller, N. *et al.* DNA polymorphisms of the apolipoprotein AII and AI–CIII–AIV genes. A study in men selected for differences in high density lipoprotein cholesterol concentration. *Am. J. Hum. Genet.*, **42**, 458–467 (1988)

124. Fager, G., Wiklund, O., Olofsson, S-O *et al.* Multivariate apolipoproteins and risk factors in relation to acute myocardial infarction. *Arteriosclerosis*, **1**, 273–279 (1981)

125. Castellani, L.W. and Lusis, A.J. Atherosclerosis in transgenic mice overexpressing apolipoprotein AII. *Science*, **262**, 469–472 (1993)

126. Deeb, S.S., Takata, W., Peng, R., Kajiyama, G. and Albers, J.J. A splice-mutation responsible for familial apolipoprotein AII deficiency. *Am. J. Hum. Genet.*, **46**, 822–827 (1990)

127. Knott, T.J., Pease, R.J., Powell, L.M., Wallis, S.C., Rall, S.C. *et al.* Complete protein sequence and identification of structural domains of human apolipoprotein B-100. *Nature*, **323**, 734–738 (1986)

128. Yang, C-Y., Chen S-H., Gianturco, S.H., Bradley, W.A., Sparrow, J.T. *et al.* Sequence, structure, receptor-binding domains and internal repeats of human apolipoprotein B-100. *Nature*, **328**, 738–742 (1986)

129. Soria, L.F., Ludwig, E.H., Clarke, H.R., Vega, G.L., Grundy, S.M. and McCarthy, B.J. Association between a specific apolipoprotein B mutation and familial defective apolipoprotein B-100. *Proc. Nat. Acad. Sci. USA.*, **86**, 587–591 (1989)

130. Vega, G.L. and Grundy, S.M. In vivo evidence for reduced binding of low density lipoproteins to receptors as a cause of primary moderate hypercholesterolaemia. *J. Clin. Invest.*, **78**, 1410–1414 (1986)

131. Allison, A.C. and Blumber, B.S. An isoprecipitation reaction distinguishing human serum-protein types. *Lancet*, **i**, 634–637 (1961)

132. Berg, K., Hames, C., Dahlen, G., Frick, M.H. and Krisham, I. Genetic variation in serum low density lipoproteins and lipid levels in man. *Proc. Natl Acad. Sci. USA.*, **73**, 937–940 (1976)

133. Humphries, S. E. DNA polymorphisms of the apolipoprotein genes – their use in the investigation of the genetic component of hyperlipidaemia and atherosclerosis. *Atherosclerosis*, **72**, 89–108 (1988)

134. Demant, T., Houlston, R.S., Caslake, M.J., Series, J.J., Shepherd, J. *et al*. Catabolic rate of low density lipoprotein is influenced by variation in the apolipoprotein B gene. *J. Clin. Invest.*, **82**, 797–802 (1988)

135. Houlston, R.S., Turner, P.R., Revill, J., Lewis, B. and Humphries, S.E. The fractional catabolic rate of low density lipoprotein is influenced by variation in the apolipoprotein Be gene. *Atherosclerosis*, **71**, 81–85 (1988)

136. Series, J., Cameron, I., Caslake, M., Gaffney, D., Packard, C.J. and Shepherd, J. The Xba I polymorphisms of the apolipoprotein B gene influences the degradation of low density lipoprotein in vivo. *Biochim. Biophys. Acta*, **1003**, 183–188 (1989)

137. Breslow, J. L. Genetic regulation of apolipoproteins. *Am. Heart J.*, **113**, 422–427 (1987)

138. Utermann, G., Feussner, G., Franceschini, G., Haas, J. and Steinmetz, A. Genetic variants of group A apolipoproteins. Rapid methods for screening and characterisation without ultracentrifugation. *J. Biol. Chem.*, **257**, 501–507 (1982)

139. Nichols, W.C., Gregg, R.E., Brewer, H.B. and Benson, M.D. A mutation in the apolipoprotein A-I gene in the Iowa type of familial amyloidotic polyneuropathy. *Genomics*, **8**, 313–323 (1990)

140. Galton, D.J. Molecular genetics of coronary heart disease. *Eur. J. Clin. Invest.*, **18**, 219–225 (1988)

141. Assmann, G., von Eckardstein, A. and Funke, H. Mutations in apolipoprotein genes and HDL metabolism. Chapter 4 in *Structure and Function of Apolipoproteins* (ed. M. Rosseneu), CRC Press Inc., Boca Raton, pp. 85–122 (1992)

142. Davignon, J., Sing, C.F., Lussier-Cacan, S., Nestruck, A.C. and Bouthillier, D. Importance of apolipoprotein E polymorphism in determining plasma lipid levels and atherosclerosis. In *Atherosclerosis*, vol. VII (eds N.H. Fidge and P.J. Nestel), Elsevier, Amsterdam, pp. 171–175 (1986)

143. Utermann, G. Apolipoprotein E polymorphism in health and disease. *Am. Heart J.*, **113**, 433–440 (1987)

144. Wincour, P.H., Tetlow, L., Durrington, P.N., Ishola, M., Hillier, V. and Anderson, D.C. Apolipoprotein E polymorphism and lipoproteins in insulin treated diabetes mellitus. *Atherosclerosis*, **75**, 167–173 (1989)

145. Eto, M., Watanabe, K., Iwashima, Y., Morikawa, A., Chonan, N. *et al*. Increased frequency of apolipoprotein E4 allele in type II diabetes with hypercholesterolaemia. *Diabetes*, **36**, 1301–1306 (1987)

146. James, R.W., Boemi, M., Giansanti, R., Furnelli, P. and Pometta, D. Underexpression of the apolipoprotein E4 isoform in an Italian population. *Arterioscler. Thomb.*, **13**, 1456–1459 (1993)

147. Kesaniemi, Y. A., Ehnholm, C. and Miettinen, T. A. Intestinal cholesterol absorption efficiency in man is related to apoprotein E phenotype. *J. Clin. Invest.*, **80**, 578–581(1987)

148. Dreon, D.M. and Krauss, R.M. Gene-diet interactions in lipoprotein metabolism. In *Molecular Genetics of Coronary Artery Disease. Candidate Genes and Processes in Atherosclerosis* (eds A.I. Lsis, J.E. Rotter and R.S. Sparkes), Karger, Basle, pp. 325–349 (1992)

149. Menzel, H.J., Kladetzky, R.G. and Assmann, G. Apolipoprotein E polymorphism and coronary artery disease. *Arteriosclerosis*, **3**, 310–315 (1983)

150. Cumming, A.M. and Robertson, F.R. Polymorphism at the apoprotein-E locus in relation to risk and coronary disease. *Clin. Genet.*, **25**, 310–313 (1984)

151. Katzel, L.I., Fleg, J.L., Paidi, M., Ragoobarsingh, N. and Goldberg, A.P. Apo E4 polymorphism increases the risk for exercise-induced silent myocardial ischaemia in older men. *Arterioscler. Thomb.*, **13**, 1495–1500 (1993)

152. Bockxmeer, F.M. and Mamotte, C.D.S. Apolipoprotein E4 homozygosity in young men with coronary heart disease. *Lancet*, **340**, 879–880 (1992)

153. Eto, M., Watanabe, K., Chonan, N. and Ishii, K. Familial hypercholesterolaemia and apolipoprotein E4. *Atherosclerosis*, **72**, 123–128 (1988)

154. Mahley, R.W. Apolipoprotein E: cholesterol transport protein with expanding role in cell biology. *Science*, **240**, 622–630 (1988)

155. Handelmann, G.E., Boyles, J.K., Weisgraber, K.H., Mahley, R.W. and Pitas, R.E. Effects of apolipoprotein E, β-very low density lipoproteins, and cholesterol on the extension of neurites by rabbit dorsal root ganglion neurons in vitro. *J. Lipid Res.*, **33**, 1677–1688 (1992)

156. Popko, B., Goodrum, J.F., Bouldin, T.W. Zhang, S.H. and Maeda, N. Nerve regeneration occurs in the absence of apolipoprotein E in mice. *J. Neurochem.*, **60**, 1155–1158 (1993)

157. Saunders, A.M., Schmader, K., Breitner, J.C.S., Genson, M.D., Brown, W.T. *et al.* Apolipoprotein E and 4 allele distributions in late-onset Alzheimer's disease and in other amyloid-forming diseases. *Lancet,* **342**, 710–711 (1993)
158. Corder, E.H., Saunders, A.M., Strittmatter, W.J., Schmechel, D.E., Gaskell, P.C. *et al.* Gene dose of apolipoprotein E type 4 allele and the risk of Alzheimer's disease in the late onset families. *Science,* **261**, 921–923 (1993)
159. Mayeux, R., Stern, Y. Ottman, R., Tatemichi, T.K., Tang, M.X. *et al.* The apolipoprotein E4 allele in patients with Alzheimer's disease. *Ann. Neurol.,* **34**, 752–754 (1993)
160. Poirier, J., Davignon, J., Boulthillier, D., Kogan, S., Bertrand, P. and Gauthier, S. Apolipoprotein E polymorphism and Alzheimer's disease. *Lancet,* **342**, 697–699 (1993)
161. Strittmatter, W.J., Weisgraber, K.H., Huang, D.Y., Dong, L-M., Salvesen, G.S. *et al.* Binding of human apolipoprotein E to synthetic amyloid B peptide: isoform-specific effects and implications for late-onset Alzheimer's disease. *Proc. Natl Acad. Sci USA.,* **90**, 8098–8102 (1993)
162. Strittmatter, W.J., Weisgraber, K.H., Goedert, M., Saunders, A.M., Huang, D. *et al.* Microtubule instability and paired helical filament formation in the Alzheimers disease brain as a function of apolipoprotein E genotype. *Exp. Neurol* (in press)

# Chapter 13

# The lipid clinic laboratory

## Cholesterol and triglyceride

It is often said that the diagnosis of hyperlipidaemia is a purely biochemical one. Although it is true that the biochemical determination of serum lipids is the usual starting point in the diagnosis, information gleaned from the history, examination and other clinical investigations is generally essential if the patient is to receive any sensible treatment or counselling. Diagnosis in medicine almost invariably, if it is to be of any value to the patient, is not simply a matter of disease classification (see Chapter 4), but is the acquisition of an 'all-the-way-through knowledge' (the original meaning of the word diagnosis) which allows decisions about therapy to be made and specific advice to be given. That is why there can be no single level of cholesterol which for all individuals necessitates a particular course of action.

In fact, very little specialist biochemistry is required to run a lipid clinic or to manage the great majority of patients with hyperlipidaemia. Methods for the accurate measurement of serum cholesterol and triglycerides are obviously essential. The determination of HDL cholesterol is also desirable. Visual inspection of the plasma should never be neglected. Lipoprotein electrophoresis, which at one time was thought to be the *sine qua non* of the lipid laboratory, rarely adds any information beyond that from the tests already mentioned and is too time-consuming to be worth preserving.

For screening purposes, non-fasting cholesterol is probably acceptable since in most people it is very close to fasting values. This enormously increases the ease with which screening can be undertaken, particularly in general practice and industry. Portable cholesterol analysers potentially have much to contribute in screening. It is essential, however, that their use does not entail any substantial deterioration in the precision of cholesterol measurement. Even the performance of many clinical laboratory methods for the determination of serum cholesterol is not good enough, if guidelines for the management of people whose cholesterol levels are in the middle range are to be reliably instituted. An error of 5% in measuring cholesterol values around 260 mg/dl (6.5 mmol/l) will, for example, mean that large numbers of people would be wrongly classified as hypercholesterolaemic or normocholesterolaemic. Laboratories should be aiming for a coefficient of variation for analytical error of 3% or less. It should also be remembered that biological variation (Chapter 3, page 88) will add a further element of imprecision (equivalent to a coefficient of variation of around 5%). Sensible clinical management therefore involves repeated measurements before any major therapeutic decision is taken. This allows the true mean value to be established and overcomes imprecision and biological variation to a large extent. Occasionally people writing about imprecisions in cholesterol measurements create the feeling that the whole business is so inaccurate it would be best not to bother about measuring it in the first place. This is to insult the intelligence of clinicians who are well versed in making only cautious interpretations of single laboratory or blood pressure measurements.

Consistent biases towards over- or under-reading, which characterize some of the methods in use today, pose a more difficult problem to overcome. Most of the methods for cholesterol currently employed are enzymic and were not the methods used in the studies upon which present recommendations about the management of hyperlipidaemia are based. These problems are fortunately increasingly recognized and laboratory quality control programmes in the UK and the USA are under way to improve matters. Undoubtedly the UK laboratories have been using standards which give higher levels than the US standards. It is difficult to make a precise estimate of the difference over recent years, but it has probably been at least 4%. It is part of the reason why the Reflotron portable analyser has generally been reported to give lower readings than wet chemistry in British laboratories: the Reflotron is standardized through the US Center for Disease Control, Atlanta. It is to be hoped that standardization will be more uniform henceforth. The facts about the prevalence of hypercholesterolaemia, the cost of intervention programmes and the comparison of USA and UK guidelines which has aroused much controversy may have been seriously distorted by differences in the standardization of cholesterol assays used in population surveys and clinical trials.

Accuracy in the determination of triglycerides is less of an issue, since we can be less precise about their importance as a risk factor. It is essential that every patient with a raised cholesterol, however, does have a fasting serum triglyceride measurement made before instituting drug therapy. Since the dietary modification for most patients with hypercholesterolaemia will be similar whether triglycerides are raised or not, it is not essential to measure fasting triglycerides before introducing diet in, for example, general practice. If this does not produce a satisfactory cholesterol response, then serum fasting triglycerides as well as cholesterol are necessary before giving more specific dietary advice tailored to the individual patient and certainly, if after this a lipid-lowering drug is to be introduced, such a knowledge is essential. A fibric acid derivative would, for example, be a more logical therapy in a patient with hypercholesterolaemia whose triglycerides are also raised than a bile-acid sequestrant (Chapter 10). Before escalating therapy beyond simply dietary recommendations to more restrictive diets or to drug therapy, it is also essential to exclude secondary hyperlipidaemia and coincidental diseases, which might lead to drug side-effects. Every patient should by that stage have had urinalysis (for protein and glucose), measurement of fasting blood glucose, creatinine and liver function tests (bilirubin, albumin, globulin, alkaline phosphatase, transaminase). Serum thyroid function tests are expensive. Generally they should only be performed when there is a suspicion from the history, clinical examination or ECG that hypothyroidism may be the cause of the hyperlipidaemia. Occasionally patients with hypothyroidism and hypercholesterolaemia have no other clinical features of the disorder. This is by no means as frequent as some authorities claim. However, hypothyroidism is an 'important diagnosis not to miss' and I certainly send off a great deal more requests for serum thyroxine which yield results in the normal range than abnormally low values. Certainly every middle-aged women with serum cholesterol >320 mg/dl (>8.0 mmol/l) is tested for hypothyroidism. Occasionally, too, other laboratory investigations such as the mean corpuscular volume, blood ethanol, immunoglobulins, Bence–Jones protein and so on are required. Inseparable from the lipid clinic is, of course, access to cardiological expertise and investigations, particularly the resting electrocardiogram and not infrequently exercise electrocardiography and coronary angiography.

## HDL cholesterol

In addition to serum cholesterol and triglycerides most laboratories also provide some measurement of HDL cholesterol. The justification for this is that:

1. Some patients with borderline hypercholesterolaemia may not have any increase in their LDL cholesterol at all, but have a high level of HDL cholesterol and thus not require lipid-lowering therapy.
2. It allows the calculation of LDL cholesterol by the Friedewald formula (see Chapter 3, page 99) which may provide a better assessment of therapeutic response than the total cholesterol, especially if the serum triglyceride level or HDL cholesterol are influenced by the treatment.
3. HDL cholesterol itself is an indicator of risk and may thus influence the rigour with which therapy is pursued. Thus a more critical approach to the acceptable LDL cholesterol level in a patient with a low HDL might be taken, certainly if HDL cholesterol levels are 35 mg/dl (0.9 mmol/l) or less. The use of the LDL : HDL ratio or the total cholesterol : HDL ratio has been advocated, not least because it may make therapeutic decisions easier for practitioners whose knowledge of hyperlipidaemia is not great. In prospective epidemiological studies the total cholesterol to HDL cholesterol ratio has often emerged as the most discriminating indicator of IHD risk (Chapter 6, page 170). A personal view, however, is that such ratios in clinical practice can be misleading and that they should rarely, if ever, be the only consideration in making important therapeutic decisions. How can it be seriously suggested that a man with a cholesterol of 200 mg/dl (5 mmol/l) and an HDL cholesterol of 32 mg/dl (0.8 mmol/l), giving him a cholesterol : HDL ratio of 6, has the same outlook as one with a cholesterol of 420 mg/dl (10.5 mmol/l) and an HDL of 70 mg/dl (1.8 mmol/l) also having a ratio of 6?

The major difficulty with HDL is that there is very little laboratory quality control. It must be performed on serum or plasma before freezing and this poses the main difficulty in standardization. Also, of course, HDL is a mixture of molecular complexes of different origins, composition and physical properties and thus different methods for its isolation may give different results and its particular physical or chemical properties, to which different methods are sensitive, may vary with different diseases independently of the actual lipid concentrations in HDL. Most of the epidemiological studies establishing HDL as a risk factor for IHD have relied on some modification of the heparin/manganese method and have employed non-enzymatic methods for cholesterol determination. It should be remembered that if EDTA plasma rather than serum is used for this method, then the manganese concentration must be increased. Furthermore, if an enzymic method for cholesterol measurement is used, the manganese must later be chelated or it will be precipitated, interfering with the optical density determination. A fundamental difficulty is also that the most popular method for HDL in the routine laboratory is by phosphotungstate/magnesium precipitation. This tends to give lower values than heparin/manganese and thus results obtained with it must be interpreted with caution, since present guidelines relate to the heparin/manganese isolation procedure.

A wide range of other precipitation methods have been developed and critical evaluation and inter-laboratory standardization is important if HDL is to realize its full potential in clinical practice.

The advent of immunoassays for apolipoprotein AI seemed to offer the potential for a more definitive clinical test, which would make their further development and laboratory evaluation more fruitful than that of HDL. However, many of them are affected by freezing and thawing and standardization procedures are still underdeveloped. Furthermore several studies have not shown apo AI to be more closely related to the development of IHD than serum HDL cholesterol and some have shown it to be less discriminating. The determination of HDL subfractions has attracted much attention and, without denying their importance in the research laboratory, it is nevertheless the case that none of the methods currently employed is suitable for routine clinical use. There is considerable variation in the reference ranges for HDL subfractions with different methods and from various laboratories, indicating that quite apart from technical considerations there is not even a universal definition of what constitutes $HDL_2$ or $HDL_3$. The component of HDL which contains apo AI, but no AII has also attracted considerable interest because of the possibility that it may be more strongly predictive of IHD risk than the whole of HDL. Prospective studies and the development of robust assays are needed to establish the place of such measurement in clinical practice.

## Other investigations of lipoproteins which are occasionally useful

In the diagnosis of type III hyperlipoproteinaemia access to ultracentrifugation or to an apolipoprotein E isoelectric focusing technique is valuable (Chapter 8, page 220). Such facilities do not need to be available in every laboratory servicing a lipid clinic. The diagnosis can often be made on clinical grounds and even when only suspected, so far as the patient is concerned, a satisfactory therapeutic response is more valuable than a precise laboratory diagnosis. The distinction between familial lipoprotein lipase deficiency, apolipoprotein CII deficiency or other causes of severe hypertriglyceridaemia may also be impossible without access to specialist laboratory investigations (Chapter 8). Again, clinical experience in the management of such patients, particularly in the exclusion of secondary causes and the institution of the most appropriate diet by an experienced dietitian, is generally more important than precise laboratory diagnosis, which may, in any case, be difficult even in centres where lipoprotein lipase assays are available.

## Potentially valuable laboratory methods

The apolipoproteins and the clotting factors are two important areas of research which, when translated into practical terms, may improve our ability to assess an individual patient's risk more accurately and thus assist in making important therapeutic decisions. Particularly in its middle range, cholesterol is a poor indicator of individual prognosis and the introduction of HDL into the routine clinical laboratory has improved this to only a limited extent. On the other hand, immunoassay of apolipoprotein B and apo (a) (Chapter 6, page 179, and Chapter 12, page 364) may provide a more accurate indication of risk than cholesterol, HDL cholesterol, triglycerides and apolipoprotein AI. Whilst case-control studies strongly support such a view prospective studies have given conflicting results. Furthermore, laboratory standardization and quality control present major problems as is the case with immunoassays for all apolipoproteins. Some of the problems they present may add a new dimension to clinical chemistry. The reason is that some methods or antisera may be more sensitive to certain apolipoprotein molecular conformations produced by different isoforms (or polymorphisms) or their presence in different lipoprotein particles. These molecular variations may be more closely linked to their role in atheroma than their absolute concentration. Thus an assay which may give the most accurate estimate of mass may not give as much information of clinical importance than one which is more sensitive to certain molecular variants.

Immunoassay of apo B does have an established place in the investigation of patients with hypertriglycerideaemia in assessing their cardiovascular risk (Chapter 7, page 191). It can also be valuable in other situations where the serum or LDL cholesterol is a misleading indicator of whether the concentration of whole LDL particles is increased, such as phytosterolaemia (Chapter 12, page 368), and some families in whom IHD risk is increased without obvious risk factors.

Because of the clinical promise of laboratory methods for apolipoprotein determination and thus their enormous commercial potential, a large array of such methods are already in production. It should be realized that many of these have not undergone adequate evaluation against reference methods, nor often have they been the methods used in epidemiological investigations.

The smaller molecular weight subfractions of LDL are increasingly being recognized as being closely associated with IHD risk even when the whole LDL cholesterol is not increased. If methods easier than the present ones for the determination of the smaller LDL subfractions can be developed they may have great clinical utility. Potentially important too may be methods for measuring lipoproteins modified by such processes as oxidation and glycation and for determining lipid transfer proteins and rates of transfer of cholesteryl ester between lipoproteins.

Fibrinogen has also been shown in epidemiological investigations to be an important predictor of cardiovascular risk. It might thus prove useful in the assessment of risk in patients with hyperlipidaemia and help decide whether to introduce lipid-lowering drugs, for example. The difficulty in practice is that fibrinogen levels vary considerably within the same patient and a series of values must thus be obtained before fibrinogen can be used to predict individual risk. There is no reason why this should in itself be an obstacle, however, in a clinical practice in which blood samples are already taken regularly, such as in the lipid clinic. The further practical evaluation of serum fibrinogen and other clotting factors is therefore likely to be of importance.

## Further reading

LIPID METHODS AND GENERAL REFERENCES

Belsey, R., Vandenbark, M., Goitein, R.K. and Baer, D.M. Evaluation of a laboratory system intended for use in physicians' offices. II. Reliability of results produced by health care workers without formal or professional laboratory training. *J. Am. Med. Assoc.*, **258**, 357–363 (1987)

Bhatnagar, D. and Durrington, P.N. An evaluation of the Roflotron for the determination of plasma cholesterol in capillary blood: effect of operator variability. *Occup. Med.*, **43**, 69–71 (1993)

Blank, D.W., Hoeg, J.M., Kroll, M. H. and Ruddell, M.E. The method of determination must be considered in interpreting blood cholesterol levels. *J. Am. Med. Assoc.*, **256**, 2867–2870 (1986)

Broughton, P.M.G. and Buckley, B.M. The need for better plasma cholesterol assays. *Ann. Clin. Biochem.*, **22**, 547–549 (1985)

Broughton, P.M.G., Bullock, D.G. and Cramb, R. Quality of plasma cholesterol measurements in primary care. *Br. Med. J.*, **298**, 297–298 (1989)

Cooper, G.R., Myers, G.L., Smith, S.J. and Sampson, E J. Standardization of lipid, lipoprotein, and apolipoprotein measurements. *Clin. Chem.*, **34**, B95–B105 (1988)

Durrington, P.N. Biological variation in serum lipid concentrations. *Scand. J. Clin. Lab. Invest.*, **50** (Suppl. 198), 86–91 (1990)

Mackness, M.I. and Durrington, P.N. Lipoprotein separation and analysis for clinical studies. Chapter 1 in *Lipoprotein Analysis* (eds C.A. Converse and E.R. Skinner), Oxford University Press, Oxford, pp. 1–42 (1991)

Naito, H.K. Reliability of lipid, lipoprotein, and apolipoprotein measurements. *Clin. Chem.*, **34**, B84–B94 (1988)

Naito, H.K. and David, J.A. Laboratory considerations. Determination of cholesterol, triglyceride, phospholipid, and other lipids in blood and tissues. In *Lipid Research Methodology* (ed. J. A. Storey), Alan R. Liss Inc., New York, pp 1–76 (1984)

Packard, C.J., Bell, M.A., Eaton, R.H., Dagen, M.M., Cassidy, M. and Shepherd, J. A pilot scheme for improving the accuracy of serum cholesterol measurement in Scotland and Northern Ireland. *Ann. Clin. Biochem.*, **30**, 387–393 (1993)

Phillips, S., Wyndham, L., Shaw, J. and Walker, S.F. How accurately does the Reflotron dry-chemistry system measure total cholesterol levels when used as a community-screening device? *Med. J. Aust.*, **149**, 122–125 (1988)

von Schenk, H., Treichl, L., Tilling, B. and Olsson, A.G. Laboratory and field evaluation of three desktop instruments for assay of cholesterol and triglyceride. *Clin. Chem.*, **33**, 1230–1232 (1987)

Warnick, G.R. Enzymatic methods for quantification of lipoprotein lipids. In *Methods in Enzymology*, vol. 129, *Plasma Lipoproteins: Part B: Characterization, Cell Biology and Metabolism* (eds J.J. Albers and J.P. Segrest.), Academic Press, Orlando, Ca, pp. 101–123 (1986)

Zak, B. Cholesterol methodologies. A review. *Clin. Chem.*, **23**, 1201–1214 (1977)

## LIPOPROTEINS

Albers, J.J., Warnick, G.R. and Nichols, A.V. Laboratory measurement of HDL. In *Clinical and Metabolic Aspects of High-Density Lipoprotein* (eds N.E. Miller and G.J. Miller), Elsevier, Amsterdam, pp. 381–414 (1984)

Albers, J.J., Warnick, G.R., Wiebe, D., King, P., Steiner, P., Smith, L. *et al.* Multi-laboratory comparison of three heparin $Mn^{2+}$ precipitation procedures for estimating cholesterol in high-density lipoprotein. *Clin. Chem.*, **24**, 853–856 (1978)

Bachorik, P.S. and Albers, J.J. Precipitation methods for quantification of lipoproteins. In *Methods in Enzymology*, vol. 129, *Plasma Lipoproteins: Part B: Characterization, Cell Biology and Metabolism* (eds J.J. Albers and J.P. Segrest), Academic Press, Orlando, Ca, pp. 78–100 (1986)

Burstein, M. and Legmann, P. Lipoprotein precipitation. In *Monographs on Atherosclerosis*, vol. II (eds T.B. Clarkson and O.J. Pollak), S. Karger, Basle (1982)

Carlson, K. Lipoprotein fractionation. *J. Clin. Pathol.*, **26** (Suppl. 5), 32–37 (1973)

Hatch, F.T. and Lees, R.S. Practical methods for plasma lipoproteins analysis. *Adv. Lipid Res.*, **6**, 1–68 (1968)

Havel, R.J., Eder, H.A. and Bragdon, J.H. The determination and chemical composition of ultracentrifugally separated lipoproteins in human serum. *J. Clin. Invest.*, **34**, 1345–1353 (1955)

Lindgren, F.T., Jensen, L.C. and Hatch, F.T. The isolation and quantitative analysis of serum lipoproteins. In *Blood Lipids and Lipoproteins: Quantitation, Composition and Metabolism* (ed. G.J. Nelson), Wiley Interscience, New York, pp. 181–274 (1972)

Steele, B.W., Koehler, D.F., Azar, M.M., Blaszkowski, T.P., Kuba, K. and Dempsey, M.E. Enzymatic determinations of cholesterol in high-density-lipoprotein fractions prepared by a precipitation technique. *Clin. Chem.*, **22**, 98–101 (1976)

Wallentin, L., and Fahreaus, L. HDL3 and HDL2 determination by a combined ultracentrifugation and precipitation procedure. *Clin. Chim. Acta*, **116**, 199–208 (1981)


## APOLIPOPROTEINS AND LIPOPROTEIN (a)

Bhatnagar, D. and Durrington, P.N. Clinical value of apolipoprotein measurements. *Ann. Clin. Biochem.*, **28**, 427–437

Bhatnagar, D. and Durrington, P.N. Does measurement of apolipoproteins add to the clinical diagnosis and management of dyslipidaemia? *Curr. Opin. Lipidol.*, **4**, 299–304 (1993)

Henderson, L.O., Hannon, W.H., Smith, S.J. and Cooper, G.R. An international collaborative study on standardization of apolipoproteins AI and B. Part II: Evaluation of contributions of antisera to among-laboratory variance components. *Clin. Chem.*, **3**, 2250–2256 (1987)

Kane, J.W. and Gowland, E. A method for the identification of apolipoprotein E isoforms employing chemical precipitation and flat bed isoelectric focusing in agarose. *Ann. Clin. Biochem.*, **23**, 509–513 (1986)

Kostner, G.M. Standardization of Lp(a) assays. *Clin. Chim. Acta*, **221**, 191–194 (1992)

Mackness, M.I. and the Multicentre Lipoprotein (a) Methods Study Group Report on the Lp(a) Workshop. *Comm. Lab. Med.*, **2**, 49–51

Marcoriva, S.M. and Albers, J.J. International Federation of Clinical Chemistry study on the standardization of apolipoproteins AI and B. *Curr. Opin. Lipidol.*, **2**, 355–361 (1991)

Smith, S. J., Cooper, G. R., Henderson, L. O., Hannon, W. H. and the Apolipoprotein Standardization Collaborating Group. An international collaborative study on standardization of apolipoproteins AI and B. Part 1: Evaluation of a lyophilized candidate reference and calibration material. *Clin. Chem.*, **33**, 2240–2249 (1987)

Stampfer, M.J., Sacks, F.M., Salvini, S., Willet, W.C. and Hennekens, C.H. A prospective study of cholesterol, apolipoproteins, and the risk of myocardial infarction. *N. Engl. J. Med.*, **325**, 373–381 (1991)

Sigurdsson, G., Baldursdottir, A., Sigvaldson, H., Agnarsson, U., Throgeirsson, G. and Sigfusson, N. Predictive value of apolipoproteins in a prospective survey of coronary artery disease in men. *Am. J. Cardiol.*, **69**, 1251–1254 (1992)

Wald, N.J., Law, M., Watt, H.C., Wu, T., Bailey, A. *et al.* Apolipoproteins and ischaemic heart disease: implications for screening. *Lancet*, **343**, 75–79 (1994)

Zannis, V.I. Genetic polymorphism in human apolipoprotein E. In *Methods in Enzymology*, vol. 128, *Plasma Lipoprotein. Part A: Preparation, Structure and Molecular Biology* (eds J.P. Segrest and J.J. Albers), Academic Press, Orlando, Ca, pp. 823–851 (1986)


## LIPOPROTEIN SUBFRACTIONS

Austin, M.A., Breslow, J.L., Hennekens, C.H., Buring, J.E., Willett, W.C. and Krauss, R.M. Low-density lipoprotein subclass patterns and risk of myocardial infarction. *J. Am. Med. Assoc.*, **260**, 1917–1921 (1988)

Fruchart, J.C. and Bard, J.M. Lipoprotein particle measurement: an alternative approach to the classification of lipoprotein disorders. *Curr. Opin. Lipidol.*, **2**, 362–366 (1991)

Krauss, R.M. and Blanche, P.J. Detection and quantitation of LDL subfractions. **3**, 377–383 (1992)


## LIPOPROTEIN MODIFICATION

Chait, A. Methods for assessing lipid and lipoprotein oxidation. *Curr. Opin. Lipidol.*, **3**, 389–394 (1992)

Tames, T.J., Mackness, M.I., Arrol, S., Laing, I. and Durrington, P.N. Non-enzymatic glycation of apolipoprotein B in the sera of diabetic and non-diabetic subjects. *Atherosclerosis*, **93**, 237–244 (1992)

## TRIGLYCERIDE CLEARANCE AND LIPOPROTEIN LIPASE ACTIVITY

Bengtsson-Olivecrona, G. and Olivecrona, T. Assay of lipoprotein lipase and hepatic lipase. Chapter 7a in *Lipoprotein Analysis* (eds C.A. Converse and E.R. Skinner), Oxford University Press, Oxford, pp. 169–185 (1992)

Gibson, J.C., Paterniti, J.R. and Goldberg, I.J. Measurement of heparin-releasable triacylglycerol lipases. In *Lipid Research Methodology* (ed. J.A. Story), Alan R. Liss Inc., New York, pp. 241–286 (1984)

Rossner, S. Studies on an intravenous fat tolerance test. Methodological, experimental and clinical experience with Intralipid. *Acta Med. Scand.* (Suppl. 564), 1–24 (1974)


## FIBRINOGEN

Desrignes, P. and Bonnet, P. Direct determination of plasma fibrinogen levels by heat precipitation. A comparison of the technique against thrombin clottable fibrinogen with spectrophotometry and radial immunodiffusion. *Clin. Chim. Acta*, **110**, 9–17 (1981)

# Index